A
ESSENTIALS

MW01520314

Cheston B. Cunha, MD, FACP

Director, Antimicrobial Stewardship Program
Rhode Island Hospital and The Miriam Hospital
Infectious Disease Division
Assistant Professor of Medicine
Brown University Alpert School of Medicine
Providence, Rhode Island

Burke A. Cunha, MD, MACP

Chief, Infectious Disease Division*
Winthrop-University Hospital
Mineola, New York
Professor of Medicine
State University of New York
School of Medicine,
Stony Brook, New York

Seventeenth Edition
2020

JAYPEE BROTHERS MEDICAL PUBLISHERS
The Health Sciences Publisher
New Delhi | London

* formerly

Pharmaceuticals edition: 2021

 Jaypee Brothers Medical Publishers (P) Ltd

Headquarter

Jaypee Brothers Medical Publishers (P) Ltd
4838/24, Ansari Road, Daryaganj
New Delhi 110 002, India
Phone: +91-11-43574357
Fax: +91-11-43574314
Email: jaypee@jaypeebrothers.com

Overseas Office

J.P. Medical Ltd
83 Victoria Street, London
SW1H 0HW (UK)
Phone: +44 20 3170 8910
Fax: +44 (0)20 3008 6180
Email: info@jpmedpub.com

Website: www.jaypeebrothers.com

Website: www.jaypeedigital.com

Antibiotic Essentials / *Cheston B. Cunha, Burke A. Cunha*

Seventeenth Edition: **2020**

ISBN: 978-93-89776-31-7

Printed at: Sterling Graphics Pvt. Ltd. India.

ABOUT THE EDITORS

Cheston B. Cunha, MD, FACP Medical Director of the Antimicrobial Stewardship Program at Rhode Island Hospital and The Miriam Hospital in Providence, Rhode Island, USA. He is also an attending in adult infectious disease in the Division of Infectious Diseases at The Miriam Hospital and Rhode Island Hospital. He is Assistant Professor of Medicine at Brown University Alpert School of Medicine. Dr. Cunha obtained his medical degree from the Pennsylvania State University College of Medicine in Hershey, Pennsylvania. He completed his residency in Internal Medicine at Brown University. He also completed his Infectious Disease Fellowship at Brown University. Dr. Cunha's clinical and research interests include general infectious disease, antimicrobial therapy, ancient plagues, fever of unknown origin (FUO), and zoonoses. He has written/edited 51 articles, 50 book chapters and 8 books on antimicrobial stewardship, antibiotic therapy, and hospital epidemiology. He is an Editor of the books Antibiotic Stewardship and Antibiotic Essentials. He has been an annual recipient of the Dean's Excellence in Teaching Award from the Alpert Medical School of Brown University.

Burke A. Cunha, MD, MACP formerly Chief, Infectious Disease Division at Winthrop-University Hospital, Mineola, New York and Professor of Medicine, State University of New York School of Medicine, Stony Brook, New York. He is one of the world's leading authorities on antimicrobial therapy and infectious diseases. He has written/edited 1355 articles, 222 book chapters, and 37 books. He has received numerous teaching awards, including the Aesculapius Award for teaching excellence and the Spatz Award for clinical excellence. Dr. Cunha is a Master of the American College of Physicians, awarded for lifetime achievement as a Master Clinician and Master Teacher.

DEDICATION

for Marie

"Grace in her steps,
Heaven in her eye,
In every gesture, dignity and love"

Milton

TABLE OF CONTENTS

EDITORS

Cheston B. Cunha, MD, FACP   **Burke A. Cunha, MD, MACP**

CONTRIBUTORS*

Cheston B. Cunha, MD, FACP
Director, Antimicrobial Stewardship Program
Rhode Island Hospital and The Miriam Hospital
Infectious Disease Division
Assistant Professor of Medicine
Brown University Alpert School of Medicine
Providence, Rhode Island
Infectious Disease Differential Diagnosis
Overview of Antimicrobial Therapy
Empiric Therapy Based of Clinical Syndromes
Antimicrobial Drug Summaries

Jeffrey Baron, PharmD
Clinical Pharmacist
Hematology/Oncology Service
Roswell Park Cancer Center
Buffalo, New York
HBV, HCV, and HIV Guidelines
Antimicrobial Drug Summaries

Sharon Blum, PharmD
Infectious Disease Clinical Pharmacist
Antimicrobial stewardship
Department of Pharmacy
NYU Winthrop Hospital
Mineola, New York

Edward J. Bottone, PhD
Professor of Microbiology
Mount Sinai School of Medicine
New York, New York
Medical Microbiology; Parasites,
Fungi, Unusual Organisms

Amy Brotherton, PharmD
Infectious Disease Clinical Pharmacist
The Miriam Hospital
Providence
Rhode Island
HBV, HCV, and HIV Guidelines

Burke A. Cunha, MD, MACP
Chief, Infectious Disease Division
Winthrop-University Hospital
Mineola, New York
Professor of Medicine
State University of New York
School of Medicine
Stony Brook, New York
All chapters except HIV Infection & Pediatric ID

John L. Brusch, MD
Associate Chief of Medicine
Infectious Disease Service
Cambridge Health Alliance
Assistant Professor of Medicine
Harvard Medical School
Boston, Massachusetts
Endocarditis: Therapy & Prophylaxis

Daniel Caplivski, MD
Infectious Disease Division
Assistant Professor of Medicine
Mt. Sinai School of Medicine
New York, New York
Fungal Stain Atlas

Jamie Chin, MS, PharmD
Hematology/Oncology
Pharmacy Resident
National Institutes of Health (NIH)
Bethesda, Maryland
Mineola, New York
Antimicrobial Drug Summaries

Dennis J. Cleri, MD
St. Francis Medical Center
Professor of Medicine
Seton Hall University
School of Graduate Medical Education
Trenton, New Jersey
Bioterrorism

Staci A. Fischer, MD
Director, Transplant Infectious Diseases
Rhode Island Hospital
Infectious Disease Division
Associate Professor of Medicine
Brown University Alpert School of Medicine
Providence, Rhode Island
Transplant Infections: Therapy & Prophylaxis

Pierce Gardner, MD
Senior Advisor, Clinical Research and Training
National Institutes of Health
John E. Fogarty International Center for
Advanced Study in the Health Sciences
Bethesda, Maryland
Prophylaxis and Immunization

John Gian, MD
Infectious Disease Division
Winthrop-University Hospital
Mineola, New York
HIV

Arthur Gran, MD
Infectious Disease Division
Winthrop-University Hospital
Mineola, New York
Antimicrobial Drug Summaries

Jean E. Hage, MD
Infectious Disease Division
Winthrop-University Hospital
Mineola, New York
Empiric Therapy of Clinical Syndromes;
Prophylaxis & Immunization;
Parasitic & Fungi; Unusual Organisms;
Antimicrobial Drug Summaries

Mark H. Kaplan, MD
Professor of Medicine
Infectious Diseases
University of Michigan School of Medicine
Ann Arbor, Michigan
HIV Drug Summaries

Douglas S. Katz, MD
Vice Chairman, Clinical Research and Education
Director, Body CT
Winthrop-University Hospital
Mineola, New York
Professor of Clinical Radiology
State University of New York School of Medicine
Stony Brook, New York
Chest X-ray Atlas

Raymond S. Koff, MD
Clinical Professor of Medicine
University of Connecticut School of Medicine
Farmington, Connecticut
Viral Hepatitis: Therapy & Prophylaxis

Leonard R. Krilov, MD
Chief, Pediatric Infectious Disease Division
Winthrop-University Hospital
Mineola, New York
Professor of Pediatrics
State University of New York
School of Medicine
Stony Brook, New York
Pediatric Infectious Diseases

David W. Kubiak, PharmD
Infectious Disease Clinical Pharmacist
Brigham and Women's Hospital
Boston, Massachusetts
HIV Drug Summaries

Brian R. Malone, BS, MS, RPh
Director, Pharmaceutical Services
Winthrop-University Hospital
Mineola, New York
Adjunct Affiliate Professor
College of Pharmacy St. John's University
Queens, New York
Pediatric Drug Summaries

George H. McCracken, Jr., MD
Distinguished Professor of Pediatric Infectious
Disease and the Sarah M. and Charles E. Seay
Chair in Pediatric Infectious Disease
University of Texas Southwestern Medical Center
Dallas, Texas
Pediatric Infectious Diseases

James H. McGuire, MD
Master Clinician, Division of Infectious Diseases
Brigham and Women's Hospital
Professor of Medicine
Harvard Medical School
Boston, Massachusetts
Parasites, Fungi, Unusual Organisms

Nardeen Mickail, MD
Infectious Disease Division
Winthrop-University Hospital
Mineola, New York
Antimicrobial Drug Summaries

Maria D. Mileno, MD
Director, Travel Medicine
The Miriam Hospital
Infectious Disease Division
Associate Professor of Medicine
Brown University Alpert School of Medicine
Providence, Rhode Island
Prophylaxis and Immunizations

Robert Moore, MD
Chairman, Department of Radiology
Stony Brook University Hospital
Professor of Radiology
State University of New York School of Medicine
Stony Brook, New York
Chest X-ray Atlas

Sigridh Muñoz-Gomez, MD
Infectious Disease Division
Winthrop-University Hospital
Mineola, New York
Antimicrobial Drug Summaries

Ronald L. Nichols, MD
William Henderson Professor of Surgery
Professor of Microbiology and Immunology
Tulane University School of Medicine
New Orleans, Louisiana
Surgical Prophylaxis and Therapy

Asif Noor, MD
Attending Physician, Pediatric Infectious
Disease Division
Winthrop-University Hospital
Mineola, New York
Pediatric Infectious Diseases

Genovefa Papanicolaou, MD
Attending Physician, Infectious Disease Service
Memorial Sloan Kettering Cancer Center
Associate Professor of Medicine
Weill Cornell Medical College
New York, New York
Transplant Infections: Therapy & Prophylaxis

Diane M. Parente, PharmD
Infectious Disease Clinical Pharmacist
Antimicrobial Stewardship Team
The Miriam Hospital
Providence, Rhode Island
Drug Summaries

Muhammed Raza, MBBS
Infectious Disease Division
Winthrop-University Hospital
Mineola, New York
Antimicrobial Drug Summaries

Michael F. Rein, MD
Professor of Medicine
University of Virginia Health System
Charlottesville, Virginia
Sexually Transmitted Diseases

John H. Rex, MD
Adjunct Professor of Medicine
University of Texas Medical School
Houston, Texas
Medical Director for Infection
AstraZeneca Pharmaceuticals
Macclesfield, UK
Antifungal Therapy

Paul E. Sax, MD
Clinical Director
Division of Infectious Diseases and HIV
Brigham and Women's Hospital
Professor of Medicine
Harvard Medical School
Boston, Massachusetts
HIV

David Schlossberg, MD
Tuberculosis Control Program
Philadelphia Department of Health
Professor of Medicine
Temple University School of Medicine
Philadelphia, Pennsylvania
Tuberculosis

Paul E. Schoch, PhD
Director, Clinical Microbiology Laboratory
Winthrop-University Hospital
Mineola, New York
Medical Microbiology

Julia Sessa, PharmD
Pharmacy Resident
Pharmacy Department
Winthrop-University Hospital
Mineola, New York
Antimicrobial Drug Summaries

Daniel S. Siegal, MD
Department of Radiology
Mount Auburn Hospital
Harvard Medical School
Boston, Massachusetts
Chest X-ray Atlas

Rodger P. Silletti, PhD
Director, Clinical Microbiology Laboratory
Winthrop-University Hospital
Mineola, New York
Medical Microbiology

Stephanie Strollo, MD
Infectious Disease Division
Winthrop-University Hospital
Mineola, New York
Susceptibility Testing

Uzma Syed, DO
Infectious Disease Division
Winthrop-University Hospital
Mineola, New York
Susceptibility Testing

Samad Tirmizi, PharmD
Infectious Disease Clinical Pharmacist
Antibiotic Stewardship Team
Department of Pharmacy
NUV Winthrop Hospital
Mineola, New York
Post Antibiotic Effects

Damary C. Torres, PharmD
Clinical Pharmacy Specialist
Winthrop-University Hospital
Mineola, New York
Associate Clinical Professor
College of Pharmacy St. John's University
Queens, New York
Antimicrobial Drug Summaries

Kenneth F. Wagner, DO
Infectious Disease Consultant
National Naval Medical Center
Associate Professor of Medicine
Uniformed Services, University of
the Health Sciences
F. Edward Hebert School of Medicine
Bethesda, Maryland
Parasites, Fungi, Unusual Organisms

Shan Wang, PharmD
Director, Clinical Pharmacy Residency
Winthrop-University Hospital
Mineola, New York
Associate Clinical Professor
College of Pharmacy St. John's University
Queens, New York
Antimicrobial Drug Summaries

Debra Willner, PharmD
Pharmacy Resident
Pharmacy Department
Winthrop-University Hospital
Mineola, New York
Antimicrobial Drug Summaries

Gina L. Wu, MD
Infectious Disease Division
Winthrop-University Hospital
Mineola, New York
HIV

Veronica B. Zafonte, PharmD
Infectious Disease Pharmacy Resident
University of Rochester Medical Center
Rochester, New York
Antimicrobial Drug Summaries

---

* Author affiliations are indicative of their positions at the time of their initial contributions.

NOTICE

- *Not all recommendations in this book are approved indications by the U.S. Food and Drug Administration, and antimicrobial recommendations are not limited to indications in the package insert.*
- *The use of any drug should be preceded by careful review of the package insert, which provides indications and dosing approved by the U.S. Food and Drug Administration.*
- The information provided in this book is essential not exhaustive, and the reader is referred to the manufacturer's product literature for further information.
- *Clinical use of the information provided and any consequences that may arise from its use is the responsibility of the prescribing physician.*
- *The authors, editors, and publisher do not warrant or guarantee the information herein contained and do not assume and expressly disclaim any liability for errors or omissions or any consequences that may occur from use of this information.*

BASIS OF RECOMMENDATIONS

The therapeutic recommendations in Antibiotic Essentials are based on evidence and experience as assessed by the contributor's clinical expertise.

ABBREVIATIONS

ABE	acute bacterial endocarditis	CSD	cat scratch disease
ABM	acute bacterial meningitis	CSF	cerebrospinal fluid
ADA	adenosine deaminase	CT	computerized tomography
ADV	Adenovirus	cUTI	Complicated UTIs
AFB	acid fast bacilli	CVA	costovertebral angle
AGEP	acute generalized exanthematous pustulosis	CVC	central venous catheter
AIH	autoimmune lupoid hepatitis	CVID	common variable immune deficiency
AIHA	autoimmune hemolytic anemia	CVVH	continuous veno venous hemofiltration
AML	acute myelogenous leukemia	CXR	chest x-ray
ANA	antinuclear antibody	DFA	direct fluorescent antibody
ARDS	adult respiratory distress syndrome	DI	diabetes insipidus
AST/ALT	serum transaminases	DIC	disseminated intravascular coagulation
A-V	atrio-ventricular	DM	diabetes mellitus
β-lactams	penicillins, cephalosporins, cephamycins (not monobactams or carbapenems)	DOT	directly observed therapy
		e.g.	for example
		EBV	Ebstein-Barr virus
BAL	bronchoalveolar lavage	EEE	Eastern equine encephalitis
BG	β 1, 3 D-glucan	EEG	electroencephalogram
BMT	bone marrow transplant	EIA	enzyme immunoassay
BPH	benign prostatic hypertrophy	EIEC	enteroinvasive E. coli
CAB	catheter associated bacteriuria	ELISA	enzyme-linked immunosorbent assay
CABG	coronary artery bypass grafting	EM	erythema migrans
CAC	catheter associated candiduria	EMB	ethambutol
CAH	chronic active hepatitis	Enterobacteria-ceae:	Citrobacter, Edwardsiella, Enterobacter, E. coli, Klebsiella, Proteus, Providencia, Shigella, Salmonella, Serratia, Hafnia, Morganella, Yersinia
CA-MRSA	community-acquired MRSA		
CAP	community-acquired pneumonia		
CD₄	CD₄ T-cell lymphocyte		
CE	California encephalitis virus		
CFS	chronic fatigue syndrome	ESBLs	extended spectrum β-lactamases
CGD	chronic granulomatous disease	esp	especially
CHIKV	Chikungunya fever	ESR	erythrocyte sedimentation rate
CIE	counter immunoelectrophoresis	ESRD	end stage renal disease
cIAI	Complicated intra-abdominal infections	ET	endotracheal
		ETEC	enterotogenic E. coli
CLL	chronic lymphocytic leukemia	EV	enterovirus
CML	chronic myelogenous leukemia	EVD	external ventricular drain
CMV	Cytomegalovirus	FTA-ABS	fluorescent treponemal antibody absorption test
CNS	central nervous system		
CO-MRSA	community onset MRSA	FUO	fever of unknown origin
CoNS	coagulase negative staphylococci	G6PD	glucose-6-phosphate dehydrogenase
CoV	coronavirus	GC	gonococcus/gonorrhea
CPH	chronic persistent hepatitis	GCA	giant cell arteritis
CPK	creatine phosphokinase	GI	gastrointestinal
CrCl	creatinine clearance	gm	gram
CRE	carbapenemase resistant Enterobacteriaceae	GM	galactomannan
		GNB	Gram negative bacilli (aerobic)

GU	genitourinary
GVHD	graft versus host disease
HA-MRSA	hospital acquired MRSA
HAP	hospital acquired pneumonia
HAV	hepatitis A virus
HBcAb	hepatitis B core antibody
HBoV	human bocavirus
HBsAg	hepatitis B surface antigen
HBV	hepatitis B virus
HCV	hepatitis C virus
HD	hemodialysis
HDV	hepatitis D virus
HEV	hepatitis E virus
HFHD	high flux hemodialysis
HFV	hepatitis F virus
HFM	hand foot mouth disease
HGA	human granulocytic anaplasmosis
HHV-6,7,8	human herpes virus 6,7,8
HME	human monocytic ehrlichiosis
hMPV	human metapneumovirus
HPS	Hanta virus pulmonary syndrome
HPV	human papilloma virus
HTLV-1	human T-cell leukemia virus
HRIG	human rabies immune globulin
HRTV	heartland virus
HSV	herpes simplex virus
HZ	herpes zoster
I & D	incision and drainage
IFA	immunofluorescent antibody
IgA	immunoglobulin A
IgG	immunoglobulin G
IgM	immunoglobulin M
IM	intramuscular
INH	isoniazid
IP	intraperitoneal
IT	intrathecal
ITP	idiopathic thrombocytopenic purpura
IV	intravenous
IV/PO	IV or PO
IVDA	intravenous drug abuser
IVIG	intravenous immunoglobulin
IVT	intraventricular
JE	Japanese encephalitis
kg	kilogram
L	liter
LAM	lipoarabinomannan
LCM	lymphocytic choriomeningitis
LDH	lactate dehydrogenase
LFTs	liver function tests
LGV	lymphogranuloma venereum

LTB	latent TB
MAI	Mycobacterium avium-intracellulare
MAYV	Mayaro virus
MBC	minimum bactericidal concentration
MCD	multicentric Castleman's disease
mcg	microgram
mcL	microliter
MDR	multidrug resistant
MDRO	multidrug resistant organism
MDRSP	multidrug resistant S. pneumoniae
MERS	middle east respiratory syndrome
mg	milligram
mL	milliliter
MIC	minimum inhibitory concentration
min	minute
MMR	measles, mumps, rubella
MPD	myeloproliferative disorder
MRI	magnetic resonance imaging
MRSA	methicillin resistant S. aureus
MRSE	methicillin resistant S. epidermidis
MS	multiple sclerosis
MSSA	methicillin susceptible S. aureus
MSSE	methicillin susceptible S. epidermidis
MTT	methlytetrathiazole
MU	million units
MVP	mitral valve prolapse
NDM	New Delhi metallo-β-lactamase
NHAP	nursing home acquired pneumonia
NNRTI	non-nucleoside reverse transcriptase inhibitor
NP	nosocomial pneumonia
NRTI	nucleoside reverse transcriptase inhibitor
NSAIDs	nonsteroidal anti-inflammatory drugs
NTM	non-tuberculous mycobacteria
OI	opportunistic infection
OPAT	outpatient parenteral antibiotic therapy
PAN	polyarteritis nodosa
PBC	primary biliary cirrhosis
PBS	protected brush specimen
PCEC	purified chick embryo cells
PCN	penicillin
PCP	Pneumocystis (carinii) jiroveci pneumonia
PCR	polymerase chain reaction
PD	peritoneal dialysis
PDA	patent ductus arteriosus
PE	Powassan encephalitis
PEP	post-exposure prophylaxis
PI	protease inhibitor

PID	pelvic inflammatory disease	TA	temporal arteritis
PML	progressive multifocal leukoencephalopathy	TAA	teichoic acid antibody titers
PMN	polymorphonuclear leucocytes	TAH/BSO	total abdominal hysterectomy/ bilateral salpingoophorectomy
PO	oral	TB	M. tuberculosis
PPD	tuberculin skin test	TEE	transesophageal echocardiogram
PPIs	proton pump inhibitors	TEN	toxic epidermal necrolysis
PPNG	penicillinase producing N. gonorrhoeae	TID	three times per day
PRSP	penicillin resistant S. pneumoniae	TMP	trimethoprim
PTBM	partially treated bacterial meningitis	TMP–SMX	trimethoprim-sulfamethoxazole
PVE	prosthetic valve endocarditis	TOSV	Toscana virus
PVL	Panton-Valentine leukocidin	TPN	total parenteral nutrition
PZA	pyrazinamide	TRNG	tetracycline resistant N.gonorrhoeae
q__d	every __ days	TSS	toxic shock syndrome
q__h	every __ hours	TTE	transthoracic echocardiogram
q month	once a month	TTP	thrombotic thrombocytopenic purpura
q week	once a week	TTPC	time to positive blood cultures
RA	rheumatoid arthritis	TURP	transurethral resection of prostate
RBC	red blood cells	UC	ulcerative colitis
RE	regional ileitis (Crohn's disease)	UTI	urinary tract infection
RMSF	rocky mountain spotted fever	VA	ventriculoatrial
RSV	respiratory syncytial virus	VAP	ventilator associated pneumonia
RUQ	right upper quadrant	VCA	viral capsid antigen
RVA	rabies vaccine absorbed	VEE	Venezuelan equine encephalitis virus
RZV	recombinant zoster vaccine	VISA	vancomycin intermediate susceptible S. aureus
SARS	severe acute respiratory syndrome	VLM	visceral larval migrans
SBE	subacute bacterial endocarditis	VP	ventriculoperitoneal
SCID	severe combined immune deficiency	VRE	vancomycin resistant enterococci
SFTS	severe fever thrombocytopenia syndrome	VRSA	vancomycin resistant S. aureus
SLE	systemic lupus erythematosus	VSE	vancomycin susceptible enterococci
St. LE	Saint Louis encephalitis	VZV	varicella zoster virus
SOT	solid organ transplant	WBC	white blood cells
sp.	species	WEE	western equine encephalitis
SPB	spontaneous bacterial peritonitis	WNE	west nile encephalitis
SPEP	serum protein electrophoresis	XDR	extensively drug resistant
SQ	subcutaneous	yrs	years
STD	sexually transmitted diseases	ZIKV	zika virus

Chapter 1

Overview of Antimicrobial Therapy

Cheston B. Cunha, MD, Burke A. Cunha, MD

Overview of Antimicrobial Therapy

FACTORS IN ANTIBIOTIC SELECTION

Spectrum
- Antibiotic spectrum refers to the range of microorganisms an antibiotic is usually effective against, and is the basis for empiric antibiotic therapy.
- *In vitro* susceptibility does not always predict *in vivo* effectiveness.

Tissue Penetration
- **Antibiotics unable to reach the site of infection will be ineffective. Antibiotic tissue penetration depends on antibiotic properties, e.g., lipid solubility, molecular size, adequacy of blood supply and presence of inflammation.**
- Antibiotics cannot be expected to eradicate organisms from difficult to penetrate areas. Abscesses usually require surgical drainage for cure.
- Device associated infections usually need device removal for cure.

Antibiotic Resistance
- **Bacterial resistance to antimicrobial therapy may be classified as natural/ intrinsic or acquired relative or absolute.**
- Pathogens not covered by the usual spectrum of an antibiotic are termed *naturally/intrinsically* resistant, e.g., 25% of S. pneumoniae are *naturally resistant* to macrolides.
- *Acquired* resistance refers to a previously susceptible pathogen that is no longer susceptible to an antibiotic, e.g., ampicillin resistant H. influenzae. **Organisms with intermediate level (relative) resistance manifest as an increase in minimum inhibitory concentrations (MICs), but are susceptible if achievable serum/tissue concentrations > MIC, e.g., penicillin resistant S. pneumoniae and PCN.**
- Organisms with *high level (absolute) resistance cannot be overcome by higher-than-usual antibiotic doses*, e.g., gentamicin resistant P. aeruginosa.
- **Most acquired antibiotic resistance is agent specific, not class related resistance (usually limited to one or two species).**
- **Resistance is not related, per se, to volume or duration of use, e.g., doxycycline, ceftriaxone.**
- Some antibiotics have little resistance potential, i.e., "low resistance" potential even when used in high volume. Other antibiotics can induce resistance, e.g., **"High resistance potential" antibiotics may induce resistance even with limited use.**

Table 1.1 Resistance Potential of Selected Antibiotics

"High Resistance Potential" Antibiotics to Avoid	Usual Organism(s) Resistant to Each Antibiotic	Preferred "Low Resistance Potential" Antibiotic Alternatives in Same Class	Preferred "Low Resistance Potential" Antibiotic Alternatives in Different Classes
Aminoglycosides			
Gentamicin or Tobramycin	P. aeruginosa	Amikacin	Levofloxacin, Colistin, Cefepime
Cephalosporins			
Ceftazidime	P. aeruginosa	Cefepime	Levofloxacin, Colistin, Polymyxin B
Tetracyclines			
Tetracycline	S. pneumoniae S. aureus	Doxycycline, Minocycline	Levofloxacin, Moxifloxacin
Quinolones			
Ciprofloxacin	S. pneumoniae	Levofloxacin, Moxifloxacin	Doxycycline
Ciprofloxicin	P. aeruginosa	Levofloxacin	Amikacin, Colistin, Cefepime
Glycopeptides			
Vancomycin	MSSA MRSA	None	Linezolid, Daptomycin, Minocycline, Tigecycline
Carbapenems			
Imipenem	P. aeruginosa	Meropenem, Doripenem	Amikacin, Cefepime, Colistin, Polymyxin B
Macrolides			
Azithromycin	S. pneumoniae	None	Doxycycline, Levofloxacin, Moxifloxacin
Dihydrofolate Reductase Inhibitors			
TMP-SMX	S. pneumoniae	None	Doxycycline, Levofloxacin, Moxifloxacin

Safety Profile
- Whenever possible, avoid antibiotics with serious/frequent side effects.

Mode of Antibiotic and Excretion/Excretory Organ Toxicity
- *The mode of elimination/excretion does not predispose to excretory organ toxicity per se,* e.g., nafcillin (hepatically eliminated) is not hepatotoxic, and it's main side effect is nephrotoxicity (interstitial nephritis). In contrast, oxacillin (renally eliminated), is not nephrotoxic, it's main side effect is hepatotoxicity (hepatitis).
- The primary route of antibiotic elimination is protective and does not predispose to excretory organ toxicity.

Cost
- *Switching early from IV to PO antibiotics is the single most important cost saving strategy in hospitalized patients.*
- Institutional cost of IV administration (~$10/dose) may exceed the cost of the antibiotic.
- *Antibiotic costs can also be minimized by using antibiotics with long half-lives, by choosing monotherapy over combination therapy, and decreasing duration of therapy.*

HEMODIALYSIS (HD) DOSING STRATEGIES

Intra-HD Dosing
- For renally eliminated antibiotics, begin therapy with the usual initial dose, then *decrease the maintenance doses/intervals for a CrCl < 10 mg/min* (for specific antibiotics, *see* Chapter 11, Drug Summaries).
- *For antibiotics partially/totally removed by HD, a post-HD is needed* (for specific antibiotics, *see* Chapter 11, Drug Summaries).

Post-HD Dosing
- For selected antibiotics with the requisite PK/PD properties, *treatment may be given after each HD* (Table 1.2).

Table 1.2 Selected Antibiotics for Dialysis Dosing
(*Regimens that do not require Intra-HD Dosing*)

Antibiotic	ESRD (t½h)	Clinical Spectrum	Resistance Potential	Post-Dialysis Dosing
Cefazolin	40 hours	MSSA, Klebsiella pneumoniae, E. coli	Low	2 gm (IV) q HD
Cefepime	18 hours	P. aeruginosa, Aerobic GNBs	Low	2 gm (IV) q HD

(cont'd)

Table 1.2 Selected Antibiotics for Dialysis Dosing *(cont'd)*

Antibiotic	ESRD (t½h)	Clinical Spectrum	Resistance Potential	Post-Dialysis Dosing
Ceftazidime	21 hours	P. aeruginosa, Aerobic GNB	High (P. aeruginosa)	2 gm (IV) q HD
Daptomycin	30 hours	MSSA, MRSA, VSE, VRE	Low	6-12 mg/kg (IV) q HD*
Levofloxacin	40 hours	P. aeruginosa, Aerobic GNBs, MSSA	Low	500 mg (IV/PO) q HD
Meropenem	7 hours	P. aeruginosa, Aerobic GNBs, MSSA, VSE	Low	2 gm (IV) q HD
Ertapenem	14 hours	Aerobic GNBs, MSSA	Low	1 gm (IV) q HD

* For bacteremia due to MSSA/MRSA use 6 mg/kg, for VSE/VRE use 12 mg/kg.

MICROBIOLOGY AND SUSCEPTIBILITY TESTING

Limitations of Microbiology Susceptibility Testing
- *In vitro* data do not differentiate between colonizers and pathogens.
- ***In vitro* data do not necessarily translate into *in vivo* efficacy.**
- *Antibiotic activity-effectiveness depends on body site concentrations local pH, degree of inflammation, cellular debris, local oxygen levels, blood supply and penetrability.*
- ***In vitro* susceptibility testing is dependent on the microbe, methodology, pH, and antibiotic concentration.**
- *In vitro susceptibility testing assumes the isolate was recovered from blood, using serum concentrations of an antibiotic given in the usual dose.*
- **Since some body site, e.g., bladder urine contains higher antibiotic concentrations than found in serum, and other body site, e.g., CSF levels may be lower than in serum, i.e., *in vitro* susceptibility may be misleading for non-bloodstream infections.**
- Antibiotics should be prescribed at the usual recommended doses; attempts to lower cost by reducing dosage may decrease antibiotic efficacy, e.g., cefoxitin 2 gm IV inhibits ~ 85% of B. fragilis, whereas 1 gm IV inhibits only ~ 20%.

Table 1.3 Antibiotic-Organism Combinations for Which *In Vitro* Susceptibility Testing Does Not Predict *In Vivo* Effectiveness

Antibiotic	"Susceptible" Organism
Penicillin	H. influenzae, Yersinia pestis, VSE*
TMP–SMX	Klebsiella, VSE, Bartonella
Polymyxin B	Proteus, Salmonella
Imipenem	Stenotrophomonas maltophilia
Vancomycin	Erysipelothrix rhusiopathiae
Gentamicin	Mycobacterium tuberculosis
Aminoglycosides	Streptococci, Salmonella, Shigella
Clindamycin	Fusobacteria, Clostridia, Listeria
Macrolides	P. multocida
1st, 2nd generation cephalosporins	Salmonella, Shigella, Bartonella
3rd, 4th generation cephalosporins	Listeria, Bartonella, MRSA†
Quinolones	MRSA†

† In spite of apparent *in vitro* susceptibility of antibiotics against MRSA, only vancomycin, minocycline, quinupristin/dalfopristin, linezolid, tedizolid, daptomycin, ceftaroline, telavancin, dalbavancin, oritavancin, eravacycline and tigecycline are effective *in vivo*.

* Effective penicillin therapy for systemic enterococcal infections due to VSE requires an aminoglycoside, e.g., gentamicin.

PK/PD AND OTHER CONSIDERATIONS IN ANTIMICROBIAL THERAPY

Antibiotic Dosing: Concentration vs. Time Dependent Kinetics

Table 1.4 Pharmacokinetic/Pharmacodynamic (PK/PD) Considerations
(also see Appendix)

Antibiotics		Optimal Dosing Strategies
Concentration Dependent Antibiotics (Cmax: MIC)		
• Quinolones • Aminoglycosides • Vancomycin (if MIC ≥ 1 mcg/ml) use 2 gm (IV) q12h	• Doxycycline • Tigecycline • Colistin/ Polymyxin B	**Use highest effective dose (without toxicity)**

(cont'd)

Table 1.4 Pharmacokinetic/Pharmacodynamic (PK/PD) *(cont'd)*

Antibiotics	Optimal Dosing Strategies
Time Dependent Antibiotics (T > MIC)	
• PCN: maintain concentrations > MIC for ≥ 60% of the dosing interval • β-lactams: maintain concentrations > MIC for ≥ 75% of the dosing interval • Carbapenems: maintain concentrations > MIC for ≥ 40% of the dosing interval • Vancomycin (if MIC ≤ 1 mcg/mL) use 1 gm (IV) q12h	**Use high doses (which increase serum concentrations which also increase T > MIC for more of the dosing interval)**
Other Antibiotics (Cmax: MIC/T>MIC and or AUC $_{0-24}$/MIC)	

• Quinolones
    > 125 (effective)
    > 250 (more effective)
	Use highest effective dose (without toxicity)

Bactericidal vs. Bacteriostatic Therapy (also see Appendix)
- For most infections, bacteriostatic and bactericidal antibiotics inhibit/kill organisms at the same rate, and **should not be a factor in antibiotic selection.**
- Bactericidal antibiotics have an advantage in certain infections, such endocarditis, meningitis, and febrile leukopenia, but there are exceptions even in these cases.

Monotherapy vs. Combination Therapy
- **Monotherapy is preferred to combination therapy for nearly all infections.**
- In addition to cost savings, monotherapy results in less chance of medication error and fewer missed doses/drug interactions.
- Combination therapy may be useful for drug synergy or for extending spectrum beyond what can be obtained with a single drug.
- **Combination therapy is not effective in preventing antibiotic resistance, except in very few situations (anti-TB therapy).**

IV to PO Switch Therapy
- Patients admitted to the hospital are usually started on IV antibiotic therapy, then switched to equivalent oral therapy after clinical improvement/defervescence (usually within 72 hours).
- **Advantages of early IV-to-PO switch programs include reduced cost, early hospital discharge, less need for home IV therapy, and virtual elimination of IV line infections**.
- Drugs well-suited for IV-to-PO switch or for treatment entirely by the oral route have high bioavailibility, e.g., doxycycline, minocycline, clindamycin, metronidazole, chloramphenicol, amoxicillin, trimethoprim-sulfamethoxazole, quinolones, and linezolid.

Table 1.5 Bioavailability of Oral Antimicrobials

Bioavailability	Antimicrobials		
Excellent (> 90%)	Amoxicillin Cephalexin Cefprozil Cefadroxil Clindamycin Quinolones Chloramphenicol	TMP TMP–SMX Doxycycline Minocycline Fluconazole Metronidazole Cycloserine	Linezolid Tedizolid Isavuconazole Voriconazole Rifampin Isoniazid Pyrazinamide
Good (60–90%)	Cefixime Cefpodoxime Ceftibuten Cefuroxime Cefaclor Delafloxacin	Valacyclovir Famciclovir Valganciclovir Macrolides Nitrofurantoin	Ethambutol 5-Flucytosine Posaconazole Itraconazole (solution) Nitazoxanide (with food)
Poor (< 60%)	Vancomycin Acyclovir	Cefdinir Lefamulin	Omadacycline Fosfomycin

Oral Antibiotic Therapy for Serious Systemic Infections

- Most infectious diseases should be treated orally unless the patient is critically ill, cannot take antibiotics by mouth, or there is no equivalent oral antibiotic.
- If the patient is able to take/absorb oral antibiotics, there is no difference in clinical outcome using equivalent IV or PO antibiotics.
- It is more important to think in terms of antibiotic spectrum, bioavailability and tissue penetration, rather than route of administration.
- **Nearly all non-critically ill patients may be treated in part or entirely with oral antibiotics.**
- When switching from IV to PO therapy, **oral antibiotic chosen should have the same spectrum/degree of activity against the presumed/known pathogen and achieve the same blood and tissue levels as the equivalent IV antibiotic.**

OPAT (outpatient parenteral antibiotic therapy)

- OPAT has been used to treat infections IV on an outpatient basis or to complete IV therapy begun during hospitalization. Preferred OPAT antibiotics are those with few adverse effects and those with a long serum half life. The most frequently used OPAT antibiotics are ceftriaxone and vancomycin.

- The preferred alternative to OPAT is oral antibiotic therapy, e.g., for MRSA, minocycline or linezolid are equally efficacious as OPAT regimens.
- Other agents with long $t_{1/2}$ ideal for OPAT of Gram positive cSSSIs due to MRSA are telavancin 10 mg (IV) q 24 h, dalbavancin 1 gm (IV) × 1 doses then 500 mg (IV) × 1 dose 7 days later; tedizolid 200 mg (IV)q 24 h × 6 days, then 200 mg (PO) q 24 h × 6 days; and oritavancin 1200 mg (IV) × 1 dose.

Duration of Therapy

- Most bacterial infections in normal hosts are treated with antibiotics for 1–2 weeks.
- The duration of therapy may need to be extended in patients with impaired immunity, e.g., diabetes, SLE, alcoholic liver disease, neutropenia, diminished splenic function, etc., chronic bacterial infections e.g., endocarditis, osteomyelitis, chronic viral and fungal infections, or certain bacterial intracellular pathogens.

COLONIZATION VS. INFECTION

Table 1.6 Urinary Tract: Infection vs. Colonization

Acute Uncomplicated Cystitis (AUC) = Infection	
Dysuria + Bacteriuria (cc: > 100 K cfu/mL)	Treat with PO antibiotic* (see p. 111)
Asymptomatic Bacteriuria (AB) = Colonization	
No rationale for UC if no dysuria	
AB = Bacteriuria (< 100 K cfu/mL) + no dysuria	*Do not treat* (If treated, AB usually returns)
Catheter Associated Bacteriuria (CAB) = Infection vs. Colonization	
<u>Asymptomatic CAB</u> (*bacteriuria without dysuria*) = **colonization**	
Replace Foley and repeat UC (bacteriuria eliminated)	*Do not treat*
<u>Symptomatic CAB</u> (*bacteriuria with dysuria*) = **infection** (*if dysuria is not due to irritation*)	Treat with PO antibiotic*

*Repeat UC/UA after 1-3 days on therapy to verify antibiotic response in AUC (urine colony counts rapidly decrease with effective therapy)

COLONIZATION VS. INFECTION

Table 1.7 Nosocomial Pneumonia: Colonization vs. Infection

- Colonization of respiratory secretions in ventilated patients is the rule and a function of time (days intubated).
- GNB from the ICU milieu colonize respiratory secretions.
- Common GNB colonizers include *Klebsiella, Enterobacter, Serratia, S. maltophilia, B. cepacia* and *P. aeruginosa.*
- Most GNB colonizing organisms rarely, if ever, cause NP/VAP, e.g., *Enterobacter, S. maltophilia, B. cepacia.*
- In ventilated patients with fever, leukocytosis, and infiltrates on CXR unless accompanied by the characteristic clinical features of the pathogen, *organisms cultured from respiratory secretions should be considered as airway colonizers* and not the cause of NP/VAP.
- *Klebsiella sp.* pneumonia presents with fevers and cavitation (3-5 days after infiltrates) *P. aeruginosa* pneumonia presents with high spiking fevers, elastin fibers in respiratory secretions, hemoptysis and rapid cavitation (<3 days after infiltrates).

- Ventilated patients treated with antibiotics with minimal *S. aureus* activity, e.g., ciprofloxacin, ceftazidime are often colonized with MSSA or MRSA, but do not progress to *S. aureus* NP/VAP.
- *S. aureus* (MSSA or MRSA) CAP may complicate influenza pneumonia, but rarely, if ever, causes NP/VAP.
- Reports of *S. aureus* in ventilated patients with fever, leukocytosis and infiltrates on CXR is based on respiratory secretion cultures and represents colonization and not the cause of NP.
- Without the distinctive clinical features of MSSA or MRSA CAP, e.g., high fevers, cyanosis, elastin fibers in respiratory secretions, hemoptysis, clinical deterioration and rapid cavitation (<3 days) on CXR, patients should be considered as being colonized with MSSA or MRSA (or may have tracheobronchitis) but not MSSA/MRSA NP/VAP.

GNB = Gram negative bacilli
NP = nosocomial pneumonia
VAP = ventilator associated pneumonia

COLONIZATION VS. INFECTION

Table 1.8 Colonization vs. Infection: Draining Wounds

Wound drainage	Wound Gram stain	Wound culture	Diagnosis
Clear	Few or some WBCs	+	Colonization
Serous	Few or some WBCs	+	Colonization
Serosanguineous	Few or some WBCs	+	Colonization
Purulent	Abundant WBCs	+	Infection

Table 1.9 Chronic Osteomyelitis: Colonization vs. Infection
Sacral Decubitus Ulcers (Stage III/IV) or Chronic/Deep Diabetic Foot Ulcers

- **Always treat the usual pathogens related to body site flora rather than "covering the cultured organism" from deep ulcers (since the culture specimen is not representative of the underlying pathogen in the infected bones).**
  - **Diabetic foot ulcers with chronic osteomyelitis:**
    Cover the usual osteomyelitis pathogens: GAS, GBS, common coliforms, *S. aureus*, and *B. fragilis* (not *P. aeruginosa*)
- **Do not cover surface ulcer colonizers cultured** *P. aeruginosa*, *Acinetobacter sp.*, VSE/VRE, *Enterobacter sp.*, *Burkholderia sp.*, *Stenotrophomonas sp.*
  - Do not rely on deep ulcer/fistula cultures (which represent skin flora) and are not reflective of bone pathogens, i.e., osteomyelitis.
  - If *P. aeruginosa* is cultured from deep ulcer/fistula, do not cover for *P. aeruginosa*. Over 95% of diabetic foot ulcers/fistulas will be culture positive from *P. aeruginosa* (due to *P. aeruginosa* colonization from wet socks, wet dressings, whirlpool baths). In aseptically collected bone specimens in the OR.
- *P. aeruginosa* is NOT a bone pathogen in diabetics with chronic osteomyelitis.
  - **Sacral decubitus ulcers (stage III/IV) = chronic osteomyelitis**
    Cover the usual chronic osteomyelitis pathogens:
    GAS, GBS, *S. aureus*, coliforms, and *B. fragilis*.
- **Do not cover ulcer surface colonizers cultured ("water organisms"):**
  - *Stenotrophomonas sp.*, *Acinetobacter sp.*, *Enterobacter sp.*, *P. aeruginosa sp.*, *Burkholderia sp.*

GAS = group A streptococci	VSE = vancomycin susceptible enterococci
GBS = group B streptococci	VRE = vancomycin resistant enterococci

Table 1.10 Positive Blood Cultures vs. Bacteremia (MSSA, MRSA, CoNS)

Factors Favoring + Blood Cultures (not bacteremia)	Factors Favoring Bacteremia (not BC skin contaminants)
MSSA/MRSA + BCs (skin contamination likely) with:	**MSSA/MRSA Bacteremia** with:
• Intermittently positive BCs • Low level/low grade BC positivity (1/4 - 2/4 BCs +) • TTPC = > 2 days • No clinical source of MSSA/MRSA bacteremia (CVC, abscesses, osteomyelitis, ABE)	• Persistently positive BCs • High level/high grade bacteremia (3/4 4/4 BCs +) • TTPC = < 2 days • Clinical source of MSSA/MRSA bacteremia clinically apparent (CVC, abscesses, osteomyelitis, ABE)
CoNS (skin contamination likely) with: • Intermittently positive BCs • Low level/low grade BC positivity (1/4 - 2/4 + BCs) • TTPC = > 2 days • No clinical source of CoNS + BCs (CVC, implanted orthopedic/cardiac devices, prosthetic materials, severe/prolonged neutropenia)	**CoNS Bacteremia** (infection likely) with: • Persistently positive BCs • High level/high grade bacteremia (3/4 – 4/4 BCs +) • TTPC = < 2 days • Clinical source of + BCs for CoNS apparent (CVC, implanted orthopedic/cardiac devices, prosthetic materials, severe/prolonged neutropenia)

Implanted/prosthetic device associated: Dx = gallium or indium scan. ABE: Dx = cardiac vegetation. Abscess Dx = Gallium scan or CT scan. CVC associated: Dx = SQ removed CVC tip culture with > 15 col of same organism as in BCs not drawn from the CVC. TTPC = time to positive culture

Table 1.11 Clinical Features of Drug Fever

History
- Many, but not all patients are atopic
- Most patients have been on a "sensitizing medication" for years "without a problem"
- Less likely due to new or recent medications

Physical exam
- Unexplained/persistent fevers with relative bradycardia
- Fevers usually between 102°–104° F, but may exceed 106°F
- Patient appears "inappropriately well" for degree of fever

Laboratory tests
- Elevated WBC count (usually with left shift) mimicking an infectious etiology
- Eosinophils almost always present, but eosinophilia is uncommon
- Elevated erythrocyte sedimentation rate over baseline
- Commonly transient, mild elevations of serum transaminases
- Negative blood cultures (excluding skin contaminants)

COMMONEST SENSITIZING MEDICATIONS CAUSING DRUG FEVER

Common	Less Common
Amphotericin B	Allopurinol
Barbituates	Hydralazine
Methyldopa	Iodides
Penicillins	Isoniazid
Cephalosporins	Rifampin
Procainamide	NSAIDs
Quinidine	Anti-seizure medications
Sulfonamides	Sedatives
Opiates	Sleep medications
Colace	
Lasix	

Table 1.12 Relative Bradycardia: Pulse/Temperature-Pulse Relationships*

Temperature	Appropriate Pulse Response (beats/min)	If Relative Bradycardia Pulse (beats/min)
106°F (41.1°C)	150/min	< 140/min
105°F (40.6°C)	140/min	< 130/min
104°F (40.7°C)	130/min	< 120/min
103°F (39.4°C)	120/min	< 110/min
102°F (38.9°C)	110/min	< 100/min

- Exloading second/third-degree heart block, pacemaker rhythms, or those taking beta-blockers, diltiazem, or verapamil.

ANTIBIOTIC FAILURE

Table 1.13 Apparent and Actual Causes Persistent Fevers on Appropriate Antibiotic Therapy

Microbiologic Factors
- *In vitro* susceptibility but ineffective *in vivo*
- Treating coloniztation (no fever) vs. infection (fever)

Antibiotic Factors
- Inadequate antimicrobial spectrum (for site of infection)
- Inadequate antibiotic tissue levels (relative to serum levels)
- Decreased antibiotic activity (pH dependent)

Antibiotic Penetration Factors
- Undrained/inadequate abscess
- Device associated infections (no blood supply)
- Organ hypoperfusion/diminished blood supply, e.g. DM, PVD

Non-infectious Diseases
- Disorders mimicking infections, e.g., SLE, malignancies
- Drug fever

Antibiotic Unresponsive Infectious Diseases
- Viral or fungal infections

Table 1.14 Infections Not Curable with Antimicrobial Therapy Alone

- Chronic sinusitis, otitis, mastoiditis*
- PVE[†], Intracardiac abscess*
- Intra-abdominal/Pelvic abscesses*
- Chronic prostatitis (if calcifications[¥])
- Chronic osteomyelitis sacral decubitus (Stage III/IV)[§]
- Foot osteomyelitis[§]

* Surgical drainage required for cure
[†] Removal of device needed for cure
[§] Bone debridement (bone, not just skin)
[¥] Surgical removal (TURP)

ANTIMICROBIAL STEWARDSHIP: PRINCIPLES AND PRACTICE

Antimicrobial Stewardship: Principles and Practice

Colonization vs. Infection (see also Tables 1.6–1.10)
- Treat infection, not colonization.
- Provide empiric coverage primarily directed against the most probable pathogens causing the infection at the body site.
- Avoid "covering" or "chasing" multiple organisms cultured that are (pathogens and non-pathogens) at the body site cultured.
- Selectively treat CAB in immunocompromised hosts. Avoid treating CAB in normal hosts.
- Colonization of respiratory secretions, wounds, or urine with "water" (S. maltophilia, B. cepacia, P. aeruginosa) or skin organisms (MSSA, MRSA, CoNS, VSE, VRE) is the rule.

Narrow vs. Broad Spectrum Therapy
- Narrow vs broad spectrum doesn't prevent resistance, e.g., in treating E. coli urosepsis switching from a carbapenem (broad spectrum) to ampicillin (narrow spectrum) may actually increase resistance potential.
- Narrow spectrum vs broad spectrum is not clinically superior to well chosen broad spectrum therapy, e.g., switching from ceftriaxone (broad spectrum) to penicillin (narrow spectrum in treating S. pneumoniae has no clinical rationale or clinical advantage and has no effect on controlling resistance.
- Antibiotic resistance potential is related to individual antibiotics and not antibiotics class, e.g., meropenem (low resistance potential) vs. imipenem (high resistance potential).
- Antibiotic resistance is not related to spectrum narrowness or broadness, e.g., levofloxacin (broad spectrum but "low resistance potential") vs ampicillin (narrow spectrum but "high resistance potential").

Antibiotic Resistance (see also Table 1.1)
- The best way to control resistance is a *selectively restricted formulary*; restricted only to "high resistance potential" antibiotics, e.g., ciprofloxacin (not levofloxacin or moxifloxacin), imipenem (not meropenem or ertapenem), cefazidime (not other 3rd of 4th GC), gentamicin/tobramycin (not amikacin).
- Some antibiotics may be restricted for other reasons, e.g., excessive vancomycin (IV not PO) use predisposes to VRE emergence and vancomycin may cause cell wall thickening in S. aureus resulting in permeability related resistance (to vancomycin and other antibiotics, e.g., daptomycin).
- *Over-restriction of antibiotics may impair timely effective therapy and does not, per se, control or decrease resistance.*
- Preferentially select antibiotics (all other things being equal) with a "low resistance potential". Avoid, if possible, "high resistance potential" antibiotics, e.g., macrolides (for respiratory infections), TMP-SMX (for UTIs).
- Except for TB therapy, *combination therapy doesn't prevent resistance.* The only examples of combination therapies that prevent resistance are carbenicillin + gentamicin and FC + amphotericin B.
- Since resistance is, in part, concentrations dependant, subtherapeutic or low antibiotic tissue concentrations, (all other things being equal) predisposes to resistance.

- Suboptimal dosing or usual dosing with inadequate tissue penetration, e.g., into the body fluids or undrained abscesses (source control is key) also predisposes to resistance.
- Treat for the shortest duration of therapy that is effective in eliminating the infection.

Monotherapy vs. Combination Therapy

- Preferably use monotherapy whenever possible to cover the most likely pathogen or cultured pathogen clinically relevant to the site of infection.
- Combination therapy should be avoided if possible. Always tty to preferentially use monotherapy.
- Monotherapy is usually less expensive than combination therapy and has less potential for adverse effects and drug-drug interactions.
- Combination therapy is often used for potential synergy (rarely occurs and if used must be based on microbiology laboratory synergy studies), to increase spectrum (preferable to use monotherapy with same spectrum), or to prevent resistance (except for TB, ineffective in nearly all contributors).

PO and IV-to-PO Switch Antibiotic Therapy (see also Table 1.5)

- Wherever possible, treat with entirely oral antibiotic therapy instead of IV therapy.
- Switch from IV-to-PO antibiotic therapy after clinical defervescence (usually < 72 hours).
- Early IV-to-PO switch therapy eliminates phlebitis and IV line associated infections.

Antibiotic De-escalation

- De-escalation is problematic if based on microbiology data alone without site-pathogen correlation.
- De-escalation is appropriate in the setting of broad spectrum coverage of "presumed urosepsis" which can be narrowed after the uropathogen is identified in blood/urine.
- In intubated/ventilate patients, microbiology data from respiratory secretion cultures are usually misleading and not representative of NP or VAP lung pathogens.
- In patients with NP or VAP, it is more prudent to treat the most likely pathogen, e.g., P. aeruginosa (even if not cultured from respiratory secretions) than to be misguided into treating multiple colonizing organisms in respiratory secretions.
- De-escalation can be harmful if microbiology data is misleading, e.g., represents colonization rather than being reflective of the pathogen (underlying bone pathogen, not ulcer organisms), e.g., diabetic foot ulcers/chronic osteomyelitis or sacral ulcers/chronic osteomyelitis.

C. difficile Diarrhea/Colitis

- Preferentially select antibiotics (all other things being equal) with low C. difficile potential.
- Predisposing factors to C. difficile include relatively few antibiotics, e.g., clindamycin, β-lactams, ciprofloxacin.
- Most antibiotics have little/no C. difficile potential, e.g., aminoglycosides, aztreonam, maerolides, TMP-SMX, colistin, polymyxin B, daptomycin, Q/D, doxycycline, minocycline, tigecycline, vancomycin, linezolid.
- Some antibiotics are protective against C. difficile, e.g., doxycycline, tigecycline.
- Always consider non-antibiotic factors that may predispose to C. difficile, e.g., cancer chemotherapy, anti-depressants, statins, PPIs.
- Also consider person to person spread or acquisition from the environment.

Empiric Antibiotics for Fever and Leukocytosis
- Avoid treating unexplained fever/leukocytosis. If due to infection, let the infection declare itself and then initiate early therapy.
- Try to diagnose the many non-infectious causes of fever/leukocytosis rather than treating empirically with antibiotics.
- Avoid prolonged antibiotic therapy of fever/leukocytosis in the presence of a device associated infection or undrained/inadequately drained abscesses.
- Avoid antibiotic therapy of non-infectious fevers or non-antibiotic responsive infections, e.g., drug fevers, malignancies, hematomas, rheumatic/inflammatory disorders, viral infections.

Pharmacoeconomic Considerations
- The least expensive therapy is usually not the best therapy.
- The least expensive antibiotic (acquisition cost) may, in fact, be expensive (re: total cost) when considering the cost implications to the institution of dosing frequency, C. difficile potential, resistance potential, and degree of activity against the known or likely pathogen, and the cost of potential therapeutic failure vis-à-vis ↑ LOS and medicolegally.
- Stewardship savings are best achieved by decreasing duration of antibiotic therapy, and by treating entirely with oral antibiotic therapy or early IV-to-PO switch therapy.

REFERENCES

Bennett JE, Dolin R, Blaser MJ (eds). Mandell, Douglas, and Bennett's Principles and Practice of Infectious Diseases (9th Ed). Philadelphia Elsevier Churchill Livingstone, 2019.

Bryskier A (ed). Antimicrobial Agents. ASM Press, Washington, D.C., 2005.

Cohen J, Powderly WG, Opal S (eds). Infectious Diseases (4th Ed). Philadelphia: Elsevier, 2016.

Cunha CB. Antibiotic Stewardship Programs (ASP) Perspective: Oral Antibiotic Therapy of Common Infectious Diseases. Medical Clinics of North America. 102:947-954, 2018.

Cunha CB. Antimicrobial Stewardship: Principles and Practice. Medical Clinics of North America. 102:797-803, 2018.

Cunha CB. Principles of Stewardship. In: LaPlante K, Cunha C, Morrill H, Rice L, Mylonakis E (eds). Antimicrobial Stewardship: Principles and Practice, CABI Publishers, London, 2017.

Cunha CB, Cunha BA (eds). Infectious Diseases in Critical Care Medicine (4th Ed.) CRC Press, New York, 2020.

Cunha CB, Opal SM. Antimicrobial Stewardship: Strategies to Minimize antibiotic Resistance While Maximizing Antibiotic Effectiveness. Medical Clinics of North America. 102:831-843, 2018.

Cunha CB, Schlossberg D (eds). Clinical Infectious Disease (3rd Ed), Cambridge University Press, Cambridge, 2020.

Finch RG, Greenwood D, Norrby SR, Whitley RJ (eds). Antibiotic and Chemotherapy (8th Ed). Churchill Livingstone, Edinburgh, 2003.

Gorbach SL, Bartlett JG, Blacklow NR (eds). Infectious Diseases (3rd Ed). Philadelphia, Lippincott, Williams & Wilkins, 2004.

Grayson ML (ed). Kucer's The Use of Antibiotics (6th Ed), ASM Press, Washington, DC, 2010.

O'Grady F, Lambert HP, Finch RG, Greenwood D (eds). Antibiotic and Chemotherapy (2nd Ed). Churchill Livingstone, New York, 1997.

Ristuccia AM, Cunha BA (eds). Antimicrobial Therapy. Raven Press, New York, 1984.

Scholar EM Pratt WB (eds). The Antimicrobial Drugs (2nd Ed), Oxford University Press, New York, 2000.

Yu V, Edwards G, McKinnon PS, Peloquin C, Morse G (eds). Antimicrobial Therapy and Vaccines, Volume II: Anti-microbial Agents (2nd Ed), Esun Technologies, Pittsburgh, 2005.

Chapter 2

Empiric Therapy Based on Clinical Syndrome

**Cheston B. Cunha, MD, Burke A. Cunha, MD, John L. Brusch, MD,
Ronald L. Nichols, MD, Genovefa Papanicolaou, MD,
Jean E. Hage, MD, Raymond S. Koff, MD,
John H. Rex, MD, Dennis J. Cleri, MD, Staci A. Fischer, MD,
Jeffrey Baron, PharmD, David Schlossberg, MD**

- *Clinical summaries immediately follow each treatment grid.*
- **Therapeutic recommendations are based on antimicrobial effectiveness, resistance potential, and clinical experience.**
- Antimicrobial dosages in this section represent the usual dosages for normal renal and hepatic function in adults.
- **In any given grid category, drug choices are equivalent alternatives.**
- Dosage adjustments, side effects, drug interactions, and other prescribing information are described in individual Drug Summaries (Chapter 11).

- *Use of any drug should be preceded by careful review of the package insert, which provides indications and dosing approved by the U.S. Food and Drug Administration.*
- "PO Therapy or IV-to-PO Switch" entry in the treatment grids indicates the clinical syndrome can be treated, PO therapy alone, or IV followed by PO therapy.
- *Most patients on IV therapy should be switched to equivalent PO therapy after clinical improvement.*

Empiric Therapy of CNS Infections

Acute Bacterial Meningitis (ABM) (see Color Atlas for CSF Gram stains)

Subset	Usual Pathogens	Preferred IV Therapy	Alternate IV Therapy	IV-to-PO Switch
Normal host	N. meningitidis H. influenzae S. pneumoniae	Ceftriaxone 2 gm (IV) q12h × 2 weeks	Meropenem 2 gm (IV) q8h × 2 weeks	Chloram-phenicol 500 mg (PO) q6h × 2 weeks
Elderly or malig-nancy	Listeria monocyto-genes N. meningitidis H. influenzae S. pneumoniae	<u>Before culture results</u> Ceftriaxone 2 gm (IV) q12h **plus** Ampicillin 2 gm (IV) q4h <u>*Listeria present* after culture results</u> Ampicillin 2 gm (IV) q4h × 3 weeks <u>*Listeria not present*</u> Ceftriaxone 2 gm (IV) q12h × 2 weeks	<u>After culture results</u> *Listeria present* TMP–SMX 5 mg/kg (IV) q6h × 3 weeks **or** Meropenem 2 gm (IV) q8h × 3 weeks **or** Chloramphenicol 500 mg (IV) q6h × 2 weeks **or** Linezolid 600 mg (IV) q12h × 3 weeks <u>*Listeria not present*</u> Ceftriaxone 2 gm (IV) q12h × 2 weeks	<u>For Listeria meningitis only</u> TMP–SMX 5 mg/kg (PO) q6h × 3 weeks **or** Chloram-phenicol 500 mg (PO) q6h × 3 weeks **or** Linezolid 600 mg (PO) q12h × 3 weeks <u>For usual meningeal pathogens</u> Chloram-phenicol 500 mg (PO) q6h × 2 weeks

Acute Bacterial Meningitis (ABM) (see Color Atlas for CSF Gram stains) *(cont'd)*

Subset	Usual Pathogens	Preferred IV Therapy	Alternate IV Therapy	IV-to-PO Switch
CNS shunt infections (VA shunts)	S. aureus S. epidermidis (CoNS)	<u>MSSA/MSSE</u> Meropenem 2 gm (IV) q8h* <u>MRSA/MRSE</u> Linezolid 600 mg (IV) q12h*	<u>MSSA/MSSE</u> Cefepime 2 gm (IV) q8h* <u>MRSA/MRSE</u> Vancomycin 2 gm (IV) q12h* **plus** Vancomycin 20 mg (IT) q24h (until shunt removal)	<u>MSSE/MRSE</u> Linezolid 600 mg (PO) q12h* <u>MSSA/MRSA</u> 200 mg (PO) × 1, then 100 mg (PO) q12h* **or** Linezolid 600 mg (PO) q12h*
CNS shunt infections (VP shunts)	E. coli K. pneumoniae Enterobacter S. marcescens	Ceftriaxone 2 gm (IV) q12h × 2 weeks (after shunt removal)	TMP–SMX 5 mg/kg (IV) q6h × 2 weeks (after shunt removal)	TMP–SMX 5 mg/kg (PO) q6h × 2 weeks (after shunt removal)
Ventriculitis (EVD associated)	MDR P. aeruginosa	Meropenem 2 gm (IV) q8h ± Colistin 5 mg/kg (IV) q8h **plus** Colistin 10 mg (IT) q24h × 2 weeks (after shunt removal)	Meropenem 2 gm (IV) q8h ± Amikacin 1 gm (IV) q24h **plus** Amikacin 10 mg (IT) q24h × 2 weeks (after shunt removal)	
	MDR Acinetobacter	Ampicillin/ Sulbactam 4.5 gm (IV) q6h × 2 weeks (after shunt removal) **plus either** Meropenem 2 gm (IV) q8h × 2 weeks (after shunt removal) **or** Colistin 10 mg (IT) q12h × 2 weeks (after shunt removal)	Meropenem 2 gm (IV) q8h × 2 weeks (after shunt removal) **or** Ampicillin/ Sulbactam 4.5 gm (IV) q6h × 2 weeks (after shunt removal) **plus** Colistin 10 mg (IT) q12h × 2 weeks (after shunt removal)	

MSSA/MRSA = methicillin-sensitive/resistant S. aureus; MSSE/MRSE = methicillin-sensitive/resistant S. epidermidis.
* Treat until 1 week after shunt removal.

Clinical Presentation: Abrupt onset of fever, headache, stiff neck.
Diagnosis: CSF gram stain/culture.

Acute Bacterial Meningitis (Normal Hosts)

Diagnostic Considerations: Gram stain of centrifugated CSF is still the best diagnostic test. CSF antigen/CIE are unhelpful in establishing the diagnosis (many false-negatives). In ABM, typical CSF findings include a WBC count of 100–5000 cells/mm^3, elevated opening pressure, variably elevated protein and CSF lactic acid levels (> 6 mmol/L). After the Gram stain, the single most important CSF Dx test is the CSF lactic acid level. In ABM, CSF LA levels >6 mmol/L. In partially treated ABM, CSF LA levels 4-6 mmol/L. ABM is effectively ruled out with CSF LA <4 mmol/L. If the WBC is extremely high (> 20,000 cells/mm^3), suspect brain abscess with rupture into the ventricular system, and obtain a CT/MRI to confirm.

Pitfalls: If ABM is suspected, always perform lumbar puncture (LP) before obtaining a CT scan, since early antibiotic therapy is critical. A CT/MRI should be obtained before LP only if a mass lesion is a primary concern. A stiff neck on physical examination has limited diagnostic value in the elderly, since nuchal rigidity may occur without meningitis (e.g., cervical arthritis) and meningitis may occur without nuchal rigidity. Recurrence of fever during the first week of H. influenzae meningitis is commonly due to subdural effusion, which usually resolves spontaneously over several days. Meningococcal meningitis may occur with or without meningococcemia. On Gram stain, S. pneumoniae may be mistaken for H. influenzae, and Listeria may be mistaken for S. pneumoniae.

Therapeutic Considerations: Do not reduce "meningeal" antibiotic dosing as the patient improves. Repeat LP if the patient is not responding to antibiotics after 48 hours; lack of response may be due to therapeutic failure, relapse, or noninfectious CNS disorder. For S. pneumoniae meningitis, penicillin-resistant strains are susceptible to meningeal doses of beta-lactam antibiotics e.g., ceftriaxone. Highly resistant pneumococcal strains (rare in the CSF) may be treated for 2 weeks with meropenem 2 gm (IV) q8h or linezolid 600 mg (IV) q12h. Dexamethasone 0.15 mg/kg (IV) q6h × 4 days may be given to reduce the incidence/severity of neurologic sequelae, although the value of steroids in adults is unclear. If used, give dexamethasone 30 minutes before the initial antibiotic dose.

Prognosis: Often fatal without treatment. Case-fatality rates in treated adults are 10–20%. Neurological deficits on presentation are associated with a poor prognosis. Permanent neurological deficits are more frequent with S. pneumoniae than H. influenzae, even with early therapy. In meningococcal meningitis, there are no neurological deficits in survivors.

Acute Bacterial Meningitis (Elderly/Malignancy)

Diagnostic Considerations: Diagnosis by CSF Gram stain/culture and CSF LA (see above). ABM pathogens include usual pathogens in normal hosts plus Listeria monocytogenes, a gram-positive, aerobic, bacillus. Listeria is the most common ABM pathogen in patients with malignancies, and is a common pathogen in the elderly. With Listeria meningitis, CSF cultures are positive in 100%, but CSF gram stain is negative in 50%. Meningeal carcinomatosis is suggested by multiple cranial nerve abnormalities.

Pitfalls: "Diphtheroids" isolated from CSF should be speciated to rule out Listeria. Listeria are motile and hemolytic on blood agar, but diphtheroids are not.

Therapeutic Considerations: Elderly patients and cancer patients with ABM require empiric coverage of Listeria plus other ABM pathogens in normal hosts (N. meningitidis, H. influenzae, S. pneumoniae). Third-generation cephalosporins are not active against Listeria.

Prognosis: Related to underlying immunocompetence of the host.

Acute Bacterial Meningitis (CNS Shunt Infections)/Ventriculitis (EVD infections)
Diagnostic Considerations: Diagnosis by CSF Gram stain/culture and ↑ CSF lactic acid levels >6 nmol/L.
Pitfalls: Blood cultures are usually negative shunt pathogens. VA shunt infections usually due to skin organisms. VP shunt infections may be due to GNB from GI tract.
Therapeutic Considerations: In addition to systemic antibiotics in meningeal doses, adjunctive intraventricular (IVT)/intrathecal (IT) antibiotics are sometimes given to control shunt infections before shunt removal. Cure requires VA/VP shunt or EVD removal.
Prognosis: Good if EVD or CNS shunt is removed.

Acute Nonbacterial Meningitis/Chronic Meningitis

Subset	Usual Pathogens	Preferred IV Therapy	Alternate IV Therapy	PO Therapy or IV-to-PO Switch
Viral (aseptic)	EBV, LCM, Parvo B19, mumps, enteroviruses, WNE. No effective therapy for most. For HIV*			
	HSV-1* HSV-2*	<u>IV Therapy:</u> Acyclovir 10 mg/kg (IV) q8h × 10 days Ganciclovir 5 mg/kg (IV) q12h × 10 days <u>PO Therapy:</u> Valacyclovir 1 gm (PO) q8h × 10 days		
	VZV	<u>IV Therapy:</u> Acyclovir 10 mg/kg (IV) q8h × 10 days. <u>PO Therapy:</u> Valacyclovir 2 gm (PO) q6h × 10 days		
	HHV-6	Gangciclovir: 5 mg/kg (IV) q12h × 2 weeks **or** Foscarnet 90 mg/kg (IV) q12h × 2 weeks		
Primary amebic meningo-encephalitis (PAM)	Naegleria fowleri	Amphotericin B 1 mg/kg (IV) q24h until cured **plus** Amphotericin B 1 mg (IVT) via Ommaya reservoir q24h until cured		
Granuloma-tous amebic meningo-encephalitis (GAM)	Acanth-amoeba	Amphotericin B 1 mg/kg (IV) q24h until cured		
Lyme neuro-borreliosis	Borrelia burgdorferi	Ceftriaxone 2 gm (IV) q24h × 2 weeks **or** Minocycline 200 mg (IV) × 1, then 100 mg (IV) q12h × 2 weeks **or** Doxycycline 200 mg (IV) q12h × 3 days, then 100 mg (IV) q12h × 4 days		Minocycline 200 mg (PO) × 1, then 100 mg (PO) q12h × 2 weeks **or** Doxycycline 200 mg (PO) q12h × 3 days, then 100 mg (PO) q12h × 11 days

* Therapy optional depending on severity.

Acute Nonbacterial Meningitis/Chronic Meningitis *(cont'd)*

Subset	Usual Pathogens	Preferred IV Therapy	Alternate IV Therapy	PO Therapy or IV-to-PO Switch
Leptospirosis	Leptospira interrogans	Ceftriaxone 2 gm (IV) q12h × 1 weeks **or** Doxycycline 200 mg (IV) q12h × 3 days, then 100 mg (IV) q12h × 4 days		Doxycycline 200 mg (PO) q12h × 3 days, then 100 mg (PO) q12h × 11 days
Neuro-brucellosis	Brucella sp.	Ceftriaxone 2 gm (IV) q12h **plus** Doxycycline 100 mg (PO) q12h **plus** Rifampin 600 mg (PO) q24h × 4 weeks, then Doxycycline **plus** Rifampin (same doses) × 4 weeks		
TB	M. tuberculosis	INH 300 mg (IV/PO) q24h × 6 months **plus** Rifampin 600 mg (IV/PO) q24h × 6 months **plus** PZA 25 mg/kg (PO) q24h × 2 months **plus** EMB 15 mg/kg (PO) q24h (until susceptibilities known)		
		Treat with 4 drugs, as for pulmonary TB, but extend treatment for 9–12 months. Corticosteroids tapered over 1–2 months helpful.		
Fungal *Non-HIV*	Cryptococcus neoformans, C. gatti	Isavuconazole 200 mg (IV) q8h × 48 h, then 200 mg (IV/PO) q24h × 4–6 weeks **or** Liposomal amphotericin (L-amb) 6 mg/kg (IV) q24h × 4–6 weeks **followed by** Fluconazole 800 mg (IV or PO) × 1 dose, then 400 mg (PO) q24h × 8 weeks*	Amphotericin B 0.7–1 mg/kg (IV) q24h × 4–6 weeks* **plus** Flucytosine 25 mg/kg (PO) q6h × 6 weeks* **followed by** Fluconazole 800 mg (IV or PO) × 1 dose, then 400 mg (PO) q24h × 8 weeks* **or** Liposomal amphotericin (L-amb) 6 mg/kg (IV) q24h × 4–6 weeks	PO therapy alone Fluconazole may be given PO*
HIV	Cryptococcus neoformans (see Chapter 5)			
Chronic meningitis	Coccidioidomycosis, Histoplasmosis, Neurocysticercosis (see Chapter 4)			Do not treat empirically

* May need suppressive fluconazole 200 mg (PO) q24h × 12 months.
‡ Levofloxacin 500 mg or Moxifloxacin 400 mg.

Viral (Aseptic) Meningitis

Clinical Presentation: Headache, low-grade fever, mild meningismus, photophobia. Natalizumab (NTZ) predisposes to HSV and VZV meningitis or meningoencephalitis.

Diagnostic Considerations: Diagnosis by specific serological tests, or CSF viral PCR. CSF LA levels are < 4 mmol/L. HSV-1, usually more severe than HSV-2. HSV, HHV-6, and WNE meningitis is indistinguishable clinically from other causes of viral meningitis. EBV meningitis is usually associated with clinical/laboratory features of EBV infectious mononucleosis; suspect the diagnosis in a patient with a positive monospot and unexplained meningoencephalitis. VZV meningitis is typically associated with cutaneous vesicular lesions (H. zoster). VZV meningitis may later (weeks/months) be followed by a CVA. LCM meningitis begins as a "flu-like" illness usually in the fall after hamster contact, and may have low CSF glucose. Enterovirus meningitis is often associated with a maculopapular rash, non-exudative pharyngitis, diarrhea, and rarely low CSF glucose. Aseptic meningitis due to mumps may present without parotid swelling ± acute deafness and decreased CSF glucose. Drug-induced aseptic meningitis usually have eosinophils in the CSF and little/no fever.

Pitfalls: Consider NSAIDs, TMP–SMX, and IV immunoglobulin as causes of drug induced aseptic meningitis.

Therapeutic Considerations: Usually no need to treat mild HSV-1 or HSV-2 meningitis in normal hosts.

Prognosis: Without neurological deficits, full recovery is the rule.

Primary Amebic Meningoencephalitis (PAM) (Naegleria fowleri)

Clinical Presentation: Acquired by freshwater exposure containing the protozoa, often by jumping into a lake/pool. Affects healthy children/young adults. Organism penetrates cribriform plate and enters CSF. Symptoms occur within 7 days of exposure and may be indistinguishable from fulminant bacterial meningitis, including headache, fever, anorexia, vomiting, signs of meningeal inflammation, altered mental status, coma. May complain of unusual smell/taste sensations early in infection. CSF has RBCs and low glucose.

Diagnostic Considerations: Diagnosis by demonstrating organism in CSF. Worldwide distribution. Free-living freshwater amoeba flourish in warmer climates. Key to diagnosis rests on clinical suspicion based on history of freshwater exposure in previous 1–2 weeks.

Pitfalls: CSF findings resemble bacterial meningitis, but RBCs present.

Therapeutic Considerations: Often fatal despite early treatment.

Prognosis: Frequently fatal.

Granulomatous Amebic Meningoencephalitis (GAM) (Acanthamoeba sp.)

Clinical Presentation: Insidious onset with focal neurologic deficits ± mental status changes, seizures, fever, headache, hemiparesis, meningismus, ataxia, visual disturbances. May be associated with Acanthamoeba keratoconjunctivitis, skin ulcers, or disseminated disease. Usually seen only in immunocompromised/debilitated patients.

Diagnostic Considerations: Diagnosis by demonstrating organism in brain biopsy specimen. CT/MRI shows mass lesions. "Stellate cysts" characteristic of Acanthamoeba. Worldwide distribution. Strong association with extended wear of contact lenses. Differentiate from N. fowleri by culture.

Pitfalls: Not associated with freshwater exposure, unlike primary amebic meningoencephalitis (Naegleria fowleri). Resembles subacute/chronic meningitis. No trophozoites in CSF. Skin lesions may be present for months before onset of CNS symptoms.

Therapeutic Considerations: No proven treatment. Often fatal despite early treatment.

Prognosis: Usually fatal.

Neuroborreliosis (CNS Lyme Disease)

Clinical Presentation: May have mild neck stiffness not frank nucal rigidity. Low grade fever < 102°F usually ~ 100–101°F. Recent tick exposure. Often without rash. Sore throat in some, WBC count WNL, mildly ↑ AST/ALT in some.

Diagnostic Considerations: Diagnosed by demonstrating B. burgdorferi antibody production in the CNS. A CSF : serum IgM ELISA Lyme titer ratio > 1:1 is diagnostic.

Pitfalls: If CNS symptoms present with acute Lyme disease, rash may be absent and serology may be negative early. Neuroborreliosis cannot be reliably diagnosed using CSF : serum IgM if antibiotics given before the LP (antibiotics change the CSF : serum ratio and render the test useless).

Therapeutic Considerations: Preferred Oral Options: doxycycline or minocycline.

Prognosis: Related to underlying health of host. Prognosis with neuroborreliosis is good even with delayed treatment.

Leptospirosis Meningitis (Leptospira interrogans)

Clinical Presentation: Abrupt onset of fever, no chills, severe headache, conjunctival suffusion, cough, intense myalgias (gastroc/back). Meningitis (early) CSF + for leptospires; aseptic meningitis (late) → CSF – for leptospires.

Diagnostic Considerations: Diagnosis by blood/urine culture, PCR or ↑ MAT IgM titers.

Pitfalls: CSF glucose normal and WBCs < 500/hpf. Only ID with CSF bilirubin > serum.

Therapeutic Considerations: β-lactam or doxycycline may result in a Jarish-Herxheimer reaction.

Prognosis: Excellent if treated early.

TB Meningitis (Mycobacterium tuberculosis)

Clinical Presentation: Subacute onset of nonspecific symptoms. Fever usually present ± headache, nausea, vomiting. Acute presentation and cranial nerve palsies uncommon.

Diagnostic Considerations: Diagnosis by CSF AFB smear/culture; CSF PCR is specific but not very sensitive. CSF may be normal, but if TB suspected, obtain serial LPs. CSF in TB typically shows a mild lymphocytic pleocytosis, ↓ glucose, highly ↑ protein, and few RBCs. CSF lactic acid levels slightly elevated ↑ CSF adenosine deaminase (ADA) levels diagnostically helpful. ADA levels more highly elevated in TB than in ABM, listeria ABM or neurobrucellosis.

Pitfalls: CSF may have PMN predominance early, before developing typical lymphocytic predominance. Eosinophils in CSF is not a feature of TB, and should suggest another diagnosis. Chest x-ray, PPD, and CSF smear/culture may be negative.

Therapeutic Considerations: Dexamethasone 4 mg (IV or PO) q6h × 4–8 weeks is useful to reduce CSF inflammation if given early. Proteinaceous TB exudates may obstruct ventricles and cause hydrocephalus, which is diagnosed by CT/MRI and may require shunting.
Prognosis: Poor prognostic factors include delay in treatment, neurologic deficits, or hydrocephalus.

Fungal (Cryptococcal) Meningitis (Cryptococcus neoformans)

Clinical Presentation: Insidious onset of nonspecific symptoms. Headache most common. Chronic cases may have CNS symptoms for weeks to months with intervening asymptomatic periods. Acute manifestations are more common in AIDS, chronic steroid therapy, lymphoreticular malignancies. 50–80% of patients are abnormal hosts.
Diagnostic Considerations: C. neoformans is the most common cause of fungal meningitis, and the only encapsulated yeast in the CSF to cause meningitis. Diagnosis by CSF India ink preparations showing encapsulated yeasts/cryptococcal latex antigen by latex agglutination/culture. Consider HIV.
Pitfalls: False + crytococcal antigen may occur with BBL Port-A-Cul transport vials. CSF latex antigen titer may not return to zero. Continue treatment until titers decline/do not decrease further, and until CSF culture is negative for cryptococci. India ink preparations showing encapsulated yeasts of CSF are useful for initial infection, but should not be relied on to diagnose recurrent episodes, since smears may be positive despite negative CSF cultures (dead cryptococci may remain in CSF for years). Diagnosis of recurrences rests on CSF culture.
Therapeutic Considerations: Treat until CSF is sterile or CSF latex antigen titer is zero or remains near zero on serial lumbar punctures. After patient defervesces on amphotericin B/5FC, switch to oral fluconazole × 10 weeks. Lipid amphotericin may be used if amphotericin B cannot be tolerated. HIV patients require life-long suppressive therapy with fluconazole 200 mg (PO) q24h.
Prognosis: Good. Poor prognostic factors include no CSF pleocytosis, many organisms in CSF, and altered consciousness on admission.

Encephalitis

Subset	Usual Pathogens	IV-to-PO Switch
Herpes simplex	HSV-1 HSV-2	<u>IV Therapy:</u> Acyclovir 10 mg/kg (IV) q8h × 10 days* **or** Ganciclovir 5 mg/kg (IV) q12h × 10 days.* <u>PO Therapy:</u> Valacyclovir 1 gm (PO) q8h × 10 days*
Herpes zoster (VZV)	VZV	<u>IV Therapy:</u> Acyclovir (IV) q8h 10 mg/kg × 10 days.* <u>PO Therapy:</u> Valacyclovir 2 gm (PO) q6h × 10 days*

Encephalitis *(cont'd)*

Subset	Usual Pathogens	IV-to-PO Switch	
	HHV-6	Ganciclovir 5 mg/kg (IV) q12h × 2 weeks **or** Foscarnet 90 mg/kg (IV) q12h × 2 weeks	
Arboviral	<u>Mosquito borne:</u> California encephalitis (CE), La Crosse encephalitis (LE) Western equine encephalitis (WEE), Venezuelan equine encephalitis (VEE), Eastern equine encephalitis (EEE), St. Louis encephalitis (St. LE), Japanese encephalitis (JE), Jamestown canyon virus (JCV), Nipah virus, West Nile encephalitis (WNE) dengue, chikungunya, zika virus <u>Tick borne:</u> Powassan (POWV), TBE (RSSE/CCE) <u>IV/PO Therapy:</u> None		
Mycoplasma	M. pneumoniae	Doxycycline 200 mg (IV) q12h **or** Azithromycin 500 mg (IV) × 1, then 250 mg (IV) q24h × 2 weeks	Doxycycline 200 mg (PO) q12h **or** Azithromycin 500 mg (PO) × 1, then 250 mg (PO) q24h × 2 weeks
Rickettsial	R. rickettsii (RMSF) Candidatus Rickettsia tarasevichiae (CRT)	Doxycycline 200 mg (IV) q12h × 3 days, then 100 mg (IV) q12h × 2 weeks	Doxycycline 200 mg (PO) q12h × 3 days, then 100 mg (PO) q12h × 2 weeks
Listeria	L. monocytogenes	Treat as for Listeria meningitis (see p. 18) but treat for 6 weeks	
HIV	see Chapter 5		
Transplants, HIV	CMV HHV-6 Toxoplasma	Transplants (see p. 174), HIV (see Chapter 5)	

*   Severe HSV encephalitis may require a longer duration of therapy, i.e., 14-21 days.

Herpes Encephalitis (HSV-1)

Clinical Presentation: Acute onset of fever and change in mental status without nuchal rigidity. Natalizumab (NTZ) predisposes to HSV meningitis, meningoencephalitis, or encephalitis.

Diagnostic Considerations: EEG is best early (< 72 hours) presumptive test, showing unilateral temporal lobe abnormalities. Brain MRI is abnormal before CT scan, which may require several days before a temporal lobe focus is seen. Definitive diagnosis is by CSF PCR for HSV-1 DNA. Usually presents as encephalitis or meningoencephalitis; RBCs in CSF ~ CNS damage Early/mild HSE may have no RBCs in CSF. CSF may have PMN predominance and low glucose levels, unlike other viral causes of meningitis.

Pitfalls: HSV-2 HSE rare in young adults; HSV-2 aseptic menigitis common HSV-2 HSE occurs in the elderly/immunosuppres. In normal hosts, HHV-6 may mimic HSV-1 encephalitis with a frontal/temporal focus on EEG.

Therapeutic Considerations: HSV is treatable. Treat as soon as possible, since neurological deficits may be mild and reversible early on, but severe and irreversible later.

Prognosis: Related to extent of brain injury and early anti-HSV therapy.

Rickettsial Encephalitis

Clinical Presentation: RMSF: Acute onset of fever (with relative bradycardia), headache, change/decrease in mental status days after tick bite. RMSF suggested by wrist/ankle MP rash that later becomes petechial with periorbital edema with edema of the dorsum of hands/feet, normal WBC count with thrombocytopenia encephalitis. Candidatus Rickettsia tarasevichiae (CRT): Presents with a flu-like illness in china. Fever/chills, malaise, myalgias, dry cough. CNS symptoms include headache, dizziness, mental confusion. N/V/D common generalized adenopathy common; rash rare. Eschar in some, bleeding in some hemoptysis, hematuria, epistaxis, petechiae/ecchymoses. ↑ LDH, CPK, AST/ALT. Leukopenia, relative lymphopenia, thrombocytopenia. Many (2/3) co-infected with SFTS (severe fever with thrombocytopenia syndrome).

Diagnostic Considerations: RMSF: Diagnosis by specific serology. CRT: PCR.

Pitfalls: Usually occurs in summer/fall. Easily confused with enteroviral exauthems.

Therapeutic Considerations: Doxycycline should be started immediately before dx test results reported.

Prognosis: Good if treated early.

Mycoplasma Encephalitis

Clinical Presentation: Acute onset of fever and change in mental status without nuchal rigidity.

Diagnostic Considerations: Diagnosis suggested by CAP with sore throat, otitis, E. multiforme, soft stools/diarrhea, with elevated IgM mycoplasma titers, and very high (≥ 1:512) cold agglutinin titers. CSF shows mild mononucleosis/pleocytosis and normal/low glucose.

Pitfalls: CNS findings may overshadow pulmonary findings.

Therapeutic Considerations: Among macrolides, only azithromycin effective in encephalitis. Doxycycline rapidly ↓ mycoplasma shedding in oropharyngeal secretions (vs. prolonged shedding with macrolides). "High dose" doxycycline more effective than with usual doses.

Prognosis: With early treatment, prognosis is good without neurologic sequelae.

Listeria Encephalitis

Clinical Presentation: Fever/mental confusion (encephalitis/cerebritis) ± nuchal rigidity (meningoencephalitis).

Diagnostic Considerations: Diagnosis by LP. Suspect Listeria if CSF with "purulent profile" plus RBCs. Listeria seen on CSF Gram stain in 50%; but CSF cultures positive in 100%.

Pitfalls: Not to be confused with other Gram-positive bacilli (GPB) isolated from CSF (diphtheroids). Listeria are motile and hemolytic on blood agar vs. other GPB from the skin.

Therapeutic Considerations: 3rd generation cephalosporins not active against Listeria. In penicillin-tolerant patients, use (meningeal dosed) ampicillin. TMP-SMX, meropenem, or linezolid.

Prognosis: Good with early/adequate treatment. Related to degree of T-lymphocyte dysfunction.

CMV Encephalitis (see Chapter 5)

Toxoplasma Encephalitis (see Chapter 5)

**Brain Abscess/Subdural Empyema/Cavernous Vein
Thrombosis/Intracranial Suppurative Thrombophlebitis**

Subset	Usual Pathogens	Preferred IV Therapy	Alternate IV Therapy	IV-to-PO Switch
Brain Abscess (Single Mass Lesion)				
Open trauma	S. aureus (MSSA) GNB P. aeruginosa	Meropenem 2 gm (IV) q8h × 2 weeks **or** Cefepime 2 gm (IV) q8h × 2 weeks	Not applicable	
Neurosurgical procedures	S. aureus S. epidermidis (CoNS)	<u>MSSA</u> Nafcillin 2 gm (IV) q4h × 2 weeks **or** <u>MRSA/MSSE/MRSE</u> Linezolid 600 mg (IV) q12h × 2 weeks **or** Minocycline 200 mg (IV) × 1, then 100 mg (IV) q12h × 2 weeks		<u>MSSA/MRSA/MSSE/ MRSE</u> Linezolid 600 mg (PO) q12h × 2 weeks **or** Minocycline 200 mg (PO) × 1, then 100 mg (PO) q12h × 2 weeks
Mastoid/otitic source	Enterobacter Proteus	Treat the same as for open trauma (see above)		
Dental source	Oral anaerobes Actinomyces	Ceftriaxone 2 gm (IV) q12h × 2 weeks		Doxycycline 200 mg (PO) q12h × 3 days, then 100 mg (PO) q12h × 2 weeks
Subdural empyema/ sinus source	Oral anaerobes H. influenzae	Treat the same as for dental source (see above)		
Cardiac source (ABE; right-to-left shunt)	S. aureus (MSSA) S. pneumoniae H. influenzae	Ceftriaxone 2 gm (IV) q12h × 2 weeks **or** Meropenem 2 gm (IV) q8h × 2 weeks		
	S. aureus (MRSA)	Linezolid 600 mg (IV) q12h × 2 weeks **or** Minocycline 200 mg (IV) × 1, then 100 mg (IV) q12h × 2 weeks		Minocycline 200 mg (PO) × 1, then 100 mg (PO) q12h × 2 weeks
Pulmonary source	Oral anaerobes Actinomyces	Ceftriaxone 2 gm (IV) q12h × 2 weeks		Ceftizoxime 3 gm (IV) q6h × 2 weeks
Bacteremic source	Listeria monocytogenes	TMP–SMX 5 mg/kg (IV) q6h × 6 weeks **or** Meropenem 2 gm (IV) q8h × 6 weeks **or** Linezolid 600 mg (IV) q12h × 6 weeks		TMP–SMX 5 mg/kg (PO) q6h × 6 weeks **or** Linezolid 600 mg (PO) q12h × 6 weeks

Clinical Presentation: Variable presentation, with fever, change in mental status, cranial nerve abnormalities ± headache.

Diagnostic Considerations: Diagnosis by CSF gram stain/culture. If brain abscess is suspected, obtain head CT/MRI. Lumbar puncture may induce herniation.

Pitfalls: CSF analysis is negative for bacterial meningitis unless abscess ruptures into ventricular system.

Therapeutic Considerations: Treatment with meningeal doses of antibiotics is required. Large single abscesses may be surgically drained; multiple small abscesses are best treated medically.

Prognosis: Related to underlying source and health of host.

Brain Abscess (Dental Source)

Diagnostic Considerations: Diagnosis by Panorex x-rays/gallium scan of jaw demonstrating focus in mandible/erosion into sinuses.

Pitfalls: Apical root abscess may not be apparent clinically.

Therapeutic Considerations: Large single abscess may be surgically drained. Multiple small abscesses are best treated medically. Treat until lesions on CT/MRI resolve or do not become smaller on therapy.

Prognosis: Good if dental focus is removed.

Brain Abscess (Subdural Empyema/Sinus Source/Mastoid/Otitic Source)

Diagnostic Considerations: Diagnosis by sinus films/CT/MRI to confirm presence of sinusitis/bone erosion (cranial osteomyelitis/epidural abscess or mastoiditis).

Pitfalls: Do not overlook underlying bone infection, which may need surgical drainage.

Therapeutic Considerations: Obtain ENT consult for possible surgical debridement of sinuses or mastoid.

Prognosis: Good prognosis if properly treated/drained.

Brain Abscess (Cardiac Source: Acute Bacterial Endocarditis)

Diagnostic Considerations: Blood cultures often positive if brain abscess due to acute bacterial endocarditis (ABE) pathogen. Head CT/MRI shows multiple mass lesions.

Pitfalls: Do not overlook right-to-left cardiac shunt (e.g., patent foramen ovale, atrial septal defect) as source of brain abscess. Cerebral embolization results in aseptic meningitis in SBE, but septic meningitis/brain abscess in ABE (due to high virulence of pathogens).

Therapeutic Considerations: Multiple lesions suggest hematogenous spread. Use susceptibility of blood culture isolates to determine coverage. Meningeal doses are the same as endocarditis doses.

Prognosis: Related to location/size of CNS lesions and extent of cardiac valvular involvement.

Brain Abscess (Pulmonary Source)
Diagnostic Considerations: Diagnosis suggested by underlying bronchiectasis, empyema, cystic fibrosis, or lung abscess in a patient with a brain abscess.
Pitfalls: Brain abscesses are most often due to chronic suppurative lung disease (e.g., bronchiectasis, lung abscess/empyema), not chronic bronchitis/AECB.
Therapeutic Considerations: Lung abscess may need surgical drainage.
Prognosis: Related to extent/location of CNS lesions, drainage of lung abscess/empyema, and control of lung infection.

Brain Abscess (Bacteremia Source)
Diagnostic Considerations: Diagnosis by head CT/MRI demonstrating focus in brain.
Pitfalls: If patient doesn't have a cardiopulmonary disorder predisposing to brain abscess, look for a clinically silent dental (apical root) abscess by gallium scan of jaws/Panorex dental x-rays.
Therapeutic Considerations: Treat Listeria rhomboencephalitis or brain abscess for at least 6 weeks.
Prognosis: Good.

Empiric Therapy of HEENT Infections

Facial/Periorbital Cellulitis

Subset	Usual Pathogens	Preferred IV Therapy	Alternate IV Therapy	PO Therapy or IV-to-PO Switch
Facial cellulitis	Group A streptococci (GAS) H. influenzae	Ceftriaxone 1 gm (IV) q24h × 2 weeks **or** Respiratory quinolone* (IV) q24h × 2 weeks	Ceftizoxime 2 gm (IV) q8h × 2 weeks	Any oral 2nd or 3rd gen. cephalosporin × 2 weeks **or** Respiratory quinolone* (PO) q24h × 2 weeks

* Levofloxacin 500 mg or Moxifloxacin 400 mg.

Clinical Presentation: Acute onset of warm, painful, facial rash without discharge, swelling, pruritus.

Diagnostic Considerations: Diagnosis by clinical appearance. May spread rapidly across face. Purplish hue suggests H. influenzae.

Pitfalls: If periorbital cellulitis, obtain head CT/MRI to rule out underlying sinusitis/CNS involvement. If secondary to an abrasion after contact with a saliva-contaminated surface, consider Herpes gladiatorum; lesions are painful/edematous and do not respond to antibiotic therapy for cellulitis.

Therapeutic Considerations: May need to treat × 3 weeks in compromised hosts (chronic steroids, diabetics, SLE, etc.).

Prognosis: Good with early treatment; worse if underlying sinusitis/CNS involvement.

Bacterial Sinusitis

Sub-set	Usual Pathogens	IV Therapy (Hospitalized)	PO Therapy or IV-to-PO Switch (Ambulatory)
Acute	S. pneumoniae H. influenzae M. catarrhalis	Respiratory quinolone[†] (IV) q24h × 1–2 weeks **or** Ceftriaxone 1 gm (IV) q24h × 1–2 weeks **or** Doxycycline 200 mg (IV) q12h × 3 days, then 100 mg (IV) q12h × 11 days	Respiratory quinolone[†] (PO) q24h × 1–2 weeks **or** Amoxicillin 1 gm (PO) q8h × 10 days **or** Doxycycline 200 mg (PO) q12h × 3 days, then 100 mg (PO) q12h × 11 days* **or** Cephalosporin[‡] (PO) × 2 weeks
Chronic	S. pneumoniae H. influenzae M. catarrhalis	May require prolonged antimicrobial therapy (4–6 weeks) Do not use oral cephalosporins for chronic sinusitis (Poor penetration into sinus fluid)	

† Moxifloxacin 400 mg × 7 days or Levofloxacin 750 mg × 5 days.

‡ Cefdinir 300 mg q12h or Cefditoren 400 mg q12h or Cefixime 400 mg q12h or Cefpodoxime 200 mg q12h.

Acute Bacterial Sinusitis

Clinical Presentation: Nasal discharge and cough frequently with headache, facial pain, and low-grade fever lasting > 10–14 days. Can also present acutely with high fever (≥ 104°F) and purulent nasal discharge ± intense headache lasting for ≥ 3 days. Other manifestations depend on the affected sinus: <u>maxillary sinus</u>: percussion tenderness of molars; maxillary toothache; local extension may cause osteomyelitis of facial bones with proptosis, retroorbital cellulitis, ophthalmoplegia; direct intracranial extension is rare; <u>frontal sinus</u>: prominent headache; intracranial extension may cause epidural/brain abscess, meningitis, cavernous sinus/superior sagittal sinus thrombosis; orbital extension may cause periorbital cellulitis; <u>ethmoid sinus</u>: eyelid edema and prominent tearing; extension may cause retroorbital pain/periorbital cellulitis and/or cavernous sinus/superior sagittal sinus thrombosis; <u>sphenoid sinus</u>: severe headache; extension into cavernous sinus may cause meningitis, cranial nerve paralysis [III, IV, VI], temporal lobe abscess, cavernous sinus thrombosis). Cough and nasal discharge are prominent in children.

Diagnostic Considerations: Diagnosis by sinus x-rays or CT/MRI showing complete sinus opacification, air-fluid levels, mucosal thickening. Consider sinus aspiration in immunocompromised hosts usually in children, acute sinusitis is a clinical diagnosis; imaging studies are not necessary.

Pitfalls: May present as periorbital cellulitis (obtain head CT/MRI to rule out underlying sinusitis). If CT/MRI demonstrates "post-septal" involvement, treat as acute bacterial meningitis. In children, transillumination, sinus tenderness to percussion, and color of nasal mucus are not reliable indicators of sinusitis.

Therapeutic Considerations: Treat for full course to prevent relapses/complications. Macrolides and TMP SMX may predispose to drug-resistant S. pneumoniae (DRSP), and ≥ 30% of S. pneumoniae are naturally resistant to macrolides. Consider local resistance rates before making empiric antibiotic selections.

Prognosis: Good if treated for full course. Relapses common with suboptimal treatment. For frequent recurrences, obtain ENT consultation.

Chronic Bacterial Sinusitis

Clinical Presentation: Generalized headache, fatigue, nasal congestion, post-nasal drip lasting > 3 months with little/no sinus tenderness by percussion. Local symptoms often subtle. Fever is uncommon.

Diagnostic Considerations: Sinus films and head CT/MRI are less useful than for acute sinusitis (chronic mucosal abnormalities may persist after infection is treated). Some cases of chronic maxillary sinusitis are due to a dental cause; obtain dental panorex x-rays if suspected.

Pitfalls: Clinical presentation is variable/nonspecific. Malaise and irritability may be more prominent than local symptoms. May be mistaken for allergic rhinitis. Head CT/MRI can rule out sinus tumor.

Therapeutic Considerations: Therapeutic failure/relapse is usually due to inadequate antibiotic duration, dose, or tissue penetration. Treat for full course. If sinusitis persists after 4 weeks of optimal antibiotic therapy, refer to ENT for surgical drainage procedure.

Prognosis: Good if treated for full course. Relapses may occur with suboptimal treatment. For persistence after 4 weeks of therapy, obtain ENT consultation.

Keratitis

Subset	Pathogens	Topical Therapy
Bacterial	S. aureus S. pneumoniae M. catarrhalis	Antibacterial eyedrops (ciprofloxacin, ofloxacin, or tobramycin/bacitracin/polymyxin B) hourly while awake × 2 weeks
Viral	HSV-1	Trifluridine 1% solution 1 drop hourly while awake × 2 days, then 1 drop q6h × 14–21 days **or** viral ophthalmic topical ointment (e.g., vidarabine) at bedtime × 14–21 days
Amebic	Acanthamoeba	Propamidine (0.1%), neomycin, gramicidin, or polymyxin B eyedrops hourly while awake × 1–2 weeks **or** polyhexamethylene biguanide (0.02%) eyedrops hourly while awake × 1–2 weeks

Clinical Presentation: Corneal haziness, infiltrates, or ulcers.
Diagnosis: Appearance of corneal lesions/culture.

Bacterial Keratitis
Diagnostic Considerations: Usually secondary to eye trauma. Always obtain ophthalmology consult.
Pitfalls: Be sure to culture ulcer. Unusual organisms are common in eye trauma.
Therapeutic Considerations: Treat until lesions resolve. Ointment easier/lasts longer than solutions. Avoid topical steroids.
Prognosis: Related to extent of trauma/organism. S. aureus, B. cereus, P. aeruginosa have worst prognosis.

Viral Keratitis (HSV-1)
Diagnostic Considerations: "Dendritic" corneal ulcers characteristic. Obtain ophthalmology consult.
Pitfalls: Small corneal ulcers may be missed without fluorescein staining.
Therapeutic Considerations: Treat until lesions resolve. Oral acyclovir is not needed. Avoid ophthalmic steroid ointment.
Prognosis: Good if treated early (before eye damage is extensive).

Amebic Keratitis (Acanthamoeba)
Diagnostic Considerations: Usually associated with extended use of soft contact lenses. Corneal scrapings are positive with calcofluor staining. Acanthamoeba keratitis is painful with typical circular, hazy, corneal infiltrate. Always obtain ophthalmology consult.
Pitfalls: Do not confuse with HSV-1 dendritic ulcers. Avoid topical steroids.

Therapeutic Considerations: If secondary bacterial infection, treat as bacterial keratitis.
Prognosis: No good treatment. Poor prognosis.

Conjunctivitis

Subset	Usual Pathogens	PO/Topical Therapy
Bacterial	M. catarrhalis H. influenzae S. pneumoniae	Antibacterial eyedrops (ciprofloxacin, ofloxacin, moxi-floxacin, or tobramycin/bacitracin/polymyxin B) q12h × 1 week plus antibacterial ointment (same antibiotic) at bedtime × 1 week
Viral	Adenovirus	Not applicable
	VZV	Valacyclovir 1 gm (PO) q8h × 10–14 days **or** Famciclovir 500 mg (PO) q8h × 10–14 days
Chlamydial	C. trachomatis (trachoma)	Doxycycline 100 mg (PO) q12h × 1–2 weeks **or** Azithromycin 1 gm (PO) × 1 dose

Bacterial Conjunctivitis
Clinical Presentation: Profuse, purulent exudate from conjunctiva.
Diagnostic Considerations: Reddened conjunctiva; culture for specific pathogen.
Pitfalls: Do not confuse with allergic conjunctivitis, which itches and has a clear discharge.
Therapeutic Considerations: Obtain ophthalmology consult. Ointment lasts longer in eye than solution. Do not use topical steroids without an antibacterial.
Prognosis: Excellent when treated early, with no residual visual impairment.

Viral Conjunctivitis
Adenovirus
Clinical Presentation: Reddened conjunctiva, watery discharge, negative bacterial culture.
Diagnostic Considerations: Diagnosis by cloudy/steamy cornea with negative bacterial cultures. Clue is punctate infiltrates with a cloudy cornea. Extremely contagious; careful handwashing is essential. Obtain viral culture of conjunctiva for diagnosis.
Pitfalls: Pharyngitis a clue to adenoviral etiology (pharyngoconjunctival fever).
Therapeutic Considerations: No treatment available. Usually resolves in 1–2 weeks.
Prognosis: Related to degree of corneal haziness. Severe cases may take weeks to clear.

VZV Ophthalmicus
Diagnostic Considerations: Vesicles on tip of nose predict eye involvement (Hutchinson's sign).
Pitfalls: Do not miss vesicular lesions in external auditory canal in patients with facial palsy (Ramsey-Hunt Syndrome).
Therapeutic Considerations: Obtain ophthalmology consult. Topical steroids may be used if given with anti-VZV therapy.
Prognosis: Good if treated early with systemic antivirals.

Trachoma (C. trachomatis) Conjunctivitis
Diagnostic Considerations: Diagnosis by direct fluorescent antibody (DFA)/culture of conjunctiva.
Pitfalls: Do not confuse bilateral, upper lid, granular conjunctivitis of Chlamydia with viral/bacterial conjunctivitis, which involves both upper and lower eyelids.
Therapeutic Considerations: Ophthalmic erythromycin treatment is useful for neonates. Azithromycin 1 gm (PO) × 1 dose or Doxycycline 100 mg (PO) q12h × 7 days curative. Single-dose azithromycin may be associated with recurrence.
Prognosis: Excellent with early treatment.

Chorioretinitis

Subset	Usual Pathogens	Preferred IV Therapy	Alternate IV Therapy	PO Therapy or IV-to-PO Switch
Viral	CMV	See p. 174		
Fungal[†]	Candida albicans	Fluconazole 800 mg (IV) × 1 dose, then 400 mg (IV) q24h × 2 weeks[‡] **or** Voriconazole 6 mg/kg (IV) q12h × 1 day, then 4 mg/kg (IV) q12h × 2 weeks[‡]	Amphotericin B 0.6 mg/kg (IV) q24h × (total of 1 gm) **or** Liposomal amphotericin (L-amb) (IV) q24h × 3 weeks[†*]	Fluconazole 800 mg (PO) × 1 dose, then 400 mg (PO) q24h × 2 weeks[‡]
Protozoal	Toxoplasma gondii	<u>IV Therapy</u> Not applicable	<u>PO Therapy</u> Pyrimethamine 75 mg (PO) × 1 dose, then 25 mg (PO) q24h × 6 weeks **plus either** Sulfadiazine 1 gm (PO) q6h × 6 weeks **or** Clindamycin 300 mg (PO) q8h × 6 weeks	

‡ Therapy should be continued until resolution of infection. Close follow-up with an ophthalmologist is required.

* For usual dose, see Chapter 11 (Drug Summaries)

CMV Chorioretinitis (see p. 345)

Candida Chorioretinitis
Clinical Presentation: Small, raised, white, circular lesions on retina.
Diagnostic Considerations: Fundus findings similar to white, raised colonies on blood agar plates.
Pitfalls: Candida endophthalmitis signifies invasive/disseminated candidiasis.
Therapeutic Considerations: Treat as disseminated candidiasis.
Prognosis: Good with early treatment.

Toxoplasma Chorioretinitis
Clinical Presentation: Grey/black pigmentation of macula.
Diagnostic Considerations: Diagnosis by IgM IFA toxoplasmosis titers.
Pitfalls: Unilateral endophthalmitis usually indicates acquired toxoplasmosis; congenital toxoplasmosis is usually bilateral.
Therapeutic Considerations: Obtain ophthalmology consult. Treat only acute/active toxoplasmosis with visual symptoms; do not treat chronic chorioretinitis. Add folinic acid 10 mg (PO) q24h to prevent folic acid deficiency.
Prognosis: Related to degree of immunosuppression.

Endophthalmitis

Subset	Usual Pathogens	Preferred IV Therapy	Alternate IV Therapy	PO Therapy or IV-to-PO Switch
Bacterial	H. influenzae S. aureus (MSSA)	**Intravitreal injection:** Cefepime 2.25 mg/0.1 mL sterile saline × 1 dose; repeat × 1 if needed in 2–3 days **plus** **Subconjunctival injection:** Cefepime 100 mg/0.5 mL sterile saline q24h × 1–2 weeks **plus** Levofloxacin 500 mg (IV/PO) q12h × 1–2 weeks		
	S. aureus (MRSA) S. epidermidis (CoNS)	**Intravitreal injection:** Vancomycin 1 mg/0.1 mL sterile saline × 1 dose; repeat × 1 if needed in 2–3 days **plus** **Subconjunctival injection:** Vancomycin 2.5 mg/0.5 mL sterile saline q24h × 1–2 weeks **plus** Linezolid 600 mg (IV/PO) q12h × 1–2 weeks		
Fungal[‡]	C. albicans	Fluconazole 800 mg (IV) × 1 dose, then 400 mg (IV) q24h × 2 months	Voriconazole (IV) × 2 months	Fluconazole (PO) same as IV dose **or** Voriconazole (PO)* × 2 months

* For usual dose, see Chapter 11 (Drug Summaries).

Endophthalmitis *(cont'd)*

Subset	Usual Pathogens	Preferred IV Therapy	Alternate IV Therapy	PO Therapy or IV-to-PO Switch
	A. fumigatus A. flavus	Amphotericin B (intravitreal) 10 mg (in 0.1 mL of saline) q2–3 days	Voriconazole (IV)* × 2 months	Voriconazole (PO)* × 2 months
TB	M. tuberculosis	Treat the same as for TB pneumonia (see p. 55)		
Infected lens implant*	GNB S. aureus (MSSA)	Meropenem 1 gm (IV) q8h × 2 weeks **or** Cefepime 2 gm (IV) q8h × 2 weeks	Chloramphenicol 500 mg (IV) q6h × 2 weeks	Chloramphenicol 500 mg (PO) q6h × 2 weeks
	S. aureus (MRSA)	Linezolid 600 mg (IV) q12h × 2 weeks	Minocycline 100 mg (IV) q12h × 2 weeks	Linezolid 600 mg (PO) q12h × 2 weeks **or** Minocycline 100 mg (PO) q12h × 2 weeks

‡ Duration of therapy is approximate and should be continued until resolution of disease. Close follow-up with an ophthalmologist is required.
* For usual dose, see Chapter 11 (Drug Summaries).

Bacterial Endophthalmitis

Clinical Presentation: Ocular pain/sudden vision loss.

Diagnosis: Post-op endophthalmitis occurs 1–7 days after surgery. Hypopyon seen in anterior chamber.

Pitfalls: Delayed-onset endophthalmitis may occur up to 6 weeks post-op. White intra-capsular plaque is characteristic.

Therapeutic Considerations: Use steroids (dexamethasone 0.4 mg/0.1 mL intravitreal and 10 mg/1 mL subconjunctival) with antibiotics in post-op endophthalmitis. Also use systemic antibiotics for severe cases. Vitrectomy is usually necessary.

Prognosis: Related to pathogen virulence.

Fungal Endophthalmitis

Clinical Presentation: Slow deterioration in visual acuity ± eye pain. N fever. Antecedent/concomitant TPN, central IV line, prolonged antibiotic/immunosuppressive therapy, steroids, IVDA, or post-cataract surgery.

Diagnostic Considerations: Blood cultures frequently positive in Candida endophthalmitis. Small/round white lesions near retinal vessels. Cultures of aqueous/vitreous humors diagnostic.

Pitfalls: Symptoms develop insidiously with little/no eye pain or fever. Blood cultures negative with Aspergillus endophthalmitis.

Therapeutic Considerations: Penetration of antibiotic into vitreous humor requires high lipid solubility and inflammation. IV/intravitreous/subconjunctival antimicrobial choice depends on physiochemical properties of drug selected. Vitrectomy preferred by some.

If using intravitreal amphotericin B, there is no benefit in adding systemic IV therapy. Voriconazole penetrates CSF/eye, but clinical experience is limited. Based on limited data, caspofungin appears to have poor penetration into the vitreous and should not be relied upon to treat fungal endophthalmitis.

Prognosis: Best results with vitrectomy plus intravitreal antifungal therapy.

Tuberculous (TB) Endophthalmitis

Clinical Presentation: Raised retinal punctate lesions ± visual impairment.

Diagnostic Considerations: Signs of extraocular TB are usually present. Confirm diagnosis of miliary TB by liver/bone biopsy.

Pitfalls: TB endophthalmitis is a sign of disseminated TB.

Therapeutic Considerations: Treat as disseminated TB. Systemic steroids may be used if given with anti-TB therapy.

Prognosis: Related to degree of immunosuppression.

Infected Lens Implant

Diagnostic Considerations: Diagnosis by clinical appearance and culture of anterior chamber. Obtain ophthalmology consult.

Pitfalls: Superficial cultures are inadequate. Anterior chamber aspirate may be needed for culture.

Therapeutic Considerations: Infected lens must be removed for cure.

Prognosis: Good with early lens removal and recommended antibiotics.

External Otitis

Subset	Usual Pathogens	Preferred IV Therapy	Alternate IV Therapy	Topical Therapy or IV-to-PO Switch
Benign	P. aeruginosa	Use otic solutions only (ofloxacin 0.3%, tobramycin, polymyxin B); apply ear drops q6h × 1 week		
Malignant	P. aeruginosa	Meropenem 1 gm (IV) q8h × 4–6 weeks **or** Cefepime 2 gm (IV) q8h × 4–6 weeks **or** Levofloxacin 750 mg (IV) q24h × 4–6 weeks		Levofloxacin 750 mg (PO) q24h × 4–6 weeks

Benign External Otitis (Pseudomonas aeruginosa)

Clinical Presentation: Acute external ear canal drainage without perforation of tympanic membrane or bone involvement.

Diagnostic Considerations: Diagnosis suggested by external ear drainage after water exposure. Usually acquired from swimming pools ("swimmers ear"). Not an invasive infection.

Pitfalls: Be sure external otitis is not associated with perforated tympanic membrane, which requires ENT consultation and systemic antibiotics.

Therapeutic Considerations: Treat topically until symptoms/infection resolve.

Prognosis: Excellent with topical therapy.

Malignant External Otitis (Pseudomonas aeruginosa)

Clinical Presentation: External ear canal drainage with bone involvement.

Diagnostic Considerations: Diagnosis by demonstrating P. aeruginosa in soft tissue culture from ear canal plus bone/cartilage involvement on x-ray. Usually affects diabetics. CT/MRI of head shows bony involvement of external auditory canal.

Pitfalls: Rare in non-diabetics.

Therapeutic Considerations: Requires surgical debridement plus antibiotic therapy for cure.

Prognosis: Related to control of diabetes mellitus.

Acute Otitis Media

Subset	Usual Pathogens	IM Therapy	PO Therapy
Initial uncomplicated	S. pneumoniae H. influenzae M. catarrhalis	Ceftriaxone 50 mg/kg (IM) × 1 dose	Amoxicillin 1 gm or 10 mg/kg (PO) q8h × 10 days **or** Clarithromycin 7.5 mg/kg (PO) q12h × 10 days **or** Azithromycin 10 mg/kg (PO) × 1 dose, then 5 mg/kg (PO) q24h × 4 days

Acute Otitis Media

Clinical Presentation: Fever, otalgia, hearing loss. Nonspecific presentation is more common in younger children (irritability, fever). Key to diagnosis is examination of the tympanic membrane. Uncommon in adults.

Diagnostic Considerations: Diagnosis is made by finding an opaque, hyperemic, bulging tympanic membrane with loss of landmarks and decreased mobility on pneumatic otoscopy.

Pitfalls: Failure to remove cerumen (inadequate visualization of tympanic membrane) and reliance on history of ear tugging/pain are the main factors associated with overdiagnosis of otitis media. Otitis media with effusion (i.e., tympanic membrane retracted or in normal position with decreased mobility or mobility with negative pressure; fluid present behind the drum but normal in color) usually resolves spontaneously and should not be treated with antibiotics.

Therapeutic Considerations: Risk factors for infection with PRSP or MDR S. pneumoniae include antibiotic therapy in past 30 days, failure to respond within 48–72 hours of therapy, day care attendance, and antimicrobial prophylaxis. Macrolides and TMP–SMX may predispose to DRSP, and 25% of S. pneumoniae are naturally resistant to macrolides.

Prognosis: Excellent, but tends to recur. Chronic otitis, cholesteatomas, mastoiditis are rare complications. Tympanostomy tubes/adenoidectomy for frequent recurrences of otitis media are the leading surgical procedures in children.

Mastoiditis

Subset	Usual Pathogens	Preferred IV Therapy	Alternate IV Therapy	PO Therapy or IV-to-PO Switch
Acute	S. pneumoniae H. influenzae S. aureus (MSSA)	Ceftriaxone 1 gm (IV) q24h × 2 weeks **or** Cefepime 2 gm (IV) q12h × 2 weeks	Levofloxacin 500 mg (IV) q24h × 2 weeks **or** Doxycycline 200 mg (IV) q12h × 3 days, then 100 mg (PO) q12h × 2 weeks	Moxifloxacin 400 mg (PO) q24h × 2 weeks **or** Levofloxacin 500 mg (PO) q24h × 2 weeks **or** Doxycycline 100 mg (PO) q12h × 2 weeks
Chronic	S. pneumoniae H. influenzae P. aeruginosa S. aureus (MSSA)	Meropenem 1 gm (IV) q8h × 4 weeks **or** Cefepime 2 gm (IV) q8h × 4 weeks	Moxifloxacin 400 mg (IV) × 4–6 weeks **or** Levofloxacin 750 mg (IV) q24h	Moxifloxacin 400 mg (PO) × 4–6 weeks **or** Levofloxacin 500 mg (PO) q24h × 4–6 weeks

Acute Mastoiditis

Clinical Presentation: Pain/tenderness over mastoid with fever.

Diagnostic Considerations: Diagnosis by CT/MRI showing mastoid involvement.

Pitfalls: Obtain head CT/MRI to rule out extension into CNS presenting as acute bacterial meningitis.

Prognosis: Good if treated early.

Chronic Mastoiditis

Clinical Presentation: Subacute pain/tenderness over mastoid with low-grade fever.

Diagnostic Considerations: Diagnosis by CT/MRI showing mastoid involvement. Rarely secondary to TB (diagnose by AFB smear/culture of bone biopsy or debrided bone).

Pitfalls: Obtain head CT/MRI to rule out CNS extension.

Therapeutic Considerations: Usually requires surgical debridement for cure. Should be viewed as chronic osteomyelitis. If secondary to TB, treat as skeletal TB.

Prognosis: Progressive without surgery. Poor prognosis with associated meningitis/brain abscess.

Suppurative Parotitis

Subset	Usual Pathogens	Preferred IV Therapy	Alternate IV Therapy	PO Therapy or IV-to-PO Switch
Parotitis (bacterial)	S. aureus (MSSA) GNB	Meropenem 1 gm (IV) q8h × 2 weeks **or** Respiratory quinolone* (IV) q24h × 2 weeks	Ceftriaxone 1 gm (IV) q24h × 2 weeks	Respiratory quinolone* (PO) q24h × 2 weeks

* Levofloxacin 500 mg or Moxifloxacin 400 mg.

Clinical Presentation: Unilateral parotid pain/swelling with discharge from Stensen's duct ± fever.

Diagnostic Considerations: Diagnosis by clinical presentation, ↑ amylase, CT/MRI demonstrating stone in parotid duct/gland involvement.

Pitfalls: Differentiate from unilateral mumps by purulent discharge from Stensen's duct.

Therapeutic Considerations: If duct is obstructed, remove stone.

Prognosis: Good with early therapy/hydration.

Pharyngitis

Subset	Usual Pathogens	PO Therapy
Bacterial	Group A streptococci (GAS)	Amoxicillin 1 gm (PO) q8h × 7–10 days **or** Cefprozil 500 mg (PO) q12h × 7–10 days **or** Clindamycin 300 mg (PO) q8h × 7–10 days **or** Azithromycin† 500 mg (PO) q24h × 5 days

Pharyngitis *(cont'd)*

Subset	Usual Pathogens	PO Therapy
Membranous	Arcanobacterium (Corynebacterium) hemolyticum	Doxycycline 100 mg (IV or PO) q12h × 1–2 weeks **or** Azithromycin 500 mg (IV or PO) × 1 dose then 250 mg (IV or PO) q24h × 1–2 weeks **or** Cephalosporin (IV or PO) × 1–2 wks
	C. diphtheriae C. ulcerans	Diphtheria antitoxin ± penicillin or macrolide
Viral	Respiratory viruses EBV CMV HHV-6	Not applicable. EBV/CMV cause pharyngitis in infectious mononucleosis syndrome, along with hepatitis and lymph node involvement.
Other	M. pneumoniae C. pneumoniae	Respiratory quinolone* (PO) q24h × 1 week **or** Doxycycline 100 mg (PO) q12h × 1 week **or** Azithromycin 500 mg (PO) q24h × 5 days

*   Levofloxacin 500 mg or Moxifloxacin 400 mg.
†   Increasing group A streptococcal resistance.

Bacterial Pharyngitis

Clinical Presentation: Acute sore throat with fever, bilateral anterior cervical adenopathy, and elevated ASO titer. No hoarseness.

Diagnostic Considerations: Diagnosis of Group A streptococcal pharyngitis by elevated ASO titer after initial sore throat and positive throat culture. Rapid strep tests unnecessary, since delay in culture results (~1 week) still allows adequate time to initiate therapy and prevent acute rheumatic fever. Group A streptococcal pharyngitis is rare in adults > 30 years.

Pitfalls: Gram stain of throat exudate differentiates Group A streptococcal colonization (few or no PMNs) from infection (many PMNs) in patients with a positive throat culture or rapid strep test. Neither throat culture nor rapid strep test alone differentiates colonization from infection.

Therapeutic Considerations: Benzathine penicillin 1.2 mu (IM) × 1 dose can be used as an alternative to oral therapy. Penicillin, erythromycin, and ampicillin fail in 15% of cases due to poor penetration into oral secretions or beta-lactamase producing oral organisms.

Prognosis: Excellent. Treat within 10 days to prevent acute rheumatic fever.

Membranous Pharyngitis

Clinical Presentation: A. hemolyticum presents with a scarlet fever-like rash and membranous pharyngitis. C. diphtheriae pharyngitis has no fever/rash.

Diagnostic Considerations: Diagnosis by throat culture/recovery of organism in patients with scarlatiniform rash.

Pitfalls: A. hemolyticum must be differentiated from C. diphtheriae on culture.

Therapeutic Considerations: For A. hemolyticum, doxycycline or erythromycin are more active than beta-lactams. Penicillin or macrolides are preferred for C. diphtheriae. C. diphtheriae should be treated with antitoxin ASAP since antibiotic therapy is adjunctive.

Prognosis: Related to degree of airway obstruction. Good with early treatment of A. hemolyticum. Diphtheria prognosis related to early antitoxin treatment and to presence/severity of toxic myocarditis.

Viral Pharyngitis

Clinical Presentation: Acute sore throat. Other features depend on specific pathogen.

Diagnostic Considerations: Most cases of viral pharyngitis are caused by respiratory viruses, and are frequently accompanied by hoarseness, but not high fever, pharyngeal exudates, palatal petechiae, or posterior cervical adenopathy (EBV). Other causes of viral pharyngitis (CMV, HHV-6) are usually associated with ↑ SGOT/SGPT. EBV infectious mononucleosis (IM) may present with exudative or non-exudative pharyngitis, and is diagnosed by a positive mono spot test or elevated EBV IgM viral capsid antigen (VCA) titer. Before mono spot test becomes positive (may take up to 8 weeks), a presumptive diagnosis of EBV infections mono nucleosis can be made by ESR and SGOT/SGPT which are elevated in EBV and not in Group A streptococcal pharyngitis. If EBV mono spot is negative, retest weekly × 8 weeks; if still negative, obtain IgM CMV HHV-6 and toxoplasmosis titers to diagnose the cause of "mono spot negative" pharyngitis.

Pitfalls: 30% of patients with EBV pharyngitis have Group A streptococcal colonization.

Therapeutic Considerations: Symptomatic care only. Short-term steroids should only be used in EBV infection if airway obstruction is present/imminent. Since many patients with viral pharyngitis are colonized with Group A streptococci, do not treat throat cultures positive for Group A streptococci if non-streptococcal pharyngitis features are present.

Prognosis: Related to extent of systemic infection. Post-viral fatigue is common. CMV IM may present with prolonged fatigue for 6–12 months with mildly elevated serum transaminases.

Mycoplasma/Chlamydophilia (Chlamydia) Pharyngitis

Clinical Presentation: Acute sore throat ± laryngitis. Usually non-exudative.

Diagnostic Considerations: Diagnosis by elevated IgM M. pneumoniae or C. pneumoniae titers. Consider diagnosis in patients with non-exudative pharyngitis without viral or streptococcal pharyngitis. Mycoplasma pharyngitis is often accompanied by otitis/bullous myringitis.

Pitfalls: Patients with C. pneumoniae frequently have laryngitis, which is not a feature of EBV, CMV, Group A streptococcal, or M. pneumoniae pharyngitis.

Therapeutic Considerations: Treatment of C. pneumoniae laryngitis results in rapid (~ 3 days) return of normal voice, which does not occur with viral pharyngitis.
Prognosis: Excellent.

Chronic Fatigue Syndrome (CFS)

Clinical Presentation: Fatigue > 1 year with cognitive impairment and minimal or no pharyngitis.
Diagnostic Considerations: Rule out other causes of chronic fatigue (cancer, adrenal/thyroid disease, etc.) before diagnosing CFS. HHV-6/Coxsackie B titers are often elevated. Some have ↓ natural kill (NK) cells/activity. Subnormal ESR approaching 0 mm/h. Crimson crescents on both tonsillar pillars in the posterior pharynx are non-specific but common.
Pitfalls: ↑ VCA IgG EBV titers is common in CFS, but EBV does not cause CFS. Do not confuse CFS with fibromyalgia, which has muscular "trigger points" and no cognitive impairment. CFS and fibromyalgia may coexist. In presumed CFS, if there is pharyngitis or if the ESR is elevated, consider an alternate diagnosis.
Therapeutic Considerations: No specific therapy is available. Patients with ↓ NK cells may benefit from β-carotene 50,000 U (PO) q24h × 3 weeks. Patients with ↑ C. pneumoniae IgG titers may benefit from doxycycline 100 mg (PO) q24h × 3 weeks.
Prognosis: Cyclical illness with remissions (precipitated by exertion, stress, or sleep lack). Avoid exercise.

Thrush (Oropharyngeal Candidiasis)

Subset	Pathogens	PO Therapy
Fungal	C. albicans	Fluconazole 200 mg (PO) × 1 dose, then 100 mg (PO) q24h ×† weeks **or** Posaconazole 100 mg (PO) q12h × 1 day, then 100 mg (PO) q24h × 13 days **or** Clotrimazole 10 mg troches (PO) 5x/day ×† weeks **or** Itraconazole 200 mg (PO) q24h ×† weeks
	Fluconazole-resistant or non-albicans Candida	Posaconazole 400 mg (PO) q12h × weeks* **or** Voriconazole 200 mg (PO) q12h × weeks* **or** Caspofungin 70 mg (IV) × 1, then 50 mg (IV) q24h × weeks* **or** Itraconazole 200 mg (PO) q12h × weeks*

*   Duration of therapy depends on underlying disease and clinical response.

Thrush (Oropharyngeal Candidiasis)

Clinical Presentation: White coated tongue or oropharynx. White adherent plaques may be on any part of the oropharynx.
Diagnostic Considerations: Gram stain/culture of white plaques demonstrates yeasts (Candida). Culture and susceptibility testing of causative fungus is useful in analyzing failure to respond to therapy.

Pitfalls: Lateral, linear, white, striated tongue lesions may resemble thrush but really represent hairy leukoplakia. Hairy leukoplakia should suggest HIV. Thrush may occur in children, alcoholics, diabetics, those receiving steroids/antibiotic therapy, or HIV.

Therapeutic Considerations: Almost all infections are caused by C. albicans, a species that is usually susceptible to fluconazole. Fluconazole-unresponsive infections may be caused by infection with fluconazole-resistant C. albicans (most common explanation), infection with a fluconazole-resistant non-albicans species (rare), noncompliance with therapy (common), or drug interactions (e.g., concomitant usage of rifampin, which markedly reduced azole blood levels). For suspected fluconazole-resistance, a trial with another azole is appropriate as cross-resistance is not universal.

Prognosis: Non-HIV patients respond well to therapy, particularly when the predisposing factor is eliminated/decreased (i.e., antibiotics discontinued, steroids reduced, etc.). HIV patients may require longer courses of therapy and should be treated until cured. Relapse is frequent in HIV patients, and institution of effective antiretroviral therapy is the most effective general strategy.

Mouth Ulcers/Vesicles

Subset	Usual Pathogens	Preferred IV Therapy	Alternate IV Therapy	PO Therapy or IV-to-PO Switch
Vincent's angina	Borrelia Fusobacterium	Any β-lactam (IV) × 2 weeks **or** Ceftizoxime 2 gm (IV) q8h × 2 weeks	Clindamycin 600 mg (IV) q8h × 2 weeks	Clindamycin 300 mg (PO) q8h × 2 weeks **or** Amoxicillin/ Clavulanic acid 500/125 mg (PO) q8h × 2 weeks
Ludwig's angina	Group A streptococci (GAS)	Any β-lactam (IV) × 2 weeks **or** Ceftizoxime 2 gm (IV) q8h × 2 weeks	Clindamycin 600 mg (IV) q8h × 2 weeks	Clindamycin 300 mg (PO) q8h × 2 weeks **or** Amoxicillin/ Clavulanic acid 500/125 mg (PO) q8h × 2 weeks
Stomatitis	Normal mouth flora	Not applicable		
Herpangina	Coxsackie A	Not applicable		

Mouth Ulcers/Vesicles *(cont'd)*

Subset	Usual Pathogens	Preferred IV Therapy	Alternate IV Therapy	PO Therapy or IV-to-PO Switch
Herpes gingivo-stomatitis	HSV-1	<u>PO Therapy</u> Valacyclovir 500 mg (PO) q12h × 1 week **or** Acyclovir 400 mg (PO) 5x/day × 1 week		
Herpes labialis (cold sores/fever blisters)	HSV-1 (recurrent)	<u>PO Therapy</u> Valacyclovir 2 gm (PO) q12h × 1 day (2 doses) started at onset of symptoms (tingling/burning) **or** Acyclovir 400 mg (PO) 5x/day × 1 week		

Vincent's Angina (Borrelia/Fusobacterium)

Clinical Presentation: Painful/bleeding gums without fever.

Diagnostic Considerations: Foul breath, poor dental hygiene/pyorrhea.

Pitfalls: Do not attribute foul breath to poor dental hygiene without considering other serious causes (e.g., lung abscess, renal failure).

Therapeutic Considerations: After control of acute infection, refer to dentist.

Prognosis: Excellent with early treatment.

Ludwig's Angina (Group A streptococci)

Clinical Presentation: Painful floor of mouth with fever.

Diagnostic Considerations: Elevated floor of mouth is diagnostic. Massive neck swelling may be present.

Pitfalls: C_{1q} deficiency has perioral/tongue swelling, but no fever or floor of mouth elevation. Rarely, Ludwig's, angina may be due to F. necrophorum.

Therapeutic Considerations: Surgical drainage is not necessary. May need airway emergently; have tracheotomy set at bedside.

Prognosis: Early airway obstruction has adverse impact on prognosis.

Stomatitis (normal mouth flora)

Clinical Presentation: Painful mouth ulcers with fever.

Diagnostic Considerations: Diagnosis based on clinical appearance.

Pitfalls: Do not miss a systemic cause (e.g., acute leukemia).

Therapeutic Considerations: Painful; treat symptomatically.

Prognosis: Related to severity of underlying systemic disease.

Herpangina (Coxsackie A)

Clinical Presentation: Painful mouth ulcers/vesicles with fever.

Diagnostic Considerations: Ulcers located posteriorly in pharynx. No gum involvement or halitosis.

Pitfalls: Do not confuse with anterior vesicular lesions of HSV.

Therapeutic Considerations: No good treatment available. Usually resolves spontaneously in 2 weeks.

Prognosis: Good, but may be recurrent.

Herpes Gingivostomatitis (HSV-1)

Clinical Presentation: Painful gums with fever.

Diagnostic Considerations: Anterior ulcers in pharynx. Associated with bleeding gums, not halitosis.

Pitfalls: Do not miss a systemic disease associated with bleeding gums (e.g., acute myelogenous leukemia). Periodontal disease is not usually associated with oral ulcers.

Therapeutic Considerations: Oral analgesic solutions may help in swallowing.

Prognosis: Excellent with early treatment.

Herpes labialis (Cold Sores/Fever Blisters) (HSV-1)

Clinical Presentation: Painful vesicles along vermillion border of upper or lower lip with fever.

Diagnostic Considerations: Caused by recurrent HSV-1 infection, which appears as painful vesicular lesions on/near the vermillion border of lips. Attacks may be triggered by stress, sun exposure, menstruation, and often begin with pain or tingling before vesicles appear. Vesicles crust over and attacks usually resolve by 1 week. "Fever blisters" are not triggered by temperature elevations per se, but may accompany malaria, pneumococcal/meningococcal meningitis. Diagnosis is clinical.

Pitfalls: Do not confuse with perioral impetigo; impetigo has crusts (not vesicles), is itchy (not painful), and does not involve the vermillion border of the lips.

Therapeutic Considerations: Treatment is not always needed. If valacyclovir if used, it should be started when pain/tingling appear to decrease symptoms/vesicles/duration of attack. Valacyclovir is of no proven value once vesicles have appeared. Non-prescription topical products (docosanol 10%, tetracaine cream) may decrease pain/itching. Once-daily suppressive therapy may be considered for frequent recurrences or during times of increased risk (e.g., sun exposure). Sun screen may be helpful.

Prognosis: Tends to be recurrent in normal hosts. May be severe in compromised hosts.

Aphthous Ulcers

Clinical Presentation: Painful mouth ulcers/vesicles without fever.

Diagnostic Considerations: Usually an isolated finding. Ulcers are painful.

Pitfalls: May be a clue to systemic disorder, e.g., Behcet's syndrome. Mouth ulcers in SLE are painless.

Therapeutic Considerations: Usually refractory to all treatment and often recurrent. Steroid ointment (Kenalog) may be helpful.

Prognosis: Good, but tends to recur.

Deep Neck Infections, Lemierre's Syndrome, Severe Dental Infections

Subset	Usual Pathogens	Preferred IV Therapy	Alternate IV Therapy	IV-to-PO Switch
Deep neck infections (lateral pharyngeal, retro-pharyngeal, space)	Oral anaerobes	Meropenem 1 gm (IV) q8h × 2 weeks **or** Tigecycline 100 mg (IV) × 1 dose, then 100 mg (IV) q24h or 50 mg (IV) q12h × 2 weeks	Clindamycin 600 mg (IV) q8h × 2 weeks **or** Piperacillin/ Tazobactam 3.375 mg (IV) q6h × 2 weeks **or** Ertapenem 1 gm (IV) q24h × 2 weeks	Clindamycin 300 mg (PO) q8h × 2 weeks **or** Doxycycline 200 mg (PO) q12h × 3 days, then 100 mg (PO) q12h × 11 days*
Lemierre's Syndrome	Fusobacterium necrophorum	Treat as deep neck infection (see above)		
Severe dental infections	Oral anaerobes	Clindamycin 600 mg (IV) q8h × 2 weeks **or** Piperacillin/ Tazo-bactam 3.375 mg (IV) q6h × 2 weeks	Ertapenem 1 gm (IV) q24h × 2 weeks **or** Meropenem 1 gm (IV) q8h × 2 weeks	Clindamycin 300 mg (PO) q8h × 2 weeks **or** Doxycycline 200 mg (PO) q12h × 3 days, then 100 mg (PO) q12h × 11 days*

Deep Neck Infections
(lateral pharyngeal, retropharyngeal)

Diagnostic Considerations: Lateral pharyngeal space infection: Anterior → fever/chills, trismus, dysphagia, swelling or angle of mandible, ± parotid swelling, and bulging of lateral pharyngeal wall. Posterior pharyngeal space infection → bacteremic septic, no trismus/pain, and no pharyngeal wall bulging. Retropharyngeal space infection: fever/chills, dysphagia, dyspnea, ± mucal rigidity, esophageal regurgitation, and bulging of posterior pharyngeal wall.

Pitfalls: Retropharyngeal "danger space" infection may extend to mediastinum and present as mediastinitis.

Therapeutic Considerations: Obtain ENT consult for surgical drainage.

Prognosis: Worst prognosis with posterior lateral and retropharyngeal space infections.

Lemierre's Syndrome

Clinical Presentation: Severe sore throat with fever, toxemic appearance, and tenderness over jugular vein. Jugular vein septic thrombophlebitis and septic pulmonary emboli.

Diagnostic Considerations: May present as multiple septic pulmonary emboli. Usually follows recent dental infection. Jugular vein tenderness diagnostic. Blood cultures positive for F. necrophorum or F. nucleatum; rarely MSSA/MRSA.

Pitfalls: Suspect Lemierre's syndrome in patients with concurrent/antecedent dental/oropharyhngeal infection with severe sore throat and jugular vein tenderness.

Therapeutic Considerations: If unresponsive to antibiotic therapy, may need venotomy.

Prognosis: Good with prompt treatment. May be more severe with concurrent M. pneumoniae or EBV pharyngitis.

Severe Dental Infections

Diagnostic Considerations: Obtain CT/MRI of jaws to rule out osteomyelitis or abscess.

Pitfalls: Chronic drainage in a patient with an implant is diagnostic of chronic osteomyelitis/abscess until proven otherwise.

Therapeutic Considerations: Abscesses should be drained for cure.

Prognosis: Poor prognosis and recurrent without adequate surgical drainage.

Epiglottitis

Subset	Usual Pathogens	Preferred IV Therapy	Alternate IV Therapy	IV-to-PO Switch
Epiglottitis	S. pneumoniae H. influenzae Respiratory viruses	Ceftriaxone 1 gm (IV) q24h × 2 weeks **or** Meropenem 1 gm (IV) q8h × 2 weeks	Moxifloxacin 400 mg (IV) q24h × 2 weeks **or** Levofloxacin 500 mg (IV) q24h × 2 weeks	Moxifloxacin 400 mg (PO) q24h × 2 weeks **or** Levofloxacin 500 mg (PO) q24h × 2 weeks **or** Cefprozil 500 mg (PO) q12h × 2 weeks

Clinical Presentation: Stridor with upper respiratory infection.

Diagnostic Considerations: Lateral film of neck shows epiglottic edema. Neck CT/MRI may help if neck films are non-diagnostic.

Pitfalls: Do not attempt to culture the epiglottis (may precipitate acute upper airway obstruction).

Therapeutic Considerations: Treat empirically as soon as possible. Obtain ENT consult.

Prognosis: Early airway obstruction is associated with an adverse prognosis.

Empiric Therapy of Lower Respiratory Tract Infections

Acute Exacerbation of Chronic Bronchitis (AECB)

Subset	Pathogens	PO Therapy
AECB	S. pneumoniae H. influenzae M. catarrhalis	Respiratory quinolone* (PO) q24h × 5 days **or** Doxycycline 100 mg (PO) q12h × 5 days **or** Amoxicillin/clavulanic acid 875 mg (PO) q12h × 5 days **or** Azithromycin† 500 mg (PO) q24h × 5 days **or** Clarithromycin XL 1 gm (PO) q24h × 5 days

*   Moxifloxacin 400 mg Levofloxacin 500 mg, or Delafloxacin 450 mg (PO) q12h.
†   Increasing S. pneumoniae resistance.

Clinical Presentation: Productive cough and negative chest x-ray in a patient with chronic bronchitis.

Diagnostic Considerations: Diagnosis by productive cough, purulent sputum, and chest x-ray negative for pneumonia. H. influenzae is relatively more common than other pathogens.

Pitfalls: Do not obtain sputum cultures in chronic bronchitis; cultures usually reported as normal/mixed flora and should not be used to guide therapy.

Therapeutic Considerations: Treated with same antibiotics as for community-acquired pneumonia, since pathogens are the same (even though H. influenzae is relatively more frequent). Respiratory viruses/C. pneumoniae may initiate AECB, but is usually followed by bacterial infection, which is responsible for symptoms and is the aim of therapy. Bronchodilators are helpful for bronchospasm. Macrolide-resistant S. pneumoniae is an important clinical problem (prevalence ≥ 30%).

Prognosis: Related to underlying cardiopulmonary status.

Mediastinitis

Subset	Usual Pathogens	IV Therapy	IV-to-PO Switch
Following esophageal perforation or thoracic surgery	Oral anaerobes	<u>Preferred:</u> Piperacillin/Tazobactam 3.375 gm (IV) q6h × 2 weeks **or** Ampicillin/Sulbactam 3 gm (IV) q6h × 2 weeks <u>Alternate:</u> Meropenem 1 gm (IV) q8h × 2 weeks **or** Ertapenem 1 gm (IV) q24h × 2 weeks	Amoxicillin/ Clavulanate 500/125 mg (PO) q8h × 2 weeks **or** Respiratory quinolone* (PO) q24h × 2 weeks

* Moxifloxacin 400 mg or Levofloxacin 500 mg.

Diagnostic Considerations: Chest x-ray usually shows perihilar infiltrate in mediastinitis. Pleural effusions from esophageal tears have elevated amylase levels.

Pitfalls: Do not overlook esophageal tear in mediastinitis with pleural effusions.

Therapeutic Considerations: Obtain surgical consult if esophageal perforation is suspected.

Prognosis: Related to extent, location, and duration of esophageal tear/mediastinal infection.

Community Acquired Pneumonia (CAP) (see Color Atlas for Sputum Gram stains and Chapter 8 for Differential Diagnosis of CXR patterns)

Subset	Usual Pathogens*	Alternate IV Therapy	PO Therapy or IV-to-PO Switch
Pathogen unknown	S. pneumoniae¶ H. influenzae M. catarrhalis B. pertussis Legionella Mycoplasma pneumoniae	**Monotherapy** Respiratory quinolone† (IV) q24h **or** Doxycycline‡ (IV) × 1–2 weeks **Combination Therapy** Ceftriaxone 1 gm (IV) q24h × 1–2 weeks **plus either** Doxycycline‡ (IV) × 1–2 weeks **or** Azithromycin¶ 500 mg (IV) q24h × 1–2 weeks	Respiratory quinolone† (PO) q24h **or** Doxycycline‡ (PO) × 1–2 weeks

† Moxifloxacin 400 mg × 1–2 weeks or Levofloxacin 750 mg × 5 days (or 500 mg × 1–2 weeks) or Delafloxacin 300 mg (IV) q12h or 450 mg (PO) q12h × 1–2 weeks.

¶ Macrolide monotherapy should be avoided in areas where *macrolide resistant S. pneumoniae (MRSP)* strains are prevalent.

‡ Doxycycline 200 mg (IV or PO) q12h × 3 days, then 100 mg (IV or PO) q12h × 4–11 days.

Community Acquired Pneumonia (CAP) *(cont'd)*

Subset	Usual Pathogens*	Preferred IV Therapy	Alternate IV Therapy	PO Therapy or IV-to-PO Switch
Typical bacterial pathogens	S. pneumoniae H. influenzae M. catarrhalis	Ceftriaxone 1 gm (IV) q24h × 5 days **or** Respiratory quinolone[†] (IV) q24h × 5 days **or** Doxycycline[‡] 200 mg (IV) q12h × 3 days, then 100 mg (IV) q12h × 4 days	Tigecycline** 200 mg (IV) × 1 dose, then 100 mg (IV) q24h × 4 days **or** Lefamulin 150 mg (IV) q12h × 5 days **or** Omadacycline 200 mg (IV) × 1 dose, then 100 mg (IV) q24h × 4 days	Lefamulin 600 mg (PO) q12h × 5 days **or** Doxycycline 100 mg (PO) q12h × 5 days **or** Omadacycline 300 mg (PO) q24h × 5 days
	K. pneumoniae	Meropenem 1 gm (IV) q8h × 5 days **or** Ceftriaxone 1 gm (IV) q24h × 5 days **or** Respiratory quinolone[§] (IV) q24h × 5 days	Ertapenem 1 gm (IV) q24h × 5 days **or** Doripenem 1 gm (IV) q8h × 5 days	Respiratory quinolone[§] (PO) q24h × 5 days
	MDR K. pneumoniae CRE	Ceftazidime/ Avibactam 2.5 gm (IV) q8h × 5 days **or** Tigecycline** 200 mg (IV) × 1 dose, then 100 mg (IV) q24h × 4 days**	Polymyxin B 1.25 mg/kg (IV) q12h[¥] × 5 days **or** Colistin 2.5 mg/kg (IV) q12h[¶] × 5 days **or** Fosfomycin 6 gm (IV) q12h × 5 days	Fosfomycin 3 gm (PO) q24h × 5 days

† Moxifloxacin 400 mg × 1–2 weeks or Levofloxacin 750 mg × 5 days (or 500 mg × 1–2 weeks) or Delafloxacin 300 mg (IV) q12h or 450 mg (PO) q12h × 1–2 weeks

§ Moxifloxacin 400 mg or Levofloxacin 500 mg.

¥ 1 mg Colistin = 12,500 IU; 1 mg Polymyxin B = 10,000 IU.

‡ Doxycycline 200 mg (IV or PO) q12h × 3 days, then 100 mg (IV or PO) q12h × 4–11 days.

** **Depending on the MIC, higher doses of tigecycline (LD: 400 mg (IV) × 1 dose, then MD: 200 mg (IV) q24h) may be necessary for some (relatively resistant, non-susceptible) MDR GNBs.**

Community Acquired Pneumonia (CAP) *(cont'd)*

Subset	Usual Pathogens*	Preferred IV Therapy	Alternate IV Therapy	PO Therapy or IV-to-PO Switch
Pneumonias Atypical *(Zoonotic)*	C. psittaci (psittacosis) Coxiella burnetii (Q fever) Francisella tularensis (tularemia)	Doxycycline 200 mg (IV) q12h × 3 days, then 100 mg (IV) q12h × 2 weeks	Respiratory quinolone† (IV) q24h × 2 weeks	Doxycycline 200 mg (PO) q12h × 3 days, then 100 mg (PO) q12h × 11 days **or** Quinolone† (PO) q24h × 2 weeks
Atypical Pneumonias *(Non-zoonotic)*	Legionella‡ Mycoplasma pneumoniae‡ C. pneumoniae‡	Levofloxacin 500 mg (IV) q24h × 1–2 weeks **or** Moxifloxacin 400 mg (IV) q24h × 1–2 weeks **or** Doxycycline 200 mg (IV) q12h × 3 days, then 100 mg (IV) q12h × 4–11 days	Tigecycline 200 mg (IV) × 1 dose, then 100 mg (IV) q24h × 1–2 weeks **or** Azithromycin** 500 mg (IV) q24h × 1–2 weeks (minimum of 2 doses before switching to PO) **or** Delafloxacin 300 mg (IV) q12h × 1–2 weeks	Doxycycline 200 mg (PO) q12h × 3 days, then 100 mg (PO) q12h × 4–11 days **or** Respiratory quinolone† (PO) q24h × 1–2 weeks **or** Azithromycin** 500 mg (PO) q24h × 1–2 weeks **or** Delafloxacin 450 mg (PO) q12h × 1–2 weeks
Viral Pneumonias	Adenovirus	Cidofovir 5 mg/kg (IV) q × 2 weeks (severe cases)	Ribavirin 30 mg/kg (IV) × 1, then 8 mg/kg (IV) q6h × 3-6 days	
Influenza (mild or moderate) without bacterial CAP	Influenza A	Baloxavir 40 mg (40–80 kg) or 80 mg (>80 kg) tablets (PO) × 1 dose **or** Oseltamivir 75 mg (PO) q24h × 5 days	Laninamivir 40 mg (via inhaler) × 1 dose **or** Zanamivir 10 mg (via inhaler) q12h × 5 days	Oseltamivir may be ineffective against avian influenza (H_5N_1), but effective against swine influenza (H_1N_1)

*   Compromised hosts may require longer courses of therapy.

** Increasing M. pneumoniae resistance.

†   Moxifloxacin 400 mg or Levofloxacin 500 mg.

‡   May require prolonged therapy: Legionella (2–3 weeks); Mycoplasma (2 weeks); Chlamydia (2 weeks).

Community Acquired Pneumonia (CAP) *(cont'd)*

Subset	Usual Pathogens*	Preferred IV Therapy	Alternate IV Therapy	PO Therapy or IV-to-PO Switch
Influenza *(severe)* pneumonia	Influenza A	Peramivir 600 mg (IV) q24h × 1 dose **or** Oseltamivir 75 mg (PO) q12h × 5 days **plus** Amantadine 200 mg (PO) q24h × 7–10 days¶¶		Start within 3 days. Rimantadine/ amantadine inactive against Influenza B.
Influenza with <u>simultaneous</u> *bacterial CAP*¶	MSSA/MRSA	<u>MSSA</u> Nafcillin 2 gm (IV) q4h × 2 weeks **or** Cefazolin 1 gm (IV) q8h × 2 weeks **or** Meropenem 1 gm (IV) q8h × 2 weeks <u>MRSA</u> Vancomycin 1 gm (IV) q12h × 2 weeks **or** Tigecycline 200 mg (IV) × 1 dose then 100 mg (IV) q24h × 2 weeks **or** Linezolid 600 mg (IV) q12h × 2 weeks		<u>MSSA</u> Cephalexin 1 gm (PO) q6h × 2 weeks **or** Minocycline 200 mg (PO) × 1, then 100 mg (PO) q12h × 2 weeks <u>MRSA</u> Minocycline 200 mg (PO) × 1, then 100 mg (PO) q12h × 2 weeks **or** Linezolid 600 mg (PO) q12h × 2 weeks
Post-influenza *recovering from influenza (with* <u>subsequent</u> *bacterial CAP).*	S. pneumoniae H. influenzae	Respiratory quinolone‡ (IV) q24h × 2 weeks **or** Ceftriaxone 1 gm (IV) q24h × 2 wks	Doxycycline 200 mg (IV) × 3 days, then 100 mg (IV) q12h × 11 days	Respiratory quinolone‡ (PO) q24h × 2 weeks **or** Doxycycline 200 mg (IV) × 3 days, then 100 mg (PO) (IV) q12h × 11 days
Chickenpox pneumonia	VZV	Acyclovir 5–10 mg/kg (IV) q8h × 10 days		Valacyclovir 1–2 gm (PO) q8h × 10 days

* Compromised hosts predisposed to organisms listed, but may be infected by usual pathogens in normal hosts.

‡ May require prolonged therapy: Legionella (2–3 weeks); Mycoplasma (2 weeks); Chlamydia (2 weeks).

¶ If CXR shows multiple rapidly cavitating infiltrates < 72 hours, begin empiric anti-MSSA/CA-MRSA therapy with anti-influenza therapy.

¶¶ Resistance common, but may improve oxygenation in severe influenza A.

§ Dose for CrCl > 30 ml/min = 30 mg (PO) q12h; for CrCl > 10–30 ml/min = 30 mg (PO) q24h.

Community Acquired Pneumonia (CAP) *(cont'd)*

Subset	Usual Pathogens*	Preferred IV Therapy	Alternate IV Therapy	PO Therapy or IV-to-PO Switch
Aspiration	Oral anaerobes§	Ceftriaxone 1 gm (IV) q24h × 2 weeks **or** Respiratory quinolone‡ (IV) q24h × 2 weeks	Doxycycline 200 mg (IV) q12h × 3 days, then 100 mg (IV) q12h × 11 days	Respiratory quinolone‡ (PO) q24h × 2 weeks **or** Doxycycline 200 mg (PO) q12h × 3 days, then 100 mg (PO) q12h × 4–11 days** **or** Amoxicillin 1 gm (PO) q8h × 2 weeks
Tuberculosis (TB)	M. tuberculosis	INH 300 mg (PO) q24h (and pyridoxine 50 mg (PO) q24h) × 6 months **plus** RIF 600 mg (PO) q24h × 6 months **plus** PZA 25 mg/kg (PO) q24h × 2 months **plus** EMB 15 mg/kg (PO) q24h (until susceptibilities known)††		
	XDR-TB	Pretomanid 200 mg (PO) daily × 26 weeks **plus** Bedaquiline 400 mg daily × 2 weeks, then 200 mg (PO) thrice weekly × 24 weeks (total of 26 weeks) **plus** Linezolid 1200 mg (PO) daily × 26 weeks		
Non-tuberculous (atypical Mycobacteria)	M. avium – intracellulare (MAI)/complex (MAC)	<u>Treat for 12 months after sputum negative for MAI:</u> EMB 15 mg/kg (PO) q24h **plus either** Clarithromycin 500 mg (PO) q12h or Azithromycin 500 mg (PO) q24h **plus either** (Rifampin **or** Rifabutin). May substitute a quinolone (PO)‡ q24h for rifamycin		
	M. kansasii	RIF 600 mg (PO) q24h **plus** INH 300 mg (PO) q24h **plus** pyridoxine 50 mg (PO) q24h **plus** EMB 15 mg/kg (PO) q24h. Treat × 12 months after negative sputum		

‡   Moxifloxacin 400 mg or Levofloxacin 500 mg.

†† **If isolate is sensitive, discontinue EMB and continue as above to complete 6 months. If INH-resistant, continue EMB, RIF and PZA to complete 6–9 months. If any other resistance is present, obtain infectious disease or pulmonary consult.**

§   Oral anaerobes susceptible to all antibiotics. No need for below the waist (B. fragilis) anerobe coverage, e.g., clindamycin, moxifloxacin, metronidazole, cefoxitin. Any CAP antibiotic effective against oral anerobes.

Community Acquired Pneumonia (CAP) *(cont'd)*

Subset	Usual Pathogens*	Preferred IV Therapy	Alternate IV Therapy	PO Therapy or IV-to-PO Switch
Chronic alcoholics	K. pneumoniae S. pneumoniae	Meropenem 1 gm (IV) q24h × 2 weeks **or** Ertapenem 1 gm (IV) q24h × 2 weeks **or** Tigecycline 200 mg (IV) × 1, then 100 mg (IV) q24h × 1–2 weeks	Ceftriaxone 1 gm (IV) q24h × 2 weeks **or** Respiratory quinolone‡ (IV) q24h × 2 weeks	Respiratory quinolone (PO)‡ q24h × 2 weeks
	MDR K. pneumoniae CRE	Ceftazidime/ Avibactam 2.5 gm (IV) q8h × 1-2 weeks **or** Tigecycline 200 mg (IV) × 1 dose, 100 mg (IV) q24h × 1–2 weeks	Polymyxin B 1.25 mg/kg (IV) q12h × 1-2 weeks **or** Colistin 2.5 mg/ kg (IV) q12h × 1-2 weeks **or** Fosfomycin 6 gm (IV) q6h¶	Fosfomycin 3 gm (PO) q24h × 1–2 weeks
Bronchiec- tasis, cystic fibrosis	S. maltophilia B. cepacia Achromo- bacter (Alcaligenes) xyloxidans	<u>Preferred:</u> TMP–SMX 2.5 mg/kg (IV) q6h¶ **or** Minocycline 200 mg (IV) × 1, then 100 mg (IV) q12h¶ <u>Alternate:</u> Doxycycline 100 mg (IV) q12h¶		TMP–SMX 1 SS tablet (PO) q6h¶ **or** Minocycline 100 mg (PO) q12h¶
	P. aeruginosa	Meropenem 2 gm (IV) q8h¶ **or** Levofloxacin 750 mg (IV) q24h¶	Fosfomycin 6–12 gm (IV) q12h¶ **or** Cefepime 2 gm (IV) q8h¶ ± Amikacin 1 gm (IV) q24h¶	Levofloxacin 750 mg (PO) q24h¶ **or** Ciprofloxacin 750¶ mg (PO) q12h
	MDR P. aeruginosa CRE	Ceftazidime/ Avibactam 2.5 gm (IV) q8h¶ **or** Doripenem 1 gm (IV) q8h¶	Polymyxin B 1.25 mg/kg (IV) q12h¶ᵛ **or** Colistin 2.5 mg/kg (IV) q12h¶ **or** Fosfomycin 6–12 gm (IV) q12h¶	Fosfomycin¶ 3 gm (PO) q24h × 1–2 weeks

* Compromised hosts predisposed to organisms listed but may be infected by usual pathogens in normal hosts.

¶ Treat until cured.

‡ Moxifloxacin 400 mg or Levofloxacin 500 mg.

Community Acquired Pneumonia (CAP) *(cont'd)*

Subset	Usual Pathogens*	Preferred IV Therapy	Alternate IV Therapy	PO Therapy or IV-to-PO Switch
Chronic steroid therapy†	Aspergillus	Isavuconazole 200 mg (IV) q8h × 48h, then 200 mg (IV/PO) q24h**¶ **or** Voriconazole (IV)**¶	Liposomal amphotericin (L-amb) (IV)**¶ **or** Itraconazole 200 mg (IV) q12h × 2 days then 200 mg (PO) q12h*¶	Voriconazole (PO)** **or** Posaconazole 200 mg (PO) q6h initially, then 400 mg (PO) q12h¶
	P. (carinii) jiroveci (PCP)	TMP–SMX 5 mg/kg (IV) q6h × 3 weeks‡	Pentamidine 4 mg/kg (IV) q24h × 3 weeks‡	TMP–SMX 5 mg/kg (PO) q6h × 3 weeks **or** Atovaquone 750 mg (PO) q12h × 3 weeks **or** Dapsone 100 mg (PO) q24h × 3 weeks
	CMV	Valganciclovir 900 mg (PO) q12h until cured		
HIV	Typical/atypical CAP pathogens	see Chapter 5		
	P. (carinii) jiroveci (PCP)	see Chapter 5		
Other pathogens	For Cryptococcus neoformans, Blastomyces, Histoplasma, Coccidioides, Paracoccidioides (see Isavuconazote, above). For Actinomyces, Nocardia, Pseudallescheria boydii, Sporothrix, Mucor (see Chapter 4).			

¶   Treat until cured.

†   Treat IV or IV-to-PO switch.

*   Compromised hosts predisposed to organisms listed, but may be infected by usual pathogens of normal hosts.

** For usual dose, see Chapter 11 (Drug Summaries).

‡   **Steroid dosage: prednisone 40 mg (PO) q12h on days 1–5, then 40 mg (PO) q24h on days 6–10, then 20 mg (PO) q24h on days 11–21. Methylprednisolone (IV) can be substituted at 75% of prednisone dose.**

†† Moxifloxacin 400 mg or Levofloxacin 500 mg.

Clinical Presentation: Fever, cough, respiratory symptoms, chest x-ray consistent with pneumonia. Typical CAPs present only with pneumonia without extrapulmonary findings.

Diagnosis: Identification of organism on sputum gram stain/culture. Same organism is found in blood if blood cultures are positive. Also see Chapter 8 for typical chest x-ray patterns.

Community Acquired Pneumonia (Typical Bacterial Pathogens)

Diagnostic Considerations: Sputum is useful if a single organism predominates and is not contaminated by saliva. Purulent sputum, pleuritic chest pain, pleural effusion favor typical pathogens.

Pitfalls: Obtain chest x-ray to verify the diagnosis and rule out noninfectious mimics (e.g., heart failure).

Therapeutic Considerations: CAP most commonly due to S. pneumoniae or H. influenzae. After pathogen identified, no benefit in narrowing spectrum e.g., ceftriaxone as effective as PCN, but also is effective against PRSP, and the advantage of q24h dosing. Severity of CAP is related to the degree of cardiopulmonary/immune dysfunction and impacts the length of hospital stay, not the therapeutic approach or antibiotic choice.

Prognosis: Related to cardiopulmonary status and splenic function.

Community Acquired Pneumonia (Pertussis)

Clinical Presentation: Rhinorrhea over 1–2 weeks (catarrhal stage) progressing to paroxysms of cough (paroxysmal stage) lasting 2–4 weeks, often without a characteristic inspiratory whoop, followed by a convalescent stage lasting 1–2 weeks during which cough paroxysms decrease in frequency/severity. Fever is low grade or absent. In children < 6 months, whoop is frequently absent and apnea may occur. Older children/adults may present with persistent cough (without whoop) lasting 2–6 weeks.

Diagnostic Considerations: A positive PCR or DFA for Bordetella pertussis from a nasopharyngeal swab (NP). May be cultured by beside inoculation from NP swab of Bordet-Gengou media. "Shaggy heart" on chest x-ray is characteristic. The only CAP with lymphocytosis > 60%.

Pitfalls: Consider pertussis in older children and adults with prolonged coughing. Hoarseness uncommon, but may be misleading by mimicking viral laryngitis or C. pneumoniae.

Therapeutic Considerations: By the paroxysmal stage, antibiotics have minimal effect on the course of the illness but are indicated to decrease transmission.

Prognosis: Good, despite the prolonged course.

Community Acquired Pneumonia (Atypical Pathogens)

Clinical Presentation: CAP with extrapulmonary symptoms, signs, or laboratory abnormalities.

Diagnosis: Confirm by specific serological tests.

Non-Zoonotic Atypical CAPs

Legionnaire's Disease (Legionella sp.)

Epidemiology: Legionella organisms live in a fresh water environment and survive in a symbiotic relationship with freshwater amoeba. Legionella infection may be introduced into humans via droplet aerosolization of Legionella-contaminated water supplies (e.g., cooling towers, water systems, whirlpools, showers, air conditioners, respiratory therapy devices). LD can occur in isolated cases or in outbreaks (community-acquired or nosocomial). Legionella has a seasonal predisposition and is most common in the late summer/early fall. LD is rare in young children, uncommon in young adults, but is most common in adult/elderly patients. Individuals with impaired cell-mediated immunity ($\downarrow$ T-lymphocyte function) e.g., TNF-$\propto$ antagonists are predisposed to LD, but normal hosts can be infected as well.

Clinical Presentation: LD is more severe than M. pneumoniae or C. pneumoniae CAP. Onset is usually acute, with high fever ($\geq$ 102°F) and relative bradycardia Myalgias and chills are not uncommon. Like other atypical pneumonias, LD has a characteristic pattern of extrapulmonary manifestations, which is the key to presumtive clinical diagnosis. On chest x-ray, LD is suggested not by the appearance of the infitrate, but by its rapid, asymmetric progression. With LD, bilateral involvement is usual, consolidation/pleural effusion are not uncommon, and cavitation is rare. Extrapulmonary LD findings include, otherwise unexplained, mental confusion, watery diarrhea, abdominal pain, relative lymphopenia $\uparrow$ ESR/CRP, mild/transient $\uparrow$ AST/ALT, early/transient $\downarrow$ serum phosphorus, $\uparrow$ ferritin levels (> 2 × n) $\uparrow$ CPK, and early microscopic hematuria.

Diagnostic Considerations: Lack of response to beta-lactam therapy in a CAP patient suggests the possibility of LD and should prompt specific testing. Diagnosis is confirmed by Legionella DFA of sputum/respiratory secretions, Legionella IgM/IgG titers (a single titer $\geq$ 1:256 or $\geq$ 4 fold increase between acute and convalescent titers) is diagnostic. Legionella may also be cultured on BCYE agar from sputum/ respiratory secretions, pleural effusion, or lung tissue. Legionella pneumophila (serotypes 01-06) may also be diagnosed by urinary antigen test.

Pitfalls: As no individual finding is pathognomonic the constellation of signs/symptoms of LD are often overlooked. The characteristic pattern of extrapulmonary organ involvement differentiates LD from other CAPs. Hyponatremia is common but nonspecific, but serum phosphorus is a more specific for LD. Findings suggestive of an alternate (non-Legionella) cause of CAP include $\uparrow$ cold agglutinin titer, normal AST/ALT, normal serum phosphorus, normal CPK level, upper respiratory tract involvement (non-exudative pharyngitis, laryngitis, otitis) or splenomegaly. Legionella DFA of sputum/ respiratory secretions is positive early, but rapidly becomes negative with treatment. Legionella titers, may be negative if ordered early (usually at the time of presentation). Antimicrobial therapy may eliminate/blunt a titer rise. Legionella urinary antigen testing is useful but has limitations, as it is not always positive early when the patient presents, and detects only Legionella pneumophila (serotypes 01-06), but not other Legionella species.

Therapeutic Considerations: Antimicrobial agents with a high degree of anti-Legionella activity are quinolones, doxycycline, tigecycline, and macrolides. Rifampin has in vitro anti-Legionella activity, but as part of combination therapy (erythromycin + rifampin) has not been shown to offer any advantage over well selected monotherapy (quinolone, doxycycline). LD does not respond to beta-lactams and only somewhat to erythromycin. Patients treated with a quinolone, doxycycline, or tigecycline typically defervesce slowly (5–7 days). Therapy is usually continued for 2–3 weeks depending upon clinical severity/host factors.

Prognosis: In immunocompetent hosts with good cardiopulmonary function, prognosis is good. Prognosis is guarded in the elderly and those with impaired CMI (HIV, organ transplants, corticosteroid therapy) and in those severe cardiopulmonary disease (CAD, valvular heart disease, COPD, chronic bronchiectasis).

Mycoplasma pneumoniae

Epidemiology: M. pneumoniae primarily affects young adults and the elderly. M. pneumoniae is spread from person-to-person via aerosolized droplets.

Clinical Presentation: Onset is subacute with a characteristic dry/nonproductive cough that lasts for weeks, low-grade fever (< 102°F) /chills, and mild myalgias. As with other atypical CAPs, M. pneumoniae is characterized by its pattern of extrapulmonary organ involvement, which may include sore throat (non-exudative pharyngitis), bullous myringitis, otitis media, and/or watery loose stools/diarrhea (Table 2.1). Features that argue against the diagnosis of M. pneumoniae CAP include high fevers (>102°F), relative bradycardia, laryngitis, abdominal pain, ↑ AST/ALT, low serum phosphorus, or renal abnormalities. Chest x-ray typically shows ill-defined unilateral infiltrates without pleural effusion, consolidation or cavitation. M. pneumoniae may present as severe CAP in compromised hosts, the elderly, and those with advanced COPD.

Diagnostic Considerations: M. pneumoniae testing is recommended for patients with otherwise unexplained protracted nonproductive cough, low-grade fevers, loose stools/ watery diarrhea, and an ill-defined infiltrate on chest x-ray. Cold agglutinin titers are elevated early/transiently (75%) and provide a rapid presumptive diagnosis; titers ≥ 1:64 are due to M. pneumoniae. An elevated M. pneumoniae IgM ELISA titer suggests acute infection, but an elevated IgG titer indicates only past exposure; M. pneumoniae may be cultured from respiratory secretions on viral media (requires 1–2 weeks for growth).

Pitfalls: A dry, nonproductive cough also suggests an ILI or C. pneumoniae. Before ascribing E. multiforme to M. pneumoniae, be sure that it is not due to other causes (e.g., drug induced). Features that argue against the diagnosis of M. pneumoniae include temperature > 102°F, relative bradycardia, moderate/large pleural effusion, consolidation/

cavitation, otherwise unexplained abdominal pain, ↑ AST/ALT or low serum phosphorus. Suspect M. pneumoniae in chronic dry cough/new onset asthma.

Therapeutic Considerations: Doxycycline, macrolides, quinolones, or tigecycline result in rapid clinical response: in < 72 hours, but dry cough usually persists for weeks. Because Mycoplasma organisms reside on/in the bronchial epithelium, antimicrobial therapy should be continued for 2 weeks to eliminate carriage from oropharyngeal secretions and reduce the risk of transmission via aerosolized droplets.

Prognosis: M. pneumoniae is usually a mild, self-limiting illness in immunocompetent adults. M. pneumoniae may be severe in compromised hosts, the elderly, and those with advanced lung disease. Patients with M. pneumoniae and meningoencephalitis (headaches/stiff neck, mental confusion, very high cold agglutinin titers [often ≥ 1:1024]) have a good prognosis. M. pneumoniae may be complicated by transverse myelitis, brain stem/cerebellar ataxia, or Guillain-Barré syndrome after M. pneumoniae some patients develop permanent asthma.

Chlamydophilia (Chlamydia) pneumoniae

Epidemiology: C. pneumoniae is may occur as sporadic cases part of an outbreak NHAP. C. pneumoniae is spread from person-to-person via aerosolized droplets. C. pneumoniae has no seasonal predisposition. Some patients with C. pneumoniae CAP develop permanent asthma.

Clinical Presentation: C. pneumoniae presents as a "mycoplasma-like" illness. Like other atypical CAPs, C. pneumoniae CAP is characterized by extrapulmonary findings, particularly nasal discharge, sore throat, and hoarseness. Temperature is usually ≤ 102°F. Chest x-ray findings typically show a unilateral ill-defined infiltrate without consolidation, cavitation, or pleural effusion. C. pneumoniae testing is recommended in a patient with a "mycoplasma-like" illness and hoarseness.

Diagnostic Considerations: The diagnosis of C. pneumoniae CAP requires a single IgM titer of ≥ 1:16 or an IgG titer > 1:512 (ELISA or MIF). C. pneumoniae may be cultured from respiratory secretions using viral culture media.

Pitfalls: IgG titers indicate past exposure, not current infection. ↑ IgM and ↑ IgG titers may be delayed for more than 3 and 6 weeks, respectively. False negatives may occur if IgM titers are obtained too early. Recovery of C. pneumoniae from respiratory secretions does not differentiate carriage from infection. In a CAP patient with otherwise unexplained wheezing should suggest the possibility of C. Pneumoniae.

Therapeutic Considerations: Doxycycline, or quinolones are effective. C. pneumoniae is sensitive to erythromycin in vitro, but erythromycin is often ineffective in vivo. C. pneumoniae also responds to newer macrolides.

Prognosis: C. pneumoniae CAP is usually a mild/moderate pneumonia with an excellent prognosis. Severe CAP may occur in compromised hosts, the elderly, or those with severe lung disease some develop permanent asthma.

Table 2.1 Diagnostic Features of Non-Zoonotic Atypical Pneumonias

Key Characteristics	Mycoplasma pneumoniae	Legionnaire's Disease	C. pneumoniae
Symptoms			
Mental confusion	–†	+	–
Prominent headache	–	±	–
Meningismus	–	–	–
Myalgias	±	±	±
Ear pain	+	–	±
Pleuritic pain	–	±	–
Abdominal pain	–	±	–
Loose stools/watery diarrhea	±	⊕	–
Signs			
Rash	± a	–	–
Non-exudative pharyngitis	+	–	+
Hemoptysis	–	±	–
Wheezing	–	–	+
Lobar consolidation	–	±	–
Cardiac involvement	± b	– c	–
Splenomegaly	–	–	–
Relative bradycardia	–	+	–
Laboratory Abnormalities			
WBC count	↑/N	↑	N
Thrombocytosis	±	–	–
Hyponatremia	–	+	–
Hypophosphatemia (early)	–	+	–
↑ AST/ALT	–	+	–
↑ CPK	–	±	–
↑ ESR (> 100 mm/h)	–	+	–
↑ Ferritin (> 2 x n)	–	+	–
↑ Cold agglutinins (≥ 1:64)	+	–	–
Microscopic hematuria (early)	–	±	–
Chest X-Ray			
Infiltrate	Patchy	Patchy/multifocal	Circumscribed lesions
Bilateral hilar adenopathy	–	–	–
Pleural effusion	± (small)	±	–

+ = usually present; ± = sometimes present; – = usually absent.
↑ = increased; ↓ = decreased; ↑↑↑ = markedly increased.
ALT = alanine aminotransferase; AST = aspartate aminotransferase; N = normal; WBC = white blood cell.
a = erythema multiforme; b = myocarditis, heart block, or pericarditis; c = unless endocarditis.
† = mental confusion only if meningoencephalitis.
†† = often not positive early, but antigenuria persists for weeks. Useful only to diagnose L. pneumophila (serogroup 1), not other species/serogroups.

Zoonotic Atypical CAPs

Subset	Usual Pathogens*	Preferred IV Therapy	Alternate IV Therapy	PO Therapy or IV-to-PO Switch
Zoonotic pathogens	C. psittaci (psittacosis) C. caviae Coxiella burnetii (Q fever) Francisella tularensis (tularemia)	Doxycycline 200 mg (IV) q12h × 3 days, then 100 mg (IV) q12h × 11 days	Levofloxacin 500 mg (IV) × 2 weeks **or** Moxifloxacin 400 mg (IV) × 2 weeks	Doxycycline 200 mg (PO) q12h × 3 days, then 100 mg (PO) q12h × 11 days **or** Levofloxacin 500 mg (PO) × 2 weeks

* Compromised hosts may require longer courses of therapy.

Zoonotic Atypical Pneumonias

Chlamydophila (Chlamydia) psittaci (Psittacosis)

Clinical Presentation: Recent close contact with a psittacine bird followed by non-productive cough and prominent headache suggests psittacosis. Fever with relative bradycardia present in most. Epistaxis may be present early. Horder's spots (on face) are pathognomonic. Splenomegaly is frequent. Obscure phlebitis is rare. Serum transaminases are usually mildly elevated.

Diagnostic Considerations: CAP presenting with splenomegaly limits DDx possibilities to psittacosis or Q fever. Diagnosis by ↑ C. psittaci CF or MIF titers.

Pitfalls: C. psittaci titers may XR with C. pneumoniae. In a severe CAP patient with presumed psitticosis, lack of bird contact, but recent guinea pig contact should suggest possible C. caviae CAP (send PCR C. psittaci for further typing).

Therapeutic Considerations: Doxycycline preferred. Macrolides less effective.

Prognosis: Good, if uncomplicated by CNE.

Coxiella burnetii (Q fever)

Clinical Presentation: Recent exposure to sheep, goats, cattle, or parturient cats. Acutely presents as a zoonotic atypical CAP with headache, malaise, nonproductive cough, and fever with relative bradycardia. Splenomegaly common. ↑ serum transaminases usual. Thrombocytosis and ↑ cold agglutinins in some. Subclinical or acute CAP may later be complicated by chronic Q fever usually manifested as CNE which may affect native or prosthetic valves.

Diagnostic Considerations: Q fever pneumonia (acute) diagnosed by ↑ phase II titers. Chronic Q fever CNE diagnosed by ↑ phase I titers (> 1:800). Q fever (phase I) titers may XR with other Chlamydia sp., Legionella sp., Ehrlichia/Anaplasma, or Bartonella.

Pitfalls: Be sure to ask in depth about appropriate vector contact. Often the patient denies having a cat but fails to mention the neighbor's parturient cat. With chronic Q fever, CNE valvular vegetations are often flat and may not be visible on TTE/TEE but are detectable on PET scan.

Therapeutic Considerations: Doxycycline alone optimal for Q fever CAP. For chronic Q fever CNE, doxycycline plus hydroxychloroquine is preferred therapy.

Prognosis: Excellent with acute Q fever. Problematic with chronic Q fever CNE.

Tularemia (F. tularensis)

Clinical Presentation: Acute onset of fever, chills, myalgias, headache (encephalopathy absent), dyspnea and a nonproductive cough. Zoonotic atypical CAP following recent tick, rabbit, deer exposure. CXR in tularemic pneumonia usually accompanied by hilar adenopathy (unilateral > bilateral) with serosanguinous or bloody pleural effusion. Relative bradycardia is not present and serum transaminases are not elevated. Tularemic pneumonia may accompany any of the six clinical types of tularemia (ulceroglandular, glandular, oculoglandular, oropharyngeal, typhoidal).

Diagnostic Considerations: Tularemic pneumonia can resemble other atypical zoonotic pneumonias but hilar adenopathy with pleural effusion should suggest tularemia on Gram stain of sputum or bloody effusion shows small, bipolar staining GNB. Diagnosis is confirmed serologically.

Pitfalls: In sputum may resemble Y. pestis without bipolar staining.

Therapeutic Considerations: Streptomycin preferred but gentamicin may be substituted. Doxycycline, chloramphenicol, or a quinolone are also effective.

Prognosis: Mortality rates for severe untreated infection can be as high as 30%.

Other Zoonotic CAPs

Severe Acute Respiratory Syndrome (SARS)

Clinical Presentation: Fever, dry cough, myalgias, diarrhea in some. Auscultation of the lungs resembles viral influenza (i.e., quiet, no rales). Biphasic infection: fever decreases after few days, patient improves, then fever recurs in a few days and patients become short of breath/hypoxic. Chest x-ray shows bilateral interstitial (diffuse) infiltrates. WBC and platelet counts are usually normal or slightly decreased. Relative lymphopenia present early. Mild increases in AST/ALT, LDH, CPK are common.

Diagnostic Considerations: Diagnosis by viral isolation or specific SARS serology. Important to exclude influenza A, Legionnaires' disease and tularemic pneumonia.

Pitfalls: Should not be confused with viral influenza (a 3-day illness). Patients with SARS deteriorate during week 2 when influenza patients are recovering. Early, chest x-ray in SARS has discrete infiltrates (unlike influenza unless superimposed CAP) that may be ovoid. Late, ARDS on chest x-ray.

Therapeutic Considerations: Most patients are severely hypoxemic and require oxygen/ventilatory support. In a preliminary study, some patients benefitted from corticosteroids (pulse-dosed methylprednisolone 500 mg [IV] q24h × 3 days followed by taper/step down with prednisone [PO] to complete 20 days) plus Interferon alfacon-1 (9 mcg [SQ] q24h × at least 2 days, increased to 15 mcg/d if no response) × 8–13 days. Ribavirin of no benefit.

Prognosis: Related to underlying cardiopulmonary/immune status/ARDS. Frequently fatal.

Middle East Respiratory Syndrome (MERS)

Clinical Presentation: Presents as an influenza like illness (ILI) with acute onset of fever, chills, dry cough/SOB, myalgias ± N/V/D. Headache/sore throat common. Hemoptysis in some. Rapidly progressive respiratory failure/ARDS is typical (~ 1 week). WBC counts usually normal, thrombocytopenia, ↑AST/ALT, ↑LDH, relative lymphopenia, but lymphocytosis in some. CXR: basilar unilateral (initially) or bilateral dense interstitial/nodular infiltrates (later). Consolidation common ± pleural effusions.

Diagnostic Considerations: MERS resembles an ILI clinically (unlike SARS-CoV). Contact with dromedary camels (MERS reservoir). Dx is by RT-PCR of MERS-CoV virus in respiratory secretions (lower > upper). MERS, in respiratory secretions (lower > upper), but not in stools/urine (unlike SARS-CoV).

Pitfalls: Resembles severe influenza A. Not a biphasic illness (like SARS-CoV).

Therapeutic Considerations: Ventilatory support, but no effective treatment available. No bacterial co-infections, i.e., no antibiotics for superimposed bacterial CAP. IC measures important to prevent person-to-person/nosocomial spread.

Prognosis: High mortality rate with rapidly progressive severe respiratory failure/ARDS especially with comorbidities.

Coronavirus Disease - 19 (COVID-19)

Clinical Presentation: COVID-19 (caused by the novel beta coronavirus SARS-CoV-2) presents as an influenza-like illness (ILI) or a viral pneumonia resembling influenza. SARS and MERS are zoonotic viral pneumonias, caused by two other beta-CoVs, differ from the COVID-19 novel beta coronavirus (SARS-CoV-2). SARS-CoV-2 has been identified as a new cause of viral zoonotic pneumonia (COVID-19). Initially, SARS-CoV-2 was acquired from wild animals. SARS-CoV-2 is spread by droplet/airborne transmission. Person-to-person (including nosocomial) spread is common. Myocarditis and diarrhea frequent, unlike with SARS or MERS. However, like SARS and particularly MERS, ARDS may complicate severe cases. Usual COVID-19 lab abnormalities include leukopenia, relative lymphopenia, thrombocytopenia. Mild elevations of AST/ALT, LDH, CPK are common.

Diagnostic Considerations: SARS-CoV-2 RT-PCR of respiratory secretions/specimens diagnostic. In symptomatic cases where COVID-19 is likely, early false negatives may require serial testing (× 2–3) before becoming RT-PCR +. COVID-19 patients may remain RT-PCR + for 1–2 weeks post-recovery.

Pitfalls: Clinically, COVID-19 most closely resembles influenza A. Typical clinical course of COVID-19 is unlike the biphasic course of SARS or the frequently fulminant course of MERS.

Therapeutic Considerations: Remdesivir 200 mg (IV) × 1, then 100 mg (IV) q24h × 5–10 days. Alternately, hydroxychloroquine 400 mg (PO) q12h × 1 day, then 200 mg (PO) q12h × 4 days plus azithromycin 500 mg (PO) x 1 dose, then 250 mg (PO) q24h × 4 days (synergistic).

Prognosis: Spectrum of COVID-19 ranges from a mild flu-like illness to fatal CAP. Prognosis worse when complicated by myocarditis, ARDS.

Table 2.2 Diagnostic Features of Zoonotic Atypical Pneumonias

Key Characteristics	Psittacosis	Q Fever	Tularemia
Symptoms			
Mental confusion	–	±	–
Prominent headache	+	+	+
Meningismus	–	–	–
Myalgias	+	+	+
Ear pain	–	–	–
Pleuritic pain	±	±	+
Abdominal pain	–	–	–
Diarrhea	–	–	–
Signs			
Rash	± a	–	–
Nonexudative pharyngitis	–	–	±
Hemoptysis	–	–	±
Lobar consolidation	+	+	+
Cardiac involvement	± b	± c	–
Splenomegaly	±	+	–
Relative bradycardia	±	±	–
Chest X-Ray			
Infiltrate	Patchy/Lobar consolidation	"Round" infiltrates/ Lobar consolidation –	"Ovoid infiltrates"
Bilateral hilar adenopathy	–	–	±
Pleural effusion	–	–	Bloody
Laboratory Abnormalities			
WBC count	↓	↑/N	↑/N
Thrombocytosis	–	±	–
Hyponatremia	±	±	±
Hypophosphatemia	–	–	–
↑ AST/ALT	+	+	–
↑ Cold agglutinins	–	±	–
Anti-smooth muscle antibodies (anti-SMA)	–	±	–
Microscopic hematuria	–	–	–

+ = usually present; ± = sometimes present; – = usually absent.
↑ = increased; ↓ = decreased; ↑↑↑ = markedly increased.
ALT = alanine aminotransferase; AST = aspartate aminotransferase; N = normal; WBC = white blood cell.
a = Horder's spots (facial spots), resemble the (truncal spots) of typhoid fever (rose spots)
b = Mycocarditis; c = Endocarditis.

Influenza A Pneumonia

Clinical Presentation: Acute onset of fever, headache, myalgias/arthralgias, sore throat, prostration, dry cough. Myalgias most pronounced in lower back/legs. Eye pain is common. Rapid high fever initially, which decreases in 2–3 days. Severity ranges from mild flu to life-threatening pneumonia. Chest x-ray in early influenza is normal/near normal without focal/segmental infiltrates or pleural effusion.

Diagnostic Considerations: Mild cases with headache, sore throat, and rhinorrhea resemble the common cold/respiratory viruses (influenza-like illnesses) and can be caused by type A or B. Severe flu is usually due to type A. Rapid diagnosis by PCR of respiratory secretions (nasopharyngeal swabs).

Pitfalls: Influenza pneumonia has no chest auscultatory findings and the chest x-ray is normal/near normal. Severe influenza pneumonia is accompanied by an oxygen diffusion defect ($\uparrow$ A-a gradient), and patients are hypoxemic/cyanotic. Pleuritic chest pain may be present. Influenza can invade the intercostal muscles to mimic pleuritic chest pain. Labor/segmental infiltrates on CXR with influenza pneumonia indicate simultaneous or subsequent bacterial CAP. If CAP presents with fulminant/severe necrotizing pneumonia in a normal host look for antecedent or concomitant influenza pneumonia.

Therapeutic Considerations: Mild/moderate influenza can be treated with neuraminidase inhibitors (Tamiflu/Relenza), which reduce symptoms by 1–2 days. Peramivir may be given in severe cases. Flu with simultaneous bacterial CAP is due to MSSA/MRSA and post-influenza CAP usually due to S. pneumoniae or H. influenzae (Table 2.3).

Prognosis: Good for mild/moderate flu. Severe flu may be fatal due to profound hypoxemia with influenza pneumonia. Prognosis is worse if presents with simultaneous MSSA/MRSA. Influenza with necrotizing community-acquired (CA) MSSA/MRSA CAP is frequently fatal. Prognosis is worst for CA-MRSA Panton-Valentine Leukocidin (PVL)-positive strains. Dry cough/fatigue may persist for weeks after influenza.

Avian Influenza (H_5N_1, H_7N_9) Pneumonia

Clinical Presentation: Influenza following close contact with infected poultry. Recent outbreaks in humans in Asia. Human-to-human transmission reported. Often fulminant respiratory illness rapidly followed by ARDS/death.

Diagnostic Considerations: Often acute onset of severe influenza illness ± diarrhea/conjunctival suffusion with leukopenia, lymphopenia, mildly $\uparrow$ AST/ALT and $\uparrow$ LDH. Diagnosis by hemagglutin-specific RT-PCR for avian influenza or culture of respiratory secretions. Not complicated by bacterial CAP.

Pitfalls: Influenza A HI test insensitive to avian influenza hemagglutinins resulting in false negatives.

Therapeutic Considerations: Antivirals must be given early to be effective. Avian influenza strains may be resistant to oseltamivir and amantadine/rimantadine.

Prognosis: Often fulminant with ARDS/death. Unlike human/swine influenza, avian influenza is often rapidly/highly lethal, but not complicated by MSSA/MRSA CAP.

Swine Influenza (H_1N_1) Pneumonia

Clinical Presentation: Swine influenza (H_1N_1) may present with a mild illness with fever, cough, and loose stools/diarrhea to severe viral pneumonia requiring ventilation that may rapidly progress to ARDS/death. Patients with swine influenza (H_1N_1) pneumonia as well as other viral pneumonias typically present as influenza-like illnesses (ILIs). Swine influenza (H_1N_1) pneumonia affects primarily young healthy adults. In admitted adults, swine influenza (H_1N_1) pneumonia typically presents with high fevers > 102°F often with shaking chills and myalgias. Patients may also complain of headache or sore throat. Dry cough is characteristic. Patients are variably short of breath. Conjunctival suffusion is rare. Lungs are clear to auscultation. Patients often have loose stools/diarrhea but not abdominal pain. CXR early (< 48 hours) typically is clear or may show accentuated bibasilar lung markings resembling basilar atelectasis. CXR later (> 48 hours) typically shows bilateral patchy interstitial infiltrates. Degree of hypoxemia is related to the severity of pneumonia. In adults, nonspecific laboratory clues include otherwise unexplained relative lymphopenia, thrombocytopenia, elevated CPKs or mildly elevated serum transaminases. Atypical lymphocytes are not present in adults. Unlike in human seasonal and avian influenza (H_5N_1), leukopenia is uncommon in swine influenza (H_1N_1) pneumonia in adults. Serum LDH is variably elevated. Elevated cold agglutinin titers are not elevated.

Diagnostic Considerations: Definitive diagnosis is by RT-PCR of oropharyngeal/respiratory secretions/lung. All respiratory secretion diagnostic tests may be negative in autopsy proven cases of swine influenza (H_1N_1) pneumonia whose lungs are RT-PCR positive.

Pitfalls: While human seasonal influenza may present simultaneously with MSSA/MRSA CAP, this and has been uncommon with swine influenza (H_1N_1) pneumonia. Cold agglutinins and atypical lymphocytes may occur in pediatric cases but in adults should suggest an alternate diagnosis, e.g., adenoviral or CMV pneumonia.

Therapeutic Considerations: Swine influenza (H_1N_1) appears to respond to oseltamivir. If the CXR in swine influenza (H_1N_1) pneumonia has no lobar/focal infiltrates, there is no need to treat with empiric antimicrobial therapy.

In patients unable to take oral oseltamivir, IV peramivir may be given.

Prognosis: Prognosis is directly related to the severity of pneumonia (degree/duration of severe hypoxemia) and degree/persistence of relative lymphopenia.

Non-Zoonotic Viral Pneumonias

Influenza-like Illness (ILIs)
(hMPV, RSV, HPIV, R/E, Coronaviruses)

Clinical Presentation: Admitted adults present as an ILI with viral CAP. Viral ILIs important due to their potential to mimic influenza or Legionnaire's disease, e.g., HPIV-3. Viral ILIs implicated in nosocomial and nursing home outbreaks. May be severe in normal hosts/elderly.

Diagnostic Considerations: CXR typically unremarkable early. Later, bilateral patchy interstitial infiltrates ± small pleural effusions. Presumptive diagnosis by lymphocyte; monocyte (L:M) ratios > 2 (influenza L:M ratio <2). All ILI viruses have L:M > 2 (except HPIV-3). Definitive diagnoses by PCR of respiratory secretions.

Pitfalls: Atypical lymphocytes may be present > 3 days with viral ILIs. In adults admitted with an ILI, atypical lymphocytes effectively rule out Dx of influenza.

Therapeutic Considerations: Aside from supportive care, nitazoxanide has activity against influenza and some ILI viruses, (RSV, HPIV, coronaviruses) and may be useful in some cases.

Prognosis: Viral ILIs have protracted LOS predisposing to nosocomial infections.

Adenovirus

Clinical Presentation: Following recent URI onset begins with fever, dry cough and short-ness of breath (± diarrhea). Adenoviral CAP is frequently severe in immunocompetent hosts. Progression to respiratory failure in hours – days. The only viral CAP with unilateral focal/segmental infiltrates.

Diagnostic Considerations: Features pointing to an adenoviral CAP are bilateral conjunc-tivitis (± hemorrhagic). Headache/myalgias less prominent than with ILIs. Diagnosis by viral culture/PCR of respiratory secretions or conjunctivae (if conjunctivitis). Serological diag-nosis by ↑ IgM adenoviral titres. Leukopenia, relative lymphopenia, thrombocytopenia, unelevated ESR, mildly ↑ serum transaminases, ↑ CPK are typical findings. Cold agglutinins present in some. Adenovirus present in stool (± diarrhea) and excreted in feces for weeks.

Pitfalls: Adenoviral CAP may mimic bacterial CAP or Legionnaire's disease. CXR usually presents as an unilateral lower lobe focal/segmental infiltrate (± pleural effusion). Later, progression to bilateral patchy interstitial infiltrates. Unlike LD, ESR is unelevated, no hypo-phosphatemia, and ferritin levels not highly ↑ in adenoviral CAP. If cold agglutinins present titers than with mycoplasma CAP.

Prognosis: Ribavirin or cidofovir may be of benefit in BMT/SOTs, but effectiveness in immunocompetent hosts uncertain.

Miscellaneous Other CAPs

S. aureus (MSSA/MRSA) Pneumonia

Clinical Presentation: Only occurs with an antecedent ILI or concurrent influenza pneu-monia. Does not occur in DM or those on chronic steroids/immunosuppressive therapy. Presents as a fulminant necrotizing CAP with high fevers, hemoptysis, cyanosis, and hypo-tension. CXR shows unilateral/bilateral rapid cavitation of pulmonary infiltrates < 72 hrs.

Diagnostic Considerations: Patient severely hypoxemic with ↑ A-a gradient (>35) due to underlying influenza pneumonia. Blood/sputum cultures + for MSSA/MRSA.

Pitfalls: Culture of MSSA/MRSA from sputum in CAP without rapid cavitation < 72 hrs on CXR, represents colonization, not diagnostic of MSSA/MRSA CAP. Patients CAP due to MSSA/MRSA are critically ill with high spiking fevers, hemoptysis, cyanosis, and hypoten-sion. Diagnosis not supported by MSSA/MRSA in sputum/blood cultures unless accompa-nied by the clinical features of MSSA/MRSA pneumonia

Therapeutic Considerations: Treat underlying influenza as well as the superimposed MSSA/MRSA pneumonia with an antibiotic with a high degree of anti- MSSA/MRSA activity, e.g., linezolid (avoid daptomycin). Resection of necrotic lung segments may be life saving.

Prognosis: Poor (independent of host factors). Worst prognosis is with PVL + strains.

Aspiration Pneumonia

Diagnostic Considerations: Sputum not diagnostic. No need for transtracheal aspi-rate culture.

Pitfalls: Lobar location varies with patient position during aspiration.

Therapeutic Considerations: Oral anaerobes are sensitive to all beta-lactams and most antibiotics used to treat CAP. Additional anaerobic (B. fragilis) coverage is not needed.

Prognosis: Related to severity of CNS/esophageal disease.

HIV with CAP (*Sputum Negative for AFB*)

Clinical Presentation: Bacterial CAP in HIV patient with focal infiltrate(s) and normal/slightly depressed CD_4.

Diagnostic Considerations: Diagnosis by sputum gram stain/culture $\pm$ positive blood cultures (bacterial pathogens) or Legionella/Chlamydia serology (atypical pathogens).

Pitfalls: Bacterial CAP (focal/segmental infiltrates) in HIV does not resemble PCP (bilateral patchy interstitial infiltrates). PCP presents with profound hypoxemia and $\uparrow$ LDH and β 1,3 D-glucan +, aspergillus galactomannan –. S. pneumoniae CAP relatively uncommon in HIV, but if present usually occurs in early/well controlled HIV. Unlike in normal hosts, in HIV S. pneumoniae CAP may present as necrotizing/cavitating pneumonia.

Therapeutic Considerations: R/O TB/MAI with negative sputum AFB stain.

Prognosis: Same as bacterial CAP in normal hosts.

Tuberculous (TB) Pneumonia

Clinical Presentation: Community-acquired pneumonia with single/multiple infiltrates.

Diagnostic Considerations: Diagnosis by sputum AFB smear/culture. Primary TB is lower lobe usually with hilar adenopathy and or pleural effusion. Reactivation TB is usually bilateral/apical $\pm$ old, healed Ghon complex; cavitation/fibrosis are common, but adenopathy or pleural effusions uncommon. TB reactivation $\uparrow$ with steroids, immunosuppressive drugs, HIV, gastorectomy, jejunoileal bypass, silicosis, DM, renal insufficiency, advanced age. Urinary lipoarabinomannan glycan (LAM) test useful for pulmonary TB. In HIV negative patients, levels ~ disease severity.

Pitfalls: Primary TB may present as CAP and improve transiently with quinolone therapy. Primary TB patients with large pleural effusion usually anergic.

Therapeutic Considerations: Usually sputum becomes smear negative in 1–2 weeks of therapy.

Prognosis: Related to underlying health status.

Mycobacterium avium-intracellulare (MAI)/avium complex (MAC) Pneumonia

Clinical Presentation: Community-acquired pneumonia in normal hosts with bronchietasis or immunosuppressed/HIV patient with focal single/multiple infiltrates indistinguishable from TB.

Diagnostic Considerations: Diagnosis by AFB culture. In HIV, MAI/MAC may disseminate, resembling miliary TB. MAI/MAC typically lingular with tree in bud appearance on chest CT. BHA more frequent than with TB.

Pitfalls: May mimic reactivation TB. Must differentiate TB from MAI/MAC by AFB culture, since therapy for MAI/MAC differs from TB.

Therapeutic Considerations: Should be treated until sputum cultures are negative × 1 year.

Prognosis: Good in normal hosts. In HIV related to degree of immunosuppression/CD_4 count.

Mycobacterium kansasii Pneumonia

Clinical Presentation: Subacute CAP resembling reactivation TB.

Diagnostic Considerations: Chest x-ray infiltrates/lung disease plus M. kansasii in a single sputum specimen. M. kansasii can cause disseminated infection, like TB, and is diagnosed by culturing M. kansasii from sputum, blood, liver, or bone marrow.

Pitfalls: M. kansasii in sputum with a normal chest x-ray and no symptoms does not indicate infection.

Therapeutic Considerations: Should be treated until sputum cultures are negative × 1 year.

Prognosis: Good in normal hosts. May be rapidly progressive/fatal without treatment in HIV patients.

Pneumonia in Chronic Alcoholics

Diagnostic Considerations: Klebsiella pneumoniae usually occurs only in chronic alcoholics, and is characterized by blood-flecked currant jelly sputum and cavitation (typically in 3–5 days).

Pitfalls: Suspect Klebsiella pneumonia that cavitates. S. pneumoniae necrotizing pneumonia with cavitation rarely occurs in alcoholics (also rarely in HIV and compromised hosts), but not in normal hosts. Empyema is more common than pleural effusion.

Therapeutic Considerations: Monotherapy with newer anti-Klebsiella agents, e.g., 3rd GC, carbapenems, colistin, tigecycline, are as effective or superior to double-drug therapy with older agents.

Prognosis: Related to degree of hepatic/splenic dysfunction.

Bronchiectasis/Cystic Fibrosis

Diagnostic Considerations: Cystic fibrosis/bronchiectasis is characterized by viscous secretions ± low grade fevers; less commonly may present as lung abscess. Colonization common of "water commensals", e.g., S maltophilia, B. cepacia, but onset of pneumonia heralded by cough, increase in viscosity/volume of sputum, and a decrease in pulmonary function.

Pitfalls: Sputum colonization is common (e.g., S. maltophilia, B. cepacia, P. aeruginosa); may not reflect the actual pneumonia pathogens, but may decrease pulmonary function.

Therapeutic Considerations: Important to select antibiotics with low resistance potential and good penetration into respiratory secretions (e.g., quinolones, meropenem).

Prognosis: Related to extent of underlying lung disease/severity of infection.

Pneumonia in Organ Transplants

CMV Pneumonia

Clinical Presentation: CAP with perihilar infiltrates and hypoxemia.

Diagnostic Considerations: CMV pneumonia is diagnosed by stain/culture of lung biopsy or by demonstrations of CMV CPE in BAL cytology specimens.

Pitfalls: ↑ CMV PCR (viral load) indicative of reactivation of CMV in peripheral WBCs, but diagnostic of CMV CAP is CMV CPE in BAL cytology specimens.

Therapeutic Considerations: Treat as CMV pneumonia if CMV is predominant pathogen on lung biopsy. CMV may progress despite ganciclovir therapy.

Prognosis: Related to degree of immunosuppression.

Pneumonia on Chronic Steroid Therapy

If fungal infection is suspected, obtain lung biopsy to confirm diagnosis/identify causative organism. Non-responsiveness to appropriate antibiotics should suggest fungal infection. Avoid empirically treating fungi; due to the required duration of therapy, it is advantageous to confirm the diagnosis by lung biopsy first. Prognosis related to degree of immunosuppression.

Acute Aspergillus Pneumonia

Clinical Presentation: Chest x-ray shows progressive necrotizing pneumonia (bilateral in half) unresponsive to antibiotics. Characteristic of early Apsergillus pneumonia is the halo sign. A few days later the halo decreases in size. After a week after the appearance of the halo sign, the air crescent sign is typically present. Only in compromised hosts.

Diagnostic Considerations: Diagnosis by lung biopsy (not bronchoalveolar lavage) demonstrating hyphae invading lung parenchyma/blood vessels. Usually occurs only in patients on chronic steroids, cancer chemotherapy, organ transplants, leukopenic compromised hosts, or with chronic granulomatous disease (CGD) aspergillus CAP: β 1,3 D-glucan (BG) +, aspergillus galactomannan (GM) +. Aspergillus galactomannan (GM) may XR with Geotrichum, Blastomyces, Penicillium, or Alternaria. ↑ GM levels with cyclophosphamide and if enteritis/colitis (↑ absorption of GM).

Pitfalls: Invasive Aspergillus pneumonia does not occur in normal/non-immunosuppressed hosts. PCP has ↑ LDH and β 1,3 D-glucan (BG) +, but aspergillus galactomannan (GM) −.

Prognosis: Cavitation is a good prognostic sign. Prognosis related to degree of immunosuppression.

Lung Abscess/Empyema

Subset	Usual Pathogens	Preferred IV Therapy	Alternate IV Therapy	PO Therapy or IV-to-PO Switch
Lung abscess/ empyema	Oral anaerobes S. aureus K. pneumoniae S. pneumoniae	Meropenem 1 gm (IV) q8h* **or** Piperacillin/ Tazobactam 3.375 gm (IV) q8h*	Ertapenem 1 gm (IV) q24h* **or** Clindamycin 600 mg (IV) q8h*	Clindamycin 300 mg (PO) q8h* **or** Respiratory quinolone† (PO) q24h*

*   Treat until resolved. Duration of therapy represents total time IV, PO, or IV + PO. Most patients on IV therapy able to take PO meds should be switched to PO therapy soon after clinical improvement (usually < 72 hours).

†   Moxifloxacin 400 mg or Levofloxacin 500 mg.

Clinical Presentation: Lung abscess presents as single/multiple cavitary lung lesion(s) with fever. Empyema presents as persistent fever/pleural effusion without layering on lateral decubitus chest x-ray.

Diagnostic Considerations: In lung abscess, plain film/CT scan demonstrates cavitary lung lesions appearing > 1 week after pneumonia. Most CAPs are not associated with pleural effusion, and few develop empyema. In empyema, pleural fluid pH is ≤ 7.2; culture purulent exudate for pathogen.

Pitfalls: Pleural effusions secondary to CAP usually resolve rapidly with treatment. Suspect empyema in patients with persistent pleural effusions with fever.

Therapeutic Considerations: Chest tube/surgical drainage needed for empyema. Treat lung abscess until it resolves (usually 3–12 months).

Prognosis: Good if adequately drained.

Nursing Home Acquired Pneumonia (NHAP)

Subset	Usual Pathogens*	Preferred IV Therapy	Alternate IV Therapy	PO Therapy or IV-to-PO Switch
Nursing home-acquired pneumonia (NHAP)	H. influenzae S. pneumoniae M. catarrhalis	Ceftriaxone 1 gm (IV) q24h × 2 weeks **or** Respiratory quinolone†† (IV) q24h × 2 weeks **or** Doxycycline 200 mg (IV) q12h × 3 days; then 100 mg (IV) q12h × 2 weeks	Ertapenem 1 gm (IV) q24h × 2 weeks **or** Cefepime 2 gm (IV) q12h × 2 weeks	Respiratory quinolone†† (PO) q24h × 2 weeks **or** Doxycycline 200 mg (PO) q12h × 3 days, then 100 mg (PO) q12h × 11 days

Diagnostic Considerations: The term "healthcare associated pneumonia" (HCAP) should be avoided since it does not describe the pathogens or LOS of NHAP. Resembles community-acquired pneumonia in terms of pathogens and length of stay, more than nosocomial pneumonia. NHAP outbreaks may be due to influenza a ILIs, H. influenzae, C. pneumoniae, or Legionnaire's disease.

Pitfalls: No need to cover P. aeruginosa or GNB which are common colonizers of nursing home patients, but not causes of NHAP.

Therapeutic Considerations: Treat as community-acquired pneumonia, not nosocomial pneumonia.

Prognosis: Related to underlying cardiopulmonary status.

Nosocomial Pneumonia (NP)/Hospital Acquired Pneumonia (HAP)/
Ventilator Associated Pneumonia (VAP)[§]

Subset	Usual Pathogens	Preferred IV Therapy	Alternate IV Therapy	IV-to-PO Switch
Empiric therapy	P. aeruginosa* E. coli K. pneumoniae S. marcescens (S. aureus)[†]	Meropenem 1 gm (IV) q8h × 1–2 weeks **or** Levofloxacin 750 mg (IV) q24h × 1–2 weeks		Levofloxacin 750 mg (PO) q24h × 1–2 weeks **or** Ciprofloxacin 750 mg (PO) q12h × 1–2 weeks
Specific therapy	P. aeruginosa*[‡]	Meropenem 1 gm (IV) q8h × 2 weeks **or** Levofloxacin 750 mg (IV) q24h × 2 weeks **or** Cefepime 2 gm (IV) q12h × 1–2 weeks ± Amikacin 1 gm (IV) q24h × 2 weeks		Levofloxacin 750 mg (PO) q24h × 2 weeks **or** Ciprofloxacin 750 mg (PO) q12h × 2 weeks
	MDR Klebsiella Acinetobacter	Meropenem 1 gm (IV) q8h × 2 weeks **or** Tigecycline 200 mg (IV) × 1 dose, then 100 mg (IV) q24h × 2 weeks[¶] **or** Ceftazidime/Avibactam 2.5 gm (IV) q8h × 2 weeks **or** Ceftolozane/Tazobactam 1.5 gm (IV) q8h × 2 weeks **or** Polymyxin B 1.25 mg/kg (IV) q12h × 2 weeks **or** Colistin 2.5 mg/kg (IV) q12h × 2 weeks		
	MDR P. aeruginosa	Doripenem 1 gm (IV) q8h × 2 weeks[†] **plus** Amikacin 1 gm (IV) q24h × 2 weeks **or** Meropenem 1 gm (IV) q8h × 2 weeks[§] **plus** Amikacin 1 gm (IV) q24h × 2 weeks **or** Ceftazidime/Avibactam 2.5 gm (IV) q8h × 2 weeks **or** Ceftolozane/Tazobactam 1.5 gm (IV) q8h × 2 weeks **or** Fosfomycin 6–12 gm (IV) q12h × 2 weeks		
	CRE	Eravacycline 1 mg/kg (IV) q12h × 2 weeks **or** Tigecycline 200 mg (IV) × 1 dose, then 100 mg (IV) q24h × 2 weeks[¶] **or** Ceftazidime/Avibactam 2.5 gm (IV) q8h × 2 weeks **or** Polymyxin B 1.25 mg/kg (IV) q12h × 2 weeks **or** Colistin 2.5 mg/kg (ItV) q12h × 2 weeks **or** Fosfomycin 6–12 gm (IV) q12h × 2 weeks **or** Cefiderocol 2 gm (IV) q8h × 2 weeks **or** Meropenem/Vaborbactam 4 gm (IV) q8h × 2 weeks **or** Imipenem/Relebactam (IMI = 500 mg + REL = 250 mg) q6h × 1–2 weeks		

Nosocomial Pneumonia (NP) / Hospital-Acquired Pneumonia (HAP) /

Ventilator-Associated Pneumonia (VAP)§ *(cont'd)*

*   **For empiric P. aeruginosa coverage, monotherapy is sufficient.** For lung bx proven *P. aeruginosa* NP/VAP, *combination therapy preferred.*

†   **MSSA/MRSA are common colonizers of respiratory secretions. In ventilated patients with fever, leukocytosis, and infiltrates on CXR, are *not* diagnostic of MSSA/MRSA NP/HAP/VAP. *MSSA/MRSA NP/HAP/VAP is clinically distinctive and rare.***

§   If susceptible.

‡   P. aeruginosa NP/VAP shows multiple infiltrates with rapid cavitation in <72 h on CXR ± otherwise unexplained blood cultures for P. aeruginosa (BCs negative with inhalation acquired P. aeruginosa VAP and BCs + in hematogenously acquired P. aeruginosa NP/VAP).

**   Presents late in course of VAP as "failure to wean", does *not* present as early VAP.

¶   Higher than usual doses of tigecycline may be necessary for non-susceptible/relatively resistant MDR GNBs.

Clinical Presentation: Pulmonary infiltrate compatible with a bacterial pneumonia occurring ≥ 1 week in-hospital ± fever/leukocytosis.

Diagnostic Considerations: CXR infiltrates with leukocytosis and fever are nonspecific/nondiagnostic of NP/VAP. Definitive diagnosis by lung biopsy. P. aeruginosa is a common colonizer in ventilated patients. P. aeruginosa VAP manifests as a necrotizing pneumonia with rapid cavitation (< 72 hours), microabscesses, and blood vessel invasion. S. aureus (MSSA/MRSA) NP/VAP remains rare. MSSA/MRSA common colonizers of respiratory secretions. Acinetobacter/Legionella NP/VAP usually occur in clusters/outbreaks. Acinetobacter NP/VAP occur in clusters/outbreaks not as single cases. Respiratory secretions culture + for acinetobacter represents colonization until proven otherwise.

Pitfalls: No rationale for "covering" non-pulmonary pathogens colonizing respiratory secretions in ventilated patients (Enterobacter, B. cepacia, S. maltophilia, Citrobacter, Flavobacterium, Enterococci); these organisms rarely if ever cause NP/VAP. Semi-quantitative BAL/protected brush specimens often reflect airway colonization. Characteristic clinical presentation (necrotizing pneumonia with rapid cavitation < 72 hrs) or tissue biopsy is needed for diagnosis of P. aeruginosa NP/VAP. MSSA/MRSA are common colonizers of respiratory secretions and are not uncommon causes of tracheobronchitis in ventilated patients. While MSSA/MRSA colonization of respiratory secretions is common, MSSA/MRSA necrotizing/rapidly cavitating NP/VAP remains very rare.

Therapeutic Considerations: NP (HAP/VAP) is defined as pneumonia acquired > 5 hospital days. So called "early" NP occurring < 5 days of hospitalization, usually due to S. pneumoniae or H. influenzae, represents CAP that manifests early after hospital admission. Empiric therapy recommendations cover usual NP/VAP (as well as late CAP) pathogens. Monotherapy is as effective as combination therapy for non-P. aeruginosa NP/VAP, but 2-drug therapy is recommended for confirmed P. aeruginosa NP/VAP. Treat aspiration NP/VAP the same as NP/VAP since anaerobes are not important pathogens in NP/VAP.

Prognosis: Related to underlying cardiopulmonary status.

Empiric Therapy of Cardiovascular Infections

Native Valve Subacute Bacterial Endocarditis (SBE)

Subset	Usual Pathogens	Preferred IV Therapy	Alternate IV Therapy (Penicillin allergy)	PO Therapy or IV-to-PO Switch
No obvious source or oral	Viridans streptococci (MIC < 0.5 mcg/ml) Viridans streptococci*† Groups B, C, G streptococci, S. bovis (PCN MIC > 0.5 mcg/ml)	**Monotherapy** Ceftriaxone 2 gm (IV) q24h × 4 weeks **Combination Therapy** Ceftriaxone 2 gm (IV) q24h × 2 weeks*‡ **plus** Gentamicin 120 mg **or** 2.5 mg/kg (IV) q24h × 2 weeks*	**Monotherapy** Vancomycin 1 gm (IV) q12h × 4 weeks **or** Linezolid 600 mg (IV) q12h × 4 weeks **Combination Therapy** Penicillin G 3 mu (IV) q4h × 2 weeks*‡ **plus** Gentamicin 120 mg or 2.5 mg/kg (IV) q24h × 2 weeks*	Linezolid§ 600 mg (PO) q12h × 4–6 weeks **or** Amoxicillin§ 1 gm (PO) q8h × 4–6 weeks
	Nutritionally-variant streptococci (NVS) Abiotrophia, granuli-catella**	As above, but treat × 6 weeks	As above, but treat × 6 weeks	As above§, but treat × 6 weeks
	Listeria monocyto-genes	Ampicillin 2 gm (IV) q4h × 4–6 weeks **or** TMP-SMX 5 mg/kg (IV) q6h × 4–6 weeks	Meropenem 2 gm (IV) q8h × 4–6 weeks	Amoxicillin§ 1 gm (PO) q8h × 4–6 weeks **or** Linezolid§ 600 mg (PO) q12h × 4–6 weeks

*   If *relatively* PCN resistant (MIC 0.12–0.5 mcg/ml) or if *intra/extra cardiac complications*, treat × 4 weeks.
‡   In PCN allergic patients, Vancomycin 1 gm (IV) q12h × 2 weeks.
§   IV therapy preferred. PO therapy if no IV access or if patient not a surgical candidate.
†   Groups of viridans streptococci (most common species in each group)
   S. anginosus (S. milleri group) (S. anginosus, S. constellatus, S. intermedius); **S. mitis** (S. mitis, S. oralis, S. peroris; **S. sanguinis** (S. sanguinis, S. parasanguinis, S. gordonii); **S. salivarius** (S. salivarius, S. vestibularis); **S. mutans** (S. mutans, S. sobrinus).

Native Valve Subacute Bacterial Endocarditis (SBE) *(cont'd)*

Subset	Usual Pathogens	Preferred IV Therapy	Alternate IV Therapy (Penicillin allergy)	PO Therapy or IV-to-PO Switch
GI/GU source likely	E. faecalis (VSE)[†]	Ampicillin 2 gm (IV) q4h × 4–6 weeks **plus either** Ceftriaxone 2 gm (IV) q12h × 4–6 weeks **or** Gentamicin 120 mg or 3 mg/kg (IV) q24h or 80 mg (IV) q8h × 2 weeks	Vancomycin 1 gm or 15 mg/kg (IV) q12h × 4–6 weeks **plus** Gentamicin 120 mg or 3 mg/kg (IV) q24h × 2 weeks	Amoxicillin[§] 1 gm (PO) q8h × 4–6 weeks **or** Linezolid[§] 600 mg (PO) q12h × 4–6 weeks
	E. faecium (VRE)[†]	Linezolid 600 mg (IV) q12h × ≥ 8 weeks **or** Daptomycin 12 mg/kg (IV) q24h × 6-8 weeks		Linezolid[§] 600 mg (PO) q12h × ≥ 8 weeks
GI source	(Non-enterococcal group D streptococci) S. (bovis) gallolyticus	Treat the same as "no obvious source" subset (p. 76)		
"Culture Negative" Endocarditis (CNE)	Pathogen unknown PCN resistant organisms with MIC > 0.5 mcg/ml	Ampicillin 2 gm (IV) q4h × 4–6 weeks **plus** Gentamicin 120 mg or 2.5 mg/kg (IV) q24h or 80 mg (IV) q8h × 2 weeks	Quinolone[†] (IV) q24h × 4–6 weeks	Quinolone[†§] (PO) q24h × 4–6 weeks

VRE = vancomycin resistant enterococci. Duration of therapy represents total time IV, PO, or IV + PO.

[†]   Symptoms < 3 months → treat × 4 weeks.
    Symptoms > 3 months → treat × 6 weeks.

**   NVS (*nutritionally variant streptococci*) include: Abiotrophia defectivus, Granulicatella adjacens/elegans.

[§]   IV therapy preferred. PO therapy if no IV access or if patient not a surgical candidate.

Native Valve Subacute Bacterial Endocarditis (SBE) *(cont'd)*

Subset	Usual Pathogens	Preferred IV Therapy	Alternate IV Therapy (Penicillin allergy)	PO Therapy or IV-to-PO Switch
HACEK organisms	Hemophilus sp. Aggegatibacter (Actinobacillus) actinomycetemcomitans Cardiobacterium hominis Eikenella corrodens Kingella kingae	Ceftriaxone 2 gm (IV) q24h × 4–6 weeks **or** Any 3rd generation cephalosporin (IV) × 4–6 weeks **or** Cefepime 2 gm (IV) q12h × 4–6 weeks	Ampicillin 2 gm (IV) q4h × 4–6 weeks **plus** Gentamicin[§] 120 mg or 2.5 mg/kg (IV) q24h × 2 weeks **Monotherapy** Ampicillin/Sulbactam 3 gm (IV) q6h × 4–6 weeks **or** Quinolone[†] (IV) q24h × 4–6 weeks	Quinolone[†§] (PO) q24h × 4–6 weeks
	Legionella Chlamydophilia (Chlamydia) psittaci	Doxycycline** 200 mg (IV) q12h × 3 days, then 100 mg (IV) q12h × 3 months	Quinolone[†] (IV) q24h × 3 months	Doxycycline**§ 200 mg (PO) q12h × 3 days, then 100 mg (PO) q12h × 3 months
	Coxiella burnetii (Q fever)	Doxycycline** 200 mg (IV/PO) q12h × 24 months **plus** Hydroxchloroquin 200 mg (PO) q8h × 24 months		
Brucella SBE[†]	Brucella	Doxycycline 200 mg** (IV) q12h × 3 days, then 100 mg (PO) q12h × ≥ 6 weeks **plus** Rifampin 300 mg (PO) q8h × ≥ 6 weeks **and** TMP-SMX 1 DS tablet (PO) q8h × ≥ 6 weeks		

*   Slow growing/fastidious organisms may require ↑ CO_2 and prolonged incubation.
†   Levofloxacin 500 mg or Moxifloxacin 400 mg.
** Loading dose is not needed PO if given IV with the same drug or if patient not a surgical candidate.
§   IV therapy preferred. PO therapy if no IV access or if patient not a surgical candidate.
§§ May be given as a once daily dose or given in divided doses q8h.

Native Valve SBE

Clinical Presentation: Subacute febrile illness $\pm$ localizing symptoms/signs in a patient with a heart murmur. Peripheral manifestations are commonly absent with early diagnosis/treatment.

Diagnosis: High grade/continuous bacteremia (due to a endocarditis pathogen) plus vegetation on TTE/TEE is diagnostic.

SBE (No Obvious Source)

Diagnostic Considerations: Most common pathogen is viridans streptococci. Source is usually the mouth, although oral/dental infection is usually inapparent clinically.

Pitfalls: Vegetations without positive blood cultures or peripheral manifestations of SBE are not diagnostic of endocarditis. SBE vegetations may persist after antibiotic therapy, but are sterile.

Therapeutic Considerations: In penicillin-allergic (anaphylactic) patients, vancomycin may be used alone or in combination with gentamicin. Follow ESR weekly to monitor antibiotic response. No need to repeat blood cultures unless patient has persistent fever or is not responding clinically. Two-week treatment is acceptable for uncomplicated viridans streptococcal SBE. Treat nutritionally-variant streptococci (NVS) (B_6/pyridoxal dependent streptococci) same as viridans streptococcal SBE.

Prognosis: Related to extent of embolization/severity of heart failure.

SBE (GI/GU Source Likely)

Diagnostic Considerations: Commonest pathogens from GI/GU source are Enterococci (especially) E. faecalis. If S. bovis, look for GI polyp, tumor source. Enterococcal SBE commonly follows GI/GU instrumentation.

Pitfalls: Low back pain prominent with enterococcal/S. bovis SBE, S. bovis associated with CNS embolization, Vertebral osteomyelitis, and large valvular vegetations.

Therapeutic Considerations: For penicillin-allergic patients, use vancomycin plus gentamicin. Vancomycin alone is inadequate for enterococcal (E. faecalis) SBE. Treat enterococcal PVE the same as for native valve enterococcal SBE. Treat S. bovis SBE the same as S. viridans SBE.

Prognosis: Related to extent of embolization.

"Culture Negative" Endocarditis (CNE) (Culturable Pathogens)

Diagnostic Considerations: Culture of CNE organisms may require enhanced CO_2/special media (Castaneda vented bottles) and prolonged incubation (2–4 weeks). True CNE is rare, and is characterized by peripheral signs of SBE, and a vegetation (on TTE/TEE) with negative blood cultures.

Pitfalls: Most cases of CNE are not, in fact, CNE, but are due to slow-growing organisms.

Therapeutic Considerations: Follow clinical improvement with serial ESRs, which should return to pretreatment levels with therapy. Serial TTEs/TEEs show decreasing vegetation size during effective therapy. Sterile vegetations may persist after antibiotic therapy.

Prognosis: Related to extent of embolization.

True "Culture Negative" Endocarditis (CNE): Non-Culturable/ Serologically Diagnosed Pathogens

Diagnostic Considerations: Diagnosis by specific serology in patients with negative blood cultures but signs of SBE, e.g., splenomegaly/peripheral manifestations. Large vessel emboli suggests CNE.

Pitfalls: If peripheral SBE manifestations are absent do not diagnose CNE in patients with a heart murmur and negative blood cultures. Vegetations may not be visible on TTE/TEE in Q fever SBE, but vegetations may be visualized on PET scan. The diagnosis of chronic Q fever is made by demonstrating elevated IgG (phase I) titers $\geq$ 1:800 at 6 months following acute Q fever. Since Bartonella titers may present XR with C. burnetii (Q fever) titers and vice versa, an elevation of either titer may be a clue to the other and should prompt testing for both. Phase I titers may present XR with Legionella, Ehrlichia, Rickettsia.

Therapeutic Considerations: For Q fever native valve CNE or PVE, use "high dose" doxycycline for best results 200 mg (PO) q12h plus hydroxychloroquin 200 mg (PO) q8h × 24 months.

Prognosis: Related to extent of embolization/severity of heart failure.

Native Valve Acute Bacterial Endocarditis (ABE)

Subset	Usual Pathogens	Preferred IV Therapy	Alternate IV Therapy	IV-to-PO Switch Therapy
Normal hosts*	S. aureus (MRSA)	Daptomycin 12 mg/kg (IV) q24h × 4–6 weeks **or** Linezolid 600 mg (IV) q12h × 4–6 weeks **or** Vancomycin 1 gm or 15 mg/kg (IV) q12h × 4–6 weeks **or** Minocycline 200 mg (IV) × 1, then 100 mg (IV) q12h × 4–6 weeks		Linezolid 600 mg (PO) q12h × 4–6 wks **or** Minocycline 200 mg (PO) × 1, then 100 mg (PO) q12h × 4–6 wks
	S. aureus (MSSA)	Nafcillin 2 gm (IV) q4h × 4–6 weeks **or** Cefazolin 1 gm (IV) q8h × 4–6 weeks **or** Vancomycin 1 gm or 15 mg/kg (IV) q12h × 4–6 weeks		Cephalexin 1 gm (PO) q6h × 4–6 weeks **or** Minocycline 200 mg (PO) × 1, then 100 mg (PO) q12h × 4–6 wks
	S. lugdenensis (treat as S. aureus)	Daptomycin 12 mg/kg (IV) q24h × 4–6 weeks **or** Linezolid 600 mg (IV) q24h × 4–6 weeks	Vancomycin 1 gm or 15 mg/kg (IV) q12h × 4–6 weeks	Linezolid 600 mg (PO) q12h × 4–6 wks

Native Valve Acute Bacterial Endocarditis (ABE) *(cont'd)*

Subset	Usual Pathogens	Preferred IV Therapy	Alternate IV Therapy	IV-to-PO Switch Therapy
IV drug abusers (IVDAs)[†]	S. aureus (MRSA)	<u>Before culture results</u> Vancomycin 1 gm or 15 mg/kg (IV) q12h **or** Daptomycin 12 mg/kg (IV) q24h × 4–6 weeks	<u>After culture results</u> Linezolid 600 mg (IV) q12h × 4–6 weeks **or** Vancomycin 1 gm or 15 mg/kg (IV) q12h × 4–6 weeks **or** Minocycline 200 mg (IV) × 1, then 100 mg (IV) q12h × 4–6 weeks	<u>After culture results</u> Linezolid 600 mg (PO) q12h × 4–6 weeks
	S. aureus (MSSA)	<u>Before culture results</u> Meropenem 1 gm (IV) q8h	<u>After culture results</u> Nafcillin 2 gm (IV) q4h × 4–6 weeks **or** Cefazolin 1 gm (IV) q8h × 4–6 weeks **or** Daptomycin 6 mg/kg (IV) q24h × 4–6 weeks **or** Linezolid 600 mg (IV) q12h × 4–6 weeks **or** Meropenem 1 gm (IV) q8h × 4–6 weeks	<u>After culture results</u> Linezolid 600 mg (PO) q12h × 4–6 weeks **or** Cephalexin 1 gm (PO) q6h × 4–6 weeks **or** Minocycline[†] 200 mg (PO) × 1, then 100 mg (PO) q12h × 4–6 weeks
	P. aeruginosa* S. marcesens GNB	<u>Before culture results</u> Meropenem 1 gm (IV) q8h	<u>After culture results</u> Meropenem 1 gm (IV) q8h × 4–6 weeks **or** Doripenem 1 gm (IV) q8h × 4–6 weeks **plus either** Amikacin 1 gm **or** 15 mg/kg (IV) q24h × 2 weeks **or** Aztreonam 2 gm (IV) q8h × 2–4 weeks	None

* Treat IV or with IV-to-PO switch therapy or if patient not a surgical candidate.

† ***MSSA/MRSA TV ABE may be treated IV/PO × 2 weeks if no intra-cardiac or CNS complications.*** Pulmonary septic emboli are a feature of TV ABE e.g., and are not, per se, an extracardiac complication.

Acute Bacterial Endocarditis (ABE)

Diagnostic Considerations: Clinical criteria for MRSA/MSSA ABE: continuous/high-grade bacteremia (repeatedly 3/4 or 4/4 positive blood cultures), fever (temperature usually ≥ 102°F), no, new or changing murmur, and vegetation by transesophageal/transthoracic echocardiogram.

Pitfalls: Obtain a baseline TTE. If the bacteremia continues (continuous bacteremia), × 4–5 days on appropriate therapy, a TEE should be performed for comparative purposes should ABE be complicated by valve destruction, heart failure or ring/perivalvular abscess. On TTE/TEE a vegetation may not be visible until > 1 week of ABE. In MSSA/MRSA ABE, resistance to deptomycin may occur during therapy particularly in patients initially treated with vancomycin.

Therapeutic Considerations: Treat for 4–6 weeks. Follow teichoic acid antibody titers (TAA) weekly in MSSA/MRSA ABE, which ↓ (along with the ESR) with effective therapy. If MSSA/MRSA ABE unresponsive (persistent high grade bacteremia) to appropriate MSSA/MRSA therapy or if a myocardial/paravalvular abscess present that cannot be surgically drained, "high dose" daptomycin 12 mg/kg (IV) q24h may be effective. With daptomycin resistant MSSA/MRSA strains, quinupristin/dalfopristin, linezolid or minocycline may be effective.

Prognosis: Related to extent of embolization/severity of valve destruction/heart failure.

Acute Bacterial Endocarditis (IVDAs)

Diagnostic Considerations: Clinically IVDAs with S. aureus usually have relatively mild ABE, permitting oral treatment.

Pitfalls: IVDAs with new aortic or tricuspid regurgitation should be treated IV ± valve replacement.

Therapeutic Considerations: After pathogen is isolated, may switch from IV to PO regimen to complete treatment course.

Prognosis: Prognosis is better than ABE in normal hosts if not complicated by abscess, valve regurgitation, or heart failure.

Clinical Presentation: Acute onset of fevers and chills.

Diagnosis: High-grade blood culture positivity (3/4–4/4) with endocarditis pathogen and no other source of infection.

Prosthetic Valve Endocarditis (PVE)

Early PVE (< 60 days post-PVR)

Diagnostic Considerations: Blood cultures persistently positive. Temperature usually ≤ 102°F.

Pitfalls: Obtain baseline TTE/TEE. Premature closure of mitral leaflet is early sign of impending aortic valve regurgitation. Rifampin should be given 2 days after strain shown to be susceptible.

Therapeutic Considerations: Patients improve clinically on treatment, but prosthetic valve removal may be necessary for cure.

Prognosis: Related to extent of embolization/severity of heart failure.

<u>Late PVE (> 60 days post-PVR)</u>

Pitfalls: Culture of removed valve may be negative, but valve Gram stain will be positive.

Therapeutic Considerations: Clinically, late PVE resembles viridans streptococcal SBE. Prosthetic valve removal may be necessary.

Prognosis: Related to extent of embolization/severity of heart failure.

Prosthetic Valve Endocarditis (PVE)

	Usual Pathogens	Before Culture Results	After Culture Results
Early PVE (< 60 days post-PVR)	GNB S. aureus (MSSA/MRSA) S. epidermidis (CoNS)	Meropenem 1 gm (IV) q8h Vancomycin 1 gm or 15 mg/kg (IV) q12h **or** Linezolid 600 mg (IV) q12h **or** Daptomycin 12 mg/kg (IV) q24h	<u>P. aevuginosa/GNB</u> Meropenem 1 gm (IV) q8h × 6 weeks **or** Ceftriaxone 2 gm (IV) q24h × 6 weeks <u>MSSA</u> Cefazolin 1 gm (IV) q8h × 6 weeks **or** Meropenem 1 gm (IV) q8h × 6 weeks <u>MRSA</u> Ceftaroline 600 mg (IV) q12h × 6 weeks **or** Daptomycin 12 mg/kg (IV) q24h × 6 weeks **or** Linezolid 600 mg (IV or PO) q12h × 6 weeks **or** Vancomycin 1 gm or 15 mg/kg (IV) q12h × 6 weeks **plus** Rifampin 300 mg (IV) q24h × 6 weeks*
	Candida species§	Micafungin 150 mg or 3 mg/kg (IV) q24h	Liposomal amphotericin (L-amb) (IV)** × 6 weeks **plus** 5-FC 25 mg/kg (PO) q6h × 6 weeks
Late PVE (> 60 days post-PVR)	Viridans streptococci S. epidermidis (CoNS)	Vancomycin 1 gm or 15 mg/kg (IV) q12h × 6 weeks **plus** Gentamicin 120 mg or 2.5 mg/kg (IV) q24h × 2 weeks	<u>Viridans streptococci</u> Ceftriaxone 2 gm (IV) q24h × 6 weeks <u>CoNS</u> Linezolid 600 mg (IV or PO) q12h × 6 weeks **or** Vancomycin 1 gm or 15 mg/kg (IV) q12h × 6 weeks **plus** Rifampin 300 mg (PO) q8h × 6 weeks
	VSE VRE	Daptomycin 12 mg/kg (IV) q24h × 6 weeks **or** Linezolid 600 mg (IV or PO) q12h × 6 weeks	<u>VSE</u> Ampicillin 2 gm (IV) q4h × 6 weeks **or** Meropenem 1 gm (IV) q8h × 6 weeks <u>VRE</u> Daptomycin 12 mg/kg (IV) q24h × 6 weeks **or** Linezolid 600 mg (IV or PO) q12h × 6 weeks

* If P. aeruginosa PVE.

Pericarditis/Myocarditis

Subset	Usual Pathogens	Preferred Therapy
Diphtheritic myocarditis	C. diphtheriae	Treat same as diphtheria
Lyme myocarditis	B. burgdorferi	Ceftriaxone 2 gm (IV) q24h × 2 weeks **or** Doxycycline 100 mg (IV) q12h × 2 weeks
RMSF myocarditis	R. rickettsii	Doxycycline 100 mg (IV) q12h × 2 weeks
TB pericarditis	M. tuberculosis	Treat same as pulmonary TB. Add a tapering dose of corticosteroids × 4–8 weeks
Suppurative pericarditis	S. pneumoniae S. aureus	Treat same as lung abscess/empyema

Clinical Presentation: Viral pericarditis presents with acute onset of fever/chest pain (made worse by sitting up) following a viral illness. TB pericarditis is indolent in presentation, with ↑ jugular venous distension (JVD), pericardial friction rub (40%), paradoxical pulse (25%), and chest x-ray with cardiomegaly ± left-sided pleural effusion. Suppurative pericarditis presents as acute pericarditis (patients are critically ill). Develops from contiguous (e.g., pneumonia) or hematogenous spread e.g., S. aureus bacteremia. Viral myocarditis presents with heart failure, arrhythmias ± emboli.

Diagnostic Considerations: Pericarditis/effusion manifests cardiomegaly with decreased heart sounds ± tamponade. Diagnosis by culture/biopsy of pericardial fluid or pericardium for viruses, bacteria, or acid-fast bacilli (AFB). Diagnosis of myocarditis is clinical ± myocardial biopsy.

Pitfalls: Consider other causes of pericardial effusion (malignancy, esp. if bloody effusion, uremia, etc). Excluding pulmonary emboli or infarction, otherwise unexplained tachycardia should suggest myocarditis until proven otherwise. Rule out treatable non-viral causes of myocarditis e.g., RMSF, Lyme, diphtheria. Suspect Lyme disease in any person without heart disease with exposure to endemic area who presents with otherwise unexplained heart block. Lyme IgM titers may be negative early when patients present with heart block.

Therapeutic Considerations: No specific treatment for viral myocarditis/pericarditis. TB pericarditis is treated the same as pulmonary TB ± pericardiectomy. Suppurative pericarditis is treated the same as lung abscess plus surgical drainage (pericardial window). Heart block in Lyme disease rapidly reverses with therapy, but a temporary pacemaker may be needed until heart block is reversed.

Prognosis: For viral pericarditis, the prognosis is good, but viral myocarditis may be fatal. For TB pericarditis, the prognosis is good if treated before constrictive pericarditis/adhesions develop. Suppurative pericarditis is often fatal without early pericardial window/antibiotic therapy. With Lyme myocarditis/heart block, prognosis is good if treatment is started early when diagnosis is suspected.

Central Venous Catheter (CVC) and Pacemaker/Lead Infections

Subset	Usual Pathogens	Preferred IV Therapy	Alternate IV Therapy	IV-to-PO Switch
CVC (temporary) Infections* _Bacterial_	S. aureus (MSSA) GNB	Meropenem 1 gm (IV) q8h** **or** Cefepime 2 gm (IV) q12h**	Ceftriaxone 2 gm (IV) q24h**	Quinolone‡ (PO) q24h**†
	S. aureus (MRSA/MSSA§)	Daptomycin 6 mg/kg (IV) q24h** **or** Linezolid 600 mg (IV) q12h** **or** Vancomycin 1 gm or 15 mg/kg (IV) q12h**		Linezolid 600 mg (PO) q12h**† **or** Minocycline 100 mg (PO) q12h**†
Candida¶ (Treat initially for C. albicans; if later identified as non-albicans Candida, treat accordingly).	C. albicans	Treat the same as for Candidemia		
	Non-albicans Candida	Treat the same as for Candidemia		
CVC (semi-permanent Hickman/ Broviac/Tessio) Infections* _Bacterial_	S. aureus (MSSA/MRSA)	Daptomycin 6 mg/kg (IV) q24h** **or** Linezolid 600 mg (IV) q12h** **or** Vancomycin 1 gm or 15 mg/kg (IV) q12h** **or** Minocycline 100 mg (IV) q12h**		Linezolid 600 mg (PO) q12h**† **or** Minocycline 100 mg (PO) q12h**†

† IV therapy preferred. PO therapy if no IV access

‡ Levofloxacin 500 mg or Moxifloxacin 400 mg.

* **If clinically possible, CVC should be removed if CVC suspected source of bacteremia in a septic patient. If high grade/sustained bacteremia obtain TTE/TEE to rule out ABE.**

** Treat × 2 weeks after CVC removal if no ABE.

¶ For candidemia not associated with CVCs, (see pp. 153–154).

§ MRSA drugs listed also effective against MSSA.

Central Venous Catheter (CVC) and Pacemaker/Lead Infections *(cont'd)*

Subset	Usual Pathogens	Preferred IV Therapy	Alternate IV Therapy	IV-to-PO Switch
	S. epidermidis (CoNS)	Daptomycin 6 mg/kg (IV) q24h** **or** Linezolid 600 mg (IV) q12h** **or** Vancomycin 1 gm or 15 mg/kg (IV) q12h**		Linezolid 600 mg (PO) q12h**†
Pacemaker (PPM) wire/generator infection, LVAD, ICD (Treat initially for S. aureus; if later identified as S. epidermidis, treat accordingly)	S. aureus (MSSA/MRSA)	Daptomycin 6 mg/kg (IV) q24h†§ **or** Linezolid 600 mg (IV) q12h†§ **or** Vancomycin 1 gm or 15 mg/kg (IV) q12h†		Linezolid 600 mg (PO) q12h†§ **or** Minocycline 100 mg (PO) q12h†§*
	S. epidermidis (CoNS)	Daptomycin 6 mg/kg (IV) q24h† **or** Linezolid 600 mg (IV) q12h† **or** Vancomycin 1 gm or 15 mg/kg (IV) q12h†		Linezolid 600 mg (PO) q12h†*

† IV therapy preferred. PO therapy if no IV access.

** Treat × 2 weeks after CVC removal if no IE.

* Treat × 2 weeks after wire/generator removal if no IE.

§ Obtain teichoic acid antibody titers (TAA) after 2 weeks. If titers are < 1:4, 2 weeks of therapy is sufficient. If titers are ≥ 1:4 rule out MSSA/MRSA ABE and complete 4–6 weeks of therapy.

Central Venous Catheter (CVC) and Pacemaker/Lead Infections (cont'd)

Subset	Usual Pathogens	Preferred IV Therapy	Alternate IV Therapy	IV-to-PO Switch
Septic thrombo-phlebitis	S. aureus (MSSA)	Nafcillin 2 gm (IV) q4h × 2 weeks* **or** Linezolid 600 mg (IV) q12h × 2 weeks* **or** Meropenem 1 gm (IV) q8h × 2 weeks*	Cefazolin 1 gm (IV) q8h × 2 weeks* **or** Ceftriaxone 1 gm (IV) q12h × 2 weeks* **or** Minocycline 100 mg (IV) q12h × 2 weeks	Linezolid 600 mg (PO) q12h × 2 weeks*† **or** Clindamycin 300 mg (PO) q8h × 2 weeks*† **or** Cephalexin 1 gm (PO) q6h × 2 weeks*†
	S. aureus (MRSA)	Linezolid 600 mg (IV) q12h × 2 weeks* **or** Vancomycin 1 gm or 15 mg/kg (IV) q12h × 2 weeks* **or** Minocycline 100 mg (IV) q12h × 2 weeks*		Linezolid 600 mg (PO) q12h × 2 weeks*† **or** Minocycline 100 mg (PO) q12h × 2 weeks*†

* Obtain teichoic acid antibody titers after 2 weeks. If titers are < 1:2, 2 weeks of therapy is sufficient. If titers are ≥ 1:2, TTE/TEE to rule out ABE and complete 4–6 weeks of therapy.

† IV therapy preferred. PO therapy if no IV access.

CVC (Temporary) Infections
Clinical Presentation: Temperature ≥ 102°F ± IV site erythema.

Diagnostic Considerations: Diagnosis by semi-quantitative catheter tip culture with ≥ 15 colonies plus blood cultures with same pathogen. If no other explanation for fever and line has been in place ≥ 7 days, remove line and obtain semi-quantitative catheter tip culture. Suppurative thrombophlebitis presents with hectic/septic fevers and pus at IV site + palpable venous cord.

Pitfalls: Temperature ≥ 102°F with IV line infection, in contrast to phlebitis.

Therapeutic Considerations: Line removal is usually curative, but antibiotic therapy is usually given for 1 week after IV line removal for gram-negative bacilli or 2 weeks after IV line removal for S. aureus (MSSA/MRSA). Antifungal therapy is usually given for 2 weeks after IV line removal for Candidemia.

Prognosis: Good if line is removed before endocarditis/metastatic spread.

CVC (Semi-Permanent) Hickman/Broviac Infections
Clinical Presentation: Fever ± IV site erythema.

Diagnostic Considerations: Positive blood cultures plus gallium scan pickup on catheter is diagnostic.

Pitfalls: Antibiotics will lower temperature, but patient will usually not be afebrile without line removal.
Therapeutic Considerations: Lines usually need to be removed for cure. Rifampin 600 mg (PO) q24h may be added to IV/PO regimen if pathogen is S. aureus.
Prognosis: Good with organisms of low virulence.

Pacemaker/Lead Infections
Clinical Presentation: Persistently positive blood cultures without endocarditis in a pacemaker patient.
Diagnostic Considerations: Positive blood cultures with gallium scan pickup on wire/pacemaker generator is diagnostic. Differentiate wire from pacemaker pocket infection by chest CT/MRI.
Pitfalls: Positive blood cultures are more common in wire infections than pocket infections. Blood cultures may be negative in both, but more so with pocket infections.
Therapeutic Considerations: Wire alone may be replaced if infection does not involve pacemaker generator. Replace pacemaker generator if involved; wire if uninvolved can usually be left in place.
Prognosis: Good if pacemaker wire/generator replaced before septic complications develop.

Septic Thrombophlebitis
Clinical Presentation: Temperature $\geq 102°F$ with local erythema and signs of sepsis.
Diagnostic Considerations: Palpable venous cord and pus at IV site when IV line is removed.
Pitfalls: Suspect diagnosis if persistent bacteremia and no other source of infection in a patient with a peripheral IV.
Therapeutic Considerations: Remove IV catheter. Surgical venotomy is usually needed for cure.
Prognosis: Good if removed early before septic complications develop.

Vascular Graft Infections

Subset	Usual Pathogens	Preferred IV Therapy	Alternate IV Therapy	IV-to-PO Switch
AV graft/shunt infection	S. aureus (MRSA)	Daptomycin*[†§] 6 mg/kg (IV) q24h **plus** Rifampin 300 mg (PO) q8h **or** Linezolid[†§] 600 mg (IV) q12h **plus** Rifampin[†§] 300 mg (PO) q8h	Vancomycin*[†§] 1 gm or 15 mg/kg (IV) q12h **plus** Rifampin 300 mg (PO) q8h **or** Minocycline[†§] 100 mg (IV) q12h **plus** Rifampin[†§] 300 mg (PO) q8h	Linezolid[†§] 600 mg (PO) q12h **plus** Rifampin 300 mg (PO) q8h **or** Minocycline[†§] 100 mg (PO) q12h **plus** Rifampin[†§] 300 mg (PO) q8h

*   Follow with maintenance dosing for renal failure (CrCl < 10 ml/min) and type of dialysis.
†   If ABE not present, treat for 2 weeks after graft is removed/replaced. If ABE present, treat for 6 weeks.
§   IV therapy preferred. PO therapy if no IV access.

Vascular Graft Infections *(cont'd)*

Subset	Usual Pathogens	Preferred IV Therapy	Alternate IV Therapy	IV-to-PO Switch
	S. aureus (MSSA)	Nafcillin 2 gm (IV) q4h†	Vancomycin 1 gm or 15 mg/kg (IV) q12h*†	Moxifloxacin 400 mg (IV or PO) q24h*†§
	E. faecalis (VSE) GNB	Ampicillin 2 gm (IV) q4h*† **plus** Gentamicin 240 mg or 5 mg/kg (IV) q24h*†	Vancomycin 1 gm or 15 mg/kg (IV) q24h† **plus** Gentamicin 120 mg or 1 mg/kg (IV) q24h*†	
Aortic graft infection	S. aureus (MSSA) GNB P. aeruginosa	Meropenem 1 gm (IV) q8h*** **or** Cefepime 2 gm (IV) q12h***	Levofloxacin 750 mg (IV) q24h†	Levofloxacin 750 mg (PO) q24h† **or** Ciprofloxacin 750 mg (PO) q12h†

*   Follow with maintenance dosing for renal failure (CrCl < 10 mL/min) and type of dialysis.
** Depending on susceptibilities.
†   If ABE not present, treat for 2 weeks after graft is removed/replaced. If graft not removable/replaceable, treat for 6 weeks.
§   IV therapy preferred. PO therapy if no IV access.

AV Graft Infection
Clinical Presentation: Persistent fever/bacteremia without endocarditis in a patient with an AV graft on hemodialysis.
Diagnostic Considerations: Diagnosis by persistently positive blood cultures and gallium scan pickup over infected AV graft. Gallium scan will detect deep AV graft infection not apparent on exam.
Pitfalls: Antibiotics will lower temperature, but patient will usually not become afebrile without AV graft replacement.
Therapeutic Considerations: Graft usually must be removed for cure. MRSA is a rare cause of AV graft infection; if present, treat with linezolid 600 mg (IV or PO) q12h until graft is removed/replaced.
Prognosis: Good if new graft does not become infected at same site.

Aortic Graft Infection
Clinical Presentation: Persistently positive blood cultures without endocarditis in a patient with an aortic graft.
Diagnostic Considerations: Diagnosis by positive blood cultures plus gallium scan pickup over infected aortic graft or abdominal CT/MRI scan.
Pitfalls: Infection typically occurs at anastomotic sites.

Therapeutic Considerations: Graft must be removed for cure. Operate as soon as diagnosis is confirmed (no value in waiting for surgery). MRSA is a rare cause of AV graft infection; if present, treat with linezolid 600 mg (IV or PO) q12h until graft is replaced.
Prognosis: Good if infected graft is removed before septic complications develop.

Empiric Therapy of GI Tract Infections

Esophagitis

Subset	Usual Pathogens	Preferred IV Therapy	Alternate IV Therapy	PO Therapy or IV-to-PO Switch
Fungal	Candida albicans	Fluconazole 200 mg (IV or PO) × 1 dose, then 100 mg (IV or PO) q24h × 2–3 weeks	Micafungin 150 mg (IV) q24h × 2–3 weeks **or** Caspofungin 50 mg (IV) q24h × 2–3 weeks **or** Anidulafungin 100 mg (IV or PO) × 1 dose then 50 mg (IV) q24h × 2–3 weeks **or** Itraconazole 100 mg (IV) q12h × 1 day, then 100 mg (IV) q24 h × 2 weeks	Fluconazole 200 mg (PO) × 1 dose, then 100 mg (PO) q24h × 2–3 weeks* **or** Posaconazole 100 mg (PO)q12h × 1 day, then 100 mg (PO) q24h × 2 weeks **or** Itraconazole 200 mg (PO) solution q24h × 2–3 weeks
Viral	HSV-1	Acyclovir 5 mg/kg (IV) q8h × 3 weeks	Valacyclovir 500 mg (PO) q12h × 3 weeks **or** Famciclovir 500 mg (PO) q12h × 3 weeks	
	CMV	Ganciclovir 5 mg/kg (IV) q12h × 3 weeks	Valganciclovir 900 mg (PO) q12h × 3 weeks	

* If given IV with the same drug loading dose is not needed PO.

Clinical Presentation: Pain on swallowing.
Diagnosis: Stain/culture for fungi/HSV/CMV on biopsy specimen.

Fungal (Candida) Esophagitis
Diagnostic Considerations: Rarely if ever in normal hosts. Often (but not always) associated with Candida in mouth. If patient is not alcoholic or diabetic and is not receiving antibiotics, test for HIV.
Pitfalls: Therapy as a diagnostic trial is appropriate. Suspect CMV-related disease and proceed to endoscopy if a patient with a typical symptom complex fails to respond to antifungal therapy.
Therapeutic Considerations: In normal hosts, treat for 1 week after clinical resolution. HIV patients respond more slowly than normal hosts and may need higher doses/treatment for 2–3 weeks after clinical resolution.
Prognosis: Related to degree of immunosuppression.

Viral Esophagitis

Diagnostic Considerations: Rarely in normal hosts. May occur in the immunosuppressed.

Pitfalls: Viral and non-viral esophageal ulcers look similar; need biopsy for specific viral diagnosis.

Therapeutic Considerations: In normal hosts, treat for 2–3 weeks after clinical resolution. HIV patients respond more slowly and may need treatment for weeks after clinical resolution.

Prognosis: Related to degree of immunosuppression.

Peptic Ulcer Disease (H. pylori)

Triple Therapy	Quadruple Therapy	Sequential Therapy
PPI **plus** amoxicillin 1 gm (PO) q12h **plus either** clarithromycin 500 mg (PO) q12h **or** tinidazole (or metronidazole) 500 mg (PO) q12h all × 2 weeks	PPI **plus** metronidazole 500 mg (PO) q12h **plus** doxycycline 100 mg (PO) q12h **plus** bismuth subsalicylate 525 mg tabs (PO) q6h all × 2 weeks	**5 days:** PPI **plus** amoxicillin 1 gm (PO) q12h; **next 5 days:** PPI **plus** either clarithromycin 500 (PO) q12h **or** levofloxacin 500 mg (PO) q24h

Diagnostic Considerations: Invasive: rapid urease test, histology, culture. **Noninvasive:** serum ELISA test, urea breath test, stool (monoclonal antibody) antigen test.

Pitfalls: *False negative H. pylori tests with antibiotics, bismuth, PPIs.*

Therapeutic Considerations: See above grid. **Therapeutic failure:** *substitute* bismuth (for amoxicillin) or *substitute* nitazoxanide 1 gm (PO) q12h (for clarithromycin, metronidazole or tinidazole) all × 2 weeks. *1 week of therapy often fails.*

Tests of Cure: Urea breath test → 4–6 weeks post-therapy. Stool antigen test → 6–8 weeks post-therapy. *Stop PPIs 2 weeks before re-testing.*

Gastric Perforation

Subset	Usual Pathogens	Preferred IV Therapy	Alternate IV Therapy	IV-to-PO Switch
Gastric perforation	Oral anaerobes	Cefazolin 1 gm (IV) q8h × 1–3 days	Any beta-lactam (IV) × 1–3 days	Amoxicillin 1 gm (PO) q8h × 1–3 days **or** Cephalexin 500 mg (PO) q6h × 1–3 days **or** Quinolone* (PO) q24h × 1–3 days

* Levofloxacin 500 mg or Moxifloxacin 400 mg.

Clinical Presentation: Presents acutely with fever and peritonitis.

Diagnostic Considerations: Obtain CT/MRI of abdomen for perforation/fluid collection.

Pitfalls: No need to cover B. fragilis with perforation of stomach/small intestine.

Therapeutic Considerations: Obtain surgical consult for possible repair.

Prognosis: Good if repaired.

Infectious Diarrhea/Typhoid (Enteric) Fever

Subset	Usual Pathogens	Preferred Therapy	Alternate Therapy
Acute watery bacterial diarrhea	E. coli (ETEC) Campylo- bacter Yersinia Vibrio Salmonella	Quinolone† (IV or PO) × 5 days **or** Azithromycin 1 gm (PO) × 1 dose **or** Azithromycin 1 gm (PO) × 1 dose **or** Doxycycline 300 mg (PO) × 1 dose	Doxycycline 100 mg (IV or PO) q12h × 5 days **or** TMP–SMX 1 DS tablet (PO) q12h × 5 days
Traveller's diarrhea	Campylo- bacter E. coli (ETEC)	Azithromycin 1 gm (PO) × 1 dose **or** Rifaxamin 200 mg (PO) q8h × 3 days.	Rifamycin (delayed release) 388 mg (2 tablets) q12h × 3 days.
Cholera	Vibrio cholera	Azithromycin 1 gm (PO) × 1 dose	Doxycycline 300 mg (PO) × 1 dose
C. difficile diarrhea/ colitis	Clostridium difficile	**Diarrhea** †§ **Initial episode:** Vancomycin 250 mg (PO) q6h × 7–10 days* (If no improvement in 3 days, ↑ dose to 500 mg (PO) q6h × 7 days)** **Relapse:** Vancomycin 500 mg (PO) q6h × 14 days** **Recurrence:**†† Vancomycin 500 mg (PO) q6h × 1 month (**do not taper vancomycin dose**). If another recurrence, *re-treat* with Vancomycin 500 mg (PO) q6h × 2 months. If another recurrence, re-treat with Vancomycin 500 mg (PO) q6h × 3 months. *If dose not tapered and if no colitis,* **this regimen will not fail!** If diarrhea continues, look for alternate diagnosis.	**Diarrhea** **Initial episode:** Nitazoxanide 500 mg (PO) q12h × 7–10 days **Relapse:** Nitazoxanide 500 mg (PO) q12h × 7–10 days **Recurrence:** Preferred Therapy Nitazoxanide 500 mg (PO) q12h × 7–10 days Alternate Therapy Rifaximin 400 mg (PO) q8h × 10 days **or** Fidoxamicin 200 mg (PO) q12h × 10 days **or** Bezlotoxumab 10 mg/ kg × 1 dose (plus an anti-C. difficile antibiotic) **or** FMT (potential to trans- mit enteric pathogens)

*   With C. difficile diarrhea (not colitis) **treatment failure common with Vancomycin 125 mg (PO) q6h and with Metronidazole at any dose,** (Flagyl frequently fails!).

**   *If no improvement after 3 days with Vancomycin 500 mg (PO) q6h,* **rule out *colitis* with abdominal CT scan.** If abdominal CT scan shows **colitis** treat as *C. difficile* **colitis.**

†   When treating C. difficile diarrhea or colitis, ***discontinue antibiotics with a high C. difficile potential***, e.g., **clindamycin, ciprofloxacin,** β-**lactams** (*excluding* ceftriaxone).

††   **Avoid C. difficile "prophylaxis."** Do *not* treat **"history of C. difficile."** Instead, *repeat C. difficile stool PCR to verify diagnosis.* Treat C. difficile diarrhea **only if** PCR + for C. difficile.

§   **Avoid anti-spasmatics in C. difficile diarrhea;** use may result in C. difficile **colitis.**

§§ Colectomy may be lifesaving in severe C. difficile pancolitis.

Infectious Diarrhea/Typhoid (Enteric) Fever *(cont'd)*

Subset	Usual Pathogens	Preferred Therapy	Alternate Therapy
		Colitis **Mild/Moderately severe:** Metronidazole 1 gm (IV) q24h until cured **plus** Ertapenem 1 gm (IV) 124h (until associated peritonitis resolves)	**Colitis** **Mild/Moderately severe:** Metronidazole 500 mg (PO) q6h until cured **plus either** Tigecycline 200 mg (IV) × 1 dose, then 100 mg (IV) q24h until cured **or** Nitazoxanide 500 mg (PO) q12h until cured ± Vancomycin 500 mg (PO) q6h) until cured*
		Severe Pancolitis:[§§] Metronidazole 500 mg (IV/PO) q6h–8h until cured **plus** Nitazoxanide 500 mg (PO) q12h × until cured **plus** Tigecycline 200 mg (IV) × 1 dose, then, 100 mg (IV) q24h until cured	
			Colitis Relapse or Recurrence: Nitazoxanide 500 mg (PO) q12h until cured
Cytomeg-alovirus colitis	CMV	Valganciclovir 900 mg (PO) q12h × 21 days	

* If C. difficle colitis with no associated diarrhea, oral vancomycin of questionable benefit.

Infectious Diarrhea/Typhoid (Enteric) Fever *(cont'd)*

Subset	Usual Pathogens	Preferred Therapy	Alternate Therapy
Typhoid (enteric) fever	Salmonella typhi/ paratyphi	Quinolone[†] (IV or PO) × 10–14 days **or** Ceftriaxone 1 gm (IV) q24h × 10–14 days **or** Azithromycin 1 gm (PO) q24h × 5 days[††]	Chloramphenicol 500 mg (IV or PO) q6h × 10–14 days **or** TMP–SMX 5 mg/kg (IV or PO) q6h × 10–14 days
	MDR *S. Typhi*	Meropenem 1 gm (IV) q8h × 10– × 14 days[††]	Azithromycin 1 gm (PO) q24h × 5 days
Chronic non-bacterial watery diarrhea	Giardia lamblia*	Tinidazole 2 gm (PO) × 1 dose **or** Nitazoxanide 500 mg (PO) q12h × 3 days	Albendazole 400 mg (PO) q24h × 5 days **or** Quinacrine 100 mg (PO) q8h × 5 days
	Cryptos-poridia*	Nitazoxanide 500 mg (PO) q12h × 5 days[§]	Paromomycin 500–750 mg (PO) q8h until response **or** Azithromycin 600 mg (PO) q24h × 4 weeks
	Cystoiso-spora (Iso-spora)* belli	TMP–SMX 1 DS tablet (PO) q12h × 10 days[‡]	
Acute dysen-tery	Entamoeba histolytica	<u>Preferred therapy:</u> Metronidazole 750 mg (PO) q8h × 10 days **followed by either** Iodoquinol 650 mg (PO) q8h × 20 days **or** Paromomycin 500 mg (PO) q8h × 7 days <u>Alternate therapy:</u> Tinidazole 1 gm (PO) q12h × 3 days	
	Shigella E. coli (EIEC)	Quinolone[†] (IV or PO) × 3–5 days **or** Azithromycin 500 mg (IV/PO) q24h × 3–5 days	TMP–SMX 1 DS tablet (PO) q12h × 3–5 days

*   May also present as acute watery diarrhea.
†   Ciprofloxacin 400 mg (IV) or 500 mg (PO) q12h or Levofloxacin 500 mg (IV or PO) q24h or Moxifloxacin 400 mg (IV or PO) q24h.
§   **Longer duration of therapy may be needed in immunosuppressed patients (treat until cured).**
†† Useful for XDR S. typhi (Sindh strains) in India, Oceania, SE Asia.

Acute Watery Bacterial Diarrhea

Clinical Presentation: Acute onset of watery diarrhea without blood/mucus.

Diagnostic Considerations: Profuse watery diarrhea (non-C. difficle) suggests V. cholerae. Diagnosis by culture of organism from stool specimens. V. cholerae demonstrate "shooting star" molility in wet preps of "rice water stools".

Pitfalls: Fecal WBCs negative in watery diarrheas. Stool PCR for V. cholerae without profuse watery diarrhea indicates carrier state (may persist for weeks) not infection.

Therapeutic Considerations: V. cholerae may be treated with single high dose of azithromycin or doxycycline.

Prognosis: Excellent. Most recover with supportive treatment.

Clostridium difficile Diarrhea/Colitis

Clinical Presentation: Voluminous watery diarrhea following exposure to C. difficile contaminated fomites, exposure to patients with C. difficile, recent cancer chemotherapy or antibiotic therapy with some, *but not most*, antibiotics. Most often associated with clindamycin, ciprofloxacin, and β-lactams (excluding ceftriaxone). Other drugs that predispose to C. difficile include PPIs, statins, laxatives/stool softeners and some anti-depressants.

Selective serotonin reuptake inhibitors (fluoxetine, escitalopram, citalopram, sertraline, paroxetine); Tricyclic antidepressants (nortriptyline, amitriptyline); Serotonin antagonists and reuptake inhibitors (trazodone); Seretonin-norepinephrine reuptake inhibitors (duloxetine, venlafaxine); norfepinephrine-dopamine reuptake inhibitors (bupropion); tetracyclic antidepressant (mirtazapine).

Diagnostic Considerations: Watery diarrhea with positive C. difficile stool toxin. A single positive PCR C. difficile stool toxin test is sufficiently sensitive/specific for diagnosis (endpoint is end of diarrhea, not stool toxin negativity); *If negative, no need to retest*. If C. difficile colitis suspected in C. difficile positive patients with fever/prominent leukocytosis/abdominal pain, confirm diagnosis by abdominal CT scan.

Pitfalls: C. difficile colitis is suggested by the presence of otherwise unexplained leukocytosis, ↑ ESR, abdominal pain and often temperature > 102°F; confirm diagnosis with CT/MRI of abdomen. Virulent strains of C. difficile may present with colitis with temperature ≤ 102°F, leukocytosis (often very high, i.e., 25–50 K/mm³), and little/no abdominal pain; confirm diagnosis with CT/MRI of abdomen. Radiographically C. difficile colitis typically is a pancolitis. Segmental colitis suggests a non-C. difficile etiology, i.e., ischemic colitis. C. difficile toxin test may remain positive in stools following resolution of diarrhea; In patients receiving enteral feeds, diarrhea is likely due to enteral feeds (high infusion rates/high osmotic loads) rather than C. difficile. Norovirus diarrhea may mimic C. difficile diarrhea or concurrent outbreaks may occur. Vancomycin may be *ineffective* in C. difficile *colitis*.

Therapeutic Considerations: For **C. difficile diarrhea** oral vancomycin or nitazoxanide are preferred; *Flagyl frequently fails*. Rifaxamin and Fidaxomycin have no advantage over vancomycin. With effective therapy, C. difficile diarrhea begins to improve (≤ 3 days) and usually resolves by 5–7 days, although some patients require 10 days of therapy. If no improvement with vancomycin 250 mg (PO) q6h,

$\uparrow$ dose to 500 mg (PO) q6h or use nitazoxanide. *Do not treat C. difficile negative diarrhea with oral vancomycin or metronidazole.* For **C. difficile colitis**, treat until colitis resolves (follow with serial ESRs/abdominal and or CT scans). Add aerobic GNB coverage for microscopic/gross peritonitis with ESRs ertapenem. Tigecycline highly effective monotherapy for C. difficile colitis; and also provides anti-B fragilis coverage (for associated microscopic/clinical peritonitis). ***Avoid*** *anti-motility agents, e.g., loperamide with C. difficile diarrhea which may result in C. difficile colitis/toxic megacolon.*
Prognosis: Prognosis with C. difficile diarrhea is excellent. C. difficile colitis prognosis is related to strain virulence/and extent of colitis.

Typhoid (Enteric) Fever (Salmonella typhi/paratyphi)

Clinical Presentation: Sustained high fevers (>102°F) without chills increasing in a stepwise fashion accompanied by relative bradycardia (at end of first week) "apathetic facies" with watery diarrhea/constipation, anorexia, RLQ abdominal pain, headache, epistaxis, tender tongue tip, dry cough tender hepatomegaly, ± Rose spots. Thrombocytopenia should suggest another diagnosis, e.g., malaria or viral infection, e.g., dengue.

Diagnostic Considerations: Most community acquired diarrheas are not accompanied by temperatures > 102°F with relative bradycardia. Diagnosis is confirmed by demonstrating Salmonella in blood, bone marrow, Rose spots, stool cultures or $\uparrow$ O and Vi antigen titers. Culture of bone marrow is the quickest method of diagnosis. WBC count is usually low normal/leukopenia. Leukocytosis should suggest another diagnosis. Patients have a musty/fetid body odor. Bowel perforation/hemorrhage heralded by chills, and by $\downarrow$ fever or hypothermia which may occur during 2nd week of typhoid fever. Eosinopenia characteristic of typhoid fever. In patients with suspected typhoid fever, eosinophilia should suggest an alternate diagnosis or parasitic coinfection. PPIs may predispose to or worsen invasive Salmonella infections.

Pitfalls: Rose spots are few/difficult to see and not present in all cases. Typhoid fever usually presents with constipation, not diarrhea. Rigors are not a feature of typhoid fever.

Therapeutic Considerations: 2nd generation cephalosporins, aztreonam, and aminoglycosides are ineffective. Since Salmonella strains causing enteric fever are intracellular pathogens, treat for a full 2 weeks to maximize cure rates/minimize relapses. Treat relapses with the suggested antibiotics × 2–3 weeks. Salmonella excretion into feces usually persists < 3 months. Persistent excretion > 3 months suggests a carrier state—rule out hepatobiliary/urinary calculi.

Prognosis: Good if treated early. Poor with late treatment/bowel perforation.

Chronic Non-Bacterial Watery Diarrhea

Clinical Presentation: Watery diarrhea without blood/mucus lasting > 1 month.
Diagnostic Considerations: Diagnosis by demonstrating organisms/cysts in stool specimens. Multiple fresh daily stool samples often needed for diagnosis especially for protozoan parasites.

Pitfalls: Concomitant transient lactase deficiency may prolong diarrhea if dairy products are consumed during an infectious diarrhea.

Therapeutic Considerations: Cryptosporidia and Isospora are being recognized increasingly in acute/chronic diarrhea in normal hosts.

Prognosis: Excellent in well-nourished patients. Untreated patients may develop malabsorption.

Giardia lamblia

Clinical Presentation: Acute/subacute onset of diarrhea, abdominal cramps, bloating, flatulence. Incubation period 1–2 weeks. Malabsorption may occur in chronic cases. No eosinophilia.

Diagnostic Considerations: Diagnosis by demonstrating trophozoites or cysts in stool/antigen detection assay. If stool exam and antigen test are negative and Giardiasis is suspected, perform "string test"/duodenal aspirate and biopsy.

Pitfalls: Cysts intermittently excreted into stool. Usually need multiple stool samples for diagnosis. Often accompanied by transient lactose intolerance.

Therapeutic Considerations: Nitazoxanide effective therapy. Diarrhea may be prolonged if milk (lactose-containing) products are ingested after treatment/cure. May need repeat courses of therapy.

Prognosis: Related to severity of malabsorption and health of host.

Cryptosporidia

Clinical Presentation: Acute/subacute onset of diarrhea. Usually occurs in HIV patients with CD_4 counts < 200. Biliary cryptosporidiosis is seen only in HIV; may present as acalculous cholecystitis or sclerosing cholangitis with RUQ pain, fever, ↑ alkaline phosphatase, but bilirubin is normal.

Diagnostic Considerations: Diagnosis by demonstrating organism in stool/intestinal biopsy specimen. Cholera-like illness in normal hosts. Chronic watery diarrhea in compromised hosts.

Pitfalls: Smaller than Cyclospora. Oocyst walls are smooth (not wrinkled) on acid fast staining.

Therapeutic Considerations: Nitazoxanide effective therapy.

Prognosis: Related to adequacy of fluid replacement/underlying health of host.

Cytoisospora (Isospora)/Cyclospora

Clinical Presentation: Acute/subacute onset of diarrhea. Incubation period 1–14 days.

Diagnostic Considerations: Diagnosis by demonstrating organism in stool/intestinal biopsy specimen. Clinically indistinguishable from cryptosporidial diarrhea (intermittent watery diarrhea without blood or mucus). Fatigue/weight loss common.

Pitfalls: Oocysts only form seen in stool and are best identified with modified Kinyoun acid fast staining. Acid fast fat globules stain pink with acid fast staining. "Wrinkled wall" oocysts are characteristic of Cyclospora, not Cryptosporidia. Oocysts are twice the size of similar appearing Cryptosporidia (~ 10 μm vs. 5 μm).

Therapeutic Considerations: Nitazoxanide effective therapy.

Prognosis: Related to adequacy of fluid replacement/underlying health of host.

Acute Dysentery

Entamoeba histolytica

Clinical Presentation: Acute/subacute onset of bloody diarrhea/mucus. Fecal WBC/RBCs due to mucosal invasion. E. histolytica may also cause chronic diarrhea. Colonic ulcers secondary to E. histolytica are round and may form "collar stud" abscesses.

Diagnostic Considerations: Diagnosis by demonstrating organism/trophozoites in stool/intestinal biopsy specimen. Serology is negative with amebic dysentery, but positive with extra-intestinal forms. Test to separate E. histolytica from non-pathogenic E. dispar cyst passers. On sigmoidoscopy, ulcers due to E. histolytica are round with normal mucosa in between, and may form "collar stud" abscesses. In contrast, ulcers due to Shigella are linear and serpiginous without normal intervening mucosa. Bloody dysentery is more subacute with E. histolytica compared to Shigella.

Pitfalls: Intestinal perforation/abscess may complicate amebic colitis. Rule out infectious causes of bloody diarrhea with mucus before diagnosing/treating inflammatory bowel disease (IBD). Obtain multiple stool cultures for bacterial pathogens/parasites. Do not confuse E. histolytica in stool specimens with E. hartmanni, a non-pathogen protozoa similar in appearance but smaller in size.

Therapeutic Considerations: E. histolytica cyst passers should be treated, but metronidazole is ineffective against cysts. Recommended antibiotics treat both luminal and hepatic E. histolytica. Use paromomycin 500 mg (PO) q8h × 7 days for asymptomatic cysts.

Prognosis: Good if treated early. Related to severity of dysentery/ulcers/extra-intestinal amebiasis.

Shigella

Clinical Presentation: Acute onset of bloody diarrhea/mucus.

Diagnostic Considerations: Diagnosis by demonstrating organism in stool specimens. Shigella ulcers in colon are linear, serpiginous, and rarely lead to perforation.

Therapeutic Considerations: Shigella dysentery is more acute/fulminating than amebic dysentery. Shigella has no carrier state, unlike Entamoeba.

Prognosis: Good if treated early. Severity of illness related to Shigella species: S. dysenteriae (most severe) > S. flexneri > S. boydii/S. sonnei (mildest).

Cholecystitis

Subset	Usual Pathogens	Preferred IV Therapy	Alternate IV Therapy	PO Therapy or IV-to-PO Switch
Normal host	E. coli Klebsiella E. faecalis (VSE)	Meropenem 1 gm (IV) q8h* **or** Piperacillin/ Tazobactam 3.375 gm (IV) q6h* **or** Tigecycline 200 mg (IV) × 1 dose, then 100 mg (IV) q24h*	Quinolone‡ (IV)* **or** Cefazolin 1 gm (IV) q8h* **plus** Ampicillin 1 gm (IV) q6h*	Quinolone‡ (PO)*
Emphy-sematous cholecys-titis†	Clostridium perfringens E. coli	Meropenem 1 gm (IV) q8h¶ **or** Piperacillin/ Tazobactam 3.375 gm (IV) q6h¶	Ertapenem 1 gm (IV) q24h¶ **or** Ticarcillin/ Clavulanate 3.1 gm (IV) q6h¶	Clindamycin 300 mg (PO) q8h¶

† Treat only IV or IV-to-PO switch.

‡ Ciprofloxacin 400 mg (IV) or Levofloxacin 500 mg (IV or PO) q24h or Moxifloxacin 400 mg (IV or PO) q24h.

* If no cholecystectomy, treat × 5–7 days. If cholecystectomy is performed, treat × 3–4 days post-operatively.

¶ Treat × 4–7 days after cholecystectomy.

Cholecystitis

Clinical Presentation: RUQ pain, fever usually ≤ 102°F, positive Murphy's sign, no percussion tenderness over right lower ribs.

Diagnostic Considerations: Diagnosis by RUQ ultrasound/positive HIDA scan.

Pitfalls: No need to cover B. fragilis.

Therapeutic Considerations: Obtain surgical consult for possible cholecystectomy.

Prognosis: Related to cardiopulmonary status.

Emphysematous Cholecystitis

Clinical Presentation: Clinically presents as cholecystitis. Usually in diabetics.

Diagnostic Considerations: RUQ/gallbladder gas on flat plate of abdomen.

Pitfalls: Requires immediate cholecystectomy.

Therapeutic Considerations: Usually a difficult/prolonged post-op course.

Prognosis: Related to speed of gallbladder removal.

Cholangitis

Subset	Usual Pathogens	Preferred IV Therapy	Alternate IV Therapy	IV-to-PO Switch
Normal host or above	E. coli Klebsiella E. faecalis (VSE)	Meropenem 1 gm (IV) q8h* **or** Tigecycline 200 mg (IV) × 1 dose, then 100 mg (IV) q24h* **or** Piperacillin/Tazobactam 3.375 gm (IV) q6h*	Ampicillin/ Sulbactam 3 gm (IV) q6h* **or** Cefoperazone 2 gm (IV) q12h* **or** Doripenem 1 gm (IV) q8h	Ciprofloxacin 500 mg (PO) q12h* **or** Levofloxacin 500 mg (PO) q24h* **or** Moxifloxacin 400 mg (PO) q24h*

* Treat until resolved (usually 5–7 days).

Clinical Presentation: RUQ pain, fever > 102°F, positive Murphy's sign, percussion tenderness over right lower ribs.

Diagnostic Considerations: Obstructed common bile duct on ultrasound/CT/MRI of abdomen.

Pitfalls: Charcot's triad (fever, RUQ pain, jaundice) is present in only 50%.

Therapeutic Considerations: Obtain surgical consult for urgent relief of obstruction. Continue antibiotics for 4–7 days after obstruction is relieved.

Prognosis: Related to speed of surgical relief of obstruction.

Gallbladder Wall Abscess/Perforation

Subset	Usual Pathogens	Preferred IV Therapy	Alternate IV Therapy	IV-to-PO Switch
Gallbladder wall abscess/ perforation	E. coli Klebsiella E. faecalis (VSE)	Piperacillin/Tazobactam 3.375 gm (IV) q6h* **or** Tigecycline 200 mg (IV) × 1 dose, then 100 mg (IV) q24h* **or** Meropenem 1 gm (IV) q8h*	Ampicillin/ Sulbactam 3 gm (IV) q6h* **or** Cefoperazone 2 gm (IV) q12h* **or** Doripenem 1 gm (IV) q8h	Ciprofloxacin 500 mg (PO) q12h* **or** Levofloxacin 500 mg (PO) q24h* **or** Moxifloxacin 400 mg (PO) q24h*

Duration of therapy represents total time IV or IV + PO.
* Treat until resolved (usually 1–2 weeks).

Clinical Presentation: RUQ pain, fever ≤ 102°F, positive Murphy's sign, no percussion tenderness over right lower ribs.

Diagnostic Considerations: Diagnosis by CT/MRI of abdomen. Bile peritonitis is common.

Pitfalls: Bacterial peritonitis may be present.

Therapeutic Considerations: Obtain surgical consult for possible gallbladder removal. Usually a difficult and prolonged post-op course.
Prognosis: Related to removal of gallbladder/repair of perforation.

Acute Pancreatitis

Subset	Usual Pathogens	Preferred IV Therapy	Alternate IV Therapy	IV-to-PO Switch
Edematous pancreatitis	None	Not applicable	Not applicable	Not applicable
Hemorrhagic/ necrotizing pancreatitis	GNB B. fragilis	Ertapenem 1 gm (IV) q24h* **or** Meropenem 1 gm (IV) q8h*	Piperacillin/ Tazobactam 3.375 mg (IV) q6h* **or** Ampicillin/ Sulbactam 1.5 gm (IV) q6h* **or** Ticarcillin/ Clavulanate 3.1 gm (IV) q6h*	**Monotherapy** Moxifloxacin 400 mg (PO) q24h* **or** **Combination Therapy** Clindamycin 300 mg (PO) q8h* **plus** Levofloxacin 500 mg (PO) q24h*

* Treat until resolved (usually 1–2 weeks).

Edematous Pancreatitis
Clinical Presentation: Sharp abdominal pain with fever ≤ 102°F ± hypotension.
Diagnostic Considerations: Diagnosis by elevated serum amylase and lipase levels with normal methemalbumin levels. May be drug-induced (e.g., steroids).
Pitfalls: Amylase elevation alone is not diagnostic of acute pancreatitis.
Therapeutic Considerations: NG tube is not needed. Aggressively replace fluids.
Prognosis: Good with adequate fluid replacement.

Hemorrhagic/Necrotizing Pancreatitis
Clinical Presentation: Sharp abdominal pain with fever ≤ 102°F ± hypotension. Grey-Turner/Cullen's sign present in some.
Diagnostic Considerations: Mildly elevated serum amylase and lipase levels with high methemalbumin levels.
Pitfalls: With elevated lipase, amylase level is inversely related to severity of disease.
Therapeutic Considerations: Obtain surgical consult for possible peritoneal lavage as adjunct to antibiotics. Serum albumin/dextran are preferred volume expanders.
Prognosis: Poor with hypocalcemia or shock.

Pancreatic Abscess/Infected Pancreatic Pseudocyst

Subset	Usual Pathogens	Preferred IV Therapy	Alternate IV Therapy	PO therapy or IV-to-PO Switch
Infected pancreatic pseudo-cyst/ pancreatic abscess	GNB B. fragilis	Meropenem 1 gm (IV) q8h* **or** Piperacillin/ Tazobactam 3.375 gm (IV) q6h* **or** Ertapenem 1 gm (IV) q24h*	Ampicillin/ Sulbactam 1.5 gm (IV) q6h* **or** Ticarcillin/Clavula-nate 3.1 gm (IV) q6h* **or** Doripenem 1 gm (IV) q8h	Moxifloxacin 400 mg (PO) q24h* **or** **Combination Therapy** Clindamycin 300 mg (PO) q8h* **plus** Quinolone† (PO)*

† Levofloxacin 500 mg q24h.
* Treat until resolved.

Clinical Presentation: Follows acute pancreatitis or develops in a pancreatic pseudo-cyst. An infected pancreatic pseudocyst is an abscess equivalent. Fevers usually ≥ 102°F.
Diagnostic Considerations: CT/MRI of abdomen demonstrates pancreatic abscess.
Pitfalls: Peritoneal signs are typically absent.
Prognosis: Related to size/extent of abscess and adequacy of drainage.

Liver Abscess

Subset	Usual Pathogens	Preferred IV Therapy	Alternate IV Therapy	PO Therapy or IV-to-PO Switch
Liver abscess	GNB E. faecalis (VSE) B. fragilis	Piperacillin/ Tazobactam 3.375 gm (IV) q6h* **or** Tigecycline 200 mg (IV) × 1 dose, then 100 mg (IV) q24h* **or** Meropenem 1 gm (IV) q8h*	**Monotherapy** Moxifloxacin 400 mg (IV) q24h* **or** Sulbactam/ Ampicillin 3 gm (IV) q6h **or** **Combination Therapy** Quinolone† (IV)* **plus either** Metronidazole 1 gm (IV) q24h* **or** Clindamycin 600 mg (IV) q8h*	**Monotherapy** Amoxicillin/Clavulanic acid 875/125 mg (PO) q12h* **or** Moxifloxacin 400 mg (PO) q24h* **or** **Combination Therapy** Quinolone† (PO)* **plus either** Metronidazole 500 mg (PO) q12h* **or** Clindamycin 300 mg (PO) q8h*
	E. histolytica	See Chapter 4.		

* Treat until abscess(es) are no longer present or stop decreasing in size on serial CT scans.
† Levofloxacin 500 mg (IV or PO) q24h.

Liver Abscess

Clinical Presentation: Fever, RUQ tenderness, negative Murphy's sign, and negative right lower rib percussion tenderness.

Diagnostic Considerations: Diagnosis by CT/MRI scan of liver and aspiration of abscess. CT shows multiple lesions in liver. Source is usually either the colon (diverticulitis or diverticular abscess with portal pyemia) or retrograde infection from the gallbladder (cholecystitis or gallbladder wall abscess).

Pitfalls: Bacterial abscesses are usually multiple and involve multiple lobes of liver; amebic abscesses are usually solitary and involve the right lobe of liver.

Therapeutic Considerations: Liver laceration/trauma usually requires ~ 2 weeks of antibiotics.

Prognosis: Good if treated early.

Hepatosplenic Candidiasis

Subset	Usual Pathogens	Preferred IV Therapy	Alternate IV Therapy	PO Therapy or IV-to-PO Switch
Hepato-splenic candi-diasis	Candida albicans	Fluconazole 800 mg (IV) × 1 dose, then 400 mg (IV) q24h × 2–4 weeks	Liposomal amphotericin (L-amb) (IV)† × 2–4 weeks	Fluconazole 800 mg (PO) × 1 dose, then 400 mg (PO) q24h × 2–4 weeks*
	Non-albicans Candida	Micafungin 100 mg (IV) q24h × 2–4 weeks **or** Liposomal amphotericin (L-amb) (IV)† × 2–4 weeks q24h × 2–4 weeks	Caspofungin 70 mg (IV) × 1 dose, then 50 mg (IV) q24h × 2–4 weeks **or** Amphotericin B 0.7 mg/kg (IV) q24h × 2–4 weeks	Itraconazole 200 mg (PO) solution q12h × 2–4 weeks **or** Posaconazole 400 mg (PO) q12h × 2–4 weeks

*   Loading dose is not needed PO if given IV with the same drug.
†   For usual dose, see Chapter 4 (Drug Summaries)

Hepatosplenic Candidiasis

Clinical Presentation: New high spiking fevers with RUQ/LUQ pain after 2 weeks in a patient with febrile leukopenia.

Diagnostic Considerations: Diagnosis by abdominal CT/MRI showing mass lesions in liver/spleen.

Pitfalls: Do not overlook RUQ tenderness and elevated alkaline phosphatase in leukopenic cancer patients as a clue to the diagnosis.
Therapeutic Considerations: Treat until liver/spleen lesions resolve. Should be viewed as a form of disseminated disease.
Prognosis: Related to degree/duration of leukopenia.

Bacterial Hepatitis

Subset	Pathogen	Preferred Therapy
BCG hepatitis	Bacille Calmette-Guérin (BCG) M. bovis	INH 300 mg (PO) q24h × 6 months **plus** Rifampin 600 mg (PO) q24h × 6 months
Leptospirosis	L. interrogans	Doxycycline 200 mg (IV/PO) q12h × 72 h, then 100 mg (IV/PO) q12h × 4 days **or** Ceftriaxone 1 gm (IV) q12h × 7 days

Granulomatous Hepatitis (BCG)
Clinical Presentation: Fever, chills, anorexia, weight loss, hepatomegaly ± RUQ pain days to weeks after intravesicular BCG for bladder cancer. Also may present as miliary BCG infection (FUO) without localizing signs.
Diagnostic Considerations: ↑ alkaline phosphatase > ↑ AST/ALT. Liver biopsy is negative for AFB/positive for granulomas. May also have granulomators prostatitis.
Pitfalls: Exclude other causes of symptoms.
Therapeutic Considerations: INH plus rifampin × 6 months is curative.
Prognosis: Excellent with early treatment.

Leptospirosis
Clinical Presentation: After incubation period of 1–2 weeks, abrupt onset of fever, no chills, N/V, headache ± meningismus, conjunctival suffusion, dry cough, intense myalgias (leg/lumbar tenderness) ± abdominal pain. 1st (leptospiremic) phase (4–9 days); 2nd (immune) phase (6–12 days). Leukocytosis with no thrombocytopenia usual. Hepatic (↑ bilirubin/transaminases) and renal (azotemia, proteinuria, sterile pyuria) involvement. Meningitis (early) → ABM with CSF + for leptospires; meningitis (late) → aseptic meningitis CSF – for leptospires. Progressive vomiting, epistaxis, jaundice/hepatosplenomegaly with Weil's syndrome (icteric leptospirosis). Intense myalgias with hepatic and renal involvement should suggest leptospirosis.
Diagnostic Considerations: Recent occupational or contaminated water (rat urine) exposure. Leptospiruria (after 2 weeks) seen in urine dark-field. BCs + early (– late); UCs + late. Leptospires die rapidly in acid urine (alkalinize urine before urine culture). Diagnosis by blood/urine culture or ↑ MAT IgM titers (after 1 week). Antibiotic therapy may blunt, delay or abort titer rise.

Pitfalls: Like influenza (headache, sore throat, myalgias), patients can recall exact hour of onset. Unlike influenza, no chills but conjunctival suffusion. CXR – in influenza (early) but CXR often + in leptospirosis. Differentiate from viral hepatitis (< 102°F, no conjunctival suffusion, leukopenia, highly ↑ transaminases, no ↑ CPK, no renal involvement). Differentiate from EBV, CMV, HSV hepatitis by + atypical lymphocytes (– with leptospirosis) and specific serologies. Like aseptic (viral) meningitis (normal glucose, WBCs < 500/hpf). Only ID with CSF bilirubin > serum. Clinically irrelevant serologic XR with Borrelia/treponemal titers.

Therapeutic Considerations: Penicillin or doxycycline (± Jarisch-Herxheimer reaction).

Prognosis: Excellent if treated early, 5–40% mortality for Weil's syndrome and elderly.

Viral Hepatitis

Subset	Pathogens	Therapy
Acute	HAV (none); HBV (consider nucleos(t)ides for HBV-acute liver failure); HCV (consider pegylated interferon +/– ribavirin if no viral clearance after 12–16 weeks); HDV (none); HEV (consider ribavirin for severe hepatitis)	

Chronic	HBV*	<u>Preferred:</u>
		  Tenofovir[a] (PO) q24h. Continue for at least 12 months after HBeAg seroconversion
		   or
		  Entecavir 0.5 mg (PO) q24h × ≥ 12 months
		<u>For lamivudine resistant strains</u>
		  Entecavir 1.0 mg q24h
		   or
		  Pegylated interferon alfa-2a 180 mcg (SQ)/week *without* ribavirin × 12 months
		<u>Alternate</u>: Telbivudine 600 mg (PO) q24h
		   or
		  Adefovir 10 mg (PO) q24h
		   or
		  Lamivudine 100 mg (PO) for × ≥ 12 months

* HBeAg+ with ALT > 2 × ULN and HBV DNA > 20,000 IU/mL or alternately, chronic HBV with moderate/severe inflammation or significant fibrosis on liver biopsy. Primary therapeutic response (< 2 log ↓) in HBV DNA levels ≥ 6 months of therapy. Treatment failures should be treated with an alternate regimen or additional treatment.

[a] Tenofovir atafenamide (TAF) and tenofovir disoproxil fumarate (TDF) are two forms of tenofovir approved by the FDA. TAF has fewer bone and kidney toxicities than TDF, while TDF is associated with lower lipid levels. Safety, cost and access are among the factors to consider when choosing between these drugs. TDF is dosed at 300 mg (PO) q24h. TAF is dosed at 25 mg (PO) q24h.

Viral Hepatitis (cont'd)

Subset	Pathogens	Therapy
Chronic	HCV	**Genotype 1 (Includes 1a & 1b)** **Preferred therapy:** Glecaprevir (300 mg)/pibrentasvir (120 mg) (**Mavyret**)[a] (PO) q24h × 8–12[b] weeks Ledipasvir (90 mg)/sofosbuvir (400 mg) (**Harvoni**)[c] (PO) q24h × 8[d]–12 weeks Elbasvir (50 mg)/grazoprevir (100 mg) (**Zepatier**)[e,f] (PO) q24h × 12 weeks Sofosbuvir (400 mg)/velpatasvir (100 mg) (**Epclusa**)[g] (PO) q24h × 12 weeks
		Genotype 2 **Preferred therapy:** Glecaprevir (300 mg)/pibrentasvir (120 mg) (**Mavyret**)[a] (PO) q24h × 8–12[b] weeks Sofosbuvir (400 mg)/velpatasvir (100 mg) (**Epclusa**)[g] (PO) q24h × 12 weeks)
		Genotype 3 **Preferred therapy:** Glecaprevir (300 mg)/pibrentasvir (120 mg) (**Mavyret**)[a] (PO) q24h × 8–12[b] weeks Sofosbuvir (400 mg)/velpatasvir (100 mg) (**Epclusa**)[g,h] (PO) q24h × 12 weeks **Alternate therapy** Sofosbuvir (400 mg)/velpatasvir (100 mg) (**Epclusa**)[g,h] (PO) q24h plus weight-based ribavirin (if baseline NS5A RAS Y93H for velpatasvir) × 12 weeks Sofosbuvir (400 mg)/velpatasvir (100 mg)/voxilaprevir (100 mg) (**Vosevi**)[i] (PO) q24h × 12 weeks (if baseline NS5A RAS Y93H for velpatasvir)
		Genotype 4 **Preferred therapy:** Glecaprevir (300 mg)/pibrentasvir (120 mg) (**Mavyret**)[a] (PO) q24h × 8–12[b] weeks Ledipasvir (90 mg)/sofosbuvir (400 mg) (**Harvoni**)[c] (PO) q24h × 8[d]–12 weeks Sofosbuvir (400 mg)/velpatasvir (100 mg) (**Epclusa**)[g] (PO) q24h × 12 weeks
		Genotype 5 or 6 **Preferred therapy:** Glecaprevir (300 mg)/pibrentasvir (120 mg) (**Mavyret**)[a] (PO) q24h × 8–12[b] weeks Ledipasvir (90 mg)/sofosbuvir (400 mg) (**Harvoni**)[c] (PO) q24h × 12 weeks Sofosbuvir (400 mg)/velpatasvir (100 mg) (**Epclusa**)[g] (PO) q24h × 12 weeks

[a]GLE/PIB; 3-tablet coformulated regimen; pangenotypic regimen; administer with food; regimens containing protease inhibitors should be avoided in patients with active or history of decompensated cirrhosis (Child-Turcotte-Pugh B or C); can be utilized in chronic kidney disease and end-stage-renal-disease.

[b]For patients with HCV/HIV coinfection and cirrhosis, duration of GLE/PIB should be extended to 12 weeks.

[c]LED/SOF; single-tablet coformulated regimen; avoid if CrCl <30 mL/min; add ribavirin or extend to 24 weeks in presence of decompensated cirrhosis; requires acid for absorption (avoid acid reducing medications).

[d]Consider 8 weeks of treatment in patients with Genotype 1 or 4 (non-4r) who are non-cirrhotic, HIV-uninfected, and whose HCV RNA level is <6 million IU/mL.

Viral Hepatitis *(cont'd)*

[e]ELB/GRZ; single-tablet coformulated regimen; regimens containing protease inhibitors should be avoided in patients with active or history of decompensated cirrhosis (Child-Turcotte-Pugh B or C); can be utilized in chronic kidney disease and end-stage-renal-disease.

[f]For Genotype 1a, baseline NS5A resistance testing required prior to use of ELB/GRZ; if resistance present (resistance-associated substitutions at amino acid positions 28, 30, 31, or 93), use alternative regimen.

[g]SOF/VEL; single-tablet coformulated regimen; pangenotypic regimen; avoid if CrCl <30 mL/min; add ribavirin or extend to 24 weeks in presence of decompensated cirrhosis; requires acid for absorption (avoid acid-reducing medications).

[h]For Genotype 3, NS5A resistance testing for Y93H is recommended for cirrhotic patients prior to use of SOF/VEL. If present, see alternative treatment options.

[i]SOF/VEL/VOX; single-tablet coformulated regimen; pangenotypic regimen; typically reserved for DAA-experienced individuals or in those with HCV resistance; administer with food; avoid if CrCl <30 mL/min; regimens containing protease inhibitors should be avoided in patients with active or history of decompensated cirrhosis (Child-Turcotte-Pugh B or C).

Acute Viral Hepatitis

Clinical Presentation: Asymptomatic or anorexia, malaise, nausea, serum-sickness like syndrome, ± jaundice, dark urine.

Diagnostic Considerations: Diagnosis by presence in HAV of IgM anti-HAV or in HBV of HBsAg and IgM anti-HBc or in HCV of anti-HCV and HCV RNA or in HDV of HBsAg, anti-HDV and HDV RNA or in HEV of anti-HEV and HEV RNA, with markedly elevated serum aminotransferases (ALT > 400). Serum alkaline phosphatase normal/mildly elevated; albumin normal or mildly depressed; INR normal or minimally elevated.

Pitfalls: Rule out other hepatitis-causing agents (EBV, CMV, HSV, etc) and drug-induced liver injury if serologic tests for HAV, HBV, HCV, HDV, and HEV are negative.

Therapeutic Considerations: For patients who develop encephalopathy and/or a prolonged INR (acute liver failure) admit to liver transplantation center.

Prognosis: Hepatitis A generally self-limited; Hepatitis B, C, D and rarely E may progress to chronic hepatitis/cirrhosis/hepatocellular carcinoma.

EBV/CMV Hepatitis

Clinical Presentation: Similar to acute viral hepatitis plus bilateral posterior cervical adenopathy and fatigue.

Diagnostic Considerations: EBV hepatitis is part of infectious mononucleosis and may be the presenting sign in adults. CMV hepatitis also may appear as a "mono-like" infection in normal hosts. In compromised hosts, hepatitis may be the primary manifestation of CMV infection. Diagnosis of EBV/CMV hepatitis can be made by serology (positive mono spot test, high EBV VCA IgM titer, high CMV IgM titer, CMV early antigen detection (via shell vial cultures) or molecular amplification techniques.

Pitfalls: In normal and immunocompromised hosts with unexplained aminotransferase (ALT/AST) elevations, consider CMV hepatitis and order appropriate tests.

Treatment: None effective in EBV hepatitis; CMV hepatitis in normal hosts may be treated with Valganciclovir 900 mg (PO) q12h × 12 days.

Prognosis: In normal hosts EBV and CMV hepatitis are usually self-limited. In immuno-compromised hosts, the prognosis of CMV hepatitis is related to the degree of Immuno-suppression and the rapidity of onset of treatment.

Chronic Viral Hepatitis

Clinical Presentation: Often asymptomatic with persistently or intermittently ele-vated serum aminotransferases but in some aminotransferases are normal. Some pres-ent with signs and symptoms of chronic liver disease.

Diagnostic Considerations: Chronic hepatitis B is diagnosed by presence of HBsAg and HBV DNA. Chronic hepatitis C is diagnosed by positive tests for anti-HCV and HCV RNA. Signal cutoff (SCO) >1.0 = HCV infection. SCO < 1.0 = false + test. Most HCV infec-tions have SCOs > 5-10. Chronic hepatitis D is diagnosed by positive tests for HBsAg and HDV RNA. Chronic hepatitis E is diagnosed by presence of anti-HEV and HEV RNA. Liver biopsy may be used to grade inflammation and stage fibrosis.

Pitfalls: Autoimmune hepatitis may present as an acute or chronic hepatitis but with elevated IgG levels, elevated ANAs, and anti-smooth muscle antibodies. For both HCV and HBV, rule out co-infection with HIV.

Therapeutic Considerations: In chronic hepatitis B treat until HBV DNA becomes undetectable, ALT normalizes, and for HBeAg-positive patients, HBeAg seroconversion occurs (then continue for 6–12 additional months). For chronic hepatitis C therapy is based on genotype.

Prognosis: Sustained clearance of HCV RNA (measured 24 weeks after discontinuation of treatment) results in a cure in 99% of chronic hepatitis C patients. Sustained clearance of HBV DNA is linked with an improved prognosis in chronic hepatitis B.

cIAIs/Intraabdominal or Pelvic Peritonitis or Abscess

Subset	Usual Pathogens	Preferred IV Therapy	Alternate IV Therapy	PO Therapy or IV-to-PO Switch
Mild/ moderate peritonitis	GNB B. fragilis	Moxifloxacin 400 mg (IV) q24h[¥] **or** Cefoxitin 2 gm (IV) q6h[¥] **or** Piperacillin/ Tazobactam 3.375 gm (IV) q6h[¥]	**Monotherapy** Ampicillin/ Sulbactam 1.5 gm (IV) q6h[¥] **or** **Combination Therapy** Ceftazidime/ Avibactam 2.5 gm (IV) q8h **plus** Metronidazole 500 mg (IV) q8h	**Monotherapy** Moxifloxacin 400 mg (PO) q24h[¥] **or** Amoxicillin/Clavu-lanate 875/125 mg (PO) q12h[¥] **Combination Therapy** Levofloxacin 500 mg (PO) q24h[¥] **plus** Clindamycin 300 mg (PO) q8h[¥]

cIAIs/Intraabdominal or Pelvic Peritonitis or Abscess *(cont'd)*

Subset	Usual Pathogens	Preferred IV Therapy	Alternate IV Therapy	PO Therapy or IV-to-PO Switch
Severe peritonitis[‡]	GNB B. fragilis	Ertapenem 1 gm (IV) q24h[¥] **or** Tigecycline 200 mg (IV) × 1 dose, then 100 mg (IV) q24h[¥] **or** Meropenem 1 gm (IV) q8h[¥] **or** Ampicillin/ Sulbactam 3 gm (IV) q6h[¥]	**Monotherapy** Eravacycline 1 mg/kg (IV) q12h[¥] **or** **Combination Therapy** Metronidazole 1 gm (IV) q24h[¥] **plus either** Ceftriaxone 1 gm (IV) q24h[¥] **or** Levofloxacin 500 mg (IV) q24h	Moxifloxacin 400 mg (PO) q24h[¥] **or** Amoxicillin/ Clavulanate 875/125 mg (PO) q12h[¥]
	CRE	Tigecycline 200 mg (IV) × 1 dose, then 100 mg (IV) q24h[¥] **or** Ceftazidime/ Avibactam 2.5 gm (IV) q8h[¥] **plus** Metronidazole 1 gm (IV) q24h[¥]	Meropenem/ Vaborbactam 4 gm (IV) q8h[¥] **or** Imipenem/ Relebactam 625 mg (IV) q6h[¥]	
Spontaneous bacterial peritonitis (SBP)[‡]	GNB (not B. fragilis) Ceftriaxone 1 gm (IV) q24h × 1–2 wks	Ceftriaxone 1 gm (IV) q24h × 1–2 wks **or** Levofloxacin 500 mg (IV) × 1–2 weeks	Aztreonam 2 gm (IV) q8h × 1–2 weeks **or** Any aminoglycoside (IV) q24h × 1–2 weeks	Quinolone (PO) × 1–2 weeks **or** Amoxicillin/Clavulanate 875/125 mg (PO) q12h × 1–2 weeks
CAPD-associated peritonitis[‡]	S. epidermidis (CoNS) S. aureus (MSSA) GNB	*Before culture results* Ceftriaxone 1 gm (IV) q24h × 1–2 wks initial dose* **or** Moxifloxacin 400 mg (IV/PO) initial dose*	*After culture results* *MSSA/Enterobacteriaceae* Meropenem 1 gm (IV) initial dose* *MRSA* Vancomycin 1 gm (IV) initial dose* **or** Linezolid 600 mg (IV or PO) initial dose	
Chronic TB peritonitis	M. tuberculosis	Not applicable		Treat the same as pulmonary TB

¥   Duration of therapy as clinically indicated or for 5–7 days following corrective surgery.
*   Follow with maintenance dose × 2 weeks.

Intra-abdominal or Pelvic Peritonitis/Abscess
(Appendicitis/Diverticulitis/Septic Pelvic Thrombophlebitis)

Clinical Presentation: Spiking fevers with acute abdominal pain and peritoneal signs. In diverticulitis, the pain is localized over the involved segment of colon. Appendicitis ± perforation presents as RLQ pain/rebound tenderness or mass. Peri-diverticular abscess presents the same as intraabdominal/pelvic abscess, most commonly in the LLQ. Septic pelvic thrombophlebitis presents as high spiking fevers unresponsive to antibiotic therapy following delivery/pelvic surgery.

Diagnostic Considerations: Diagnosis by CT/MRI scan of abdomen/pelvis.

Pitfalls: Tympany over liver suggests abdominal/visceral perforation. Pelvic peritonitis/abscess presents the same as intraabdominal abscess/peritonitis, but peritoneal signs are often absent.

Therapeutic Considerations: Patients with ischemic/inflammatory colitis should be treated the same as peritonitis, depending on severity. Obtain surgical consult for repair/lavage or abscess drainage. In SPT, fever rapidly falls when heparin is added to antibiotics.

Prognosis: Related to degree/duration of peritoneal spillage and rapidity/completeness of lavage. Prognosis for SPT is good if treated early and clots remain limited to pelvic veins.

Spontaneous Bacterial Peritonitis (SBP)

Clinical Presentation: Acute or subacute onset of fever ± abdominal pain.

Diagnostic Considerations: Diagnosis by positive blood cultures of SBP pathogens. For patients with abdominal pain, ascites, and a negative CT/MRI, paracentesis ascitic fluid with > 500 WBCs and > 100 PMNs predicts a positive ascitic fluid culture and is diagnostic of SBP. Some degree of splenic dysfunction usually exists, predisposing to infection with encapsulated organisms.

Pitfalls: Do not overlook GI source of peritonitis (e.g, appendicitis, diverticulitis); obtain CT/MRI.

Therapeutic Considerations: B. fragilis/anaerobes are not common pathogens in SBP, and B. fragilis coverage is unnecessary.

Prognosis: Related to degree of hepatitic/splenic dysfunction.

CAPD Associated Peritonitis

Clinical Presentation: Abdominal pain ± fever in a CAPD patient.

Diagnostic Considerations: Diagnosis by gram stain/culture and ↑ WBC count in peritoneal fluid. Lymphocytic predominance may suggest TB or fungi. Unlike SBP, there are not specific diagnostic criteria in peritoneal fluid.

Pitfalls: Fever is often absent.

Therapeutic Considerations: Treat with systemic antibiotics ± antibiotics in dialysate.

Prognosis: Good with early therapy and removal of peritoneal catheter.

Chronic Tuberculous Peritonitis (Mycobacterium tuberculosis)
Clinical Presentation: Abdominal pain with fevers, weight loss, ascites over 1–3 months.
Diagnostic Considerations: "Doughy consistency" on abdominal palpation. Diagnosis by AFB on peritoneal biopsy/culture.
Pitfalls: Chest x-ray is normal in ~ 70%. Increased incidence in alcoholic cirrhosis.
Therapeutic Considerations: Treated the same as pulmonary TB.
Prognosis: Good if treated early.

Empiric Therapy of Genitourinary Tract Infections

Dysuria-Pyuria Syndrome (Acute Urethral Syndrome)

Subset	Usual Pathogens	IV Therapy	PO Therapy
Acute urethral syndrome	S. saprophyticus C. trachomatis E. coli (< 10⁵ cfu/ml)	Not applicable	Doxycycline 100 mg (PO) q12h × 10 days **or** Levofloxacin 500 mg q24h × 7 days

Clinical Presentation: Dysuria, frequency, urgency, lower abdominal discomfort, fevers < 102°F.
Diagnostic Considerations: Diagnosis by symptoms of cystitis with pyuria and no growth or low concentration of E. coli ($\leq 10^3$ colonies/mL) by urine culture. Clue to S. saprophyticus is alkaline urinary pH and RBCs in urine.
Pitfalls: Resembles "culture negative" cystitis.
Therapeutic Considerations: S. saprophyticus is susceptible to most antibiotics used to treat UTIs.
Prognosis: Excellent.

Acute Uncomplicated Cystitis (AUC) (see Color Atlas for Urine Gram stains)

Subset	Usual Pathogens	Therapy
Bacterial	Enterobacteriaceae E. faecalis (VSE) S. agalactiae (GBS) S. saprophyticus	Amoxicillin 500 mg (PO) × q12h × 3 days **or** TMP–SMX 1 SS tablet (PO) × q12h × 3 days **or** Levofloxacin 500 mg (PO) q24h × 3 days **or** Nitrofurantoin 100 mg (PO) q12h × 3 days
	MDR GNB	Nitrofurantoin 100 mg (PO) q12h × 3 days Doxycycline 100 mg (PO) q12h × 3 days Fosfomycin 3 gm (PO) q24h × 3 days

Acute Uncomplicated Cystitis (AUC) *(cont'd)*

Subset	Usual Pathogens	Therapy
Fungal	C. albicans[†]	Fluconazole 200 mg (PO) × 1 dose, then 100 mg (PO) q24h × 4 days
	Fluconazole-resistant[‡] **or** Non-albicans Candida **or** C. auris	Micafungin 100 mg (IV) q24h × 5 days **or** Posaconazole 400 mg (PO) q24h × 5 days

†   C. albicans cystitis (see p. 103)
‡   Fluconazole-resistant (see p. 103)

Acute Uncomplicated Cystitis (AUC)
Clinical Presentation: Dysuria, frequency, urgency, lower abdominal discomfort, fevers < 102°F.
Diagnostic Considerations: Pyuria plus bacteriuria.
Pitfalls: Compromised hosts (chronic steroids, diabetes, SLE, cirrhosis, multiple myeloma) may require 3–5 days of therapy. In normal hosts, a single dose of amoxicillin or TMP–SMX is usually sufficient in acute uncomplicated cystitis.
Therapeutic Considerations: Pyridium 200 mg (PO) q8h after meals × 24–48h is useful to decrease dysuria (inform patients urine will turn orange).
Prognosis: Excellent in normal hosts.

Candida Cystitis
Diagnostic Considerations: Marked pyuria, urine nitrate negative ± RBCs. Speciate if not C. albicans.
Pitfalls: Lack of response suggests renal candidiasis or a "fungus ball" in the renal collecting system.
Therapeutic Considerations: If fluconazole fails, use amphotericin. For chronic renal failure/dialysis patients with candiduria, use amphotericin B deoxycholate bladder irrigation (as for catheter-associated candiduria, below). Removal of devices and correction of anatomic abnormalities are critical to success.
Prognosis: Patients with impaired host defenses, abnormal collecting systems, cysts, renal disease or stones are prone to recurrent UTIs/urosepsis.

Catheter Associated Bacteriuria (CAB)/Candiduria (CAC)

Subset	Usual Pathogens	Therapy
Catheter associated bacteriuria (CAB)[†*]	E. coli E. faecalis (VSE)	Amoxicillin 500 mg (PO) q12h × 3 days Nitrofurantoin 100 mg (PO) q12h × 3 days Doxycycline 100 mg (PO) q12h × 3 days
	E. faecium (VRE)	Nitrofurantoin 100 mg (PO) q12h × 3 days **or** Fosomycin 3 gm (PO) q24h × 3 days[††]
	MDR Klebsiella[††] MDR Acinetobacter[††]	Doxycycline 100 mg (PO) q12h × 3 days Nitrofurantoin 100 mg (PO) q12h × 3 days[††]
	MDR P. aeruginosa[††]	Fosomycin 3 gm (PO) q24h × 3 days[††]
	CRE	Nitrofurantoin 100 mg (PO) q12h × 3 days[††] **or** Fosomycin 3 gm (PO) q24h × 3 days[††]
Catheter associated candiduria (CAC)[†*]	C. albicans	Fluconazole 200 mg (PO) × 1 dose, then 100 mg (PO) q24h × 1 week
	C. albicans (fluconazole resistant) Non-albicans Candida C. auris	Amphotericin B 0.3–0.6 mg/kg q24h × 1 week **or** Amphotericin B bladder irrigation (continuous: 50 mg in 1 liter sterile water over 24h × 1–2 days; intermittent: 50 mg in 200–300 ml sterile water q6-8h × 1–2 days)[§]

* **Remove/replace urinary catheter before considering antibiotic therapy.**
† **No need to treat CAB in normal hosts**, pre-emptive therapy suggested in compromised hosts, e.g., cirrhosis, SLE, DM, myeloma, steroids, immunosuppressive drugs, and those with renal insufficiency.
†† Longer courses of therapy may be needed in compromised hosts. If pyuria substantially decreased after 3 days of therapy, complete 3 days of therapy. If not, continue therapy for 7 days.

Clinical Presentation: Indwelling urinary (Foley) catheter with bacteriuria and pyuria; no symptoms.

Diagnostic Considerations: Pyuria plus bacteriuria/candiduria. Usually afebrile or temperature < 101°F.

Pitfalls: Bacteriuria/candiduria usually represent colonization, not infection. Persistent candiduria after amphotericin B deoxycholate bladder irrigation suggests renal candidiasis.

Therapeutic Considerations: Avoid treating catheter-associated bacteriuria in normal hosts without GU tract abnormalities/disease. Compromised hosts (diabetes, SLE, chronic steroids, multiple myeloma, cirrhosis) may require therapy for duration of catheterization. If bacteriuria/candiduria does not clear with appropriate therapy, change the catheter. For chronic renal failure/dialysis patients with candiduria, use amphotericin B deoxycholate bladder irrigation. Efficacy of therapy of catheter-associated candiduria is limited and relapse is frequent unless the catheter can be replaced or (preferably) removed.

Prognosis: Excellent in normal hosts. Untreated bacteriuria/candiduria in compromised hosts may result in ascending infection (e.g., pyelonephritis) or bacteremia/candidemia.

Epididymitis

Subset	Usual Pathogens	Preferred IV Therapy	Alternate IV Therapy	PO Therapy or IV-to-PO Switch
Acute *Young males*	C. trachomatis	Doxycycline 200 mg (IV) q12h × 3 days, then 100 mg (IV) q12h × 4 days	Levofloxacin 500 mg (IV) q24h × 7 days	Doxycycline 200 mg (PO) q12h × 3 days, then 100 mg (PO) q12h × 7 days* **or** Levofloxacin 500 mg (PO) q24h × 10 days
Elderly males	P. aeruginosa	Cefepime 2 gm (IV) q8h × 10 days **or** Meropenem 1 gm (IV) q8h × 10 days	Ciprofloxacin 400 mg (IV) q8h × 10 days **or** Levofloxacin 750 mg (IV) q24h × 10 days	Ciprofloxacin 750 mg (PO) q12h × 10 days **or** Levofloxacin 750 mg (PO) q24h × 10 days
Chronic	M. tuberculosis Blastomyces dermatiditis	Treat the same as pulmonary TB (see p. 55) or pulmonary blastomycosis (see Chapter 4)		

Acute Epididymitis (Chlamydia trachomatis/Pseudomonas aeruginosa)

Clinical Presentation: Acute unilateral testicular pain ± fever.

Diagnostic Considerations: Ultrasound to rule out torsion or tumor.

Pitfalls: Rule out torsion by absence of fever and ultrasound.

Therapeutic Considerations: Young males respond to treatment slowly over 1 week. Elderly males respond to anti-Pseudomonal therapy within 72 hours.

Prognosis: Excellent in young males. Related to health of host in elderly.

Chronic Epididymitis (Mycobacterium tuberculosis/ Blastomyces dermatiditis)
Clinical Presentation: Chronic epididymoorchitis with epididymal nodules.
Diagnostic Considerations: Diagnosis by AFB on biopsy/culture of epididymis. TB epididymitis is always associated with renal TB. Blastomyces epididymitis is a manifestation of systemic infection.
Pitfalls: Vasculitis (e.g., polyarteritis nodosum) and lymphomas may present the same way.
Therapeutic Considerations: Treated the same as pulmonary TB/blastomycosis.
Prognosis: Good.

Acute Pyelonephritis/cUTIs (see Color Atlas for Urine Gram stains)

Subset	Usual Pathogens	Preferred IV Therapy	Alternate IV Therapy	PO Therapy or IV-to-PO Switch
Acute pyelo-nephritis/CUTIs (Treat initially based on urine gram stain; see therapeutic considera-tions, below)	GNB	Ceftriaxone 1 gm (IV) q24h × 1 week **or** Levofloxacin 500 mg (IV) q24h × 1 week **or** Meropenem 1 gm (IV) q8h × 1 week	Delafloxacin 300 mg (IV) q12h × 1 week **or** Aztreonam 2 gm (IV) q8h × 1 week **or** Plazomicin 15 mg/kg (IV) q24h × 1 week	Levofloxacin 500 mg (PO) q24h × 1 week **or** Amoxicillin 1 gm (PO) q8h × 1 week **or** Delafloxacin 450 mg (PO) q12h × 1 week
	E. faecalis (VSE)	Ampicillin 1 gm (IV) q4h × 1 week **or** Linezolid 600 mg (IV) q12h × 1 week **or** Meropenem 1 gm (IV) q8h × 1 week	Quinolone (IV) × 1 week	Amoxicillin 1 gm (PO) q8h × 1 week **or** Linezolid 600 mg (PO) q12h × 1 week **or** Levofloxacin 500 mg (PO) q24h × 1 week
	E. faecium (VRE)	Linezolid 600 mg (IV) q12h × 1 week	Quinupristin/Dal-fopristin 7.5 mg/kg (IV) q8h × 1 week **or** Minocycline 200 mg (IV) q12h × 3 days, then 100 mg q12h × 1 week	Linezolid 600 mg (PO) q12h × 1 week **or** Minocycline 200 mg (PO) q12h × 3 days, then 100 mg (PO) q12h × 1 week

Acute Pyelonephritis/cUTIs *(cont'd)*

Subset	Usual Pathogens	Preferred IV Therapy	Alternate IV Therapy	PO Therapy or IV-to-PO Switch
	MDR GNB	Meropenem 1 gm (IV) q8h × 1 week **or** Ceftazidime/ Avibactam 2.5 gm (IV) q8h × 1 week **or** Ceftolozane/ Tazobactam 1.5 gm (IV) q8h × 1 week	Polymyxin B 1.25 mg/kg (IV) q12h × 1 week **or** Colistin 2.5 mg/kg (IV) q12h × 1 week **or** Doripenem 1 gm (IV) q8h × 1 week **or** Fosfomycin 4 gm (IV) q6h × 1 week** **or** Delafloxacin 300 mg (IV) 12h × 1 week	Delafloxacin 450 mg (PO) q12h × 1 week **or** Levofloxacin 750 mg (PO) q24h × 1 week **or** Fosfomycin 3 gm (PO) q 3 days × 1 week
	CRE	Ceftazidime/Avibactam 2.5 gm (IV) q8h × 1 week **or** Meropenem/ Vaborbactam 4 gm (IV) q8h × 1 week **or** Tigecycline 200 mg (IV) × 1 dose then 100 mg (IV) q24h × 1 week* **or** Fosfomycin 4 gm (IV) q6h × 1 week**	Polymyxin B 1.25 mg/kg (IV) q12h × 1 week **or** Colistin 2.5 mg/kg (IV) q12h × 1 week **or** Plazomicin 15 mg/kg (IV) q24h **or** Cefiderocol 2 gm (IV) q8h × 1 week **or** Impenem/ Relebactam 625 mg 600 mg/125 mg (IV) q6h × 1 week	Fosfomycin 3 gm (PO) q 3 days × 1 week

*   Depending on MICs, higher doses may be necessary: (LD) 400 mg (IV) × 1 dose, (LD) then 200 mg (IV) q24h (MD).

Chronic Pyelonephritis/Renal TB

Subset	Usual Pathogens	Preferred IV Therapy	Alternate IV Therapy	PO Therapy or IV-to-PO Switch
Chronic pyelo-nephritis	GNB	IV Therapy Not applicable	Quinolone† (PO) × 4–6 weeks **or** TMP–SMX 1 DS tab (PO) q12h × 4–6 weeks **or** Doxycycline 200 mg (PO) q12h × 3 days, then 100 mg (PO) q12h × 4–6 weeks total	
Renal TB	M. tuberculosis	IV Therapy Not applicable	Treated the same as pulmonary TB	

*   May be used in combination therapy with another CRE antibiotic.

Acute Bacterial Pyelonephritis

Clinical Presentation: Unilateral CVA tenderness with fevers $\geq$ 102°F.

Diagnostic Considerations: Bacteriuria plus pyuria with unilateral CVA tenderness and temperature $\geq$ 102°F. Bacteremia usually accompanies acute pyelonephritis; obtain blood and urine cultures.

Pitfalls: Temperature decreases in 72 hours with or without antibiotic treatment. If temperature does not fall after 72 hours of antibiotic therapy, suspect renal/perinephric abscess.

Therapeutic Considerations: Initial treatment is based on the urinary gram stain: If gram-negative bacilli, treat as Enterobacteriaceae. If gram-positive cocci in chains (enterococcus), treat as E. faecalis; if enterococcus is subsequently identified as E. faecium, treat accordingly. Acute pyelonephritis is usually treated initially for 1–3 days IV, then switched to PO to complete 4 weeks of antibiotics to minimize progression to chronic pyelonephritis. Obtain a CT/MRI in persistently febrile patients after 72 hours of antibiotics to rule out renal calculi, obstruction, abscess, or xanthomatous pyelonephritis.

Prognosis: Excellent if first episode is adequately treated with antibiotics for 4 weeks.

Chronic Bacterial Pyelonephritis

Clinical Presentation: Previous history of acute pyelonephritis with same symptoms as acute pyelonephritis but less CVA tenderness/fever.

Diagnostic Considerations: Diagnosis by CT/MRI showing changes of chronic pyelonephritis plus bacteriuria/pyuria. Urine cultures may be intermittently negative before treatment. Chronic pyelonephritis is bilateral pathologically, but unilateral clinically.

Pitfalls: Urine culture may be intermittently positive after treatment; repeat weekly × 4 to confirm urine remains culture-negative.

Therapeutic Considerations: Treat × 4–6 weeks. Impaired medullary vascular blood supply/renal anatomical distortion makes eradication of pathogen difficult.

Prognosis: Related to extent of renal damage.

Renal TB (Mycobacterium tuberculosis)

Clinical Presentation: Renal mass lesion with ureteral abnormalities (pipestem, corkscrew, or spiral ureters) microscopic hematuria/sterile pyuria. Painless unless complicated by ureteral obstruction.

Diagnostic Considerations: Combined upper/lower urinary tract abnormalities ± microscopic hematuria/urinary pH $\leq$ 5.5. Diagnosis by culture of TB from urine. Urine TB PCR is specific, but not very sensitive.

Pitfalls: Chest x-ray is normal in 50%, but most patients are PPD positive. Rule out other infectious/inflammatory causes of sterile pyuria (e.g., Trichomonas, interstitial nephritis).

Therapeutic Considerations: Treat the same as pulmonary TB.

Prognosis: Good if treated before renal parenchymal destruction/ureteral obstruction occur.

Renal Abscess (Intrarenal/Perinephric)

Subset	Usual Pathogens	Preferred IV Therapy	Alternate IV Therapy	PO Therapy or IV-to-PO Switch
Cortical	S. aureus	MSSA: Nafcillin 2 gm (IV) q4h* **or** Ceftriaxone 1 gm (IV) q24h* **or** Cefazolin 1 gm (IV) q8h*	MSSA Meropenem 1 gm (IV) q8h* **or** Ertapenem 1 gm (IV) q24h* **or** Clindamycin 600 mg (IV) q8h*	MSSA/MRSA Linezolid 600 mg (PO) q12h* **or** Minocycline 200 mg (PO) × 1, then 100 mg (PO) q12h*
		MRSA: Linezolid 600 mg (IV) q12h* **or** Minocycline 200 mg (IV) × 1, then 100 mg (IV) q12h*	MRSA Vancomycin 1 gm (IV) q12h*	
Medullary	GNB	Quinolone (IV)†*	TMP–SMX 2.5 mg/kg (IV) q6h*	Quinolone (PO)†*

*   Treat until renal abscess resolves completely or is no longer decreasing in size on CT/MRI.

†   Levofloxacin 500 mg (IV/PO) q24h.

Clinical Presentation: Similar to pyelonephritis but fever remains elevated after 72 hours of antibiotics.

Diagnostic Considerations: Obtain CT/MRI to diagnose perinephric/intra-renal abscess and rule out mass lesion. Cortical abscesses are usually secondary to hematogenous/contiguous spread. Medullary abscesses are usually due to extension of intra-renal infection.

Pitfalls: Urine cultures may be negative with cortical abscesses.

Therapeutic Considerations: Most large abscesses need to be drained. Multiple small abscesses are managed medically. Obtain urology consult.

Prognosis: Related to degree of baseline renal dysfunction.

Prostatitis/Prostatic Abscess

Subset	Usual Pathogens	Preferred IV Therapy	Alternate IV Therapy	PO Therapy or IV-to-PO Switch
Acute prostatitis/ acute prostatic abscess[†]	GNB	Quinolone* (IV) × 2 weeks **or** Ceftriaxone 1 gm (IV) q24h × 2 weeks	TMP–SMX 2.5 mg/kg (IV) q6h × 2 weeks **or** Aztreonam 2 gm (IV) q8h × 2 weeks	Quinolone* (PO) × 2 weeks **or** Doxycycline 200 mg (PO) q12h × 3 days, then 100 mg (PO) q24h × 11 days **or** TMP–SMX 1 SS tablet (PO) q12h × 2 weeks
Chronic prostatitis	GNB		Quinolone* (PO) × 1–3 months **or** TMP–SMX 1 DS tablet (PO) q12h × 1–3 months	
	MDR GNB		Fosfomycin 3 gm (PO) q 3 days × 30 days ± Doxycycline 100 mg (PO) q12h × 1–3 months	
	CRE		Fosfomycin 3 gm (PO) q 3 days × 30 days	

† May need surgical drainage of abscess.
* Levofloxacin 500 mg or Moxifloxacin 400 mg (PO) q24h.

Acute Prostatitis/Acute Prostatic Abscess (Enterobacteriaceae)

Clinical Presentation: Acute prostatitis presents as an acute febrile illness in males with dysuria and no CVA tenderness. Prostatic abscess presents with hectic/septic fevers without localizing signs.

Diagnostic Considerations: Acute prostatitis is diagnosed by bacteriuria, pyuria plus mucus threads, with exquisite prostate tenderness, and is seen primarily in young males. Positive urine culture is due to contamination of urine as it passes through infected prostate. Prostatic abscess is diagnosed by transrectal ultrasound or CT/MRI of prostate.

Pitfalls: Do not overlook acute prostatitis in males with bacteriuria without localizing signs, or prostatic abscess in patients with a history of prostatitis.

Therapeutic Considerations: Treat acute prostatitis for 2 full weeks to decrease liklihood of progression to chronic prostatitis. Prostatic abscess is treated the same as acute prostatitis plus surgical drainage.

Prognosis: Excellent if treated early with full course of antibiotics (plus drainage if prostatic abscess present).

Chronic Prostatitis

Clinical Presentation: Vague urinary symptoms (mild dysuria ± low back pain), history of acute prostatitis, and little or no fever.

Diagnostic Considerations: Diagnosis by bacteriuria plus pyuria with mucus threads. Urine, semen, or prostate expressate are culture positive.

Pitfalls: Commonest cause of treatment failure is inadequate duration of therapy. Chronic prostatitis with prostatic calcifications (transrectal ultrasound) will not clear with antibiotics; transurethral resection of prostate (TURP) with removal of all calcifications curative.

Therapeutic Considerations: Prostate penetration and antibiotic activity in the prostatic problematic, e.g. antibiotic must be lipid-soluble with a low ionization potential, and be active at prostate pH of 6 (vs. serum pH of 7.4). In sulfa-allergic patients, TMP alone may be used in place of TMP–SMX. Fosfomycin ± doxycycline may be effective in some cases where prostatic calcifications cannot be removed.

Prognosis: Excellent if treated × 1–3 months. Prostatic abscess is a rare but serious complication (may cause urosepsis).

Urosepsis (see Color Atlas for Urine Gram stains)

Subset	Usual Pathogens	Preferred IV Therapy	Alternate IV Therapy	IV-to-PO Switch
Community acquired (Treat initially based on urine Gram stain)	Entero-bacteriaceae (ESBL –)	Ceftriaxone 1 gm (IV) q24h × 7 days* **or** Levofloxacin 500 mg (IV) q24h × 7 days*	Amikacin 1 gm or 15 mg/kg (IV) q24h × 7 days* **or** Aztreonam 2 gm (IV) q8h × 7 days*	Levofloxacin 500 mg (PO) q24h × 7 days* **or** TMP–SMX 1 SS tablet (PO) q12h × 7 days*
	(ESBL +)	Meropenem 1 gm (IV) of q8h × 7 days*	Doripenem 1 gm (IV) of q8h × 7 days*	Fosfomycin 3 gm (PO) q 3 days × 7 days*
	E. faecalis (VSE) Group B streptococci (GBS)	Ampicillin 2 gm (IV) q4h × 7 days*	Meropenem 1 gm (IV) q8h × 7 days*	Amoxicillin 1 gm (PO) q8h × 7 days* **or** Levofloxacin 500 mg (PO) q24h × 7 days*
(No urine Gram stain)	GNB E. faecalis (VSE) Group B streptococci (GBS)	Meropenem 1 gm (IV) q8h × 7 days*	Piperacillin/ Tazobactam 3.375 mg (IV) q6h × 7 days*	Levofloxacin 500 mg (PO) q24h × 7 days*

Urosepsis *(cont'd)*

Subset	Usual Pathogens	Preferred IV Therapy	Alternate IV Therapy	IV-to-PO Switch
Nosocomial Related to urological procedure Treat initially for P. aeruginosa (if later identified as non-aeruginosa Pseudomonas, treat accordingly)	P. aeruginosa Enterobacter Klebsiella Serratia	Meropenem 1 gm (IV) q8h × 7 days **or** Levofloxacin 750 mg (IV) q24h × 7 days **or** Cefepime 2 gm (IV) q8h × 7 days **or** Aztreonam 2 gm (IV) q8h × 7 days	Doripenem 1 gm (IV) q8h × 7 days **or** Amikacin 1 gm or 15 mg/kg (IV) q24h × 7 days **or** Ciprofloxacin 400 mg (IV) q8h × 7 days **or** Delafloxacin 300 mg (IV) q12h × 7 days	Ciprofloxacin 750 mg (PO) q12h × 7 days **or** Levofloxacin 750 mg (PO) q24h × 7 days **or** Delafloxacin 450 mg (PO) q12h × 7 days
	MDR GNB	Meropenem 1 gm (IV) q8h × 2 weeks **or** Ceftolozane/ Tazobactam 1.5 gm (IV) q8h × 7 days	Amikacin 1 gm or 15 mg/kg (IV) q24h × 7 days **or** Fosfomycin 6–8 gm (IV) q12h × 7 days	Doxacycline 200 mg (PO) q12h × 3 days, then 100 mg (PO) q12h × 4 days **or** Fosfomycin 3 gm (PO) q24h × 7 days
	CRE	Ceftazidime/ Avibactam 2.5 gm (IV) q8h × 7 days **or** Meropenem/Vabor–bactam 4 gm (IV) q8h × 7 days **or** Tigecycline 200 mg (IV) × 1 dose then 100 mg (IV) q24h × 7 days**	Polymyxin B 1.25 mg/kg (IV) q12h × 7 days **or** Colistin 2.5 mg/kg (IV) q12h × 7 days **or** Fosfomycin 6–8 gm (IV) q12h × 7 days	Fosfomycin 3 gm (PO) q24h × 7 days

* Longer duration needed if urologic/renal abnormalities present.

** Depending on MICs, higher doses may be necessary: (LD) 400 mg (IV) × 1 dose, (LD) then 200 mg (IV) q24h (MD).

Community Acquired Urosepsis

Clinical Presentation: Sepsis from urinary tract source.

Diagnostic Considerations: Blood and urine cultures positive for same uropathogen. If patient does not have diabetes, SLE, cirrhosis, myeloma, steroids, pre-existing renal disease or obstruction, obtain CT/MRI of GU tract to rule out abscess/obstruction. Prostatic abscess is rarely a cause of urosepsis.

Pitfalls: Mixed gram-positive/negative urine cultures suggest specimen contamination or enterovesicular fistula.

Therapeutic Considerations: Empiric treatment is based on urine gram stain. If urine gram stain shows pyuria and gram-positive cocci, treat as group D enterococci (E. faecalis-VSE). If gram-negative bacilli, treat as Enterobacteriaceae. S. aureus/S. pneumoniae are not uropathogens.

Prognosis: Related to severity of underlying condition causing urosepsis and health of host.

Urosepsis Following Urological Procedures

Clinical Presentation: Sepsis within 24 hours after GU procedure.

Diagnostic Considerations: Blood and urine cultures positive for same uropathogen. Use pre-procedural urine culture to identify uropathogen and guide therapy.

Pitfalls: If non-aeruginosa Pseudomonas in urine/blood, switch to TMP–SMX pending susceptibilities.

Therapeutic Considerations: Empiric P. aeruginosa monotherapy will cover most other uropathogens.

Prognosis: Related to severity of underlying condition causing urosepsis and health of host.

Pelvic Inflammatory Disease (PID), Salpingitis, Tuboovarian Abscess, Chorioamnionitis, Endometritis/Endomyometritis, Septic Abortion

Subset	Usual Pathogens	IV Therapy	PO Therapy or IV-to-PO Switch
Hospitalized patients[†]	B. fragilis GNB N. gonorrhoeae C. trachomatis C. sordelli[§] (septic abortion)	**Monotherapy** Moxifloxacin 400 mg (IV) q24h × 2 weeks **or** **Combination Therapy** Doxycycline 200 mg (IV) q12h × 3 days, then 100 mg (IV) q12h × 11 days **plus either** Piperacillin/Tazobactam 4.5 gm (IV) q8h × 2 weeks **or** Ertapenem 1 gm (IV) q24h × 3–10 days **or** Cefoxitin 2 gm (IV) q6h × 2 weeks **or** Cefotetan 2 gm (IV) q12h × 2 weeks **Alternate Combination Therapy** Doxycycline 200 mg (IV) q12h × 3 days, then 100 mg (IV) q12h × 11 days **plus** Ampicillin/Sulbactam 3 gm (IV) q6h × 2 weeks **or** Quinolone[‡] (IV) q24h × 2 weeks **plus** Metronidazole 1 gm (IV) q24h × 2 weeks	**Monotherapy** Moxifloxacin 400 mg (PO) q24h × 2 weeks
Outpatients (mild PID only)	N. gonorrhoeae C. trachomatis B. fragilis GNB	Moxifloxacin 400 mg (PO) q24h × 2 weeks** **or** Doxycycline 100 mg (PO) q12h × 2 weeks	

†   Treat only IV or IV-to-PO switch for salpingitis, tuboovarian abscess, endometritis, endomyometritis, septic abortion, or severe PID.

‡   Levofloxacin 500 mg (IV or PO) q24h or Ofloxacin 400 mg (IV or PO) q12h.

**   Increasing gonococcal resistance to quinolones requires careful follow-up during/after therapy.

§   Antibiotic therapy of septic abortion same as salpingitis/endometritis plus evacuation of uterine contents.

Clinical Presentation: PID/salpingitis presents with cervical motion/adnexal tenderness, lower quadrant abdominal pain, and fever. Endometritis/endomyometritis presents with uterine tenderness ± cervical discharge/fever. Endomyometritis is the most common postpartum infection.

Diagnostic Considerations: Unilateral lower abdominal pain in a female without a non-pelvic cause suggests PID/salpingitis.

Pitfalls: Obtain CT/MRI of abdomen/pelvis to confirm diagnosis and rule out other pathology or tuboovarian abscess.

Therapeutic Considerations: Tuboovarian abscess usually requires drainage/removal ± TAH/BSO, plus antibiotics (see p. 113) × 1–2 weeks after drainage/removal. Septic abortion is treated the same as endometritis/endomyometritis plus uterine evacuation.

Prognosis: Related to promptness of treatment/adequacy of drainage if tuboovarian abscess. Late complications of PID/salpingitis include tubal scarring/infertility.

Empiric Therapy of Sexually Transmitted Diseases

Urethritis/Cervicitis

Subset	Usual Pathogens	Preferred Therapy	Alternate Therapy
Gonococcal (GC)	N. gonorrhoeae	Ceftriaxone 250 mg (IM) × 1 dose	Cefixime[†] 400 mg (PO) × 1 dose[†] **plus** Azithromycin[†] 1 gm (PO) × 1 dose[†] **or** Doxycycline 100 mg (PO) of q12h × 7 days
Non-gonococcal (NGU)	C. trachomatis U. urealyticum M. genitalium	Doxycycline 100 mg (PO) q12h × 7 days[‡] **or** Quinolone[*†] (PO) × 7 days	Azithromycin 1 gm (PO) × 1 dose[*]
	Trichomonas vaginalis	Tinidazole 2 gm (PO) × 1 dose	Metronidazole 2 gm (PO) × 1 dose

[†]   Increased resistance with oral regimens. Should be considered as alternate second line therapy and test of cure essential.

[‡]   Doxycycline may also be given as 200 mg (PO) q24h × 7 days.

[*]   Increasing M. genitalium resistance.

Gonococcal Urethritis/Cervicitis

Clinical Presentation: Purulent penile/cervical discharge with burning/dysuria 3–5 days after contact.

Diagnostic Considerations: Rapid diagnosis in males by Gram stain of urethral discharge showing gram-negative diplococci; urethral cultures also positive. In females, diagnosis requires identification of organism by culture or DNA probe, not Gram stain. Rapid diagnosis in males/females by DNA probe. Obtain throat/rectal culture for N. gonorrhoeae. Co-infections are common; obtain syphilis and HIV serologies.

Pitfalls: Gram stain of cervical discharge showing gram-negative diplococci is not diagnostic of N. gonorrhoeae; must confirm by culture or nucleic acid amplification. N. gonorrhoeae infections are asymptomatic in 10% of men and 70% of women.

Therapeutic Considerations: Failure to respond suggests re-infection or relapse. Treat all GC with ceftriaxone. Because of frequent coinfection with agents of NGU, add oral azithromycin. Because of increasing resistance, consider using azithromycin 2 gm for dual therapy in patients with GC.

Prognosis: Good even with disseminated infection.

Non-Gonococcal Urethritis/Cervicitis

Clinical Presentation: Mucopurulent penile/cervical discharge ± dysuria ~ 1 week after contact.

Diagnostic Considerations: Diagnosis by positive chlamydial NAAT/Ureaplasma or Mycoplasma NAAT of urethral/cervical discharge. Evaluate urethral/cervical discharge to rule out N. gonorrhoeae. Co-infections are common; obtain syphilis and HIV serologies.

Pitfalls: C. trachomatis infections are asymptomatic in 25%.

Therapeutic Considerations: Failure to respond to doxycycline therapy suggests re-infection or Trichomonas/Ureaplasma/Mycoplasma infection. Failure to respond to azithromycin suggests trichomoniasis, or infection due to a resistant Mycoplasma (consider quinolone therapy).

Prognosis: Tubal scarring/infertility in chronic infection.

Trichomonas Urethritis/Cervicitis (Trichomonas vaginalis)

Clinical Presentation: Frothy, pruritic vaginal discharge.

Diagnostic Considerations: Trichomonas by wet mount/culture on special media.

Pitfalls: Classic "strawberry cervix" is infrequently seen.

Therapeutic Considerations: Use week-long regimen if single dose fails. Resistance now recognized as a cause of treatment failure.

Prognosis: Excellent if partner is also treated.

Vaginitis/Vaginosis

Subset	Usual Pathogens	PO Therapy
Bacterial vaginosis/ vaginitis	Polymicrobial (Gardnerella vaginalis, Mobiluncus, Prevotella, M. hominis, etc.)	Tinidazole 1 gm (PO) q24h × 5 days **or** Tinidazole 2 gm (PO) q24h × 2 days **or** Clindamycin 300 mg (PO) q12h × 7 days **or** Metronidazole 500 mg (PO) q12h × 7 days
Candida vaginitis/ balanitis	Candida albicans	Fluconazole 150 mg (PO) × 1 dose[†]

† Those failing to respond should be treated with Fluconazole 200 mg (PO) × 1 dose then 100 mg (PO) q24h × 1 week.

Bacterial Vaginosis/Vaginitis
Clinical Presentation: Non-pruritic vaginal discharge with "fishy" odor.
Diagnostic Considerations: Diagnosis by "clue cells" in vaginal fluid wet mount. Vaginal pH ≥ 4.5.
Pitfalls: "Fishy" odor from smear of vaginal secretions intensified when 10% KOH solution is added (positive "whiff test").
Therapeutic Considerations: As an alternative to oral therapy, clindamycin cream 2% intravaginally qHS × 7 days (avoid in pregnancy) or metronidazole gel 0.075% 1 application intravaginally q12h × 5 days can be used.
Prognosis: Complications include premature rupture of membranes, premature delivery, increased risk of PID. Recurrences very common.

Candida Vaginitis/Balanitis
Clinical Presentation: Pruritic white plaques in vagina/erythema of glans penis.
Diagnostic Considerations: Diagnosis by gram stain/culture of whitish plaques.
Pitfalls: Rule out Trichomonas, which also presents with pruritus in females.
Therapeutic Considerations: Uncomplicated vaginitis (mild sporadic infections in healthy individuals) responds readily to single-dose therapy. Complicated vaginitis (severe, recurrent, or in difficult-to-control diabetes) often requires ≥ 7 days of therapy (daily topical therapy or 2 doses of fluconazole 150 mg given 72h apart). Non-albicans infections respond poorly to azoles. Topical boric acid (600 mg/d in a gelatin capsule × 14 days) is often effective in this setting.

Prognosis: Good with systemic therapy. Diabetics/uncircumcised males may need prolonged therapy.

Genital Vesicles (HSV-2/HSV-1)

Subset	PO Therapy
Initial therapy	Acyclovir 200 mg (PO) 5×/day × 10 days **or** Famciclovir 500 mg (PO) q12h × 7–10 days **or** Valacyclovir 1 gm (PO) q12h × 3 days
Recurrent/ intermittent therapy (< 6 episodes/year)	Acyclovir 200 mg (PO) 5×/day × 5 days **or** Valacyclovir 500 mg [PO] q24h × 5 days; <u>HIV positive</u>: 1 gm [PO] q12h × 7–10 days** **or** Famciclovir 125 mg [PO] q12h × 5 days **or** 1 gm [PO] q12h × 1 day* <u>HIV-positive</u>: 500 mg [PO] q12h × 7 days
Chronic suppressive therapy (> 6 episodes/year)	Acyclovir 400 mg (PO) q12h × 1 year **or** Valacyclovir 1 gm [PO] q24h × 1 year; <u>HIV-positive</u>: 500 mg [PO] q12h × 1 year **or** Famciclovir 250 mg (PO) q12h × 1 year

*   Patient initiated therapy to be started immediately when recurrence begins.
** Short-course therapy with Valaciclovir 500 mg (PO) q12h × 3 days or Acyclovir 800 mg (PO) q8h × 2 days also effective.

Genital Herpes

Clinical Presentation: Painful vesicles/ulcers on genitals with painful bilateral regional adenopathy ± low-grade fever.
Diagnostic Considerations: Diagnosis by clinical presentation may be misleading.
Pitfalls: 70% of newly acquired gential herpes is due to HSV-1. Elevated IgG HSV-2 titer indicates past exposure, not acute infection. HSV-2 IgM titers may be negative.
Therapeutic Considerations: If concomitant rectal herpes, increase acyclovir to 800 mg (PO) q8h × 7 days. For recurrent genital herpes, use acyclovir or valacyclovir (dose same as primary infection) for 7 days after each relapse. Recurrent episodes of HSV-2 are less painful than primary infection, and inguinal adenopathy is less prominent/painful.
Prognosis: HSV-2 tends to recur, especially during the first year. HSV-1 recurrences less frequent.

Genital Ulcers

Subset	Usual Pathogens	IM Therapy	PO Therapy
Primary syphilis	Treponema pallidum	Benzathine penicillin 2.4 mu (IM) × 1 dose	Doxycycline 100 mg (PO) q12h × 2 weeks **or** Azithromycin 2 gm (PO) × 1 dose**
Chancroid	Hemophilus ducreyi	Ceftriaxone 250 mg (IM) × 1 dose **or** Any 3rd generation cephalosporin 250–500 mg (IM) × 1 dose	Azithromycin 1 gm (PO) × 1 dose **or** Quinolone* (PO) × 3 days **or** Erythromycin base 500 mg (PO) q8h × 7 days

*   Ciprofloxacin 500 mg q12h or Levofloxacin 500 mg or Moxifloxacin 400 mg q24h.
** Resistance increasing (followup essential).

Primary Syphilis (Treponema pallidum)
Clinical Presentation: Painless, indurated ulcers (chancres) with bilateral painless inguinal adenopathy. Syphilitic chancres are elevated, clean and indurated, but not undermined.
Diagnostic Considerations: Diagnosis by spirochetes on darkfield examination of ulcer exudate. Elevated non-treponemal (VDRL/RPR) titers after 1 week.
Pitfalls: Non-treponemal (VDRL/RPR) titers fall slowly within 1 year; failure to decline suggests treatment failure/HIV. Even after effective treatment some patients remain VDRL/RPR positive for life (serofast).
Therapeutic Considerations: Parenteral penicillin is the preferred antibiotic for all stages of syphilis. If treatment fails and VDRL/RPR titers do not decline, obtain HIV serology.
Prognosis: Good with early treatment.

Chancroid (Hemophilus ducreyi)
Clinical Presentation: Ragged, undermined, painful ulcer(s) + painful unilateral inguinal adenopathy.
Diagnostic Considerations: Diagnosis by streptobacilli in "school of fish" configuration on gram- stained smear of ulcer exudate/culture of H. ducreyi/NAAT.
Pitfalls: Co-infection is common; obtain Syphilis and HIV serologies.
Therapeutic Considerations: In HIV, multiple dose regimens or azithromycin is preferred. Resistance to erythromycin/ciprofloxacin has been reported.
Prognosis: Good with early treatment.

Suppurating Inguinal Adenopathy

Subset	Pathogens	PO Therapy
Lympho-granuloma venereum (LGV)	Chlamydia trachomatis (L$_{1-3}$ serotypes)	Doxycycline 100 mg (PO) q12h × 3 weeks **or** Erythromycin base 500 mg (PO) q6h × 3 weeks
Granuloma inguinale (Donovanosis)	Klebsiella (Calymmato-bacterium) granulomatis	Azithromycin 1 gm (PO) q week until cured. **or** Doxycycline 100 mg (PO) q12h until cured **or** Erythromycin 500 mg (PO) q6h until cured **or** TMP–SMX 1 DS (PO) q12h until cured **or** Ciprofloxacin 750 mg (PO) q12h until cured

Lymphogranuloma Venereum (Chlamydia trachomatis) LGV
Clinical Presentation: Unilateral inguinal adenopathy ± discharge/sinus tract.
Diagnostic Consideration: Diagnosis by very high Chlamydia trachomatis L$_{1-3}$ titers. Do not biopsy site (often does not heal and may form a fistula). May present as FUO.
Pitfalls: Initial papule not visible at clinical presentation. Biopsy shows granulomas; may be confused with perianal Crohn's disease.
Therapeutic Considerations: Rectal LGV may require additional courses of treatment.
Prognosis: Fibrotic perirectal/pelvic damage does not reverse with therapy.

Granuloma Inguinale (Klebsiella [Calymmatobacterium] granulomatis) Donovanosis
Clinical Presentation: Pseudolymphadenopathy with painless inguinal ulcers.
Diagnostic Considerations: Donovan bodies ("puffed-wheat" appearance) in tissue biopsy.
Pitfalls: No true inguinal adenopathy, as opposed to LGV infection.
Therapeutic Considerations: Doxycycline or azithromycin preferred. Continue therapy until lesions are healed.
Prognosis: Good if treated early.

Genital/Perianal Warts (Condylomata acuminata)

Subset	Pathogens	Therapy
Genital/perianal warts	Human papilloma virus (HPV)	Podophyllin 10–25% in tincture of benzoin or podofilox or imiquimod (patient applies) **or** surgical/laser removal/cryotherapy with liquid nitrogen **or** cidofovir gel (1%) QHS × 5 days every other week for 6 cycles **or** trichloracetic acid (TCA)/bichloracetic acid (BCA) **or** intralesional interferon. Sinecatechins (15% ointment) q8h × 4 months

Clinical Presentation: Single/multiple verrucous genital lesions ± pigmentation, without inguinal adenopathy.

Diagnostic Considerations: Diagnosis by clinical appearance. Genital warts are usually caused by HPV types 6, 11. Anogenital warts caused by HPV types 16,18,31,33,35 and others are associated with cervical neoplasia. Females with anogenital warts need serial cervical PAP smears to detect cervical dysplasia/neoplasia.

Pitfalls: Most HPV infections are asymptomatic.

Therapeutic Considerations: Cidofovir cures/halts HPV progression in 50% of cases.

Prognosis: Related to HPV serotypes with malignant potential (HPV types 16,18,31, 33,35). Preventative (not therapeutic) vaccines now available.

Syphilis

Subset	Pathogen	IV/IM Therapy	PO Therapy
Primary, secondary, or early latent syphilis (duration < 1 year)	Treponema pallidum	Benzathine penicillin 2.4 mu (IM) × 1 dose	Doxycycline 100 mg (PO) q12h × 2 weeks **or** Azithromycin 2 gm (PO) × 1 dose*
Late latent or tertiary syphilis (duration > 1 year)	Treponema pallidum	Benzathine penicillin 2.4 mu (IM) weekly × 3 weeks	Doxycycline 100 mg (PO) q12h × 4 weeks **or** Amoxicillin 1 gm (PO) q8h plus probenecid 1 gm (PO) q24h × 4 weeks
Neurosyphilis	Treponema pallidum	Penicillin G 3–4 mu (IV) q4h × 10–14 days **or** Ceftriaxone 2 gm (IV) q24h × 10–14 days **or** Alternate: Procaine penicillin 2.4 mu (IM) q24h × 10–14 days plus probenecid 500 mg (PO) q6h × 10–14 days	Doxycycline 200 mg (PO) q12h × 4 weeks

* Resistance increasing (careful follow up essential).

Duration of therapy represents total time IV, IM, or PO. All stages of syphilis in HIV patients usually respond to therapeutic regimens recommended for normal hosts. Syphilis in pregnancy should be treated according to the stage of syphilis; penicillin-allergic pregnant patients should be desensitized and treated with penicillin.

Primary Syphilis (Treponema pallidum)

Clinical Presentation: Painless, indurated ulcer(s) (chancre) with bilateral painless inguinal adenopathy.

Diagnostic Considerations: Diagnosis by spirochetes on darkfield or DFA examination of ulcer exudate. Reactive non-treponemal (VDRL/RPR) or treponemal (TPPA, others) test after 1 week. Patients with ↑ low titers of VDRL/RPR and – treponemal test may be BFP, e.g., SLE.

Pitfalls: VDRL/RPR titers fall slowly within 1 year; failure to decline suggests treatment failure.

Therapeutic Considerations: Parenteral penicillin is the preferred antibiotic for all stages of syphilis; if treatment fails and VDRL/RPR titers do not decline, obtain HIV serology. Some effectively treated patients remain VDRL/RPR positive in low titers eg 1:4 (serofast) for years.

Prognosis: Good with early treatment.

Secondary Syphilis (Treponema pallidum)

Clinical Presentation: Facial/truncal macular, papular, papulosquamous, non-pruritic, non-tender, symmetrical rash which may involve the palms/soles. Usually accompanied by generalized adenopathy. Typically appears 4–10 weeks after primary chancre, although stages may overlap. Alopecia, condyloma lata, mucous patches, iritis/uveitis may be present. Renal involvement ranges from mild proteinuria to nephrotic syndrome. Without treatment, spontaneous resolution occurs after 3–12 weeks.

Diagnostic Considerations: Diagnosis by clinical findings and VDRL/RPR in high titers (≥ 1:64). After treatment, RPR/VDRL titers usually ↓ × 4 < 6 months.

Pitfalls: If only undiluted serum is tested, prozone phenomenon may render VDRL/RPR falsely negative.

Therapeutic Considerations: Parenteral penicillin is the preferred antibiotic for all stages of syphilis.

Prognosis: Excellent with early treatment.

Latent Syphilis (Treponema pallidum)

Clinical Presentation: Patients are asymptomatic with elevated non-treponemal titers and reactive treponemal tests.

Diagnostic Considerations: Diagnosis by positive serology ± prior history, but no signs/symptoms of syphilis. Asymptomatic syphilis < 1 year in duration is termed "early" latent syphilis; asymptomatic syphilis > 1 year/unknown duration is termed "late" latent syphilis. Secondary syphilis may relapse in up to 25% of patients with early latent syphilis, but relapse is rare in late latent syphilis. Evaluate patients for neurosyphilis.

Pitfalls: Treponemal tests (FTA-ABS, MHA-TP, TPPA, others) usually remain positive for life, even after adequate treatment.

Therapeutic Considerations: Parenteral penicillin is the preferred antibiotic for all stages of syphilis. Repeat VDRL/RPR titers at 6, 12, and 24 months; therapeutic response is defined as a 4-fold reduction in RPR/VDRL titers (2 tube dilutions).

Prognosis: Excellent even if treated late.

Tertiary Syphilis (Treponema pallidum)

Clinical Presentation: May present with aortitis, neurosyphilis, iritis, or gummata 5–30 years after initial infection.

Diagnostic Considerations: Diagnosis by history of syphilis plus positive serological tests with signs/symptoms of late syphilis.

Pitfalls: Treat for signs of neurosyphilis on clinical exam or LP, even if VDRL/RPR are non-reactive.

Therapeutic Considerations: Parenteral penicillin is the preferred antibiotic for all stages of syphilis.

Prognosis: Related to extent of end-organ damage.

Neurosyphilis (Treponema pallidum)

Clinical Presentation: Patients are often asymptomatic, but may have ophthalmic/auditory symptoms, cranial nerve abnormalities, tabes dorsalis, paresis, psychosis, or signs of meningitis/dementia.

Diagnostic Considerations: Diagnosis by elevated CSF VDRL titers; no need to obtain CSF FTA-ABS titers. Diagnosis confirmed if CSF has pleocytosis (> 5 WBCs/hpf) or increased protein (> 50 mg/dL), and positive VDRL.

Pitfalls: Persistent CSF abnormalities suggest treatment failure. CSF VDRL (60% sensitive) may be negative in neurosyphilis.

Therapeutic Considerations: Parenteral penicillin is the preferred antibiotic for all stages of syphilis. CSF abnormalities should decrease in 6 months and return to normal after 2 years; repeat lumbar puncture 6 months after treatment. Failure rate with ceftriaxone is 20%.

Prognosis: Related to extent of end-organ damage.

Empiric Therapy of Bone and Joint Infections

Septic Arthritis/Bursitis

Subset	Usual Pathogens	Preferred IV Therapy	Alternate IV Therapy	PO Therapy or IV-to-PO Switch
Acute (Treat initially based on Gram stain of synovial fluid. If gram-positive cocci in clusters, treat initially for MRSA; if later identified as MSSA, treat accordingly)	S. aureus (MSSA)	Cefazolin 1 gm (IV) q8h × 3 weeks **or** Ceftriaxone 1 gm (IV) q24h × 3 weeks **or** Nafcillin 2 gm (IV) q4h × 3 weeks	Levofloxacin 500 mg (IV) q24h × 3 weeks **or** Ertapenem 1 gm (IV) q24h × 3 weeks **or** Clindamycin 600 mg (IV) q8h × 3 weeks	Cephalexin 1 gm (PO) q6h × 3 weeks **or** Clindamycin 300 mg (PO) q8h× 3 weeks **or** Quinolone* (PO) q24h × 3 weeks
	S. aureus (MRSA)[†]	Linezolid 600 mg (IV) q12h × 3 weeks **or** Minocycline 200 mg (IV) × 1, then 100 mg (IV) q12h × 3 weeks **or** Delafloxacin 300 mg (IV) q12h × 3 weeks **or** Quinupristin/Dalfopristin 7.5 mg/kg (IV) q8h × 3 weeks		Linezolid 600 mg (PO) q12h × 3 weeks **or** Minocycline 200 mg (PO) × 1, then 100 mg (PO) q12h × 3 weeks **or** Delafloxacin 450 mg (IV) q12h × 3 weeks
	Group A,B,C,G streptococci	Ceftriaxone 1 gm (IV) q24h × 3 weeks **or** Quinolone* (IV) q24h × 3 weeks	Cefazolin 1 gm (IV) q8h × 3 weeks **or** Clindamycin 600 mg (IV) q8h × 3 weeks	Clindamycin 300 mg (PO) q8h × 3 weeks **or** Cephalexin 500 mg (PO) q6h × 3 weeks **or** Quinolone* (PO) q24h × 3 weeks

*   Moxifloxacin 400 mg or Levofloxacin 500 mg or Delafloxacin 450 mg (PO) q12h
†   Vancomycin doesn't penetrate well into synovial fluid.

Septic Arthritis/Bursitis *(cont'd)*

Subset	Usual Pathogens	Preferred IV Therapy	Alternate IV Therapy	PO Therapy or IV-to-PO Switch
Acute	GNB	Ceftriaxone 1 gm (IV) q24h × 3 weeks **or** Cefepime 2 gm (IV) q12h × 3 weeks	Aztreonam 2 gm (IV) q8h × 3 weeks **or** Respiratory quinolone[‡] (IV) × 3 weeks	Respiratory quinolone[‡] (PO) × 3 weeks
	P. aeruginosa	Meropenem 1 gm (IV) q8h × 3 weeks **or** Levofloxacin 500 mg (IV) q24h × 3 weeks	Aztreonam 2 gm (IV) q8h × 3 weeks **or** Cefepime 2 gm (IV) q8h × 3 weeks	Ciprofloxacin 750 mg (PO) q12h × 3 weeks **or** Levofloxacin 750 mg (PO) q24h × 3 weeks
	N. gonorrhea (PSNG/PPNG)	Ceftriaxone 1 gm (IV) q24h × 2 weeks	Levofloxacin 500 mg (IV) q24h × 2 weeks **or** Moxifloxacin 400 mg (IV) q24h × 2 weeks	Levofloxacin 500 mg (PO) q24h × 2 weeks **or** Moxifloxacin 400 mg (PO) q24h × 2 weeks
	Salmonella	Ceftriaxone 2 gm (IV) q24h × 2–3 weeks **or** Respiratory quinolone* (IV) × 2–3 weeks	Aztreonam 2 gm (IV) q8h × 2–3 weeks **or** TMP–SMX 2.5 mg/kg (IV) q6h × 2–3 weeks	Respiratory quinolone* (PO) × 2–3 weeks **or** TMP–SMX 1 DS tablet (PO) q12h × 2–3 weeks

*   Levofloxacin 500 mg (IV or PO) q24h or Moxifloxacin 400 mg (IV or PO) q24h.

Septic Arthritis/Bursitis (cont'd)

Subset	Usual Pathogens	Preferred IV Therapy	Alternate IV Therapy	PO Therapy or IV-to-PO Switch
Secondary to animal bite wound	Pasteurella multocida Streptobacillus moniliformis Eikinella corrodens	Piperacillin/Tazobactam 3.375 gm (IV) q6h × 2 weeks **or** Ampicillin/Sulbactam 3 gm (IV) q6h × 2 weeks **or** Ticarcillin/Clavulanate 3.1 gm (IV) q6h × 2 weeks	Meropenem 1 gm (IV) q8h × 2 weeks **or** Ertapenem 1 gm (IV) q24h × 2 weeks **or** Doxycycline 200 mg (IV) q12h × 3 days, then 100 mg (IV) q12h × 11 days	Amoxicillin/Clavulanic acid 875/125 mg (PO) q12h × 2 weeks **or** Doxycycline 200 mg (PO) q12h × 3 days, then 100 mg (PO) q12h × 11 days[†] **or** Moxifloxacin 400 mg (PO) q24h × 2 weeks
Fungal arthritis	Coccidioides immitis	Not applicable	Itraconazole 200 mg (PO) solution q12h × 12 months or until cured* **or** Fluconazole 800 mg (PO) q24h until cured*	
	Sporothrix schenckii	Not applicable	Itraconazole 200 mg (PO) q12h until cured*	
TB arthritis	M. tuberculosis	Not applicable	Treat the same as for pulmonary TB (p. 55) except treat for 6–9 months	

* Itraconazole solution provides more reliable absorption than capsules.

Acute Septic Arthritis/Bursitis

Clinical Presentation: Acute joint pain with fever. Septic joint unable to bear weight. Septic bursitis presents with pain on joint motion, but patient is able to bear weight.

Diagnostic Considerations: Diagnosis by demonstrating organisms in synovial fluid by stain/culture. In septic bursitis (knee most common), there is pain on joint flexion (although the joint can bear weight), and synovial fluid findings are negative for septic arthritis. Except for N. gonorrhoeae, polyarthritis is not usually due to bacterial pathogens. Post-infectious polyarthritis is usually viral in origin, most commonly due to parvovirus B19, rubella, or HBV.

Pitfalls: Reactive arthritis may follow C. jejuni, Salmonella, Shigella, Yersinia, N. gonorrheae C. trachomatis, or C. difficile infections. Synovial fluid cultures are negative. Reactive arthritis is usually asymmetrical and is monoarticular/oligoarticular.

Therapeutic Considerations: See specific pathogen, below. Treat septic bursitis as septic arthritis.

Staphylococcus aureus (MSSA/MRSA)

Diagnostic Considerations: Painful hot joint; unable to bear weight. Diagnosis by synovial fluid pleocytosis and positive culture for joint pathogen. Examine synovial fluid to rule out gout (doubly birefringent crystals) and pseudogout (calcium pyrophosphate crystals). May occur in setting of endocarditis with septic emboli to joints; other manifestations of endocarditis are usually evident.

Pitfalls: Rule out causes of noninfectious arthritis (sarcoidosis, Whipple's disease, Ehlers-Danlos, etc.), which are less severe, but may mimic septic arthritis. In reactive arthritis following urethritis (C. trachomatis, Ureaplasma urealyticum, N. gonorrhoeae) or diarrhea (Shigella, Campylobacter, Yersinia, Salmonella), synovial fluid culture is negative, and synovial fluid WBCs counts are usually < 10,000/mm³ with normal synovial fluid lactic acid and glucose. Do not overlook infective endocarditis in mono/polyarticular MSSA/MRSA septic arthritis without apparent source.

Therapeutic Considerations: For MRSA septic arthritis, vancomycin penetration into synovial fluid is poor; use linezolid instead. Immobilization of infected joint during therapy is helpful. Local installation of antibiotics into synovial fluid has no advantage over IV/PO antibiotics.

Prognosis: Treat as early as possible to minimize joint damage. Repeated aspiration/ open drainage may be needed to preserve joint function.

Group A, B, C, G Streptococci

Diagnostic Considerations: Usually monoarticular. Not usually due to septic emboli from endocarditis.

Prognosis: Related to extent of joint damage and rapidity of antibiotic treatment.

Enterobacteriaceae

Diagnostic Considerations: Diagnosis by isolation of gram-negative bacilli from synovial fluid.

Pitfalls: Septic arthritis involving an unusual joint (e.g., sternoclavicular, sacral) should suggest IV drug abuse until proven otherwise.

Therapeutic Considerations: Joint aspiration is essential in suspected septic arthritis of the hip and may be needed for other joints; obtain orthopedic surgery consult. Local installation of antibiotics into joint fluid is of no proven value.

Prognosis: Related to extent of joint damage and rapidity of antibiotic treatment.

Pseudomonas aeruginosa
Diagnostic Considerations: P. aeruginosa septic arthritis/osteomyelitis may occur after water contaminated puncture wound (e.g., nail puncture of heel through shoes). Sternoclavicular/sacroiliac joint involvement is common in IV drug abusers (IVDAs).
Pitfalls: Suspect IVDA in P. aeruginosa septic arthritis without a history of trauma.
Therapeutic Considerations: If ciprofloxacin is used, treat with 750 mg (not 500 mg) dose for P. aeruginosa septic arthritis/osteomyelitis.
Prognosis: Related to extent of joint damage and rapidity of antibiotic treatment.

Neisseria gonorrhoeae
Diagnostic Considerations: Gonococcal arthritis may present as a monoarticular or polyarticular arthritis as part of gonococcal arthritis-dermatitis syndrome (disseminated gonococcal infection). Bacteremia with positive blood cultures occurs early during rash stage while synovial fluid cultures are negative. Joint involvement follows with typical findings of septic arthritis and synovial fluid cultures positive for N. gonorrhoeae; blood cultures are negative at this stage. Acute tenosynovitis is often a clue to gonococcal septic arthritis.
Pitfalls: Spectinomycin is ineffective against pharyngeal gonorrhea.
Therapeutic Considerations: GC arthritis-dermatitis syndrome is caused by very susceptible.
Prognosis: Excellent with arthritis-dermatitis syndrome; worse with monoarticular arthritis.

Salmonella sp.
Diagnostic Considerations: Occurs in sickle cell disease and hemoglobinopathies. Diagnosis by blood/joint cultures.
Pitfalls: S. aureus, not Salmonella, is the most common cause of septic arthritis in sickle cell disease.
Prognosis: Related to severity of infection and underlying health of host.

Septic Arthritis Secondary to Animal Bite Wound
Clinical Presentation: Penetrating bite wound into joint space.
Diagnostic Considerations: Diagnosis by smear/culture of synovial fluid/blood cultures.
Pitfalls: May develop metastatic infection from bacteremia.
Therapeutic Considerations: Treat for at least 2 weeks of combined IV/PO therapy.
Prognosis: Related to severity of infection and underlying health of host.

Chronic Septic Arthritis

Clinical Presentation: Subacute/chronic joint pain with decreased range of motion and little or no fever. Able to bear weight on joint.

Diagnostic Considerations: Diagnosis by smear/culture of synovial fluid/synovial biopsy.

Coccidioides immitis

Diagnostic Considerations: Must grow organisms from synovium/synovial fluid for diagnosis.

Pitfalls: Synovial fluid the same as in TB (lymphocytic pleocytosis, low glucose, increased protein).

Therapeutic Considerations: Oral therapy is preferred; same cure rates as amphotericin regimens.

Prognosis: Related to severity of infection and underlying health of host.

Sporothrix schenckii

Diagnostic Considerations: Usually a monoarticular infection secondary to direct inoculation/trauma.

Pitfalls: Polyarticular arthritis suggests disseminated infection.

Therapeutic Considerations: SSKI is useful for lymphocutaneous sporotrichosis, not bone/joint involvement.

Prognosis: Excellent for localized disease (e.g., lymphocutaneous sporotrichosis). In disseminated disease, prognosis is related to host factors.

Mycobacterium tuberculosis (TB)

Diagnostic Considerations: Clue is subacute/chronic tenosynovitis over involved joint. Unlike other forms of septic arthritis, which are usually due to hematogenous spread, TB arthritis may complicate adjacent TB osteomyelitis. Synovial fluid findings include lymphocytic pleocytosis, low glucose, and increased protein.

Pitfalls: Send synovial biopsy for AFB smear/culture in unexplained chronic monoarticular arthritis.

Therapeutic Considerations: TB arthritis is usually treated for 6–9 months.

Prognosis: Related to severity of infection and underlying health of host.

Lyme Arthritis

Subset	Usual Pathogens	Preferred IV Therapy	Alternate IV Therapy	PO Therapy or IV-to-PO Switch
Lyme arthritis		Ceftriaxone 1 gm (IV) q24h × 4 weeks **or** Doxycycline 200 mg (IV) q12h × 3 days, then 100 mg (IV) q12h × 4 weeks	Ceftizoxime 2 gm (IV) q8h × 4 weeks	Amoxicillin 1 gm (PO) q8h × 4 weeks **or** Doxycycline 200 mg (PO) q12h × 3 days, then 100 mg (PO) q12h × 4 weeks

* See p. 21 for Lyme neuroborreliosis and p. 78 for Lyme myocarditis.
† Doxycycline therapy × 10 days as effective as 2 weeks.
‡ For adult patients intolerant of Amoxicillin, Doxycycline if the patient is not pregnant, or Azithromycin (500 mg orally per day for 28 days), Clarithromycin (500 mg orally twice per day for 28 days), may be given. The recommended dosages of these agents for children are as follows: Azithromycin, 10 mg/kg per day (maximum of 500 mg per day); Clarithromycin, 7.5 mg/kg twice per day (maximum of 500 mg per dose); and Erythromycin, 12.5 mg/kg 4 times per day (maximum of 500 mg per dose).

Lyme Arthritis
Clinical Presentation: Acute Lyme arthritis presents with joint pain, decreased range of motion, ability to bear weight on joint, and little or no fever. Chronic Lyme arthritis resembles rheumatoid arthritis.
Diagnostic Considerations: Usually affects children and large weight-bearing joints (e.g., knee). Acute Lyme arthritis is diagnosed by clinical presentation plus elevated IgM Lyme titer. Chronic Lyme arthritis is suggested by rheumatoid arthritis-like presentation with negative ANA and rheumatoid factor, and positive IgG Lyme titer and synovial fluid PCR.
Pitfalls: Acute Lyme arthritis joint is red but not hot, in contrast to septic arthritis. In chronic Lyme arthritis, a negative IgG Lyme titer essentially rules out chronic Lyme arthritis, but an elevated IgG Lyme titer indicates only past exposure to B. burgdorferi and is not diagnostic of Lyme arthritis. Joint fluid in chronic Lyme disease is usually negative by culture, but positive by PCR; synovial fluid PCR, however, does not differentiate active from prior infection.
Therapeutic Considerations: IgG Lyme titers remain elevated for life, and do not decrease with treatment. Joint symptoms often persist for months/years after effective antibiotic therapy due to autoimmune joint inflammation; treat with anti-inflammatory drugs, not repeat antibiotic courses. Oral therapy as effective as IV therapy.
Prognosis: Good in normal hosts. Chronic/refractory arthritis may develop in genetically predisposed patients with DRW 2 or HLA types.

Infected Joint Prosthesis

Subset	Usual Pathogens	Preferred IV Therapy	Alternate IV Therapy	IV-to-PO Switch
Staphylococcal (Treat initially for MSSA; if later identified as MRSA/CoNS, treat accordingly)	S. epidermidis (CoNS)	Linezolid 600 mg (IV) q12h* **or** Meropenem 1 gm (IV) q8h*	Cefotaxime 2 gm (IV) q6h*† **or** Ceftizoxime 2 gm (IV) q8h*†	Linezolid 600 mg (PO) q12h*
	S. aureus (MSSA)	Nafcillin 2 gm (IV) q4h* **or** Cefazolin 1 gm (IV) q8h*	Meropenem 1 gm (IV) q8h* **or** Ceftriaxone 1 gm (IV) q24h*† **or** Clindamycin 600 mg (IV) q8h* **or** Minocycline 100 mg (IV) q12h*	Minocycline 100 mg (PO) q12h* **or** Linezolid 600 mg (PO) q12h* **or** Clindamycin 300 mg (PO) q8h*
	S. aureus (MRSA)	Linezolid 600 mg (IV) q12h* **or** Minocycline 100 mg (IV) q12h* **or** Delafloxacin 300 mg (IV) q12h* **or** Quinupristin/Dalfopristin 7.5 mg/kg (IV) q8h*		Linezolid 600 mg (PO) q12h* **or** Minocycline 100 mg (PO) q12h* **or** Delafloxacin 450 mg (PO) q12h*

* Treat for 1 week after joint prosthesis is replaced. † Only if MSSE strain susceptible.

Clinical Presentation: Pain in area of prosthesis with joint loosening/instability ± low-grade fevers.

Diagnostic Considerations: Infected prosthesis is suggested by prosthetic loosening/lucent areas adjacent to prosthesis on plain films ± positive blood cultures. Diagnosis confirmed by bone scan. Use joint aspiration to identify organism.

Pitfalls: An elevated ESR with prosthetic loosening suggests prosthetic joint infection. Mechanical loosening without infection is comon many years after joint replacement, but ESR is normal.

Therapeutic Considerations: Infected prosthetic joints usually must be removed for cure. Replacement prosthesis may be inserted anytime after infected prosthesis is removed. To prevent infection of new joint prosthesis, extensive debridement of old infected material is important. If replacement of infected joint prosthesis is not possible, chronic suppressive therapy may be used with oral antibiotics e.g., minocycline 100 mg (PO) q12h. TMP–SMX 5 mg/kg (PO) q6h may be successful in long-term suppression/cure in total hip replacement (treat × 6 months) or total knee replacement (treat × 9 months) due to susceptible strains of MSSA/MSSE; adding rifampin 300 mg (PO) q12h may be helpful.

Prognosis: Related to adequate debridement of infected material when prosthetic joint is removed.

Osteomyelitis

Subset	Usual Pathogens	Preferred IV Therapy	Alternate IV Therapy	PO Therapy or IV-to-PO Switch
Acute (Treat initially for MSSA; if later identified as MRSA or Enterobacteriaceae, treat accordingly)	S. aureus (MSSA)	Nafcillin 2 gm (IV) q4h × 4–6 weeks **or** Cefazolin 1 gm (IV) q8h × 4–6 weeks **or** Ceftriaxone 1 gm (IV) q24h × 4–6 weeks	Meropenem 1 gm (IV) q8h × 4–6 weeks **or** Tigecycline 200 mg (IV) × 1 dose, then 100 mg (IV) q24h × 4–6 weeks	Cephalexin 1 gm (PO) q6h × 4–6 weeks **or** Respiratory quinolone‡ (PO) q24h × 4–6 weeks
	S. aureus (MRSA)	Tigecycline 200 mg (IV) × 1 dose, then 100 mg (IV) q24h × 4–6 weeks **or** Linezolid 600 mg (IV) q12h × 4–6 weeks **or** Minocycline 100 mg (IV) q12h × 4–6 weeks **or** Vancomycin 2 gm (IV) q12h × 4–6 weeks **or** Ceftaroline fosamil 600 mg (IV) q12h × 4–6 weeks **or** Dalafloxacin 300 mg (IV) q12h × 4–6 weeks		Linezolid 600 mg (PO) q12h × 4–6 weeks **or** Minocycline 100 mg (PO) q12h × 4–6 weeks **or** Delafloxacin 450 mg (PO) q12h × 4–6 weeks
	GNB	Ceftriaxone 1 gm (IV) q24h × 4–6 wks **or** Tigecycline 200 mg (IV) × 1 dose, then 100 mg (IV) q24h × 4–6 weeks	Quinolone† (IV) × 4–6 weeks **or** Fosfomycin 6–12 gm (IV) q12h × 4–6 weeks	Quinolone† (PO) × 4–6 weeks **or** Fosfomycin 3 gm (PO) q24h × 4–6 weeks

Osteomyelitis *(cont'd)*

Subset	Usual Pathogens	Preferred IV Therapy	Alternate IV Therapy	PO Therapy or IV-to-PO Switch
Chronic Diabetes mellitus (DM) Peripheral vascular disease (PVD)	S. aureus (MSSA) E. coli P. mirabilis K. pneumoniae GAS GBS B. fragilis	Tigecycline 200 mg (IV) × 1 dose, then 100 mg (IV) q24h × 2–4 weeks **or** Meropenem 1 gm (IV) q8h* **or** Ertapenem 1 gm (IV) q24h* **or** Piperacillin/ Tazobactam 3.375 gm (IV) q6h*	**Monotherapy** Moxifloxacin 400 mg (IV) q24h* **or** Ceftizoxime 2 gm (IV) q8h* **or** Ampicillin/ Sulbactam 3 gm (IV) q6h* **or** **Combination Therapy** Ceftriaxone 1 gm (IV) q24h* **plus** Metronidazole 1 gm (IV) q24h*	**Monotherapy** Moxifloxacin 400 mg (PO) q24h* **or** **Combination Therapy** Clindamycin 300 mg (PO) q8h* **plus** Levofloxacin 500 mg (PO) q24h*
	S. aureus (MRSA) ± GNB B. fragilis	Minocycline 200 mg (IV) × 1, then 100 mg (IV) q12h × 2–4 weeks **or** Linezolid 600 mg (IV) q12h × 4–6 weeks **or** Tigecycline 200 mg (IV) × 1 dose, then 100 mg (IV) q24h × 2–4 weeks	Minocycline 200 mg (IV) × 1, then 100 mg (IV) q12h × 2–4 weeks **plus** Levofloxacin 500 mg (IV) q24h	Minocycline 200 mg (PO) × 1, then 100 mg (PO) q12h × 2–4 weeks **plus** Quinolone[†] (PO) q24h × 2–4 weeks
Chronic (cont'd)	Brucella	Doxycycline 200 mg (IV) q12h × 3 days, then 100 mg (IV) q12h until cured	Doxycycline 200 mg (IV) q12h × 3 days, then 100 mg (IV) q12h until cured	Doxycycline 200 mg (PO) q12h × 3 days, then 100 mg (PO) q12h until cured[†] **plus** Rifampin 600 mg (PO) q24h until cured

Osteomyelitis *(cont'd)*

Subset	Usual Pathogens	Preferred IV Therapy	Alternate IV Therapy	PO Therapy or IV-to-PO Switch
TB osteomyelitis	M. tuberculosis	Treat the same as pulmonary TB (p. 55), but extend treatment to 6–9 months		

*   Treat for 1 week after adequate debridement or amputation.
†   Moxifloxacin 400 mg or Levofloxacin 500 mg.

Acute Osteomyelitis

Clinical Presentation: Tenderness over infected bone. Fever and positive blood cultures common.

Diagnostic Considerations: Diagnosis by elevated ESR with positive bone scan. Bone biopsy is not needed for diagnosis. Bone scan is positive for acute osteomyelitis in first 24 hours.

Pitfalls: Earliest sign on plain films is soft tissue swelling; bony changes evident after 2 weeks.

Therapeutic Considerations: Treat 4–6 weeks with antibiotics. Debridement is not necessary for cure.

Prognosis: Related to adequacy/promptness of treatment.

Chronic Osteomyelitis
Diabetes Mellitus (DM)

Clinical Presentation: Afebrile or low-grade fever with normal WBC counts and deep penetrating ulcers ± draining sinus tracts.

Diagnostic Considerations: Diagnosis by elevated ESR and bone changes on plain films. Bone scan is not needed for diagnosis. Bone biopsy is preferred method of demonstrating organisms, since blood cultures are usually negative and cultures from ulcers/sinus tracts are unreliable.

Pitfalls: P. aeruginosa is a common colonizer and frequently cultured from deep ulcers/sinus tracts, but is not a pathogen in chronic osteomyelitis in diabetics.

Therapeutic Considerations: Surgical debridement is needed for cure; antibiotics alone are ineffective. Revascularization procedures usually do not help, since diabetes is a microvascular disease. Do not culture penetrating foot ulcers/draining sinus tracts; culture results reflect superficial flora. Bone biopsy during debridement is the best way to identify pathogen; if biopsy not possible, treat empirically.

Prognosis: Related to adequacy of blood supply/surgical debridement.

Peripheral Vascular Disease (PVD)

Clinical Presentation: Absent or low-grade fever with normal WBC counts ± wet/dry digital gangrene.

Diagnostic Considerations: Diagnosis by clinical appearance of dusky/cold foot ± wet/dry gangrene. Chronic osteomyelitis secondary to PVD/open fracture is often poly-microbial.

Pitfalls: Wet gangrene usually requires surgical debridement/antibiotic therapy; dry gangrene may not.

Therapeutic Considerations: Surgical debridement needed for cure. Antibiotics alone are ineffective. Revascularization procedure may help treat infection by improving local blood supply.

Prognosis: Related to degree of vascular compromise.

Brucella Osteomyelitis (Brucella sp.)

Diagnostic Considerations: May be evidence of brucellosis elsewhere (epididymoor-chitis). Suspect in patients with a history of animal/raw milk/cheese exposure. Serologic diagnosis by serum SAT, ELISA, or PCR.

Pitfalls: Brucella has predilection for vertebra, sacroiliac joints. Erosions of anterior vertebra adjacent to disc space typical vs. TB with diffuse vertebral destruction.

Therapeutic Considerations: May require 6 weeks of antibiotic therapy.

Prognosis: Joint destruction usually permanent.

TB Osteomyelitis (Mycobacterium tuberculosis)

Clinical Presentation: Presents similarly to chronic bacterial osteomyelitis. Vertebral TB (Pott's disease) affects disk spaces early and presents with chronic back/neck pain ± inguinal/paraspinal mass.

Diagnostic Considerations: Diagnosis by AFB on biopsy/culture of infected bone. T-spot PPD–positive.

Pitfalls: Chest x ray is normal in 50%. May be confused with cancer, brucella osteomyelitis or chronic bacterial osteomyelitis.

Therapeutic Considerations: Treated the same as TB arthritis.

Prognosis: Good for non-vertebral TB/vertebral (if treated before paraparesis/paraplegia).

Empiric Therapy of Skin and Soft Tissue Infections

Cellulitis, Erysipelas, Mastitis (uSSSIs)

Subset	Usual Pathogens	Preferred IV Therapy		PO Therapy or IV-to-PO Switch
Above or Below-the-waist	Group A, B streptococci (GAS) (GBS)	Ceftriaxone 1–2 gm (IV) q24h × 2 weeks **or** Cefazolin 1 gm (IV) q8h × 2 weeks	Quinolone* (IV) of q24h × 2 weeks **or** Clindamycin 600 mg (IV) q8h × 2 weeks	Cephalexin 500 mg (PO) q6h × 2 weeks **or** Clindamycin 300 mg (PO) q6h × 2 weeks **or** Quinolone* (PO) q24h × 2 weeks

uSSSIs = uncomplicated skin skin structure infections.
* Moxifloxacin 400 mg or Levofloxacin 500 mg.

Clinical Presentation: Cellulitis presents as warm, painful, flat, non-pruritic skin erythema without discharge. Erysipelas resembles cellulitis but is raised and sharply demarcated. Mastitis presents as cellulitis of the breast cellulitis caused by groups A, B, C or G streptococci. Aspiration of streptococcal cellutitis is serous/serosanguinous fluid not purulent (as with MSSA/MRSA abscesses). MSSA/MRSA causes cutaneous abscesses, not cellulitis. MSSA/MRSA abscesses raised, warm, and tender ± bullae. No regional adenopathy or lymphangitis.

Diagnostic Considerations: Diagnosis by clinical appearance ± culture of pathogen from aspirated skin lesion(s). Group B streptococci are important pathogens in diabetics. Lower extremity cellulitis tends to recur. Chronic lymphedema or edema of an extremity predisposes to recurrent/persistent cellulitis.

Pitfalls: Streptococcal cellulitis often accompanied by lymphangitis and regional adenopathy; fever/chills common.

Therapeutic Considerations: Lower extremity cellulitis requires ~ 1 week of antibiotics to improve. Patients with peripheral vascular disease, chronic venous stasis, alcoholic cirrhosis, and diabetes take 1–2 weeks longer to improve and often require 3–4 weeks of treatment. Treat mastitis as cellulitis above-the-waist, and drain surgically if an abscess is present.

Prognosis: Related to degree of micro (DM) and or macrovascular (PVD) insufficiency.

Complicated Skin/Skin Structure Infections (cSSSIs)

Subset	Usual Pathogens	Preferred IV Therapy		IV-to-PO Switch
Mixed aerobic-anaerobic deep soft tissue infection	GNB Group A streptococci (GAS) S. aureus (MSSA) Anaerobic streptococci Fusobacterium	Piperacillin/Tazobactam 3.375 gm (IV) q6h × 2 weeks **or** Ertapenem 1 gm (IV) q24h × 2 weeks	Meropenem 1 gm (IV) q8h × 2 weeks **or** Moxifloxacin 400 mg (IV) q24h × 2 weeks	**Monotherapy** Moxifloxacin 400 mg (PO) q24h × 2 weeks **or** **Combination Therapy** Levofloxacin 500 mg (PO) q24h × 2 weeks **plus** Clindamycin 300 mg (PO) q8h × 2 weeks
Clostridial myonecrosis (gas gangrene)	Clostridium sp.	Penicillin G 10 mu (IV) q4h × 2 weeks **or** Piperacillin/Tazobactam 3.375 gm (IV) q6h × 2 weeks	Clindamycin 600 mg (IV) q8h × 2 weeks **or** Ertapenem 1 gm (IV) q24h × 2 weeks	
Necrotizing fasciitis/ Fournier's gangrene*	Group A streptococci (GAS) Anaerobic streptococci (MSSA)	Piperacillin/Tazobactam 3.375 gm (IV) q6h × 2 weeks* **or** Ertapenem 1 gm (IV) q24h × 2 weeks	Tigecycline 200* mg (IV) × 1 dose, then 100 mg (IV) q24h × 2 weeks*	Clindamycin 300 mg (PO) q8h × 2 weeks **plus** Levofloxacin 500 mg (PO) q24h × 2 weeks
	MRSA	Daptomycin 6 mg/kg (IV) q24h × 2 weeks	Tigecycline 200* mg (IV) × 1 dose, then 100 mg (IV) q24h × 2 weeks*	Minocycline 200 mg (PO) × 1, then 100 mg (PO) q12h × 2 weeks **or** Delafloxacin 450 mg (PO) q12h × 2 weeks
Phlegmon, abscesses	MRSA MSSA	Tigecycline 200 mg (IV) × 1 dose, then 100 mg (IV) q24h × 2 weeks **or** Daptomycin 6 mg/kg (IV) q24h × 2 weeks **or** Linezolid 600 mg (IV) q12h × 2 weeks **or** Tedizolid 200 mg (IV) q24h × 6 days, then 200 mg (PO) q24h × 6 days **or** Telavancin 10 mg/kg (IV) q24h × 2 weeks **or** Dalbavancin 1 gm (IV) × 1 dose, then 500 mg (IV) 7 days later		Linezolid 600 mg (PO) q12h × 2 weeks **or** Minocycline 200 mg (PO) × 1, then 100 mg (PO) q12h × 2 weeks **or** Delafloxacin 450 mg (PO) q12h × 2 weeks

cSSSIs = complicated skin skin structure infections.
* if due to GAS, ± Clindamycin 600 mg (IV) q8h × 2 weeks for antitoxin effect.

Complicated Skin/Skin Structure Tissue Infection (cSSSIs) *(cont'd)*

Subset	Usual Pathogens	Preferred IV Therapy	IV-to-PO Switch
Pyomyositis/ necrotizing abscesses	Community-acquired MRSA (CA-MRSA)§	Daptomycin 6 mg/kg (IV) q24h × 2 weeks **or** Linezolid 600 mg (IV) q12h × 2 weeks	Linezolid 600 mg (PO) q12h × 2 weeks **or** Minocycline 200 mg (PO) × 1, then 100 mg (PO) q12h × 2 weeks

§   CA-MRSA PVL-positive strains.

Mixed Aerobic/Anaerobic Deep Soft Tissue Infection

Clinical Presentation: Local pain/tenderness ± gross gas deep in soft tissues and usually high fevers. More common in diabetics.

Diagnostic Considerations: Diagnosed clinically. Bacteriologic diagnosis by gram stain/culture of aspirated fluid. Patients usually have high fevers. Wound discharge is foul when present.

Pitfalls: Gross crepitance/prominent gas in soft tissues on x-ray suggests a mixed aerobic/anaerobic necrotizing infection, not gas gangrene. Gas gangrene extremely rare in diabetics.

Therapeutic Considerations: Prompt empiric therapy and surgical debridement may be lifesaving.

Prognosis: Related to severity of infection, adequacy of debridement, and underlying health of host.

Gas Gangrene (Clostridial Myonecrosis)

Clinical Presentation: Fulminant infection of muscle with little or n fever. Infected area is extremely painful, indurated, and discolored with or without bullae.

Diagnostic Considerations: Diagnosis is clinical. Aspiration of infected muscle shows few PMNs and gram-positive bacilli without spores (C. perfringens only). Gas gangrene is not accompanied by high fever. Patients are often apprehensive with relative bradycardia ± diarrhea. Wound discharge, if present, is sweetish and not foul. Rapidly progressive hemolytic anemia is characteristic.

Pitfalls: Gas gangrene (clostridial myonecrosis) has little visible gas on plain film x-rays; abundant gas should suggest a mixed aerobic/anaerobic infection, not gas gangrene. Gas gangrene extremely rare in diabetics.

Therapeutic Considerations: Surgical debridement is life saving and the only way to control infection.

Prognosis: Related to speed/extent of surgical debridement. Progression/death may occur in hours.

Necrotizing Fasciitis

Clinical Presentation: Acutely ill patient with high fevers and extreme local pain without gas in tissues. If scrotum involved (± abdominal wall involvement), the diagnosis is Fournier's gangrene.

Diagnostic Considerations: Diagnosis by CT/MRI shows infection involving the fascial planes. Skin is gray/necrotic, vessels thrombosed with no bleeding or surgery, "dishwater pus" is typical. Muscles fail to contract. A finger easily separates tissue planes.

Pitfalls: Extreme pain in patients with deep soft tissue infections should suggest a compartment syndrome/necrotizing fasciitis. No hemolytic anemia, diarrhea, or bullae as with gas gangrene.

Therapeutic Considerations: Control/cure of infection requires surgical debridement of all necrotic tissue, and antimicrobial therapy. Clindamycin may be added for its anti-exotoxin effects if due to group A streptococci.

Prognosis: Related to rapidity/extent of surgical debridement.

Phlegmon/Abscesses

Clinical Presentation: MSSA/MRSA infection often accompanied by bullae. A phlegmon is a pre-abscess before abscess wall formation. MSSA/MRSA abscesses are clinically indistinguishable from other abscesses, but remain the most common pathogens in cSSSI abscesses.

Diagnostic Considerations: Diagnosis of cellulitis and abscesses is clinical. Demonstration of fascitis, phlegmons, or abscesses are by imaging studies by CT/MRI.

Pitfalls: Bullae with cellulitis should suggest MSSA/MRSA (not group A streptococci). Bullae in DM/bullous diseases are not accompanied by fever/cellulitis.

Therapeutic Considerations: Cellulitis and phlegmons may be treated with antibiotic therapy alone. Fasciitis and abscesses usually require debridement (fasciitis) or drainage (abscesses).

Prognosis: Good if treated appropriately/early.

Pyomyositis/Necrotizing Abscesses (CA-MRSA)

Clinical Presentation: Abrupt onset of severe/deep muscle infection ± large abscesses should suggest community-acquired MRSA (CA-MRSA).

Diagnostic Considerations: The diagnosis of CA-MRSA is made on the basis of the distinctively fulminant/severe clinical presentation and by culturing MRSA from muscle/abscess. If available, test isolate for SCC mec IV ± Panton-Valentine leukocidin (PVL) gene.

Pitfalls: CA-MRSA susceptible to clindamycin, TMP–SMX, and doxycycline.

Therapeutic Considerations: Prompt/complete incision and drainage of abscesses and early use of anti-CA-MRSA drugs may be life-saving. Antibiotics effective against CA-MRSA (TMP–SMX, clindamycin, doxycycline) are ineffective against CO-MRSA/HA-MRSA; antibiotics effective against CO-MRSA/HA-MRSA are also effective against

CA-MRSA (see p. 15). Use minocycline instead of doxycline for CA-MRSA/CO-MRSA. Doxycycline resistance with CA-MRSA of concern. Minocycline more effective than doxycycline, TMP-SMX or clindamycin for CA-MRSA.

Prognosis: Related to presence of PVL gene CA-MRSA. CA-MRSA PVL negative infections are similar in severity to MSSA infections.

Skin Ulcers

Subset	Usual Pathogens	Preferred IV Therapy	Alternate IV Therapy	PO Therapy or IV-to-PO Switch
Decubitus ulcers **No osteomyetis** (stage I/II ulcers)	S. aureus (MSSA)	Cefazolin 1 gm (IV) q8h* **or** Ceftriaxone 1 gm (IV) q24h*	Cefotaxime 2 gm (IV) q6h* **or** Ceftizoxime 2 gm (IV) q8h*	Cephalexin 500 mg (PO) q6h* **or** Levofloxacin 500 mg (PO) q24h*
Chronic osteomyelitis (stage III/IV ulcers)	B. fragilis Group A streptococci (GAS) S. aureus (MSSA) S. aureus (MRSA)[†] GNB *(not P. aeruginosa[§])*	Eravacycline 1 mg/kg (IV) q12h[†] **or** Tigecycline 100 mg (IV) × 1 dose, then 50 mg (IV) q12h* **or** Piperacillin/ Tazobactam 3.375 gm (IV) q6h* **or** Moxifloxacin 400 mg (IV) q24h*	Meropenem 1 gm (IV) q8h* **or** Ertapenem 1 gm (IV) q24h*	**Monotherapy** Moxifloxacin 400 mg (PO) q24h* **or** **Combination Therapy** Clindamycin 300 mg (PO) q8h* **plus** Levofloxacin 500 mg (PO) q24h*

*   Treat Stages I/II (superficial) decubitus ulcers with local care. If no underlying chronic osteomyelitis, treat Stages III/IV (deep) decubitus ulcers with antibiotics and adequate bone debridement.

†   MRSA: Tigecycline 100 mg (IV) × 1 dose then 50 mg (IV) q12h* alone or one of above non-MRSA antibiotics plus [Daptomycin 4 mg/kg (IV) q24h* or Linezolid 600 mg (IV) q12h*] or Vancomycin 1 gm (IV) q12h* or Minocycline 100 mg (IV) q12h*. PO therapy or IV-to-PO switch if MRSA: Linezolid 600 mg (PO) q12h* or Minocycline 100 mg (PO) q12h* plus one of above antibiotics.

§   Deep penetrating ulcers (stage III/IV) in diabetics represent underlying chronic osteomyelitis and are not due to P. aeruginosa. However, P. aeruginosa (a water associated organism) can be cultured from > 90% of deep diabetic foot ulcers and only represents superficial colonization (from moist socks, moist dressings, whirlpool baths, etc.) is not a pathogen in diabetic foot ulcers with underlying chronic osteomyelitis.

Skin Ulcers *(cont'd)*

Subset	Usual Pathogens	Preferred IV Therapy	Alternate IV Therapy	PO Therapy or IV-to-PO Switch
Chronic Osteomyelitis Diabetic foot ulcers	S. aureus (MSSA) Group A, B streptococci B. fragilis GNB	Eravacycline 1 mg/kg (IV) q12h[†] **or** Tigecycline 200 mg (IV) × 1 dose, then 100 mg (IV) q24h[†] **or** Piperacillin/ Tazobactam 3.375 gm (IV) q6h[†] **or** Moxifloxacin 400 mg (IV) q24h[†] **or** Eravacycline 1 mg/kg (IV) q12h[†]	Ampicillin/ Sulbactam 3 gm (IV) q6h[†] **or** Ertapenem 1 gm (IV) q24h[†]	**Monotherapy** Moxifloxacin 400 mg (PO) q24h[†] **or** **Combination Therapy** Minocycline 200 mg (PO) × 1, then 100 mg (PO) q12h[†] **plus** Levofloxacin 500 mg (PO) q24h[†]
	S. aureus (MRSA)	Tigecycline 200 mg (IV) × 1 dose, then 100 mg (IV) q24h[†] **or** Daptomycin 4 mg/kg (IV) q24h[†] **or** Linezolid 600 mg (IV) q12h[†] **or** Minocycline 200 mg (IV) × 1, then 100 mg (IV) q12h[†]	Telavancin 10 mg/kg (IV) q24h[†] **or** Delafloxacin 300 mg (IV) q12h[†] **or** Dalbavancin 1 gm (IV) × 1 dose, then 500 mg (IV) 7 days later	Linezolid 600 mg (PO) q12h[†] **or** Minocycline 200 mg (PO) × 1, then 100 mg (PO) q12h[†] **or** Delafloxacin 450 mg (PO) q12h[†]

[†] Treat × 1 week after adequate bone debridement/amputation.

Skin Ulcers (cont'd)

Subset	Usual Pathogens	Preferred IV Therapy	Alternate IV Therapy	PO Therapy or IV-to-PO Switch
Ischemic foot ulcers	S. aureus (MRSA)	Treat the same as for deep/complicated diabetic foot ulcers (see above)		
	S. aureus (MSSA) Group A streptococci (GAS) E. coli	Cefazolin 1 gm (IV) q8h × 2 weeks **or** Ceftriaxone 1 gm (IV) q24h × 2 weeks	Quinolone* (IV) q24h × 2 weeks	Quinolone* (PO) q24h × 2 weeks

* Levofloxacin 500 mg or Moxifloxacin 400 mg.

Decubitus Ulcers/Chronic Osteomyelitis

Clinical Presentation: Painless ulcers with variable depth and infectious exudate ± fevers ≤ 102°F.

Diagnostic Considerations: Diagnosis by clinical appearance. Obtain ESR/bone scan to rule out underlying osteomyelitis with deep (Stage III/IV) decubitus ulcers.

Pitfalls: Superficial decubitus ulcers do not require systemic antibiotics.

Therapeutic Considerations: Deep decubitus ulcers require antibiotics and debridement, superficial ulcers do not. Coverage for B. fragilis is needed for deep perianal decubitus ulcers. Good nursing care is important in preventing/limiting extension of decubitus ulcers.

Prognosis: Related to fecal contamination of ulcer and bone involvement (e.g., osteomyelitis).

Diabetic Foot Ulcers/Chronic Osteomyelitis

Clinical Presentation: Ulcers/sinus tracts on bottom of foot/between toes; usually painless. Fevers ≤ 102°F and a foul smelling exudate are common.

Diagnostic Considerations: In diabetics, deep, penetrating, chronic foot ulcers/draining sinus tracts are diagnostic of chronic osteomyelitis. ESR ≥ 100 mm/hr in a diabetic with a foot ulcer/sinus tract is diagnostic of chronic osteomyelitis. Foot films confirm chronic osteomyelitis. Bone scan is needed only in acute osteomyelitis.

Pitfalls: Do not rely on culture results of deep ulcers/sinus tracts to choose antibiotic coverage, since cultures reflect skin colonization, not bone pathogens. Treat empirically.

Therapeutic Considerations: B. fragilis coverage is required in deep penetrating diabetic foot ulcers/fetid foot infection. P. aeruginosa is often cultured from diabetic foot ulcers/sinus tracts, but represents colonization, not infection. P. aeruginosa is a "water" organism that colonizes feet from moist socks/dressings, irrigant solutions, or whirlpool baths. Surgical debridement is essential for cure of chronic osteomyelitis in diabetics. Treat superficial diabetic foot ulcers the same as cellulitis in non-diabetics (see p. 132).

Prognosis: Related to adequacy of debridement of infected bone.

Ischemic Foot Ulcers

Clinical Presentation: Ulcers often clean/dry ± digital gangrene. No fevers/exudate.

Diagnostic Considerations: Diagnosis by clinical appearance/location in a patient with peripheral vascular disease. Ischemic foot ulcers most commonly affect the toes, medial malleoli, dorsum of foot, or lower leg.

Pitfalls: In contrast to ulcers in diabetics, ischemic ulcers due to peripheral vascular disease usually do not involve the plantar surface of the foot.

Therapeutic Considerations: Dry gangrene should not be treated with antibiotics unless accompanied by signs of systemic infection. Wet gangrene should be treated as a mixed aerobic/anaerobic infection. Both dry/wet gangrene may require debridement for cure/control. Do not rely on ulcer cultures to guide treatment; treat empirically if necessary. Evaluate for revascularization.

Prognosis: Related to degree of vascular insufficiency.

Skin Abscesses/Infected Cysts (Skin Pustules, Skin Boils, Furunculosis) (uSSSIs/cSSSIs)

Subset	Usual Pathogens	Preferred IV Therapy	Alternate IV Therapy	PO Therapy or IV-to-PO Switch
cSSSIs (Deep/ multiple skin abscesses) (Treat initially for MSSA; if later identified as MRSA, treat accordingly)	S. aureus (MRSA)	Tigecycline 200 mg (IV) × 1 dose, then 100 mg (IV) q24h × 2 weeks **or** Linezolid 600 mg (IV) q12h × 2 weeks **or** Daptomycin 4 mg/kg (IV) q24h × 2 weeks **or** Minocycline 200 mg (IV) × 1, then 100 mg (IV) q12h × 2 weeks **or** Ceftaroline 600 mg (IV) q12h × 2 weeks **or** Delafloxacin 300 mg (IV) q12h × 2 weeks **or** Vancomycin 1 mg (IV) q12h × 2 weeks **or** Dalbavancin 1.5 gm (IV) × 1 dose* **or** Telavancin 10 mg/kg (IV) q24h × 2 weeks **or** Oritavancin 1200 mg (IV) × 1 dose		Linezolid 600 mg (PO) q12h × 2 weeks **or** Minocycline 200 mg (PO) × 1, then 100 mg (PO) q12h × 2 weeks **or** Delafloxacin 450 mg (PO) q12h × 2 weeks
	S. aureus (MSSA)	Cefazolin 1 gm (IV) q8h × 2 weeks **or** Nafcillin 2 gm (IV) q4h × 2 weeks	Clindamycin 600 mg (IV) q8h × 2 weeks **or** Ceftriaxone 1gm (IV) q24h × 2 weeks	Cephalexin 500 mg (PO) q6h × 2 weeks **or** Clindamycin 300 mg (PO) q8h × 2 weeks

uSSSIs = uncomplicated skin skin structure infections; cSSSIs = complicated skin skin structure infections.
* 300 mL infusion may be given by peripheral IV over 30 min.

Skin Abscesses/Infected Cysts (Skin Pustules, Skin Boils, Furunculosis) (uSSSIs/cSSSIs) *(cont'd)*

Subset	Usual Pathogens	Preferred IV Therapy	Alternate IV Therapy	PO Therapy or IV-to-PO Switch
uSSSIs *Infected pilonidal cysts*	Group A strepto-cocci (GAS) S. aureus (MSSA) GNB	Cefazolin 1 gm (IV) q8h × 2 weeks **or** Ceftriaxone 1 gm (IV) q24h × 2 weeks	Levofloxacin 500 mg (IV) q24h × 2 weeks **or** Moxifloxacin 400 mg (IV) q24h × 2 weeks **or** Ceftizoxime 2 gm (IV) q8h × 2 weeks	Levofloxacin 500 mg (PO) q24h × 2 weeks **or** Moxifloxacin 400 mg (PO) q24h × 2 weeks
Hydradenitis suppurativa	S. aureus (MSSA)	Not applicable	TMP–SMX 1 SS tablet (PO) q12h × 2–4 weeks **or** Clindamycin 300 mg (PO) q8h × 2–4 weeks **or** Minocycline 200 mg (PO) × 1, then 100 mg (PO) q12h × 2–4 weeks	
	S. aureus (MRSA)	Not applicable	Minocycline 200 mg (PO) × 1, then 100 mg (PO) q12h × 2–4 weeks	

uSSSIs = uncomplicated SSSIs.
cSSSIs = complicated SSSIs.

Skin Abscesses (MSSA/MRSA)

Clinical Presentation: Warm painful nodules ± bullae, low-grade fever ± systemic symptoms, no lymphangitis. Skin boils/furunculosis present as acute, chronic, or recurrent skin pustules, and remain localized without lymphangitis.

Diagnostic Considerations: Specific pathogen diagnosed by gram stain of abscess. Recurring S. aureus abscesses are not uncommon and should be drained. Blood cultures are rarely positive. Suspect Job's syndrome if recurring abscesses with peripheral eosinophilia. Skin boils/furunculosis are diagnosed by clinical appearance (skin pustules).

Pitfalls: Recurring S. aureus skin infections may occur on immune basis but immunologic studies are usually negative.

Therapeutic Considerations: Repeated aspiration of abscesses may be necessary. Surgical drainage is required if antibiotics fail. Treat boils/furunculosis as in hydradenitis suppurativa.

Prognosis: Excellent if treated early.

Infected Pilonidal Cysts

Clinical Presentation: Chronic drainage from pilonidal cysts.

Diagnostic Considerations: Diagnosis by clinical appearance. Deep/systemic infection is rare.

Pitfalls: Culture of exudate is usually unhelpful.

Therapeutic Considerations: Surgical debridement is often necessary.

Prognosis: Good with adequate excision.

Hydradenitis Suppurativa (MSSA/MRSA)

Clinical Presentation: Chronic, indurated, painful, raised axillary/groin lesions ± drainage/sinus tracts.

Diagnostic Considerations: Diagnosis by clinical appearance/location of lesions. Infections are often bilateral and tend to recur.

Pitfalls: Surgical debridement is usually not necessary unless deep/extensive infection.

Therapeutic Considerations: Most anti-S. aureus antibiotics have poor penetration and usually fail.

Prognosis: Good with recommended antibiotics. Surgery, if necessary, is curative.

Skin Vesicles (Non-Genital)

Subset	Pathogen	Therapy
Herpes simplex	Herpes simplex virus (HSV)	Acyclovir 400 mg (PO) q8h × 10 days **or** Valacyclovir 1 gm (PO) q12h × 7–10 days **or** Famciclovir 250 mg (PO) q8h × 10 days
Chickenpox	Varicella zoster virus (VZV)	Acyclovir 800 mg (PO) q6h × 5 days **or** Valacyclovir 1 gm (PO) q8h × 5 days **or** Famciclovir 500 mg (PO) q8h × 5 days
Herpes zoster *Dermatomal zoster (shingles)*	Varicella zoster virus (VZV)	Acyclovir 800 mg (PO) 5x/day × 7–10 days **or** Valacyclovir 1 gm (PO) q8h × 7–10 days **or** Famciclovir 500 mg (PO) q8h × 7–10 days
Disseminated zoster		<u>IV therapy:</u> Acyclovir 10 mg/kg (IV) q8h × 7–10 days <u>PO therapy:</u> Valacyclovir 1 gm (PO) q8h × 7–10 days **or** Famciclovir 500 mg (PO) q8h × 7–10 days
Herpes whitlow	HSV-1	Acyclovir 400 mg (PO) q8h × 7–10 days **or** Valacyclovir 1 gm (PO) q12h × 7–10 days **or** Famciclovir 250 mg (PO) q8h × 7–10 days

Herpes Simplex (HSV)

Clinical Presentation: Painful, sometimes pruritic vesicles that form pustules or painful erythematous ulcers. Associated with fever, myalgias.

Diagnostic Considerations: Diagnosis by clinical appearance and demonstration of HSV by culture of vesicle fluid/vesicle base. May be severe in HIV.

Pitfalls: Painful vesicular lesions surrounded by prominent induration distinguishes HSV from insect bites (pruritic) and cellulitis (no induration).

Therapeutic Considerations: Topical acyclovir ointment may be useful early when vesicles erupt, but is ineffective after vesicles stop erupting. For severe/refractory cases, use acyclovir 5 mg/kg (IV) q8h × 2–7 days, then if improvement, switch to acyclovir 400 mg (PO) q8h to complete 10-day course.

Prognosis: Related to extent of tissue involvement/degree of cellular immunity dysfunction.

Chickenpox (VZV)

Clinical Presentation: Abrupt appearance of discrete/diffuse pruritic vesicles. Appear in successive crops over 3 days, then no more new lesions. Patients do not appear toxic.

Diagnostic Considerations: Chickenpox lesions are central and typically concentrated on the trunk, although vesicles may also occur in the mouth, GI or GU tract. Vesicles are seen at different stages of development, and are superficial with the classic "dew drop on a rose petal" appearance. Tzanck test is positive in chickenpox (negative in smallpox).

Pitfalls: Vesicles are not deep/umbilicated like smallpox. Smallpox patients are sick/toxic, and vesicles are at the same stage of development in each anatomical area. Vesicles begin and are concentrated on the face with smallpox.

Therapeutic Considerations: Begin therapy as early as possible before appearance of successive crops of vesicles appear. Treat VZV pneumonia early with acyclovir.

Prognosis: Children do better than adults. Worst prognosis in smokers/pregnancy (may develop chickenpox/VZV pneumonia).

Herpes Zoster (VZV)

Clinical Presentation: Painful, vesicular eruption in dermatomal distribution. Pain may be difficult to diagnose. Risk of disseminated VZV with steroids or statins.

Diagnostic Considerations: Diagnosis by appearance/positive Tzanck test of vesicle base scrapings. For VSV ophthalmicus see p. 35.

Pitfalls: Begin therapy within 2 days of vesicle eruption.

Therapeutic Considerations: Higher doses of acyclovir are required for VZV than HSV. See p. 363 for disseminated VZV, ophthalmic nerve/visceral involvement, or acyclovir-resistant strains.

Prognosis: Good if treated early. Some develop painful post-herpetic neuralgia of involved dermatomes.

Herpes Whitlow (HSV-1)

Clinical Presentation: Multiple vesicopustular lesions on fingers and hands. Lymphangitis, adenopathy, fever/chills are usually present, suggesting a bacterial infection.

Diagnostic Considerations: Common in healthcare workers giving patients oral care/suctioning.

Pitfalls: No need for antibiotics even though lesions appear infected with "pus."
Therapeutic Considerations: Never incise/drain herpes whitlow; surgical incision will flare/prolong the infection.
Prognosis: Excellent, unless incision/drainage has been performed.

Wound Infections

Subset	Usual Pathogens	Preferred IV Therapy	Alternate IV Therapy	PO Therapy or IV-to-PO Switch
Animal bite wounds[†]	Group A streptococci (GAS) P. multocida Capnocytophaga canimorsus (DF2) S. aureus (MSSA)	Ampicillin/ Sulbactam 3 gm (IV) q6h × 2 weeks **or** Tigecycline 200 mg (IV) × 1 dose, then 100 mg (IV) q24h × 2 weeks	Ertapenem 1 gm (IV) q24h × 2 weeks **or** Piperacillin/ Tazobactam 3.375 gm (IV) q6h × 2 weeks	Amoxicillin/ Clavulanic acid 500/125 mg (PO) q8h or 875/125 mg (PO) q12h × 2 weeks **or** Doxycycline 200 mg (PO) q12h × 3 days, then 100 mg (PO) q12h × 11 days
Human bite wounds	Oral anaerobes Group A streptococci (GAS) E. corrodens S. aureus (MSSA)	Same as above (for animal bite wounds)	Same as above for animal bite wounds	Same as above (for animal bite wounds)
Cat scratch disease (CSD)	Bartonella henselae (invasive)	Doxycycline 200 mg (IV) q12h × 3 days, then 100 mg (IV) q12h × 4–8 weeks **or** Azithromycin 500 mg (IV) q24h × 4–8 weeks	Chloram-phenicol 500 mg (IV) q6h × 4–8 weeks or Erythromycin 500 mg (IV) q6h × 4–8 weeks	Doxycycline 200 mg (PO) q12h × 3 days, then 100 mg (PO) q12h × 4–8 weeks* **or** Azithromycin 250 mg (PO) q24h × 4–8 weeks **or** Quinolone[‡] (PO) × 4–8 weeks
	B. henselae (lymphaden-opathy only)	PO therapy: Azithromycin 500 mg (PO) × 1 dose, then 250 mg (PO) × 4 days		

* If given IV with the same drug loading dose is not needed PO.
‡ Ciprofloxacin 400 mg (IV) or 500 mg (PO) q12h or Levofloxacin 500 mg (IV or PO) q24h or Moxifloxacin 400 mg (IV or PO) q24h.
† Rabies (see Chapter 6).

Wound Infections *(cont'd)*

Subset	Usual Pathogens	Preferred IV Therapy	Alternate IV Therapy	PO Therapy or IV-to-PO Switch
Burn wounds (severe)[†]	Group A streptococci (GAS) S. aureus (MSSA) Enterobacter P. aeruginosa	Meropenem 1 gm (IV) q8h × 2 weeks **or** Cefepime 2 gm (IV) q8h × 2 weeks	Doripenem 1 gm (IV) q8h × 2 weeks **or** Cefoperazone 2 gm (IV) q12h × 2 weeks	Not applicable
Freshwater-exposed wounds	Aeromonas hydrophilia	Quinolone[‡] (IV) × 2 weeks **or** TMP–SMX 2.5 mg/kg (IV) q6h × 2 weeks	Ceftriaxone 1 gm (IV) q24h × 2 weeks **or** Aztreonam 2 gm (IV) q8h × 2 weeks **or** Gentamicin 240 mg or 5 mg/kg (IV) q24h × 2 weeks	Quinolone[‡] (PO) × 2 weeks **or** TMP–SMX 1 SS tablet (PO) q12h × 2 weeks
Saltwater-exposed wounds	Vibrio vulnificus Vibrio sp.	Doxycycline 200 mg (IV) q12h × 3 days, then 100 mg (IV) q12h × 11 days **or** Quinolone[‡] (IV) × 2 weeks	Ceftriaxone 2 gm (IV) q12h × 2 weeks **or** Chloramphenicol 500 mg (IV) q6h × 2 weeks	Doxycycline 200 mg (PO) q12h × 3 days, then 100 mg (PO) q12h × 11 days* **or** Quinolone[‡] (PO) × 2 weeks

†   Treat only IV or IV-to-PO switch.
‡   Levofloxacin 500 mg (IV or PO) q24h or Moxifloxacin 400 mg (IV or PO) q24h.

Animal Bite Wounds

Clinical Presentation: Cellulitis surrounding bite wound.

Diagnostic Considerations: Diagnosis by culture of bite wound exudate. Deep bites may also cause tendinitis/osteomyelitis, and severe bites may result in systemic infection with bacteremia.

Pitfalls: Avoid erythromycin in penicillin-allergic patients (ineffective against P. multocida).

Therapeutic Considerations: For facial/hand bites, consult a plastic surgeon.

Prognosis: Related to adequacy of debridement and early antibiotic therapy.

Human Bite Wounds

Clinical Presentation: Cellulitis surrounding bite wound.

Diagnostic Considerations: Diagnosis by culture of bite wound exudate. Infection often extends to involve tendon/bone.

Pitfalls: Compared to animal bites, human bites are more likely to contain anaerobes, S. aureus, and Group A streptococci.

Therapeutic Considerations: Avoid primary closure of human bite wounds.

Prognosis: Related to adequacy of debridement and early antibiotic therapy.

Cat Scratch Disease (CSD) (Bartonella henselae)

Clinical Presentation: Subacute presentation of obscure febrile illness associated with cat bite/contact. Usually accompanied by adenopathy.

Diagnostic Considerations: Diagnosis by wound culture/serology for Bartonella. Cat scratch fever/disease may follow a cat scratch, but a lick from a kitten contaminating an inapparent micro-laceration is more common. May present as an FUO. Culture of exudate/node is unlikely to be positive, but silver stain of biopsy material shows organisms.

Pitfalls: Rule out lymphoma, which may present in similar fashion. Titers may cross react with C. burnetii (Q fever).

Therapeutic Considerations: For invasive disease, treat until symptoms/signs resolve. For lymphadenopathy, oral azithromycin decreases the size of nodes but may not reduce fever/systemic symptoms. Bartonella are sensitive in vitro to cephalosporins and TMP–SMX, but these antibiotics are ineffective in vivo.

Prognosis: Related to health of host.

Burn Wounds

Clinical Presentation: Severe (3rd/4th degree) burns ± drainage.

Diagnostic Considerations: Semi-quantitative bacterial counts help differentiate colonization (low counts) from infection (high counts). Burn wounds quickly become colonized.

Pitfalls: Treat only infected 3rd/4th degree burn wounds with systemic antibiotics.

Therapeutic Considerations: Meticulous local care/eschar removal/surgical debridement is key in preventing and controlling infection.

Prognosis: Related to severity of burns and adequacy of eschar debridement.

Freshwater-Exposed Wounds (Aeromonas hydrophilia)

Clinical Presentation: Fulminant wound infection with fever and diarrhea.

Diagnostic Considerations: Diagnosis by stool/wound/blood culture.

Pitfalls: Suspect A. hydrophilia in wound infection with fresh water exposure followed by diarrhea.

Therapeutic Considerations: Surgical debridement of devitalized tissue may be necessary.

Prognosis: Related to severity of infection and health of host.

Saltwater-Exposed Wounds (Vibrio vulnificus/Vibrio sp.)

Clinical Presentation: Fulminant wound infection with fever, painful hemorrhagic bullae, diarrhea.

Diagnostic Considerations: Diagnosis by stool/wound/blood culture. Vibrio vulnificus is a fulminant, life-threatening infection that may be accompanied by hypotension.

Pitfalls: Suspect V. vulnificus in acutely ill patients with fever, diarrhea, and bullous lesions after salt-water exposure.

Therapeutic Considerations: Surgical debridement of devitalized tissue may be necessary.

Prognosis: Related to extent of infection and health of host.

Superficial Fungal Infections of Skin and Nails

Subset	Usual Pathogens	Topical Therapy	PO Therapy
Mucocutaneous (local/non-disseminated) candidiasis	C. albicans	Clotrimazole 1% cream twice daily × 2 weeks	Fluconazole 400 mg (PO) × 1 dose, then 200 mg (PO) q24h × 2 weeks
Tinea corporis (body ringworm)	Trichophyton rubrum Epidermophyton floccosum Microsporum canis Trichophyton mentagrophytes	Clotrimazole 1% cream twice daily × 4–8 weeks **or** Miconazole 2% cream twice daily × 2 weeks **or** Econazole 1% cream twice daily × 2 weeks	Terbinafine 250 mg (PO) q24h × 4 weeks **or** Ketoconazole 200 mg (PO) q24h × 4 weeks **or** Fluconazole 200 mg (PO) weekly × 4 weeks
Tinea capitis (scalp ringworm)	Same as Tinea corporis, above	Selenium sulfide shampoo daily × 2–4 weeks	Same as Tinea corporis (see above)
Tinea cruris (jock itch)	T. cruris	Same as Tinea corporis, above	Same as Tinea corporis (see above)

Superficial Fungal Infections of Skin and Nails (cont'd)

Subset	Usual Pathogens	Topical Therapy	PO Therapy
Tinea pedis (athlete's foot)	Same as Tinea corporis, above	Same as Tinea corporis, above	Terbinafine 250 mg (PO) q24h × 2 weeks **or** Ketoconazole 200 mg (PO) q24h × 4 weeks **or** Itraconazole 200 mg (PO) q24h × 4 weeks*
Tinea versicolor (pityriasis)	Malasezzia furfur (Pityrosporum orbiculare)	Clotrimazole cream (1%) or miconazole cream (2%) or ketoconazole cream (2%) daily × 7 days	Ketoconazole 200 mg (PO) q24h × 7 days **or** Itraconazole 200 mg (PO) q24h × 7 days* **or** Fluconazole 400 mg (PO) × 1 dose
Onychomycosis (nail infection)	Epidermophyton floccosum Trichophyton mentagrophytes Trichophyton rubrum C. albicans	Not applicable	Fluconazole 200 mg (PO) q24h "pulse dosed", i.e., 1 week per month × 3 months (fingernail infection) or 6 months (toenail infection) **or** Itraconazole 200 mg (PO) q24h* pulse dosed, i.e., 1 week per month × 2 months (fingernail infection) or 3 months (toenail infection) **or** Terbinafine 250 mg (PO) q24h × 6 weeks (fingernail infection) or 12 weeks (toenail infection)

*   Itraconazole solution provides more reliable absorption than itraconazole capsules.

Mucocutaneous (Local/Non-disseminated) Candidiasis

Clinical Presentation: Primary cutaneous findings include an erythematous rash with satellite lesions, which may be papular, pustular, or ulcerated. Lesions can be limited or widespread over parts of body. Chronic mucocutaneous candidiasis manifests as recurrent candidal infections of skin, nails, or mucous mebranes.

Diagnostic Considerations: Diagnosis by demonstrating organism by stain/culture in tissue specimen. In HIV, Candida is very common on skin/mucous membranes.

Pitfalls: Do not confuse with the isolated, multinodular lesions of disseminated disease, which may resemble ecthyma gangrenosa or purpura fulminans.

Therapeutic Considerations: Diabetics and other compromised hosts may require prolonged therapy. In contrast to local disease, nodular cutaneous candidiasis represents disseminated disease (p. 290).

Prognosis: Related to extent of disease/host defense status.

Tinea Corporis (Body Ringworm)

Clinical Presentation: Annular pruritic lesions on trunk/face with central clearing.

Diagnostic Considerations: Diagnosis by clinical appearance/skin scraping.

Pitfalls: Do not confuse with erythema migrans, which is not pruritic.

Therapeutic Considerations: If topical therapy fails, treat with oral antifungals.

Prognosis: Excellent.

Tinea Capitis (Scalp Ringworm)

Clinical Presentation: Itchy, annular scalp lesions.

Diagnostic Considerations: Scalp lesions fluoresce with ultraviolet light. Culture hair shafts.

Pitfalls: T. capitis is associated with localized areas of alopecia.

Therapeutic Considerations: Selenium sulfide shampoo may be used first for 2–4 weeks. Treat shampoo Failures with oral ketoconazole, terbinafine, or fluconazole.

Prognosis: Excellent.

Tinea Cruris (Jock Itch)

Clinical Presentation: Groin, inguinal, perineal, or buttock lesions that are pruritic and serpiginous with scaling borders/central clearing.

Diagnostic Considerations: Diagnosis by clinical appearance/culture.

Pitfalls: Usually spares penis/scrotum, unlike Candida.

Therapeutic Considerations: In addition to therapy, it is important to keep area dry.

Prognosis: Excellent.

Tinea Pedis (Athlete's Foot)

Clinical Presentation: Painful cracks/fissures between toes.

Diagnostic Considerations: Diagnosis by clinical appearance/skin scraping.

Pitfalls: Must keep feet dry or relapse/reinfection may occur.

Therapeutic Considerations: In addition to therapy, it is important to keep area dry.

Prognosis: Excellent.

Tinea Versicolor (Pityriasis)

Clinical Presentation: Oval hypo- or hyperpigmented scaly lesions that coalesce into large confluent areas typically on upper trunk; chronic/relapsing.

Diagnostic Considerations: Diagnosis by clinical appearance and culture of affected skin lesions.

Pitfalls: M. furfur also causes seborrheic dermatitis, but seborrheic lesions are typically on the face/scalp.

Therapeutic Considerations: If topical therapy fails, treat with oral antifungals. Treat non-scalp seborrheic dermatitis with ketoconazole cream (2%) daily until cured.

Prognosis: Excellent.

<u>Dermatophyte Nail Infections</u>

Clinical Presentation: Chronically thickened, discolored nails.

Diagnostic Considerations: Diagnosis by culture of nail clippings.

Pitfalls: Nail clipping cultures often contaminated by bacterial/fungal colonizers. Green nail discoloration suggests P. aeruginosa, not a fungal nail infection; treat with ciprofloxacin 500 mg (PO) q12h × 2–3 weeks.

Therapeutic Considerations: Lengthy therapy is required. However, terbinafine and itraconazole remain bound to nail tissue for months following dosing and thus therapy with these compounds is not continued until clearance of the nail bed.

Prognosis: Excellent if infection is totally eradicated from nail bed. New nail growth takes months.

Skin Infestations

Subset	Usual Pathogens	Therapy
Scabies	Sarcoptes scabiei	Treat whole body with Permethrin cream 5% (Elimite); leave on for 8–10 hours **or** Ivermectin 18 mg (three 6-mg pills) (PO) × 1 dose
Head lice	Pediculus humanus var. capitis	Shampoo with Permethrin 5% (Elimite) or 1% (NIX) cream × 10 minutes
Body lice	Pediculus humanus var. corporis	Body lice removed by shower. Removed clothes should be washed in hot water or sealed in bags for 1 month, or treated with DDT powder 10% or malathion powder 1%
Pubic lice (crabs)	Phthirus pubis	Permethrin 5% (Elimite) or 1% (NIX) cream × 10 minutes to affected areas

<u>Scabies (Sarcoptes scabiei)</u>

Clinical Presentation: Punctate, serpiginous, intensely pruritic black spots in webbed spaces of hands/feet and creases of elbows/knees.

Diagnostic Considerations: Diagnosis by visualization of skin tracts/burrows. Incubation period up to 6 weeks after contact. Spread by scratching from one part of body to another.

Pitfalls: Mites are not visible, only their skin tracks, but mites may be scraped out of tracts for diagnosis.
Therapeutic Considerations: Permethrin cream is usually effective. If itching persists after treatment, do not retreat (itching is secondary to hypersensitivity reaction of eggs in skin burrows). Treat close contacts. Vacuum bedding/furniture.
Prognosis: Norwegian scabies is very difficult to eradicate.

Head Lice (Pediculus humanus var. capitis)
Clinical Presentation: White spots may be seen on hair shafts of head/neck, but not eyebrows.
Diagnostic Considerations: Nits on hair are unhatched lice eggs, seen as white dots attached to hair shaft. May survive away from body × 2 days.
Pitfalls: May need to retreat in 7 days to kill any lice that hatched from surviving nits.
Therapeutic Considerations: Shampoo with Permethrin 5% (Elimite) or 1% (NIX) cream kills lice/nits. Clothes and non-washables should be tied off in plastic bags × 2 weeks to kill lice. Alternately, wash and dry clothes/bed linens; heat from dryer/iron kills lice.
Prognosis: Related to thoroughness of therapy.

Body Lice (Pediculus humanus var. corporis)
Clinical Presentation: Intense generalized pruritus.
Diagnostic Considerations: Smaller than head lice and more difficult to see. May survive away from body × 1 week.
Pitfalls: Body lice live in clothes; leave only for a blood meal, then return to clothing.
Therapeutic Considerations: Can survive in seams of clothing × 1 week.
Prognosis: Good if clothes are also treated.

Pubic Lice (Phthirus pubis) Crabs
Clinical Presentation: Genital pruritus.
Diagnostic Considerations: Seen on groin, eyelashes, axilla. May survive away from body × 1 day.
Pitfalls: Smaller than head lice, but easily seen.
Therapeutic Considerations: Treat partners. Wash, dry, and iron clothes; heat from dryer/iron kills lice. Non-washables may be placed in a sealed bag × 7 days.
Prognosis: Good if clothes are also treated.

Ischiorectal/Perirectal Abscess

Subset	Pathogens	Preferred Therapy
Ischiorectal/ perirectal abscess	GNB B. fragilis	Treat the same as mild/severe peritonitis p. 108 ± surgical drainage depending on abscess size/severity

Clinical Presentation: Presents in normal hosts with perirectal pain, pain on defecation, leukocytosis, erythema/tenderness over abscess ± fever/chills. In febrile neutropenia, there is only tenderness.

Diagnostic Considerations: Diagnosis by erythema/tenderness over abscess or by CT/MRI.

Pitfalls: Do not confuse with perirectal regional enteritis (Crohn's disease) in normal hosts, or with ecthyma gangrenosum in febrile neutropenics.

Therapeutic Considerations: Antibiotic therapy may be adequate for mild cases. Large abscesses require drainage plus antibiotics × 1–2 weeks post-drainage. With febrile neutropenia, use an antibiotic that is active against both P. aeruginosa and B. fragilis e.g., meropenem.

Prognosis: Good with early drainage/therapy.

Sepsis/Septic Shock

Sepsis/Septic Shock

Subset	Usual Pathogens	Preferred IV Therapy	Alternate IV Therapy	IV-to-PO Switch
Unknown source	GNB B. fragilis E. faecalis (VSE)[†]	Meropenem 1 gm (IV) q8h × 2 weeks **or** Piperacillin/ Tazobactam 3.375 gm (IV) q6h × 2 weeks **or** Moxifloxacin 400 mg (IV) q24h × 2 weeks	Quinolone* (IV) × 2 weeks **plus either** Metronidazole 1 gm (IV) q24h × 2 weeks **or** Clindamycin 600 mg (IV) q8h × 2 weeks	Moxifloxacin 400 mg (PO) q24h × 2 weeks
Lung source *Community acquired pneumonia*[§] *(CAP)*	S. pneumoniae H. influenzae K. pneumoniae**	Respiratory quinolone[‡] (IV) q24h × 2 weeks **or** Ceftriaxone 1 gm (IV) q24h × 2 weeks	Meropenem 1 gm (IV) q8h × 2 weeks	Respiratory quinolone[‡] (PO) q24h × 2 weeks **or** Doxycycline 200 mg (PO) q12h × 3 days, then 100 mg (PO) q12h × 11 days

* Levofloxacin 500 mg (IV or PO) q24h.
† Treat initially for E. faecalis (VSE); if later identified as E. faecium (VRE), treat accordingly (urosepsis see p. 120).

Sepsis/Septic Shock *(cont'd)*

Subset	Usual Pathogens	Preferred IV Therapy	Alternate IV Therapy	IV-to-PO Switch
Nosocomial pneumonia (NP)	P. aeruginosa K. pneumoniae E. coli S. marcescens (not MSSA/ MRSA)	Meropenem 1 gm (IV) q8h × 2 weeks **plus either** Levofloxacin 750 mg (IV) q24h × 2 weeks **or** Amikacin 1 gm or 15 mg/kg (IV) q24h × 2 weeks **or** Aztreonam 2 gm (IV) q8h × 2 weeks		Levofloxacin 750 mg (PO) q24h × 2 weeks **or** Ciprofloxacin 750 mg (PO) q12h × 2 weeks
CVC source*** *Bacteremia* (Treat initially for MSSA; if later identified as MRSA, etc., treat accordingly)	S. epidermidis (CoNS) S. aureus (MSSA) Klebsiella Enterobacter Serratia	Meropenem 1 gm (IV) q8h × 2 weeks **or** Cefepime 2 gm (IV) q12h × 2 wks	Ceftriaxone 1 gm (IV) q24h × 2 wks **or** Respiratory quinolone* (IV) q24h × 2 wks	Respiratory quinolone* (PO) q24h × 2 weeks **or** Cephalexin 500 mg (PO) q6h × 2 weeks
	S. aureus (MRSA)	Daptomycin 6 mg/kg (IV) q24h × 2 weeks **or** Linezolid 600 mg (IV) q12h × 2 weeks Quinupristin/Dalfopristin 7.5 mg/kg (IV) q8h × 2 weeks **or** Vancomycin 1 gm (IV) q12h × 2 weeks		Linezolid 600 mg (PO) q12h × 2 weeks Minocycline 200 mg (PO) × 1, then 100 mg (PO) q12h × 2 weeks

ILI = Influenza like illness.

*   Moxifloxacin 400 mg or Levofloxacin 500 mg.

**   In alcoholics only

*** If clinically possible, remove CVC as soon as possible.

†   Patients with ILI/influenza A (human/swine) presenting with *simultaneous* MSSA/MRSA CAP often present in shock.

‡   Levofloxacin 750 mg (IV) q24h or Moxifloxacin 400 mg (IV) q24h.

§   **Uncomplicated by cardiopulmonary decompensation/failure, CAP does not present with hypotension/shock in normal hosts. Hyposplenia/asplenia should be suspected if CAP presents with hypotension/shock in patients with good cardiopulmonary function.**

Sepsis/Septic Shock (cont'd)

Subset	Usual Pathogens	Preferred IV Therapy	Alternate IV Therapy	IV-to-PO Switch
Candidemia (disseminated/invasive) Unless species is known, empiric therapy as for non-albicans/possibly fluconazole-resistant Candida is preferred	Non-albicans Candida¶ **or** Fluconazole-resistant	Isavuconazole 200 mg (IV) q8h × 48 hours, then 200 mg (IV/PO) q24h × 2 weeks **or** Micafungin 100 mg (IV) q24h × 2 weeks† **or** Voriconazole *if additional mould coverage is desired* **or** Liposomal amphotericin B (L-amb) (IV) q24h† **or** Amphotericin B (see C. albicans, above) × 2 weeks† **or** Voriconazole × 2 weeks¶† **or** Itraconazole (see C. albicans, above) **or** Anidulafungin 200 mg (IV) × 1 dose, then 100 mg (IV) q24h × 2 weeks† **or** Caspofungin (see C. albicans, above)		Voriconazole × 2 weeks¶† or Posaconazole 400 mg (PO) q12h × 2 weeks
Intra-abdominal/pelvic source	GNB B. fragilis	Piperacillin/Tazobactam 3.375 gm (IV) q6h × 2 weeks **or** Tigecycline 200 mg (IV) × 1 dose, then 100 mg (IV) q24h × 2 weeks **or** Ertapenem 1 gm (IV) q24h × 2 weeks **or** Meropenem 1 gm (IV) q8h × 2 weeks	**Combination Therapy** Ceftriaxone 1 gm (IV) q24h × 2 weeks **or** Levofloxacin 500 mg (IV) q24h × 2 weeks **plus** Metronidazole 1 gm (IV) q24h × 2 weeks	**Monotherapy** Moxifloxacin 400 mg (PO) q24h × 2 weeks **or** **Combination Therapy** Levofloxacin 500 mg (PO) q24h × 2 weeks **plus** Clindamycin 300 mg (PO) q8h × 2 weeks

¶ Best agent depends on infecting species. Fluconazole susceptibility varies predictably by species. (See Chapter 11 Drug Summaries) also, see Amphotericin B lipid-formulations (See Chapter 11 Drug Summaries).

† Treat candidemia for 2 weeks after negative blood cultures.

Sepsis/Septic Shock *(cont'd)*

Subset	Usual Pathogens	Preferred IV Therapy	Alternate IV Therapy	IV-to-PO Switch
Urosepsis *community-acquired*	GNB E. faecalis (VSE)	Piperacillin/ Tazobactam 3.375 gm (IV) q6h × 1–2 weeks **or** Meropenem 1 gm (IV) q8h × 1–2 weeks	Levofloxacin 500 mg (IV) q24h	Levofloxacin 500 mg (PO) q24h × 1–2 weeks
	E. faecium (VRE)	Daptomycin 12 mg/kg (IV) q24h × 1–2 weeks* **or** Linezolid 600 mg (IV) q12h × 1–2 weeks	Quinupristin/ Dalfopristin 7.5 mg/kg (IV) q8h × 1–2 weeks	Linezolid 600 mg (PO) q12h × 1–2 weeks **or** Minocycline 200 mg (PO) × 1, then 100 mg (PO) q12h × 1–2 weeks
Nosocomial	P. aeruginosa	Meropenem 1 gm (IV) q8h × 1–2 weeks **or** Cefepime 2 gm (IV) q12h × 1–2 weeks **or** Levofloxacin 750 mg (IV) q24h × 1–2 weeks	Aztreonam 2 gm (IV) q8h × 1–2 weeks **or** Doripenem 1 gm (IV) q8h × 1–2 weeks	Levofloxacin 750 mg (PO) q24h × 1–2 weeks
	CRE	Ceftazidime/ Avibactam 2.5 gm (IV) q 8 h × 1–2 weeks	Polymyxin B 1.25 mg/kg (IV) q12h × 1–2 weeks **or** Colistin 2.5 mg/kg (IV) q12h × 1–2 weeks	
Overwhelming sepsis with purpura (asplenia or hyposplenia)	S. pneumoniae H. influenzae N. meningitidis	Ceftriaxone 2 gm (IV) q24h × 2 weeks **or** Levofloxacin 500 mg (IV) q24h × 2 weeks	Cefepime 2 gm (IV) q12h × 2 weeks **or** Cefotaxime 2 gm (IV) q6h × 2 weeks	Levofloxacin 500 mg (PO) q24h × 2 weeks **or** Amoxicillin 1 gm (PO) q8h × 2 weeks

* VRE MIC = 2 × MRSA. Use double the usual bacteremia dose (6 mg/kg for VRE (12 mg/kg).

Sepsis/Septic Shock *(cont'd)*

Subset	Usual Pathogens	Preferred IV Therapy	Alternate IV Therapy	IV-to-PO Switch
Steroids (high chronic dose)	Aspergillus	Treat as Aspergillus pneumonia		
Miliary TB	M. tuberculosis	Treat as pulmonary TB (see p. 55) plus steroids × 1–2 wks		
Miliary BCG	Bacille Calmette-Guérin (BCG)	Treat with INH plus RIF × 6 months; may add steroids e.g., prednisolone 40 mg q24h × 1–2 weeks		

Duration of therapy represents total time IV or IV + PO.
* Plus surgical decompression/drainage if needed.

Sepsis (Unknown Source)

Clinical Presentation: Abrupt onset of high spiking fevers, rigors ± hypotension.

Diagnostic Considerations: Diagnosis suggested by high-grade bacteremia (2/4–4/4 positive blood cultures) with unexplained hypotension. Rule out pseudosepsis (GI bleed, myocardial infarction, pulmonary embolism, acute pancreatitis, adrenal insufficiency, etc.). Sepsis usually occurs from a GI, GU, or IV source, so coverage is directed against GI and GU pathogens if IV line infection is unlikely.

Pitfalls: Most cases of fever/hypotension are not due to sepsis. Before the label of "sepsis" is applied to febrile/hypotensive patients, first consider treatable/reversible mimics.

Therapeutic Considerations: Resuscitate shock patients initially with rapid adequate volume replacement, followed by pressors, if needed. Do not give pressors before volume replacement or hypotension may continue/worsen. Use normal saline, plasma expanders, or blood for volume replacement, not D_5W. If patient is persistently hypotensive despite volume replacement, consider relative adrenal insufficiency: Obtain a serum cortisol level, then give cortisone 100 mg (IV) q6h × 24–72h; blood pressure will rise promptly if relative adrenal insufficiency is the cause of volume-unresponsive hypotension. *Do not add/change antibiotics if patient is persistently hypotensive/febrile; look for GI bleed, myocardial infarction, pulmonary embolism, pancreatitis, undrained abscess, adrenal insufficiency, or IV line infection. Drain abscesses as soon as possible. Remove IV lines if the entry site is red or a central line has been in place for ≥ 7 days and there is no other explanation for fever/hypotension.* Early antibiotic therapy/surgical drainage of abscesses, debridement of necrotic tissue eg. necrotizing fasciitis or relief of obstruction is critical.

Prognosis: Related to severity of septic process and underlying cardiopulmonary/immune status.

Sepsis (Lung Source)

Clinical Presentation: Normal hosts with community-acquired pneumonia (CAP) do not present with sepsis. CAP with sepsis suggests the presence of impaired immunity/hyposplenic function (see "sepsis in hyposplenia/asplenia," p. 157). Nosocomial pneumonia uncommonly presents as (or is complicated by) sepsis with otherwise unexplained hypotension.

Diagnostic Considerations: Impaired splenic function may be inferred by finding Howell-Jolly bodies (small, round, pinkish or bluish inclusion bodies in red blood cells) in the peripheral blood smear. The number of Howell-Jolly bodies is proportional to the degree of splenic dysfunction.

Pitfalls: CAP with hypotension/sepsis should suggest hyposplenic function, impaired immunity, or an alternate diagnosis that can mimic CAP/shock. Be sure to exclude acute MI, acute heart failure/COPD, PE/infarction, overzealous diuretic therapy, concomitant GI bleed, and acute pancreatitis.

Therapeutic Considerations: Patients with malignancies, myeloma, or SLE are predisposed to CAP, which is not usually severe or associated with shock. Be sure patients with CAP receiving steroids at less than "stress doses" do not have hypotension/shock from relative adrenal insufficiency. In patients with SLE, try to distinguish between lupus pneumonitis and CAP; SLE pneumonitis usually occurs as part of a SLE flare, CAP usually does not.

Prognosis: Related to underlying cardiopulmonary/immune status. Early treatment is important.

Sepsis (Central Venous Catheter [CVC] Source)

Clinical Presentation: Temperature ≥ 102°F ± IV site erythema.

Diagnostic Considerations: Diagnosis by semi-quantitative catheter tip culture with ≥ 15 colonies plus blood cultures with same pathogen. If no other explanation for fever and line has been in place ≥ 7 days, remove CVC and obtain semi-quantitative catheter tip culture. Suppurative thrombophlebitis presents with hectic/septic fevers and pus at IV site ± palpable venous cord.

Pitfalls: Temperature ≥ 102°F with CVC infection, in contrast to phlebitis (temperature ≤ 102°F). Acute bacterial endocarditis (ABE) may complicate intracardiac or CVC (not peripheral) infection.

Therapeutic Considerations: Line removal is usually curative, but antibiotic therapy is usually given for 1 week after CVC removal for gram-negative bacilli or 2 weeks after CVC removal for S. aureus (MSSA/MRSA). Antifungal therapy is also usually given for 2 weeks after CVC removal for candidemia. Ophthalmologist to exclude candidal endophthalmitis following candidemia.

Prognosis: Good if CVC is removed before endocarditis/metastatic spread.

Sepsis (Intra-abdominal/Pelvic Source)

Clinical Presentation: Fever, peritonitis ± hypotension. Usually a history of an intra-abdominal disorder that predisposes to sepsis (e.g., diverticulosis, gallbladder disease, recent intra-abdominal/pelvic surgery). Signs and symptoms are referable to the abdomen/pelvis.

Diagnostic Considerations: Clinical presentation plus imaging studies (e.g., abdominal/pelvic CT or MRI to demonstrate pathology) are diagnostic.

Pitfalls: Elderly patients may have little/no fever and may not have rebound tenderness. Be sure to exclude intra-abdominal mimics of sepsis (e.g., GI bleed, pancreatitis).

Therapeutic Considerations: Empiric coverage should be directed against aerobic gram-negative bacilli plus B. fragilis. Anti-enterococcal coverage is not essential. Antibiotic therapy is ineffective unless ruptured viscus is repaired, obstruction is relieved, abscesses are drained.

Prognosis: Related to rapidity/adequacy of abscess drainage and repair/lavage of ruptured organs. The preoperative health of the host is also important.

Sepsis (Urinary Source)

Clinical Presentation: Fever/hypotension in a patient with diabetes mellitus, SLE, myeloma, pre-existing renal disease, stone disease, or partial/total urinary tract obstruction.

Diagnostic Considerations: Urine gram stain determines initial empiric coverage. Pyuria is also present. Diagnosis confirmed by culturing the same isolate from urine and blood.

Pitfalls: Pyuria without bacteriuria and bacteremia due to same pathogens is not diagnostic of urosepsis. Urosepsis does not occur in normal hosts; look for host defect (e.g., diabetes, renal disease).

Therapeutic Considerations: If stones/obstruction are not present, urosepsis resolves rapidly with appropriate therapy. Delayed/no response suggests infected/obstructed stent, stone, partial/total urinary tract obstruction, or renal abscess.

Prognosis: Good if stone/stent removed, obstruction relieved, abscess drained. Fatalities rare with urosepsis.

Sepsis (Hyposplenia/Asplenia)

Clinical Presentation: Presents as overwhelming septicemia/shock with petechiae.

Diagnostic Considerations: Diagnosis by gram stain of buffy coat of blood or by blood cultures. Organism may be stained/cultured from aspirated petechiae. Howell-Jolly bodies in the peripheral smear are a clue to decreased splenic function. Conditions associated with hyposplenism include sickle cell trait/disease, cirrhosis, rheumatoid arthritis, SLE, systemic necrotizing vasculitis, amyloidosis, celiac disease, chronic active hepatitis, Fanconi's syndrome, IgA deficiency, intestinal lymphangiectasia, intravenous gamma-globulin therapy, myeloproliferative disorders, non-Hodgkin's lymphoma, regional enteritis, ulcerative colitis, Sezary syndrome, splenic infarcts/malignancies, steroid therapy, systemic mastocytosis, thyroiditis, infiltrative diseases of spleen, mechanical compression of splenic artery/spleen, Waldenstrom's macroglobulinemia, hyposplenism of old age, congenital absence of spleen.

Pitfalls: Suspect hyposplenia/asplenia in unexplained overwhelming infection.

Therapeutic Considerations: In spite of early aggressive antibiotic therapy and supportive care, patients often die within hours from overwhelming infection, especially due to S. pneumoniae.

Prognosis: Related to degree of splenic dysfunction.

Sepsis (Chronic High Dose Steroids)

Clinical Presentation: Subacute onset of fever with disseminated infection (Candida, Aspergillus) in multiple organs.

Diagnostic Considerations: Diagnosis by positive blood cultures for fungi or demonstration of invasive fungal infection from tissue biopsy specimens. Sepsis is most commonly due to fungemia.

Pitfalls: Obtain blood cultures to diagnose fungemias and rule out bacteremias (uncommon).

Therapeutic Considerations: Empirical approach is the same as for invasive candidiasis/aspergillosis.

Prognosis: Related to degree of immunosuppression.

Miliary (Disseminated) TB (Mycobacterium tuberculosis)

Clinical Presentation: Unexplained, prolonged fevers without localizing signs.

Diagnostic Considerations: Usually presents as an FUO. Since localizing signs are not present, a key clinical clue to miliary TB are morning temperature spikes. In miliary TB which often mimics malignancy, appetite is preserved until late unlike in malignancies where anorexia typically occurs early. Non-specific laboratory test clues include an elevated (use up arrow instead) AP and or elevated (use up arrow instead) ferritin levels (may also be present with lymphoma).

Pitfalls: Chest x-ray is negative early in 1/3. Subtle miliary (2 mm) infiltrates on chest x-ray 1–4 weeks).

Therapeutic Considerations: Treated the same as pulmonary TB ± steroids initially.

Prognosis: Death within weeks without treatment.

Miliary (Disseminated) BCG (Bacille Calmette-Guérin)

Clinical Presentation: Fever, circulatory collapse, DIC days to weeks after intravesicular BCG. Common sites of disseminated BCG include lung, liver, and prostate. May present as an FVO.

Diagnostic Considerations: Common in compromised hosts but not uncommon in normal hosts.

Pitfalls: Avoid intravesicular BCG immediately after traumatic catheterization, bladder biopsy, TURP.

Therapeutic Considerations: Treat for 6 months with INH and RIF. Do not repeat BCG therapy.

Prognosis: Good with early treatment.

Febrile Neutropenia

Febrile Neutropenia

Subset	Usual Pathogens	Preferred IV Therapy	Alternate IV Therapy	IV-to-PO Switch
Febrile leukopenia **< 7 days**	P. aeruginosa GNB (*not* MSSA/MRSA *unless* CVC related)¶	Meropenem 1 gm (IV) q8h* **or** Levofloxacin 750 mg (IV) q24h*	Cefepime 2 gm (IV) q8h*	Levofloxacin 750 mg (PO) q24h*
> 7 days	C. albicans Non-albicans Candida Aspergillus	Micafungin 100 mg (IV) q24h* **or** Voriconazole†† **or** Caspofungin 70 mg (IV) × 1 dose, then 50 mg (IV) q24h* **or** Liposomal amphotericin) (L-amb) (IV) q24h*††	Amphotericin B 1.5 mg/kg (IV) q24h until 1–2 gm given	Itraconazole 200 mg (PO) q12h* **or** Voriconazole (see "usual dose")*†† **or** Posaconazole 400 mg (PO) q12h*
	MSSA (2° to CVC)†	Same as above for < 7 days of febrile neutropenia	Same as above for < 7 days of febrile neutropenia	Linezolid 600 mg (PO) q12h **or** Minocycline§ 200 mg (PO) × 1, then 100 mg (PO) q12h
	MRSA (2° to CVC)†	Daptomycin§ 6 mg/kg (IV) q24h **or** Vancomycin§ 1 gm (IV) q12h	Linezolid 600 mg (IV) q12h **or** Quinupristin/ Dalfopristin§ 7.5 mg/kg (IV) q8h	Linezolid 600 mg (PO) q12h **or** Minocycline§ 200 mg (PO) × 1, then 100 mg (PO) q12h

*   Treat until neutropenia resolves.
†   **If clinically possible, remove CVC.**
§   Treat for 2 weeks post--CVC removal.
¶   **Neutropenia, per se, does not predispose to MSSA/MRSA bacteremias. MSSA/MRSA bacteremias in febrile neutropenia are 2° to CVC associated infection, not neutropenia.**
†† For usual dose, see Chapter 11 (Drug Summaries).

Clinical Presentation: Incidence of infection rises as PMN counts fall below 1000/mm³.
Diagnostic Considerations: Febrile neutropenia < 7 days ± positive blood cultures. After blood cultures are drawn, anti-P. aeruginosa coverage should be initiated. Do not overlook ischiorectal or perirectal abscess as sources of fever.
Pitfalls: Suspect fungemia if abrupt rise in temperature occurs after 7 days of appropriate anti-P. aeruginosa antibiotic therapy. Fungemias usually do not occur in first 7 days of neutropenia. Viridans streptococci (S. mitis) may present with bacteremia, shock, ARDs, and rash in febrile neutropenia.

Therapeutic Considerations: If a patient is neutropenic for > 2 weeks and develops RUQ/LUQ pain/increased alkaline phosphatase, suspect hepatosplenic candidiasis; confirm diagnosis with abdominal CT/MRI showing mass lesions in liver/spleen and treat as systemic/invasive candidiasis (p. 79). S. aureus is not a common pathogen in neutropenic compromised hosts without central IV lines, and B. fragilis/anaerobes are not usual pathogens in febrile neutropenia. If IV line infection/perirectal abscess are ruled out, consider tumor fever or drug fever before changing antibiotic therapy.

Prognosis: Related to degree and duration of neutropenia.

Transplant Infections

Transplant Infections

Subset	Usual Pathogens	Preferred IV Therapy	Alternate IV Therapy	PO Therapy or IV-to-PO Switch
BACTEREMIA OR CANDIDEMIA				
Bacteremia Post-**BMT** (leukopenic pre-engraftment) **< 7 days**	P. aeruginosa GNB Viridans streptococci E. faecalis (VSE) S. aureus (MSSA)	Meropenem 1 gm (IV) q8h* **or** Piperacillin Tazobactam 3.375 mg (IV) q6h*	Quinolone† (IV) q24h* **or** Aztreonam 2 gm (IV) q8h* **or** Amikacin 1 gm or 15 mg/kg (IV) q24h*	Quinolone† (PO) q24h* **or** Ciprofloxacin 750 mg (PO) q12h*
	S. aureus (MRSA)	Daptomycin 6 mg/kg (IV) q24h × 2 weeks **or** Linezolid 600 mg (IV) q12h × 2 weeks **or** Quinupristin/Dalfopristin 7.5 mg/kg (IV) q8h × 2 weeks **or** Vancomycin 1 gm (IV) q12h × 2 weeks		Linezolid 600 mg (PO) q12h × 2 weeks **or** Minocycline 200 mg (PO) × 1, then 100 mg (PO) q12h × 2 weeks
	E. faecium (VRE)	Linezolid 600 mg (IV) q12h × 1–2 weeks	Daptomycin 6 mg/kg (IV) q24h × 1–2 weeks	Linezolid 600 mg (PO) q12h × 1–2 weeks **or** Minocycline 200 mg (PO) × 1, then 100 mg (PO) q12h × 1–2 weeks

BMT/SOT = bone marrow/solid organ transplant.
†   Levofloxacin 750 mg

Transplant Infections¶ *(cont'd)*

Subset	Usual Pathogens	Preferred IV Therapy	Alternate IV Therapy	PO Therapy or IV-to-PO Switch
Candidemia *Post-BMT (leukopenic pre-engraftment) > 7 days*	C. albicans Non-albicans Candida	Micafungin 100 mg (IV) q24h **or** Liposomal amphotericin (L-Amb) 3–5 mg/kg (IV) q24h **or** Voriconazole (IV)	Itraconazole 200 mg (IV) q12h × 2 days, then 200 mg (IV) q24h¶ **or** Caspofungin 70 mg (IV) × 1 dose, then 50 mg (IV) q24h **or** Anidulafungin 200 mg (IV) × 1 dose, then 100 mg (IV) q24h	Itraconazole 200 mg (PO) q12h¶ **or** Voriconazole (PO)§¶ **or** Fluconazole 800 mg (PO) × 1, then 400 mg (PO) q24h*‡ **or** Posaconazole 400 mg (PO) q12h¶
Bacteremia *Post-SOT* (Treat initially for MSSA; if later identified as MRSA, treat accordingly)	GNB S. aureus (MSSA)	Meropenem 1 gm (IV) q8h × 2 weeks **or** Ceftriaxone 1 gm (IV) q24h × 2 weeks	Quinolone† (IV) q24h × 2 weeks **or** Cefepime 2 gm (IV) q12h × 2 weeks	Quinolone† (PO) q24h × 2 weeks **or** Cephalexin 500 mg (PO) q6h × 2 weeks
	S. aureus (MRSA)	Linezolid 600 mg (IV) q12h × 2 weeks **or** Daptomycin 6 mg/kg (IV) q24h × 2 weeks **or** Vancomycin 1 gm (IV) q12h × 2 weeks **or** Quinupristin/Dalfopristin 7.5 mg/kg (IV) q8h × 2 weeks		Linezolid 600 mg (PO) q12h × 2 weeks **or** Minocycline 200 mg (PO) × 1, then 100 mg (PO) q12h × 2 weeks

BMT/SOT = bone marrow/solid organ transplant.
†   Levofloxacin 750 mg or Moxifloxacin 400 mg.
*   **Treat until neutropenia resolves.**
‡   Loading dose is not needed PO if given IV with the same drug.
¶   Significant drug interactions are possible with usual immunosuppressive agents (e.g., sirolinus, cyclosporine, tacrolimus). Review all concomitant medications for potential interactions. *Voriconazole contraindicated in patients with sirolimus.*
§   For usual dose, see chapter 11 (Drug Summaries)

Transplant Infections¶ *(cont'd)*

	Viremia	
CMV	Ganciclovir 5 mg/kg (IV) q12h until clinical/virologic response (not < 2 weeks) **or** Valganciclovir 900 mg (PO) q12h until clinical/virologic response (not < 2 weeks)	Follow therapy with 1-3 months of CMV prophylaxis (see p. 368) or frequent clinical/virologic followup. Risk of CMV disease greatest 3-6 months post-organ transplant in D+/R- patients during the period of maximum immuno-suppression. Coinfection with HHV-6/7 may increase risk of CMV disease. Risk also high where ALG is used for induction therapy to treat organ rejection. Also, CMV disease risk higher in lung, pancreas and intestine transplants (kidney, liver have lower risk). Lowest risk of CMV disease in D-/R-transplants (should be given leukodepleted blood products and CMV negative blood). Consider IVIG† in patients with CMV pneumonia or consider CMVIG†† in patients with CMV pneumonia or severe CMV infection.
HHV-6	Ganciclovir: 5 mg/kg (IV) q12h until viremia/ infection clears. **or** Foscarnet 90 mg/ kg (IV) q12h until viremia/infection clears. **or** Cidofovir 5 mg/kg (IV) q week × 2, then q other week* until viremia/ infection clears.	***Reduction of immunosuppression remains the mainstay of treatment.*** HHV-6-A may be gangcyclovir resistant. HHV-6-B variants susceptible to Ganciclovir and Foscarnet Treatment recommended for HHV-6 CNS disease with Ganciclovir, Foscarnet or a combination of both.
BK virus	Cidofovir 0.25 –1 mg/kg (IV) q2 weeks*	***Reduction of immunosuppression remains the mainstay of treatment.*** Treatment indicated for BKV viremia/BKV nephropathy. *No treatment necessary for asymptomatic BKV infection.* BV viremia predicts presence of BK nephropathy which precedes viruria. "Decoy cells" in urine indicate BK viruria. BK viruria is common and preceeds viremia and invasive infection. ALG: antilymphoayte globulin (thymoglobulin).

*   IVIG: 500 mg/kg (IV) q48h.

†† CMVIG:

    Renal Transplants: 150 mg/kg (IV) within 72 hours post-transplant, then 100 mg/kg (IV) at weeks 2, 4, 6, 8, then 50 mg/kg (IV) at weeks 12 and 16.

    Non-Renal Transplants: 150 mg/kg (IV) given within 72 hours post-transplant, then 150 mg/ kg (IV) at weeks 2, 4, 6, 8, then 100 mg/kg (IV) at weeks 12 and 16 after transplant.

Transplant Infections[¶] *(cont'd)*

	Viremia (cont'd)	
	Leflunomide (given as mycophenolate replacement) **Loading Dose:** 100 mg (PO) q24h × 5 days, then **Maintenance Dose:** 40 mg (PO) q24h until viremia/infection clears.	Measure leflunomide trough levels to ensure therapeutic concentrations (50–100 mcg/ml).
EBV/PTLD	Rituximab	***Reduction or discontinuation of immunosuppression remains the mainstay of treatment of PTLD*** (spontaneous regression in ¼ – ½ of cases).
RSV	Ribavirin 20 mg/mL (aerosol) for 12–18 hours q24h × 3–7 days.	***Reduction of immunosuppression remains the mainstay of treatment.*** Palivizumab may prevent progression from upper to lower RTI. IVIG may be added in severe cases.
Adenovirus	Cidofovir 5 mg/kg (IV) q 1–2 weeks (with saline hydration and probenecid) until viremia/infection clears.[§] **or** Ribavirin **Loading Dose:** 30 mg/kg (IV), then **Maintenance Dose:** 16 mg/kg (IV) q6h × 4 days, then 8 mg/kg (IV) q8h until viremia/infection clears.	***Reduction of immunosuppression remains the mainstay of treatment.*** Oral ribavirin may be effective, but outcomes are variable and may be adenovirus-serotype specific.

§ Probenecid 2 gm (PO) 3 hours prior to cidofovir, 1 gm at 2 hours and 8 hours after completion of infusion.
   Patient should receive 1 liter normal saline (IV) prior to each infusion of cidofovir; a second liter may be administered over 1–3 hours at the start of cidofovir infusion or immediately following infusion.
* With hydration/probenecid (see Cidofovir Drug Summary).

Transplant Infections¶ *(cont'd)*

	CNS INFECTIONS			
Encephalitis	CMV HHV-6	Ganciclovir 5 mg/kg (IV) q12h × 2–4 weeks or until resolution of symptoms and viremia IVIG or CMVIG may be beneficial in severe cases Valganciclovir 900 mg (PO) q24h × 3 months. After successful treatment, a course of 2° prophylaxis is recommended		
	CMV (ganciclovir-resistant CMV: MIC ≥ 3 mcg/mL) or UL 54 or UL 97 mutations	Cidofovir 5 mg/kg (IV) of 1–2 weeks with saline plus probenecid **or** Foscarnet 60 mg/kg (IV) q8h × 2 weeks **or** Foscarnet plus Ganciclovir (see above) **or** Cidofovir (see above) may be used in severe cases		
	Listeria, HSV, C. neoformans, M. tuberculosis treated the same as in normal/other compromised hosts (see p. 25–26)			
Brain abscess/ mass lesions	Aspergillus	Voriconazole (IV) until cured*¶	Ambisome (L-Amb) 5 mg/kg (IV) q24h until cured **or** Amphotericin B 1.5 mg/kg (IV) q24h until cured	Voriconazole (PO) until cured*¶
	Nocardia	TMP–SMX 5 mg/kg (IV) q6h **or** Minocycline 200 mg (IV) q12h until clinical improvement, then (PO) therapy for at least 9–12 months or until cured	Linezolid 600 mg (IV) q12h until clinical improvement, then (PO) therapy for at least 9–12 months or until cured **or** Meropenem 2 gm (IV) q8h for at least 9–12 months or until cured	TMP–SMX 2 DS (PO) q8h **or** Minocycline 200 mg (PO) q12h **or** Linezolid 600 mg (PO) q12h for at least 9–12 months or until cured
	T. gondii	<u>Preferred Therapy</u> Sulfadiazine 1–1.5 gm (PO) q6h + Pyrimethamine 200 mg (PO) × 1 dose then 50 mg (PO) q6h + folinic acid 10 mg (PO) q24h × 6–8 weeks until CT/MRI clinical response.		

¶   Significant drug interactions are possible with usual immunosuppressive agents (e.g., sirolimus, cyclosporine tacrolimus). Review all concomitant medications for potential interactions. *Voriconazole contraindicated in patients on sirolimus.*
*   For usual dose, see Chapter 11 (Drug Summaries)

Transplant Infections¶ *(cont'd)*

CNS INFECTIONS (cont'd)		
		Follow with sulfadiazine 1 gm (PO) q12h + Pyrimethamine 50 mg (PO) q24h + folinic acid 10 mg (PO) q24h until cured <u>Alternate Therapy</u> Clindamycin 600 mg (IV or PO) q6h + Pyrimethamine 200 mg (PO) × 1 dose then 50 mg (PO) q6h + folinic acid 10 mg (PO) q24h × 6–8 weeks until CT/MRI clinical response. Follow with Sulfadiazine 1 gm (PO) q12h + Pyrimethamine 50 mg (PO) q24h + folinic acid 10 mg (PO) q24h until cured
	C. neoformans	Treat the same as chronic meningitis
PNEUMONIAS		
Focal/ segmental/ nodular infiltrates *Acute*	Legionella sp.	Treat the same as in normal hosts (see p. 53)
	L. micdadei	Treat the same as in normal hosts (see p. 53) <u>Alternate Therapy</u> TMP-SMX (see p. 53)
Subacute	Aspergillus	<u>Preferred Therapy</u> Isavuconazole 200 mg (IV) q8h × 48 hours, then 200 mg (IV/PO) q24h until cured **or** Voriconazole (see "usual dose") until cured§¶ **or** Liposomal amphotericin (L-amb) (IV) q24h until cured <u>Alternate Therapy</u> Posaconazole 400 mg (PO) q12h until cured* **or** Itraconazole 200 mg (IV) q12h × 2 days, then 200 mg (IV) q24h × 1–2 weeks, then 200 mg (PO) solution q12h until cured¶
	M. tuberculosis C. neoformans Nocardia	For TB (see p. 55). For C. neoformans or Nocardia (see Chapter 4).
Diffuse infiltrates	S. stercoralis (hyperinfection syndrome)	<u>Preferred Therapy</u> Ivermectin 200 mcg/kg (PO) q24h until cured <u>Alternate Therapy</u> Thiabendazole 25–50 mg/kg (PO) q12h (max. 3 gm/day) until cured

Duration of therapy represents total time PO, IV, or IV + PO. Most patients on IV therapy able to take PO medications should be switched to PO therapy after clinical improvement.

*   If < 40 kg, use 100 mg (PO) maintenance dose.

¶   Significant drug interactions are possible with usual immunosuppressive agents (e.g., sirolimus, cyclosporine, tacrolimus). Review all concomitant medications for potential interactions. *Voriconazole contraindicated in patients on sirolimus.*

§   For usual dose, see Chapter 11 (Drug Summaries)

Transplant Infections¶ *(cont'd)*

PNEUMONIAS (cont'd)		
	PCP/RSV	Treat the same as in other compromised hosts
	CMV, HHV-6	Treat the same as CMV (see p. 57), HHV-6
HEPATITIS		
Viral hepatitis	CMV	Treat the same as for CMV pneumonia (see p. 57)
	HBV, HCV	Treat the same as in normal hosts (see p. 105–106)

Bacteremia/Candidemia (Bacteremia)

Clinical Presentation: Fever and shaking chills ± localizing signs. If localizing signs are present, the organ involved indicates the origin of the bacteremia (e.g., urinary tract findings suggest urosepsis).

Diagnostic Considerations: Diagnosis is clinical and is confirmed by positive blood cultures.

Pitfalls: 3/4 or 4/4 positive blood cultures indicates bacteremia. Even 1/4 positive blood cultures of an unusual pathogen may be clinically significant in BMT/SOT. The significance of 1/4 blood cultures with coagulase-negative staphylococci is less clear. S. epidermidis bacteremia is usually IV-line related, but in some compromised hosts, it may be pathogenic without an IV line focus.

Therapeutic Considerations: In SOT, coverage should be directed against S. aureus and Enterobacteriaceae. Anti-P. aeruginosa coverage is usually not needed since these patients are not neutropenic. If the source of infection is a central IV line, the line should be removed. In pre-engraftment BMT, coverage should be directed against P. aeruginosa until leukopenia resolves. Continued fever after 1 week of appropriate antibiotic therapy suggests the presence of candidemia, or another invasive fungal infection.

Prognosis: Good with early antibiotic therapy and, if appropriate, IV line removal.

Bacteremia/Candidemia (Candidemia)

Clinical Presentation: Fever and shaking chills ± localizing signs. If localizing signs are present, the organ involved indicates the origin of the fungemia (e.g., reddened central IV line site suggests IV line-related fungemia).

Diagnostic Considerations: Candida and Fusarium are the most common fungi associated with fungemia in BMT/SOT.

Pitfalls: Do not assume that all Candida are C. albicans. Non-albicans Candida are more common in SOT patients. Empiric therapy should be directed against non-albicans Candida pending speciation, which will also cover C. albicans (including fluconazole-resistant strains). Because mortality/morbidity associated with candidemia exceeds that of bacteremia, empiric therapy should be started as soon as candidemia is suspected.

Aspergillus, common after BMT/SOT, rarely grows in blood cultures.

Prognosis: Related to underlying immune status and promptness of empiric antifungal therapy, and if appropriate, CVC removal.

CNS Infections (Encephalitis)

Clinical Presentation: Typical encephalitis/meningitis presentation (fever, headache, ± stiff neck, change in mental status).

Diagnostic Considerations: CSF usually reveals a lymphocytic predominance with a normal or normal CSF lactic acid and low glucose. The diagnosis of HSV, CMV, HHV-6 encephalitis can be made by CSF PCR.

Pitfalls: Patients with Listeria encephalitis often have a negative CSF Gram stain, but Listeria nearly always grows on CSF culture. HSV and listeria encephalitis typically have RBCs in the CSF. Head CT/MRI rules out CNS mass lesions. Nuchal rigidity may be absent in meningitis.

Therapeutic Considerations: CMV encephalitis is rare but treatable, resulting in clinical/radiological improvement. However, neurological deficits usually remain. CMV retinitis, common in HIV (p. 327), is unusual in BMT/SOT.

Prognosis: Related to underlying immune status and promptness of therapy.

CNS Infections (Brain Abscess)

Clinical Presentation: BMT/SOT patients with brain abscesses/mass lesions present with seizures/cranial nerve abnormalities. Mental status is clear, in contrast to patients with encephalitis, and nuchal rigidity is absent, in contrast to most patients with meningitis.

Diagnostic Considerations: Head CT/MRI is the preferred diagnostic modality, and brain biopsy is the definitive diagnostic method. CSF analysis is not usually helpful in mass lesions, with the exception of infection due to M. tuberculosis or C. neoformans. With C. neoformans, the CSF cryptococcal antigen test is positive, and the CSF India ink preparation may be positive. With M. tuberculosis, acid fast smear of the CSF is sometimes positive, but culture has a higher yield and PCR is the preferred diagnostic modality.

Pitfalls: Patients with brain abscesses/mass lesions should have a head CT/MRI before lumbar puncture. To avoid herniation during lumbar puncture when a mass lesion is present, lumbar puncture should be performed by an experienced operator, and a minimal amount of CSF should be withdrawn.

Therapeutic Considerations: M. tuberculosis and C. neoformans are readily treatable. Be sure to use antimicrobial therapy that penetrates into CSF/brain. If TMP, TMP–SMX, or minocycline cannot be used for CNS Nocardia, linezolid or meropenem (meningeal doses) may be useful.

Prognosis: Related to underlying immune status and promptness of therapy.

Pneumonias (Focal, Segmental, or Nodular Pulmonary Infiltrates)

Clinical Presentation: Acute or subacute community-acquired pneumonia (CAP) with respiratory symptoms and fever.

Diagnostic Considerations: BMT/SOT patients with focal/segmental infiltrates are most commonly infected with the usual CAP pathogens affecting normal hosts (e.g., S. pneumoniae, H. influenzae, Legionella). The clinical presentation of CAP in organ transplants is indistinguishable from that in normal hosts. However, BMT/SOT patients presenting subacutely with focal/segmental infiltrates are usually infected with pulmonary pathogens with a slower clinical onset (e.g., Nocardia, Aspergillus). L. micdadei common in BMT/SOT, and may cavitate. Empiric therapy will not cover all possible pathogens; tissue biopsy is necessary for definitive diagnosis and specific therapy. Preferred diagnostic modalities include transbronchial lung biopsy, percutaneous thin needle biopsy, or open lung biopsy, not BAL which may be negative in tissue invasive infections, e.g., Aspergillus.

Pitfalls: Patients presenting with subacute onset of CAP have a different pathogen distribution than those presenting with acute CAP. PCP/CMV does not present with focal/segmental infiltrates. Unlike other Legionella sp., L. micdadei partially acid fast, and susceptible to TMP-SMX (as well as doxycycline and quinolones).

Therapeutic Considerations: BMT/SOT patients with acute onset of CAP are treated with the same antibiotics used to treat CAP in normal hosts. Empiric coverage is directed against both typical and atypical bacterial pathogens. If no improvement in clinical status after 72 hours, proceed to transbronchial biopsy or lung biopsy to identify nonbacterial pathogens (e.g., Nocardia, Aspergillus). Nocardia reinfection may require 6–12 months of therapy.

Prognosis: Best with acute focal/segmental infiltrates. Not as good with subacute or chronic focal/segmental infiltrates.

Pneumonias (Diffuse Pulmonary Infiltrates)

Clinical Presentation: Insidious onset of interstitial pneumonia usually accompanied by low-grade fevers. Focal/segmental infiltrates are absent.

Diagnostic Considerations: Bilateral diffuse infiltrates, which can be minimal or extensive, fall into two clinical categories: those with and without hypoxemia/↑ A-a gradient > 35. Diffuse pulmonary infiltrates without hypoxemia suggest a noninfectious etiology (e.g., CHF, pulmonary drug reaction, pulmonary hemorrhage). The differential diagnosis of diffuse pulmonary infiltrates with hypoxemia includes PCP, CMV, HSV, RSV, HHV-6, VZV. Quantitative PCR testing of BAL fluid for CMV, VZV, RSV, HHV-6 may be diagnostically helpful. For interstitial infiltrates with hypoxemia, the chest x-ray may be only minimally abnormal, but chest CT scans are more revealing. CMV/PCP may require tissue biopsy for definitive diagnosis. A highly elevated LDH suggests PCP. PCP : β 1,3 D-glucan +, aspergillus galactomannan –. Transbronchial biopsy (TBB) preferable, but BAL may be negative. The incidence of CMV pneumonia is highest in lung transplants and BMTs.

Pitfalls: Because infections in BMT/SOT are sequential, many patients with PCP pneumonia may have underlying CMV or HHV-6. In BMT, CMV found alone on lung biopsy suggests it is the primary pathogen. Serological tests are helpful for CMV ($\uparrow$ CMV IgM); $\uparrow$ CMV PCR viral loads reflective of peripheral WBC reactivation, not pneumonia. CMV pneumonia diagnosed by demonstrations CMV CPEs (intracellular inclusions) on lung BAL/biopsy. Candida pneumonia does not exist as a separate entity but only rarely as part of pre-terminal disseminated/invasive candidiasis.

Therapeutic Considerations: Among the subacute diffuse pneumonias, PCP is readily treatable. Initiate treatment for CMV pneumonia with ganciclovir IV; after clinical improvement, complete therapy with valganciclovir (PO) until cured. If after treatment, there is an $\uparrow$ in CMV antigen levels or quantitative PCR, treat pre-emptively to prevent CMV pneumonia with valganciclovir 900 mg (PO) q24h until CMV antigen levels return to previous levels or quantitative PCR becomes undetectable.

Prognosis: Related to underlying immune status, promptness of therapy, and general health of host.

Hepatitis (Viral)

Clinical Presentation: Fever with $\uparrow$ AST/ALT $\pm$ RUQ pain.

Diagnostic Considerations: Because CMV is of such critical importance in BMT/SOT, CMV testing should always be done in organ transplants with $\uparrow$ AST/ALT. Liver biopsy with immunohisto chemical staining is diagnostic; quantitative PCR may be helpful. Prior to SOT, HIV, HBV, HCV testing should be performed on donor and recipient. Other viruses causing acute viral hepatitis post-transplant include EBV, HHV-6, VZV, adenovirus, and influenza. Viral hepatitis is usually accompanied by some degree of leukopenia. A few atypical lymphocytes may be present, and serum transaminases may be mildly or markedly elevated. CMV viremia is the commonest manifestation of CMV infection in BMT/SOT patients. CMV has a predilection for infecting the organ transplanted, and CMV hepatitis is particularly common in liver transplants. Anicteric hepatitis is more common than icteric hepatitis.

Pitfalls: The diagnosis of active CMV hepatitis in organ transplant patients is critical because it is an immunomodulating virus, adding to the net immunosuppressive effect of immunosuppressive therapy. Do not rely on CMV IgM/IgG titers for diagnosis.

Therapeutic Considerations: CMV should be treated aggressively to minimize its potentiating immunoregulatory defects, which may predispose to non-viral opportunistic pathogens and $\uparrow$ risk of chronic rejection in SOT. CMV antigen levels or quantitative PCR increase before CMV infection. Therefore, when CMV antigen levels or quantitative PCR increase, begin early pre-emptive therapy with valganciclovir 900 mg (PO) q12h until CMV antigen levels or quantitative PCR return to previous levels. There is no treatment for EBV.

Prognosis: Treated early, CMV responds well to therapy. CMV is associated with chronic allograft rejection in SOT recipient so that prevention or early diagnosis/therapy are critical.

Toxin-Mediated Infectious Diseases

Toxin-Mediated Infectious Diseases

Subset	Usual Pathogens	IV Therapy	PO Therapy or IV-to-PO Switch
Toxic shock syndrome (TSS) (Treat initially for MRSA; if later identified as MSSA, treat accordingly)	S. aureus (MRSA)	<u>Preferred Therapy</u> Vancomycin 1 gm (IV) q12h × 2 weeks **or** Linezolid 600 mg (IV) q12h × 2 weeks <u>Alternate Therapy</u> Minocycline 100 mg (IV) q12h × 2 weeks **or** Daptomycin 6 mg/kg (IV) q24h × 2 weeks	Linezolid 600 mg (PO) q12h × 2 weeks **or** Minocycline 100 mg (PO) q12h × 2 weeks
	S. aureus (MSSA)	<u>Preferred Therapy</u> Cefazolin 1 gm (IV) q8h × 2 weeks <u>Alternate Therapy</u> Nafcillin 2 gm (IV) q4h × 2 weeks **or** Clindamycin 600 mg (IV) q8h × 2 weeks	Cephalexin 500 mg (PO) q6h × 2 weeks **or** Clindamycin 300 mg (PO) q6h × 2 weeks
	Clostridium sordelli	<u>Preferred Therapy</u> Penicillin G 10 mu (IV) q4h × 2 weeks **or** Clindamycin 600 mg (IV) q8h × 2 weeks **or** Piperacillin/Tazobactam 3.375 mg (IV) q8h × 2 weeks <u>Alternate Therapy</u> Meropenem 1 gm (IV) q8h × 2 weeks **or** Ertapenem 1 gm (IV) q24h × 2 weeks	Not applicable

Toxin-Mediated Infectious Diseases (cont'd)

Subset	Usual Pathogens	IV Therapy	PO Therapy or IV-to-PO Switch
Botulism (food, infant, wound)	Clostridium botulinum	<u>Preferred Therapy</u> 2 vials of type-specific trivalent (types A,B,E) or polyvalent (types A,B,C,D,E) antitoxin (IV)	<u>Alternate Therapy</u> Amoxicillin 1 gm (PO) q8h × 7 days (wound botulism only)
Tetanus	Clostridium tetani	<u>Preferred Therapy</u> Tetanus immune globulin (TIG) 3,000–6,000 units (IM) (50% into deltoid, 50% into wound site) **plus either** Penicillin G 4 mu (IV) q4h × 10 days **or** Doxycycline 200 mg (IV or PO) q12h × 3 days, then 100 mg (IV or PO) × 7 days	<u>Alternate Therapy</u> Tetanus antitoxin 1,500–3,000 units (IM/IV) **plus** Metronidazole 1 gm (IV) q12h × 10 days
Diphtheria (pharyngeal, nasal, wound, myocarditis)	Coryne-bacterium diphtheriae C. ulcerans	Diphtheria antitoxin (IV) over 1 hour (pharyngeal diphtheria = 40,000 units; nasopharyngeal diphtheria = 60,000 units; systemic diphtheria or diphtheria > 3 days duration = 100,000 units) **plus either** Penicillin G 1 mu (IV) q4h × 14 days **or** Erythromycin 500 mg (IV) q6h × 14 days	Diphtheria antitoxin (IV) over 1 hour (pharyngeal diphtheria = 40,000 units; naso-pharyngeal diphtheria = 60,000 units; systemic diphtheria or diphtheria > 3 days duration = 100,000 units) **plus** Procaine penicillin 600,000 units (IM) q24h × 14 days

Toxic Shock Syndrome (S. aureus)

Clinical Presentation: Scarlatiniform rash ± hypotension. Spectrum ranges from minimal infection to multiorgan system failure/shock. ↑ CPK common.

Diagnostic Considerations: Diagnosis by clinical presentation with mucous membrane, renal, liver, and skin involvement/culture of TSS-1 toxin-producing strain of S. aureus from mouth, nares, vagina, or wound.

Pitfalls: Toxic shock syndrome wound discharge is clear, not purulent.

Therapeutic Considerations: Remove source of toxin production if possible (e.g., remove tampon, drain collections). Clindamycin may be added for its anti-toxin effect.

Prognosis: Good in early/mild form. Poor in late/multisystem disease form.

Toxic Shock Syndrome (C. sordelli)

Clinical Presentation: Resembles clostridial myonecrosis (gas gangrene) with soft tissue necrotizing infection are local edema. Hypotension with acute onset of nausea/vomiting and weakness characteristic. Associated with IVDA (black tar heroin), trauma, parturition, abortion, cadaver graft surgery. Hemoconcentration with leukocytosis typical; leukemoid reactions common with WBC counts > 50k/mm^3.

Diagnostic Considerations: Clinical diagnosis. Culture of C. sordelli from necrotic soft tissue.

Pitfalls: Gas gangrene like clinical presentation but with hemoconcentration not hemolytic anemia. Nausea/vomiting instead of diarrhea as with gas gangrene. Shock with no/low fever and ↑ WBC should suggest the diagnosis. Muscle involvement (clostridial myonecrosis) and bullae typical of gas gangrene not a feature of C. sordelli TSS.

Therapeutic Considerations: Early/adequate debridement critical. Anti-anerobic antibiotics and supportive measures important.

Prognosis: Like gas gangrene, prognosis related to early diagnosis and early/adequate surgical debridement.

Botulism (Clostridium botulinum)

Clinical Presentation: Descending symmetrical paralysis beginning with cranial nerve involvement, induced by botulinum toxin. Onset begins with blurry vision, followed rapidly by ocular muscle paralysis, difficulty speaking, and inability to swallow. Respiratory paralysis may occur in severe cases. Mental status is unaffected. Usual incubation period is 10–12 hours. Incubation is shortest for Type E strain (hours), longest for Type A strain (up to 10 days), and is inversely proportional to the quantity of toxin consumed (food botulism). Wound botulism (Types A or B) may follow C. botulinum entry into IV drug abuser injection site, surgical or traumatic wounds. Infant (< 1 year) botulism (most commonly Type A or B) is acquired from C. botulinum containing honey. Patients with botulism are afebrile, and have profuse vomiting without diarrhea.

Diagnostic Considerations: Detection of botulinum toxin from stool, serum, or food (especially home canned foods with neutral or near neutral pH [~ 7] or smoked fish [Type E]) is diagnostic of food botulism. Wound botulism is diagnosed by culturing C. botulinum from the wound or by detecting botulinum toxin in the serum.

Pitfalls: Clinical diagnosis based on descending paralysis with cranial nerve involvement in an afebrile patient must be differentiated from Guillain-Barre (fever, ascending paralysis, sensory component) and polio (fever, pure ascending motor paralysis). Do not diagnose botulism in the absence of ocular/pharyngeal paralysis.

Therapeutic Considerations: Antitoxin neutralizes only unbound toxin, and does not reverse toxin-induced paralysis. Botulism is a toxin-mediated infection and antibiotic therapy (wound botulism) is adjunctive. Guanidine has been used with variable effect. Ventilator support is needed for respiratory paralysis. Bioterrorist botulism presents clinically and is treated the same as naturally-acquired botulism.

Prognosis: Good if treated early, before respiratory paralysis.

Tetanus (Clostridium tetani)

Clinical Presentation: Begins with jaw stiffness/difficulty chewing induced by C. tetani toxin (tetanospasmin). Trismus rapidly follows with masseter muscle spasm, followed by spasm of the abdominal/back muscles. Rigidity and convulsions may occur. Patients are afebrile unless there is hypothalamic involvement (central fever), in which case fevers may exceed 106°F. Usual incubation period is 3–21 days.

Diagnostic Considerations: Diagnosis suggested by muscle spasms/rigidity in a patient with trismus.

Pitfalls: In rabies, muscle spasms are localized and usually involve the face/neck, rather than primary involvement of the extremities, as in tetanus.

Therapeutic Considerations: Tetanus is self-limited with intensive supportive care. Sedation is important, and avoidance of all stimuli is mandatory to reduce the risk of convulsions. Avoid unnecessary handling/movement of patient. Antitoxin is effective only in neutralizing unbound toxin. Tracheostomy/respiratory support can be lifesaving in severe cases.

Prognosis: Good if not complicated by spinal fractures, aspiration pneumonia, or CNS involvement (hyperpyrexia, hyper/hypotension).

Diphtheria (Corynebacterium diphtheriae/Corynebacterium ulcerans)

Clinical Presentation: Within 1 week following insidious onset of sore throat without fever, pharyngeal patches coalesce to form a gray diphtheric membrane (surrounded by a red border), which is adherent/bleeds easily when removed. Membrane begins unilaterally; may extend to the soft palate, uvula and contralateral posterior pharynx; are accompanied by prominent bilateral anterior adenopathy; become necrotic (green/black); and have a foul odor (fetor oris). Submandibular edema ("bull neck") and hoarseness (laryngeal stridor) precede respiratory obstruction/death. Cutaneous diphtheria may follow C. diphtheriae contaminated wounds (traumatic, surgical) or insect/human bites, and is characterized by a leathery eschar (cutaneous membrane) covering a deep punched out ulcer. Serosanguineous discharge is typical of nasal diphtheria (membrane in nares). Diphtheric myocarditis may complicate any form of diphtheria (most commonly follows pharyngeal form), and usually occurs in the second week, but may occur up to 8 weeks after infection begins. Diphtheric polyneuritis is a common complication. Cardiac/neurologic complications are due to elaboration of a potent toxin.

Diagnostic Considerations: Diagnosis is suggested by unilateral membranous pharyngitis/palatal paralysis, absence of fever, and relative tachycardia. Diagnosis is confirmed by culture of C. diphtheriae from nares, membrane, or wound.

Pitfalls: Differentiated from Arcanobacterium (Corynebacterium) haemolyticum (which also forms a pharyngeal membrane) by culture and absence of scarlatiniform rash with C. diphtheriae. C.ulcerans has the same clinical features as C. diphtheriae.

Therapeutic Considerations: Antibiotic therapy treats the infection and stops additional toxin production. Antitoxin is effective against unbound toxin, but will not reverse toxin-mediated myocarditis/neuropathy. Serum sickness is common 2 weeks after antitoxin. Respiratory/cardiac support may be lifesaving. C.ulcerans is treated the same as C. diptheriae.

Prognosis: Poor with airway obstruction or myocarditis. Myocarditis may occur despite early treatment.

Bioterrorist Agents

Bioterrorist Agents in Adults[¶]

Subset	Pathogen	IV/IM Therapy	IV-to-PO Switch
Anthrax *Inhalation, oropharyngeal, gastrointestinal*	Bacillus anthracis	Quinolone* (IV) × 2 weeks **or** Doxycycline 200 mg (IV) q12h × 3 days, then 100 mg (IV) q12h × 11 days[‡] **or** Penicillin G 4 MU (IV) q4h ± Clindamycin 600 mg (IV) q8h × 2 weeks	Quinolone* (PO) × 2 weeks **or** Doxycycline 200 mg (PO) q12h × 3 days, then 100 mg (PO) q12h × 11 days (loading dose not needed PO if given IV). Duration of IV + PO therapy = 60 days
Cutaneous		Treat severe cases with same (PO) antibiotics as for inhalation anthrax	
Meningitis		If penicillin susceptible, treat with Penicillin G 4 MU (IV) q24h **or** Meropenem 2 gm (IV) q8h for at least 2 weeks or markedly improved and complete 60–100 days of therapy as described in the inhalation, oropharyngeal or gastrointestinal forms, in addition to quinolones or doxycycline. Consider adjunctive steroid therapy. Penicillin should NOT be used as a single agent. Not susceptible to cephalosporins or TMP–SMX.	

Duration of therapy represents total treatment time.

‡   Patients who remain critically ill after Doxycycline 200 mg (IV) q12h × 3 days should continue receiving 200 mg (IV) q12h for the full course of therapy. For patients who have improved after 3 days, the dose may be decreased to 100 mg (IV or PO) q12h to complete the course of therapy. Total duration of IV + PO therapy = 60 days.

*   Ciprofloxacin 400 mg (IV) q12h or 500 mg (PO) q12h or Levofloxacin 500 mg (IV or PO) q24h.

¶   Additional information can be obtained at www.bt.cdc.gov. For post-exposure prophylaxis, see Chapter 6.

Bioterrorist Agents in Adults¶ *(cont'd)*

Subset	Pathogen	IV/IM Therapy	IV-to-PO Switch
Tularemia pneumonia	Francisella tularensis	Doxycycline 200 mg (IV) q12h × 3 days, then 100 mg (IV) q12h × 11–18 days‡ **or** Quinolone* (IV) × 10 days ± Streptomycin 1 gm (IM) q12h × 10 days **or** Gentamicin 5 mg/kg (IM or IV) q24h × 10 days **or** Chloramphenicol 500 mg (IV) q6h × 14 days <u>If meningitis:</u> add Chloramphenicol	Doxycycline 200 mg (PO) q12h × 3 days, then 100 mg (PO) q12h × 11–18 days **or** Quinolone* (PO) × 10 days <u>If meningitis:</u> add Chloramphenicol
Pneumonic plague	Yersinia pestis	Doxycycline 200 mg (IV) q12h × 3 days, then 100 mg (IV) q12h × 11–18 days‡ **or** Quinolone* (IV) × 10 days ± Streptomycin 1 gm (IM) q12h × 10 days or Gentamicin 5 mg/kg (IM or IV) q24h × 10 days	
Botulism	Clostridium botulinum	Contrary to the package insert, administer 50 mg/kg up to 1 vial of type-specific trivalent (types A,B,E) or polyvalent (types A,B,C,D,E) antitoxin after skin testing. Antitoxin administration is not repeated (circulating antitoxin's half-life = 5–8 days). Treatment with 1 vial resulted in adverse effects in < 1%; treatment with 2–4 times present dose resulted in hypersensitivity reactions in 9%. Antibiotics do not neutralize toxin	
Smallpox	Variola virus	Tecovirimat (Tpoxx) 600 mg (PO) q12h x 14 days	
Ebola	Ebola virus	No specific therapy. Supportive therapy can be life saving	

Duration of therapy represents total treatment time.

*   Ciprofloxacin 400 mg (IV) q12h or 500 mg (PO) q12h or Levofloxacin 500 mg (IV or PO) q24h.

¶   Additional information can be obtained at www.bt.cdc.gov. For post-exposure prophylaxis, see Chapter 6.

‡   Patients who remain critically ill after Doxycycline 200 mg (IV) q12h × 3 days should continue receiving 200 mg (IV) q12h for the full course of therapy. For patients who have improved after 3 days, the dose may be decreased to 100 mg (IV or PO) q12h to complete the course of therapy. Total duration of IV + PO therapy = 60 days.

Anthrax (B. anthracis)

Clinical Presentation: Bioterrorist anthrax usually presents as cutaneous or inha-lational anthrax. Cutaneous anthrax has the same clinical presentation as naturally-acquired anthrax: Lesions begin as painless, sometimes mildly pruritic papules, usually on the upper extremities, neck, or face, and evolve into a vesicular lesion which may be surrounded by satellite lesions. A "gelatinous halo" surrounds the ves-icle as it evolves into an ulcer, and a black eschar eventually develops over the ulcer. Inhalational anthrax is a biphasic illness. Initially, there is a viral illness-like prodrome with fever, chills, and myalgias with chest discomfort 3–5 days after inhaling anthrax spores. Bacteremia is common. Patients often improve somewhat over the next 1–2 days, only to rapidly deteriorate and become critically ill with high fevers, dyspnea, cyanosis, crushing substernal chest pain, and shock. Oropharyngeal anthrax pres-ents with fever, soft tissue edema, painful cervical adenopathy. Lesions in orophar-ynx ulcerate in ~ 2 weeks. GI anthrax presents with fever, malaise ± syncope, followed in 24 hours by mild nausea/vomiting, severe abdominal pain, and then ascites, ↑ abdominal pain, flushed face, and shock.

Diagnostic Considerations: Cutaneous anthrax is a clinical diagnosis suggested by the lack of pain relative to the size of the lesion. A presumptive microbiologic diagnosis is made by finding gram-positive bacilli in the fluid from the gelatinous halo surrounding the ulcer or from under the eschar. Blood cultures may reveal B. anthracis. Definitive diagnosis depends on identifying B. anthracis from culture of the skin lesions or blood cultures. Inhalation anthrax is suspected in patients with fevers, chest pain, and mediastinal widening accompanied by bilateral pleural effu-sions on chest x-ray. If chest x-ray findings are equivocal, then a chest CT/MRI is recommended to demonstrate mediastinal lymph node enlargement. Inhalational anthrax presents as a hemorrhagic mediastinitis, not community-acquired pneumo-nia. The diagnosis is clinical but supported by Gram stain of hemorrhagic pleural fluid demonstrating gram-positive bacilli. Patients with inhalational anthrax often have positive blood cultures and may have associated anthrax meningitis. If men-ingitis is present, the CSF is hemorrhagic and CSF Gram stain shows gram-positive bacilli, which, when cultured, is B. anthracis.

Pitfalls: Cutaneous anthrax is most often initially confused with ringworm or a brown recluse spider bite. Subacute/chronic lesions may initially resemble ringworm, but the skin lesion in ringworm has an annular configuration, is painless, and is accompanied by prominent pruritus, particularly at the edges of the lesion. Patients with ringworm have no fever or systemic symptoms. Brown recluse spider bites produce extremely painful lesions with irregular edges, which eventually develop a necrotic center fol-lowed by eschar formation. The lesions of the brown recluse spider bite are irregu-lar, not accompanied by fever, and intensely painful. In contrast, cutaneous anthrax lesions are painless, round, and are not primarily pruritic in nature. Be alert to the possibility of smallpox following outbreaks of other bioterrorist agents such as anthrax, as the genome of smallpox is easily modified and can be incorporated into bacteria.

Therapeutic Considerations: B. anthracis is highly susceptible to nearly all antibiotics; in the U.S. bioterrorist experience, no strains were resistant to antibiotics. Traditionally, penicillin has been used to treat natural anthrax, but because of concern for resistant bioterrorist strains, doxycycline or quinolones are preferred. Because meningitis is frequently associated with inhalational anthrax, penicillin in (IV) meningeal doses may be added as a second or third antibiotic to quinolones or doxycycline. For meningeal anthrax use penicillin G or meropenem in meningeal doses. Clindamycin is active against B. anthracis and has been used in combination therapy because of its potential anti-exotoxin activity. Some patients seemed to respond somewhat better when clindamycin 600 mg (IV) q8h or 300 mg (PO) q8h plus rifampin 300 mg (PO) q12h is added to either a quinolone or doxycycline. Corticosteroids should be considered for severe mediastinal edema or meningitis. Depending upon antimicrobial susceptibility testing, rifampin, vancomycin, penicillin, ampicillin, chloramphenicol, imipenem, clindamycin or clarithromycin may be added if the need arises. Prolonged therapy of 100 days with or without anthrax vaccine has been recommended by some authors. Three doses of anthrax vaccine (BioThraxT, formerly AVA - anthrax vaccine absorbed) have been recommended by the ACIP and the John Hopkins Working Group on Civilian Bio-Defense with antimicrobials for prophylaxis after aerosolized exposure, but as it is not licensed, it must be administered under an IND application. Some B. anthracis strains produce cephalosporinase and inducible beta-lactamase that make penicillins drugs less suitable for initial therapy. In general, the organism is resistant to trimethoprim-sulfamethoxazole.

Prognosis: Prognosis of cutaneous anthrax is uniformly good. With inhalational anthrax, prognosis is related to the inhaled dose of the organism, underlying host status, and rapidity of initiating antimicrobial therapy. Inhalational anthrax remains a highly lethal infectious disease, but with early intervention/supportive care, some patients survive. Patients with associated anthrax meningitis have a poor prognosis.

Tularemic Pneumonia (F. tularensis)

Clinical Presentation: Fever, chills, myalgias, headache, dyspnea and a nonproductive cough may occur, but encephalopathy is absent. Chest x-ray resembles other causes of community-acquired pneumonia, but tularemic pneumonia is usually accompanied by hilar adenopathy and pleural effusion, which is serosanguineous or frankly bloody. Cavitation sometimes occurs. Relative bradycardia is not present and serum transaminases are not elevated.

Diagnostic Considerations: Tularemic pneumonia can resemble other atypical pneumonias, but in a patient presenting with community-acquired pneumonia, the presence of hilar adenopathy with pleural effusions should suggest the diagnosis. F. tularensis may be seen in the Gram stain of the sputum or bloody pleural effusion fluid as a small, bipolar staining, gram-negative bacillus. Diagnosis is confirmed serologically or by culture of the organism from respiratory fluid/blood.

Pitfalls: Gram-negative bacilli in the sputum may resemble Y. pestis but are not bipolar staining. Chest x-ray may resemble inhalational anthrax (hilar adenopathy/mediastinal widening). Both tularemic pneumonia and inhalational anthrax may be accompanied by bloody pleural effusions. In contrast to inhalational anthrax (which may be accompanied by anthrax meningitis), CNS involvement is not a feature of tularemic pneumonia.

Therapeutic Considerations: Streptomycin is the antibiotic traditionally used to treat tularemia. Gentamicin may be substituted for streptomycin if it is not available. Doxycycline, chloramphenicol, or a quinolone are also effective.

Prognosis: Depends on inoculum size and health of host. Mortality rates for severe untreated infection can be as high as 30%, although early treatment is associated with mortality rates < 1%.

Pneumonic Plague (Y. pestis)

Clinical Presentation: Bioterrorist plague presents as pneumonic plague and has the potential for person-to-person spread. After an incubation period of 1–4 days, the patient presents with acute onset of fever, chills, headache, myalgias and dizziness, followed by pulmonary manifestations including cough, chest pain, dyspnea. Hemoptysis may occur, and increasing respiratory distress and circulatory collapse are common. Compared to community-acquired pneumonia, patients presenting with plague pneumonia are critically ill. Sputum is pink and frothy and contains abundant bipolar staining gram-negative bacilli. Chest x-ray is not diagnostic.

Diagnostic Considerations: Yersinia pestis may be demonstrated in sputum Gram stain (bipolar staining gram-negative bacilli) and may be recovered from blood cultures. Laboratory confirmation requires isolation of Y. pestis from body fluid or tissue culture. Consider the diagnosis in any critically ill patient with pneumonia and bipolar staining gram-negative bacilli in the sputum.

Pitfalls: Plague pneumonia can resemble tularemic pneumonia, but there are several distinguishing features. Unlike plague, tularemic pneumonia is usually associated with hilar enlargement and pleural effusion. Although gram-negative bacilli may be present in the sputum of patients with tularemia, the organisms are not bipolar staining. Y. pestis may be misidentified as Pseudomonas luteola in hospital-automated systems.

Therapeutic Considerations: Streptomycin is the preferred drug for pneumonic plague. Doxycycline or a quinolone are also effective.

Prognosis: Depends on inoculum size, health of the host, and the rapidity of treatment. Left untreated, mortality rates exceed 50%. ARDS, DIC, and other manifestations of gram-negative sepsis are more common when treatment is delayed.

Smallpox

Clinical Presentation: After an incubation period of 1–12 days, typical smallpox is heralded by high fever, headache, and gastrointestinal complaints (vomiting, colicky pain). No rash is present at this time. After 1–2 days, the fever decreases to near normal level, and macules begin to appear on the head, usually at the hairline. Macules progress to papules, then vesicles, then finally pustules. The rash begins on the face/head and rapidly spreads to the extremities with relative sparing of the trunk. The mucous membranes of the oropharynx and upper/lower airways are also affected early. Lesions initially are umbilicated, then later lose their umbilication. The fully formed smallpox pustule is located deep in the dermis. The appearance of the pustules is accompanied by recrudescence of fever. Hemorrhagic smallpox is a fulminant form of smallpox that begins with petechial lesions in a "swimming trunk" distribution and results in widespread hemorrhage into the skin and mucous membranes. Patients look toxemic and have high fevers with no other signs of smallpox; death from toxemia often occurs before the typical rash appears.

Diagnostic Considerations: Smallpox is most likely to be confused with chickenpox or drug eruptions. Patients with chickenpox are less toxemic and the lesion distribution is different from smallpox. Chickenpox lesions occur in crops for the first 72 hours, then stop. The lesions of chickenpox are superficial, not deep in the dermis like smallpox, and chickenpox vesicles are predominantly centripetal rather than centrifugal. The chickenpox vesicle has been described as a "dewdrop on a rose petal" because of its fragility and superficial location on the skin. If there is any doubt, a Tzanck test should be performed by unroofing the vesicle, scraping cells from the base of the vesicle, and staining the cells. A positive Tzanck test indicates chickenpox, not smallpox. Alternatively, a monoclonal VZV test can be performed on vesicle base cells. Drug eruptions are not accompanied by toxemia and are usually accompanied by relative bradycardia if fever is present.

Pitfalls: Smallpox is easily missed before the rash and is difficult to diagnose. Look for the combination of high fever/headache with gastrointestinal symptoms (e.g., abdominal pain) that precedes the rash. GI complaints may be confused with appendicitis. A petechial rash in a swimming trunk distribution does not occur with any other infectious disease and should immediately suggest smallpox. Recently human monkeypox has occurred in the Western Hemisphere after transmission via imported African rodent pets. After an incubation period of 7–19 days, patients develop fever, headache, and malaise. Skin lesions appear on head, trunk, and extremities (including palms/soles). Rash begins like smallpox as macules, then papules, and finally umbilicated vesicles.

Some exudative pharyngitis/tonsillitis with cervical adenopathy may be present. Encephalitis is very rare. Laboratory results are nonspecific. Unlike smallpox, human monkeypox patients are not toxic, have pharyngitis/tonsillitis with cervical adenopathy, and have focal hemorrhage into some lesions (in hemorrhagic smallpox, hemorrhages are extensive/widespread). Patients immunized against smallpox are unlikely to acquire human monkeypox.

Therapeutic Considerations: Smallpox vaccination should be initiated as soon as the diagnosis is suspected. Smallpox vaccine may be given at full strength or in a 1:5 dilution, which is also protective. Cidofovir may prove useful but dose for smallpox is not established.

Prognosis: Variable in typical smallpox, with deep, permanent scarring, especially on the face. Hemorrhagic smallpox is highly lethal.

Ebola/Lassa Fever

Clinical Presentation: After an incubation period of 3–9 days, abrupt onset of high fevers, severe headache/myalgias followed by diarrhea, extreme malaise. Hemorrhagic phenomenon–GI, renal, vaginal, conjunctival bleeding-occur at 5–7 days. Patients rapidly become critically ill. Fever is biphasic. Patients usually have leukopenia, thrombocytopenia, and hepatic/renal dysfunction. Conjunctival suffusion is also an early finding in half the cases. If a patient is not a traveler from an endemic area (e.g., Africa), suspect bioterrorist Ebola/Lassa fever. Lassa fever differs from Ebola in having prominent head/neck edema. CNS finding (oculogyric crisis, seizures, deafness) are characteristic of Lassa fever.

Diagnostic Considerations: Ebola is a hemorrhagic fever clinically indistinguishable from Yellow fever and other African hemorrhagic fevers (e.g., Lassa fever, Marburg virus disease). Presumptive diagnosis is clinical; definitive diagnosis is confirmed by specific virologic/serologic studies.

Pitfalls: Patients with Ebola may complain initially of a sore throat and dry cough, with or without chest pain. Diarrhea/abdominal pain is not uncommon. The rash is maculopapular before it becomes hemorrhagic. Failure to consider the diagnosis may occur early when sore throat/GI symptoms are prominent (i.e., before hemorrhagic manifestations appear).

Therapeutic Considerations: There is no effective therapy available for Ebola infection. Supportive therapy can be life saving.

Prognosis: Varies with severity of infection and health of the host.

REFERENCES

Arikan S Rex JH (eds). Antifungal Drugs in Manual of Clinical Microbiology (8th Ed), 2003.

Baddour L, Gorbach SL (eds). Therapy of Infectious Diseases. Saunders, Philadelphia, Pennsylvania, 2003.

Bennett JE, Dolin R, Blaser MJ (eds). Mandell, Douglas, and Bennett's Principles and Practice of infectious Diseases (9th Ed), Elsevier Churchill Livingstone, 2019.

Bodey GP, Feinstein V (eds). Candidiasis. New York, Raven Press, 1985.

Bope ET, Kellerman RD (eds). Conn's Therapy, Elsevier, Philadelphia, PA, 2015.

Bowden RA, Ljungman P, Snydman DR (eds). Transplant Infections (3rd Ed), Lippincott Williams & Wilkins, Philadelphia, PA, 2010.

Brandstetter R, Cunha BA, Karetsky M (eds). The Pneumonias. Mosby, Philadelphia, 1999.

Brook I (ed). Sinusitis. Taylor & Francis Group, New York, New York, 2006.

Brusch JL Endocarditis Essentials. Jones & Bartlett, Sudbury, MA, 2010.

Brusch, JL. Infective Endocarditis: Management in the Era of Intravascular Devices. Informa Healthcare, New York 2007.

Bryskier A (ed). Antimicrobial Agents. ASM Press, Washington, D.C., 2005.

Calderone RA (ed). Candida and Candidiasis. ASM Press, Washington DC, 2002.

Cimolai N (ed). Laboratory Diagnosis of Bacterial Infections. New York, Marcel Dekker, 2001.

Cohen J, Powderly WG, Opal S (Eds), Infectious Diseases (4th Ed). Elsevier, Philadelphia 2016.

Cunha BA (ed). Infectious Disease in the Elderly. John Wright & Co., London, 1988.

Cunha BA (ed). Tick-Borne Infectious Diseases. Marcel Dekker, New York, 2005.

Cunha CB, Cunha BA (eds). Infectious Disease in Critical Care Medicine (4th Ed), CRC Press, Boca Raton, 2020.

Cunha CB, Schlossberg D (eds). Clinical Infections Diseases (3rd Ed), Cambridge University Press, London, 2020.

Despommier DD, Gwadz RW Hotez PJ, Knirsh CA (eds). Parasitic Diseases (5th Ed), Apple Tree Productions, LLC, New York, New York, 2005.

Faro S, Soper DE (eds). Infectious Diseases in Women. WB Saunders Company, Philadelphia, 2001.

Farrar J (eds). Manson's Tropical Diseases (23rd Ed). Elsevier Saunders, London, 2014.

Glauser MP, Pizzo PA (eds). Management of Infection in Immunocompromised Patients. W.B. Saunders, London, 2000.

Gorbach SL, Bartlett JG, Blacklow NR (eds). Infectious Diseases (3rd Ed), Philadelphia, Lippincott, Williams & Wilkins, 2004.

Grayson ML (ed). Kucers' The Use of Antibiotics (6th Ed), ASM Press, Washington, DC, 2010.

Guerrant RL, Walker DH, Weller PF (eds). Tropical Infectious Disease: Principles, Pathogens & Practice (3rd Ed), Elsevier, Philadelphia, 2011.

Halperin JJ. Encephalitis: Diagnosis and Treatment. Informa Healthcare, New York, 2008.

Hauser AR, Rello J (eds). Severe Infections Caused by Pseudomonas Aeruginosa. Kluwer Academic Publishers, Boston, Massachusetts, 2003.

Koff RS Hepatitis Essentials, Jones & Bartlett, Sudbury, MA, 2011.

Madkour MM (ed). Tuberculosis. Springer-Verlag, Berlin Germany, 2004.

Maertens JA, Marr KA. Diagnosis of Fungal Infections. Informa Healthcare, New York, 2007.

McMillan A, Young H, Ogilvie MM, Scott GR (eds). Clinical practice in Sexually Transmissible Infections, Saunders, London, England, 2002.

Pilch RF, Ziliinskas RA (eds). Encyclopedia of Bioterrorism Defense. Wiley-Liss, Hoboken, New Jersey, 2005.

Raoult D, Parola P. Rickettsial Diseases. Informa Healthcare, New York, 2007.

Rom WN, Garay SM (eds). Tuberculosis. Lippincott Williams & Wilkins, Philadelphia, Pennsylvania, 2004.

Scheld W, Whitley R, Marra C (eds). Infections of the Central Nervous System (3rd Ed), Lippincott Williams & Wilkins, Philadelphia, 2005.

Schlossberg D (ed). Tuberculosis & Nontuberculous Mycobacterial Infections (7th Ed), New York, McGraw-Hill, 2017.

Schlossberg D (ed). Current Therapy of Infectious Disease (3rd Ed), Mosby-Yearbook, St. Louis, 2008.

Schlossberg D (ed). Medical Interventions for Bioterrorism and Emerging Infections. Handbooks in Healthcare Co., Newtown, Pennsylvania, 2004.

Singh N, Aguado JM (eds). Infectious Complications in Transplant Patients. Kluwer Academic Publishers, Boston, 2000.

Studahl M, Cinque P, Bergstrom T (eds). Herpes Simplex Viruses. Taylor & Francis Group, New York, New York, 2006.

Wingard JR, Anaissie EL (eds). Fungal Infections in the Immunocompromised Patient. Taylor & Francis Group, Boca Raton, Florida, 2005.

Woods JB (ed). USAMRIID's Medical management of biological casualties handbook (6th Ed), US Army Medical Research Institute of Infections Disease, Fort Detrick, Frederick, Maryland, 2005.

Yoshikawa TT, Rajagopalan S (eds). Antibiotic Therapy for Geriatric Patients. Taylor & Francis Group, New York, New York, 2006.

Yu, V, Edwards G, McKinnon PS, Peloquin C, Morse G (eds). Antimicrobial Therapy and Vaccines, Volume II: Antimicrobial Agents (2nd Ed), ESun Technologies, Pittsburgh, Pennsylvania, 2005.

Chapter 3

Antibiotic Susceptibility Profiles and Initial Therapy of Isolates Pending Susceptibility Results

Cheston B. Cunha, MD, Paul E. Schoch, PhD, Edward J. Bottone, PhD, Rodger P. Silletti, PhD, John H. Rex, MD, Burke A. Cunha, MD

Table 3.1 Antibiotic Susceptibility Profiles (Penicillins, Macrolides, Tetracyclines, and Miscellaneous Others)

ORGANISMS	Penicillins						Anti-Pseudomonal Penicillins				Macrolides			Tetracyclines					Miscellaneous				
	Penicillin G/V (IV/PO)	Ampicillin (IV/PO)	Ampicillin/Sulbactam (IV)	Amoxicillin (PO)	Amoxicillin/Clavulanate (PO)	Nafcillin (IV)	Ticarcillin (IV)	Ticarcillin/Clavulanate (IV)	Piperacillin (IV)	Piperacillin/Tazobactam (IV)	Erythromycin (IV/PO)	Clarithromycin (PO)	Azithromycin (IV/PO)	Tetracycline (IV/PO)	Doxycycline (IV/PO)	Minocycline (IV/PO)	Eravacycline (IV)	Omadacycline (IV/PO)	Clindamycin (IV/PO)	Metronidazole (IV/PO)	Rifampin (PO)	TMP-SMX (IV/PO)	Chloramphenicol (IV/PO)
Aerobic Gram Positive Cocci (clusters)																							
Staphylococcus aureus (MSSA)	0	1	2	0	2	3	0	0	0	3	3	0	0	0	2	1	2	2	1	0	2	1	2
Staphylococcus aureus (HA/CO-MRSA)	0	0	0	0	0	0	0	0	0	0	0	0	0	0	2†	1	2	2	2†	0	2	3†	0
S. aureus (CA-MRSA)	0	0	0	0	0	0	0	0	0	0	0	0	0	0	2	1	2	2	2	0	0	2	0
S. epidermidis (CoNS)	0	0	0	0	0	0	0	0	0	0	0	0	0	0	2	2	2	2	2	0	2	2	0
Aerobic Gram Positive Cocci (chains)																							
Enterococcus faecalis (VSE)	0	1	2	1	1	0	3	2	2	2	3	0	0	0	0	0	2	0	0	0	0	3	3
Enterococcus faecium (VRE)††	0	0	0	0	0	0	0	0	0	0	0	0	0	0	3	2	2	0	0	0	0	0	3
Streptococci (Groups A, B, C, F, G)	1	2	2	1	2	0	2	2	2	2	3	3	3	0	0	0	2	2	1	0	0	0	3

Streptococcus (bovis) gallolyticus	1	2	2	1	2	0	2	2	2	3	0	0	0	0	0	0	0	0	3
Viridans streptococci (S. anginosus, S. mitis, S. mutans, S. sanguis, S. salivarius)	1	2	2	1	2	0	2	2	2	3	3	0	2	2	2	0	0	0	3
Aerobic Gram Positive Cocci (pairs)																			
Streptococcus pneumoniae (PSSP)	1	3*	2	1	2	0	2	2	2	3*	3*	3*	1	2	2	0	3*	3*	3
Streptococcus pneumoniae (PRSP)	1	0*	2	1	2	0	3	3	3	0	0	0	1	2	2	0	2	0	3
Streptococcus pneumoniae (MDRSP)	0	0	0	0	0	0	0	0	0	0	0	0	3	2	2	0	3	0	3
Aerobic Gram Negative Cocci (pairs)																			
Neisseria gonorrhoeae	3	0	2	0	2	0	0	2	0	3	2	3*	2	2	0	0	0	0	3
Neisseria meningitidis	1	2	2	0	2	0	2	0	2	0	0	0	3	3	0	0	2	2	2
Aerobic Gram Positive Bacilli																			
Bacillus anthracis	2	2	3	2	3	0	0	0	0	3	3	2	1	0	0	2	2	2	2
Corynebacterium diphtheriae	2	0	0	0	0	0	0	0	0	0	0	0	0	0	0	0	0	0	0

1 = Preferred antibiotic—High degree of activity against the isolate and likely to be clinically effective, most strains susceptible, has a favorable PK/PD characteristics, has a good safety profile, and has a "low resistance" potential (see Chapter 11 Drug Summaries for antibiotic dosing details). 2 = Alternate choice—With many attributes of preferred antibiotic. 3 = Acceptable, but preferably select an alternate antibiotic. 0 = No activity or no data or limited experience. * = May be effective initially but as a "high resistance" antibiotic potential, resistance may develop during/after therapy. † = Preferably use another CA-MRSA antibiotic, e.g. minocycline. †† = Same for vancomycin resistant E. faecalis.

Table 3.1 Antibiotic Susceptibility Profiles (Penicillins, Macrolides, Tetracyclines, and Miscellaneous Others) *(cont'd)*

ORGANISMS	Penicillin (G/V) (IV/PO)	Ampicillin (IV/PO)	Amoxicillin (PO)	Amoxicillin/Clavulanate (PO)	Ampicillin/Sulbactam (IV)	Nafcillin (IV)	Ticarcillin (IV)	Ticarcillin/Clavulanate (IV)	Piperacillin (IV)	Piperacillin/Tazobactam (IV)	Erythromycin (IV/PO)	Clarithromycin (PO)	Azithromycin (IV/PO)	Tetracycline (IV/PO)	Doxycycline (IV/PO)	Minocycline (IV/PO)	Eravacycline (IV)	Omadacycline (IV/PO)	Clindamycin (IV/PO)	Metronidazole (IV/PO)	Rifampin (PO)§	TMP-SMX (IV/PO)	Chloramphenicol (IV/PO)
Corynebacterium jeikeium (JK)	0	1	0	0	0	0	0	0	0	0	0	0	0	0	0	0	0	0	0	0	2	0	0
Listeria monocytogenes	3	1	1	2	2	0	2	2	2	2	3	0	0	3	3	3	0	0	0	0	2	1	1
Nocardia	0	0	0	0	0	0	0	0	0	0	0	0	0	3	1	2	0	0	0	0	0	1	0
Aerobic Gram-Negative Bacilli																							
Acinetobacter sp.	0	0	0	0	1	0	0	3	0	3	0	0	0	0	3	2	1	3	0	0	3	3	0
Aeromonas hydrophila	0	0	0	3	3	0	3	3	3	3	0	0	0	0	2	3	0	0	0	0	0	2	2
Bordetella sp.	0	0	0	0	0	0	0	0	0	0	1	1	1	3	3	3	0	0	0	0	3	2	3
Brucella sp.	0	0	0	0	0	0	0	0	0	0	0	0	0	3	2	3	0	0	0	0	3	3	3
Burkholderia (Pseudomonas) cepacia	0	0	0	2	0	0	0	0	0	0	0	0	0	0	3	2	0	0	0	0	0	3	3
Campylobacter sp.	0	0	2	0	0	0	0	0	0	0	1	3	1	0	0	0	0	0	0	0	0	0	2
Citrobacter sp.	0	0	0	0	0	0	3	3	3	3	0	0	0	0	0	0	0	0	0	0	0	3	3
Enterobacter sp.	0	0	0	0	0	0	3	3	3	3	0	0	0	0	0	0	1	1	0	0	0	3	0

Organism																			
Escherichia coli	0	3*	2	2	0	2	2	0	0	0	2	2	0	2	3	0	0	0	3	2
Francisella tularensis	0	0	2	0	0	0	0	0	0	3	0	0	2	0	0	0	0	3	3	3
Haemophilus sp.	0	3*	2	2	3	3	0	3	3	0	0	0	3*	1	3	0	3	3	3	2
Klebsiella sp.	0	0	3	3	0	3	0	0	0	0	0	0	0	2	0	0	0	0	0	3
Moraxella catarrhalis	0	0	3	3	0	2	0	0	0	0	0	0	0	1	3	0	0	0	3*	3
Morganella sp.	0	3	3	0	0	3	0	3	3	0	0	3	3	0	0	0	0	0	3*	3
P. aeruginosa	0	0	3	0	0	3	0	3	3	0	0	0	0	0	0	0	0	0	0	0
Proteus sp.	0	3	3	0	0	3	0	3	3	0	0	0	0	0	0	0	0	0	3*	3
Providencia sp.	0	0	3	0	0	3	0	3	3	0	0	0	0	0	0	0	0	0	3*	3
Salmonella sp.	0	3	3	3	0	3	0	3	3	0	2	0	3*	2	3	0	3	0	3	2
Serratia marcescens	0	0	3	0	0	3	0	0	0	0	0	0	0	0	2	0	0	0	3	0
Shigella sp.	0	3	3	3	0	3	0	3	3	0	0	0	0	3	0	0	3	0	3*	2
Stenotrophomonas (Xanthomonas) maltophilia	0	0	0	0	0	3	0	0	3	0	0	0	0	2	2	0	1	0	2	3
Vibrio vulnificus	0	0	0	0	0	0	0	0	0	0	0	3	3	1	0	0	0	0	0	3
Yersinia enterocolitica	0	0	3	3	0	2	0	2	2	0	0	3	0	0	0	0	0	0	1	2
Anaerobic Gram Positive Cocci (chains)																				
Peptostreptococcus	1	2	2	2	3	3	3	0	3	3	2	2	2	2	2	2	2	0	0	2

1 = Preferred antibiotic—High degree of activity against the isolate and likely to be clinically effective, most strains susceptible, has a favorable PK/PD characteristics, has a good safety profile, and has a "low resistance" potential (see Chapter 11 Drug Summaries for antibiotic dosing details). 2 = Alternate choice—With many attributes of a preferred antibiotic. 3 = Acceptable, but preferably select an alternate antibiotic. 0 = No activity or no data or limited experience. * = May be effective initially but as a "high resistance" antibiotic potential, resistance may develop during/after therapy.

§ Always use in combination with another antibiotic.

Table 3.1 Antibiotic Susceptibility Profiles (Penicillins, Macrolides, Tetracyclines, and Miscellaneous Others) *(cont'd)*

ORGANISMS	Penicillins						Anti-Pseudomonal Penicillins				Macrolides			Tetracyclines					Miscellaneous				
	Penicillin (G/V) (IV/PO)	Ampicillin (IV/PO)	Ampicillin/Sulbactam (IV)	Amoxicillin (PO)	Amoxicillin/Clavulanate (PO)	Nafcillin (IV)	Ticarcillin (IV)	Ticarcillin/Clavulanate (IV)	Piperacillin (IV)	Piperacillin/Tazobactam (IV)	Erythromycin (IV/PO)	Clarithromycin (PO)	Azithromycin (IV/PO)	Tetracycline (IV/PO)	Doxycycline (IV/PO)	Minocycline (IV/PO)	Eravacycline (IV)	Omadacycline (IV/PO)	Clindamycin (IV/PO)	Metronidazole (IV/PO)	Rifampin (PO)§	TMP-SMX (IV/PO)	Chloramphenicol (IV/PO)
Anaerobic Gram Positive Bacilli																							
Actinomyces sp.	1	1	2	1	2	0	0	0	0	0	2	2	2	2	2	2	3	3	2	0	0	0	0
Anaerobic Gram Negative Bacilli																							
Bacteroides fragilis group (*Parabacteroides distasonis*, *B. ovatus*, *B. thetaiotaomicron*, *B. vulgatus*)	0	0	2	0	2	0	2	2	2	2	0	0	0	3	2	2	2	2	1	1	0	0	2
Prevotella sp.	1	1	1	1	1	0	2	2	2	2	3	3	3	2	2	2	2	2	1	1	0	0	2

1 = Preferred antibiotic—High degree of activity against the isolate and likely to be clinically effective, most strains susceptible, has a favorable PK/PD characteristics, has a good safety profile, and has a "low resistance" potential (see Chapter 11 Drug Summaries for antibiotic dosing details). 2 = Alternate choice—With many attributes of a preferred antibiotic. 3 = Acceptable, but preferably select an alternate antibiotic. 0 = No activity or no data or limited experience. § = Always use in combination with another antibiotic.

Table 3.2 Antibiotic Susceptibility Profiles (Cephalosporins)

ORGANISMS	1st GC (IV)	1st GCs (PO)		2nd GCs (IV)				2nd GCs (PO)				3rd GCs (IV)			3rd GCs (PO)					Anti-MRSA Cephalosporin (IV)	Anti-Pseudomonal Cephalosporins (IV)			
	Cefazolin (IV)	Cefadroxil (PO)	Cephalexin (PO)	Cefoxitin (IV)	Cefamandole (V)	Cefuroxime (IV)	Cefotetan (IV)	Cefaclor (PO)	Loracarbef (PO)	Cefprozil (PO)	Cefuroxime axetil (PO)	Cefotaxime (IV)	Ceftizoxime (IV)	Ceftriaxone (IV)	Cefixime (PO)	Ceftibuten (PO)	Cefpodoxime (PO)	Cefdinir (PO)	Cefditoren (PO)	Ceftaroline fosamil (IV)	Cefiderocol (IV)	Cefoperazone (IV)	Ceftazidime (IV)	Cefepime (IV)
Aerobic Gram Positive Cocci (clusters)																								
Staphylococcus aureus (MSSA)	1	2	1	2	2	2	3	3	0	3	2	2	2	2	0	0	2	2	0	2	0	2	3	2
Staphylococcus aureus (HA/CO-MRSA)	0	0	0	0	0	0	0	0	0	0	0	0	0	0	0	0	0	0	0	1	0	0	0	0
S. aureus (CA-MRSA)	0	0	0	0	0	0	0	0	0	0	0	0	0	0	0	0	0	0	0	2	0	0	0	0
S. epidermidis (CoNS)	3	0	0	3	3	3	3	0	0	0	3	3	3	3	0	0	0	0	0	1	0	3	0	3

1 = Preferred antibiotic—High degree of activity against the isolate and likely to be clinically effective, most strains susceptible, has a favorable PK/PD characteristics, has a good safety profile, and has a "low resistance potential" (see Chapter 11 Drug Summaries for antibiotic dosing details). 2 = Alternate choice—With many attributes of a preferred antibiotic. 3 = Acceptable, but preferably select an alternate antibiotic. 0 = No activity or no data or limited experience.

Table 3.2 Antibiotic Susceptibility Profiles (Cephalosporins) *(cont'd)*

ORGANISMS	1st GC (IV)	1st GCs (PO)		2nd GCs (IV)				2nd GCs (PO)				3rd GCs (IV)			3rd GCs (PO)					Anti-MRSA Cephalosporin (IV)	Anti-Pseudomonal Cephalosporins (IV)			
	Cefazolin (IV)	Cefadroxil (PO)	Cephalexin (PO)	Cefoxitin (IV)	Cefamandole (IV)	Cefuroxime (IV)	Cefotetan (IV)	Cefaclor (PO)	Loracarbef (PO)	Cefprozil (PO)	Cefuroxime axetil (PO)	Cefotaxime (IV)	Ceftizoxime (IV)	Ceftriaxone (IV)	Cefixime (PO)	Ceftibuten (PO)	Cefpodoxime (PO)	Cefdinir (PO)	Cefditoren (PO)	Ceftaroline fosamil (IV)	Cefiderocol (IV)	Cefoperazone (IV)	Ceftazidime (IV)	Cefepime (IV)
Aerobic Gram Positive Cocci (chains)																								
Enterococcus faecalis (VSE)	0	0	0	0	0	0	0	0	0	0	0	0	0	0	0	0	0	0	0	0	0	3	0	0
Enterococcus faecium (VRE)	0	0	0	0	0	0	0	0	0	0	0	0	0	0	0	0	0	0	0	0	0	0	0	0
Streptococci (groups A, B, C, E, G)	1	2	1	2	2	2	2	2	2	1	2	1	1	1	2	3	2	2	2	2	0	1	3	2
Streptococcus (bovis) gallolyticus	1	2	1	2	2	2	2	2	2	2	2	1	1	1	2	3	2	2	2	0	0	1	3	2

Antibiotic	Viridans streptococci (S. anginosus, S. mitis, S. mutans, S. sanguis, S. salivarius)	Aerobic Gram Positive Cocci (pairs)	Streptococcus pneumoniae (PSSP)	Streptococcus pneumoniae (PRSP)	Streptococcus pneumoniae (MDRSP)	Aerobic Gram Negative Cocci (pairs)	Neisseria gonorrhoeae	Neisseria meningitidis
	0		2	2	2		0	0
	3		3	3	3		3	3
	2		3	3	3		3	3
	0		0	0	0		0	0
	2		2	2	2		0	0
	2		3	3	3		2	0
	2		3	2	2		2	0
	2		3	2	2		2	0
	3		0	0	0		3	3
	2		3	2	2		1	3
	1		1	1	1		1	1
	1		2	2	2		2	3
	1		2	2	2		2	2
	2		2	2	2		3	3
	2		1	1	1		3	3
	3		2	2	2		3	3
	2		2	2	2		3	3
	2		2	2	2		3	3
	2		2	2	2		2	2
	2		2	2	2		2	3
	1		1	1	1		0	0
	2		1	1	1		0	0
	1		1	1	1		2	3

1 = Preferred antibiotic—High degree of activity against the isolate and likely to be clinically effective, has a favorable PK/PD characteristics, has a good safety profile, and has a "low resistance potential" (see Chapter 11 Drug Summaries for antibiotic dosing details). 2 = Alternate choice—With many attributes of a preferred antibiotic. 3 = Acceptable, but preferably select an alternate antibiotic. 0 = No activity or no data or limited experience.

† Group A & B only.

Table 3.2 Antibiotic Susceptibility Profiles (Cephalosporins) *(cont'd)*

ORGANISMS	1st GC (IV)	1st GCs (PO)		2nd GCs (IV)				2nd GCs (PO)				3rd GCs (IV)			3rd GCs (PO)					Anti-MRSA Cephalosporin (IV)	Anti-Pseudomonal Cephalosporins (IV)			
	Cefazolin (IV)	Cefadroxil (PO)	Cephalexin (PO)	Cefoxitin (IV)	Cefamandole (IV)	Cefuroxime (IV)	Cefotetan (IV)	Cefaclor (PO)	Loracarbef (PO)	Cefprozil (PO)	Cefuroxime axetil (PO)	Cefotaxime (IV)	Ceftizoxime (IV)	Ceftriaxone (IV)	Cefixime (PO)	Ceftibuten (PO)	Cefpodoxime (PO)	Cefdinir (PO)	Cefditoren (PO)	Ceftaroline fosamil (IV)	Cefiderocol (IV)	Cefoperazone (IV)	Ceftazidime (IV)	Cefepime (IV)
Aerobic Gram Positive Bacilli																								
Bacillus anthracis	o	o	o	o	o	o	o	o	o	o	o	o	o	o	o	o	o	o	o	o	o	o	o	o
Corynebacterium diphtheriae	o	o	o	o	o	o	o	o	o	o	o	o	o	o	o	o	o	o	o	o	o	o	o	o
Corynebacterium jeikeium (JK)	o	o	o	o	o	o	o	o	o	o	o	o	o	o	o	o	o	o	o	o	o	o	o	o
Listeria monocytogenes	o	o	o	o	o	o	o	o	o	o	o	o	o	o	o	o	o	o	o	o	o	o	o	o
Nocardia sp.	o	o	o	o	o	o	o	o	o	o	o	3	o	3	o	o	o	o	o	o	o	o	o	o
Aerobic Gram-Negative Bacilli																								
Acinetobacter sp.	o	o	o	o	o	o	o	o	o	o	o	o	o	o	o	o	o	o	o	o	1	o	2	2

Organism																									
Aeromonas hydrophila	0	0	0	3	3	0	0	0	0	0	3	3	0	0	3	3	2	2	0	2	0	3	0	3	0
Bordetella pertussis	0	0	0	0	0	0	0	0	0	0	0	0	0	0	0	0	0	0	0	0	2	0	0	0	0
Brucella sp.	3	0	0	2	0	0	0	0	3	0	2	2	0	0	2	2	2	0	0	2	3	2	0	0	3
Burkholderia (Pseudomonas) cepacia	0	0	0	0	2	0	0	0	0	0	0	0	0	0	0	0	2	0	0	0	2	2	2	2	2
Campylobacter sp.	0	0	0	0	0	0	0	0	0	0	0	0	0	0	0	0	0	0	0	0	0	0	0	0	0
Citrobacter sp.	0	0	2	3	3	0	0	0	0	0	2	3	0	3	2	2	2	0	0	2	0	2	2	2	0
Enterobacter sp.	0	0	3	3	3	0	0	0	0	3	3	3	0	3	2	2	2	0	0	2	2	2	3	1	2
Escherichia coli	2	2	2	2	2	0	2	2	2	2	2	2	2	2	1	1	1	2	2	1	3	1	2	2	2
Francisella tularensis	0	0	0	0	0	0	0	0	0	0	0	0	0	0	0	0	0	0	0	0	0	0	0	0	0
Haemophilus sp.	3	1	1	2	2	3	2	2	2	3	1	1	2	1	1	1	1	2	2	1	1	1	2	1	2†
Klebsiella sp.	2	2	2	2	2	2	2	2	2	2	1	2	2	2	1	1	1	2	2	1	2	2	2	2	1
Moraxella catarrhalis	3	2	2	2	2	3	2	2	2	2	2	2	2	2	2	2	2	2	2	2	2	1	2	2	0
Morganella sp.	3	0	3	3	3	0	0	0	0	0	3	3	0	3	2	2	2	0	0	2	2	2	2	2	2
P. aeruginosa	0	0	0	0	0	0	0	0	0	0	0	0	0	0	0	0	0	2	0	0	0	1	1	1	1
Providencia sp.	3	0	3	3	3	0	0	0	0	0	3	3	0	3	2	2	2	0	0	2	2	2	2	2	2
Proteus sp.	3	0	3	3	3	0	0	0	0	0	3	3	0	3	2	2	2	0	0	2	2	2	2	2	2
Salmonella sp.	0	0	3	3	3	0	0	0	0	0	3	3	0	0	0	0	1	0	0	0	3	0	3	3	0

1 = Preferred antibiotic—High degree of activity against the isolate and likely to be clinically effective, most strains susceptible, has a favorable PK/PD characteristics, has a good safety profile, and has a "low resistance potential" (see Chapter 11 Drug Summaries for antibiotic dosing details). 2 = Alternate choice—With many attributes of a preferred antibiotic. 3 = Acceptable, but preferably select an alternate antibiotic. 0 = No activity or no data or limited experience.

† H. influenzae only.

Table 3.2 Antibiotic Susceptibility Profiles (Cephalosporins) *(cont'd)*

ORGANISMS	1st GC (IV)	1st GCs (PO)		2nd GCs (IV)				2nd GCs (PO)				3rd GCs (IV)			3rd GCs (PO)					Anti-MRSA Cephalosporin (IV)	Anti-Pseudomonal Cephalosporins (IV)			
	Cefazolin (IV)	Cefadroxil (PO)	Cephalexin (PO)	Cefoxitin (IV)	Cefamandole (IV)	Cefuroxime (IV)	Cefotetan (IV)	Cefaclor (PO)	Loracarbef (PO)	Cefprozil (PO)	Cefuroxime axetil (PO)	Cefotaxime (IV)	Ceftizoxime (IV)	Ceftriaxone (IV)	Cefixime (PO)	Ceftibuten (PO)	Cefpodoxime (PO)	Cefdinir (PO)	Cefditoren (PO)	Ceftaroline fosamil (IV)	Cefiderocol (IV)	Cefoperazone (IV)	Ceftazidime (IV)	Cefepime (IV)
Serratia marcescens	0	0	0	3	0	0	2	0	0	0	0	1	1	1	0	0	3	0	3	0	2	1	3	1
Shigella sp.	0	0	0	3	0	0	3	0	0	0	0	2	2	2	0	0	0	0	0	0	0	2	3	2
Stenotrophomonas (Pseudomonas) maltophilia	0	0	0	0	0	0	0	0	0	0	0	0	0	0	0	0	0	0	0	0	2	2	0	0
Vibrio vulnificus	0	0	0	0	0	0	0	0	0	0	0	2	0	0	0	0	0	0	0	0	0	0	2	0
Yersinia enterocolitica	0	0	0	3	3	3	3	0	0	0	3	2	2	2	2	2	0	2	0	0	0	2	3	2

Anaerobic Gram Positive Cocci (chains)																			
Peptostreptococcus	2	2	2	2	2	2	3	2	2	2	2	0	0	0	0	0	3	3	0
Anaerobic Gram Positive Bacilli																			
Parabacteroides Actinomyces sp.	0	0	0	0	0	0	3	3	0	0	2	0	0	0	0	0	0	0	0
Anaerobic Gram Negative Bacilli																			
Bacteroides fragilis group (Parabacteroides distasonis, B. ovatus, B. thetaiotaomicron, B. vulgatus)	0	0	2	0	0	2	2	3	0	0	2	0	0	0	0	0	3†	0	0
Prevotella sp.	2	2	2	2	2	2	2	2	2	2	2	2	2	2	0	0	3	3	0

1 = Preferred antibiotic—High degree of activity against the isolate and likely to be clinically effective, most strains susceptible, has a good safety profile, and has a "low resistance potential" (see Chapter 11 Drug Summaries for antibiotic dosing details).

2 = Alternate choice—With many attributes of a preferred antibiotic.

3 = Acceptable, but preferably select an alternate antibiotic.

0 = No activity or no data or limited experience.

†For intra-abdominal/pelvic infections, add metronidazole.

Table 3.3 Antibiotic Susceptibility Profiles (Aminoglycosides, Fluoroquinolones, Carbapenems, and Miscellaneous Others)

ORGANISMS	Aminoglycosides				Fluoroquinolones				Miscellaneous										Carbapenems*					
	Gentamicin (IV)	Tobramycin (IV)	Amikacin (IV)	Plazomicin (IV)	Ciprofloxacin (IV/PO)	Levofloxacin (IV/PO)	Moxifloxacin (IV/PO)	Delafloxacin (IV/PO)	Colistin (IV) / Polymyxin B (IV)	Aztreonam (IV)	Aztreonam/Avibactam (IV)	Tigecycline (IV)	Vancomycin (IV)	Q/D† (IV)	Linezolid (IV/PO)	Daptomycin (IV)	Nitrofurantoin (PO)	Fosfomycin (IV/PO)	Imipenem (IV)	Meropenem/Vaborbactam (IV)	Meropenem (IV)	Imipenem/Relebactam (IV)	Ertapenem (IV)	Doripenem (IV)
Aerobic Gram Positive Cocci (clusters)																								
Staphylococcus aureus (MSSA)	2	3	3	3	3	1	1	2	0	0	0	1	3	1	1	1	0	0	2	2	2	2	2	2
Staphylococcus aureus (HA/CO-MRSA)	0	0	0	0	0	0	0	2	0	0	0	1	2	1	1	1	0	0	0	0	0	0	0	0
S. aureus (CA-MRSA)	0	0	0	0	0	0	0	2	0	0	0	1	1	1	1	1	0	0	0	0	0	0	0	0
S. epidermidis (CoNS)	0	0	0	0	0	0	2	3	0	0	0	1	1	1	1	1	0	0	2	0	3	0	3	3
Aerobic Gram Positive Cocci (chains)																								
Enterococcus faecalis (VSE)	0	0	0	0	0	3	2	3	0	0	0	1	2	0	1	2	1	2	2	2	2	2	0	3
Enterococcus faecium (VRE)	0	0	0	0	0	0	0	3	0	0	0	1	0	1	1	2	1	3	2	0	0	0	0	0
Streptococci (groups A, B, C, E, G)	0	0	0	0	0	2	2	2	0	0	0	2	2	3	2	2	2	0	2	2	2	2	2	2
Streptococcus (bovis) gallolyticus	0	0	0	0	0	2	2	2	0	0	0	2	2	2	3	3	0	0	2	3	2	3	0	2

† Q/D: Quinupristin/Dalfopristin
* ± β-lactamase inhibitors

Organism																					
Viridans streptococci (S. anginosus, S. mitis, S. mutans, S. sanguis, S. salivarius)	0	0	0	2	2	2	2	0	0	0	2	2	2	2	0	2	0	2	2	2	2
Aerobic Gram Positive Cocci (pairs)																					
Streptococcus pneumoniae (PSSP)	0	0	0	3	1	1	1	0	0	0	2	2	2	3	0	2	2	2	2	2	2
Streptococcus pneumoniae (PRSP)	0	0	0	3	1	1	1	0	0	0	2	2	2	3	0	2	2	2	2	2	2
Streptococcus pneumoniae (MDRSP)	0	0	0	3	1	1	1	0	0	0	2	2	2	3	0	2	2	2	2	2	2
Aerobic Gram Negative Cocci (pairs)																					
Neisseria gonorrhoeae	0	0	0	1	2	2	2	0	2	2	0	0	0	0	0	3	3	3	3	3	3
Neisseria meningitidis	0	0	0	2	2	2	2	0	2	2	0	0	0	0	0	2	2	2	2	2	2
Aerobic Gram Positive Bacilli																					
Bacillus anthracis	0	0	0	1	1	1	1	0	0	0	0	0	0	0	0	0	0	0	0	0	0
Corynebacterium diphtheriae	0	0	0	0	0	0	0	0	0	0	3	0	0	0	0	0	0	0	0	0	0
Corynebacterium jeikeium (JK)	0	0	0	0	0	0	0	0	0	0	2	1	3	0	0	0	0	0	0	0	0

1 = Preferred antibiotic—High degree of activity against the isolate and likely to be clinically effective, most strains susceptible, has a favorable PK/PD characteristics, has a good safety profile, and has a "low resistance" potential (see Chapter 11 Drug Summaries for antibiotic dosing details). 2 = Alternate choice—With many attributes of a preferred antibiotic. 3 = Acceptable, but preferably select an alternate antibiotic. 0 = No activity or no data or limited experience. *May be effective initially but as a "high resistance" potential, antibiotic resistance may develop during/after therapy.

Table 3.3 Antibiotic Susceptibility Profiles (Aminoglycosides, Fluoroquinolones, Carbapenems, and Miscellaneous Others) *(cont'd)*

ORGANISMS	Gentamicin (IV)	Tobramycin (IV)	Amikacin (IV)	Plazomycin (IV)	Ciprofloxacin (IV/PO)	Levofloxacin (IV/PO)	Moxifloxacin (IV/PO)	Delafloxacin (IV/PO)	Colistin (IV)/Polymyxin B (IV)	Aztreonam (IV)	Aztreonam/Avibactam (IV)	Tigecycline (IV)	Vancomycin (IV)	Q/D† (IV)	Linezolid (IV/PO)	Daptomycin (IV)	Nitrofurantoin (PO)	Fosfomycin (IV/PO)	Imipenem (IV)	Meropenem/Vaborbactam (IV)	Meropenem (IV)	Imipenem/Relebactam (IV)	Ertapenem (IV)	Doripenem (IV)
Listeria monocytogenes	3	3	3	3	0	0	0	3	0	0	0	3	0	3	3	0	0	0	3	0	2	0	0	0
Nocardia	0	0	2	0	0	0	0	0	0	0	0	3	0	0	3	0	0	0	3	0	2	3	0	0
Aerobic Gram Negative Bacilli																								
Acinetobacter sp.	1	2	2	2	3	2	3	3	2	1	1	1	0	0	0	0	0	3	2*	3	3	3	3	1
Aeromonas hydrophila	2	2	2	2	1	1	1	1	0	3	3	3	0	0	0	0	0	0	2	2	2	2	3	0
Bordetella sp.	0	0	0	0	3	3	3	3	0	0	0	0	0	0	0	0	0	0	3	3	3	3	3	0
Brucella sp.	2	0	0	0	3	3	0	3	0	0	0	0	0	0	0	0	0	0	0	0	0	0	0	0
Burkholderia (Pseudomonas) cepacia	0	0	0	0	1	1	3	3	0	0	1	3	0	0	0	0	0	0	3	2	2	2	3	0
Campylobacter sp.	3	0	0	2	3	3	1	2	0	0	0	0	0	0	0	0	0	0	3	3	3	3	3	3
Citrobacter sp.	1	1	2	1	2	2	3	3	3	2	0	2	0	0	0	0	2	0	2	2	2	2	1	1
Enterobacter sp.	1	1	1	1	2	1	2	2	3	2	2	2	0	0	0	0	3	3	2	2	2	1	1	1
Escherichia coli	2	2	1	1	2	2	1	1	3	0	2	1	0	0	0	0	2	2	1	1	1	1	2	2
Francisella tularensis	1	3	0	3	2	2	2	2	0	0	0	0	0	0	0	0	0	0	0	0	0	0	0	0

† Q/D: Quinupristin/Dalfopristin

Haemophilus sp.	3	3	3	3	1	1	1	1	3	3		2	0	0	0	0	0	0	2	2	2	2	2	2
Klebsiella sp.	2	2	1	2	2	1	1	1	1	1	1	1	0	0	0	0	2	2	1	1	1	1	1	1
Moraxella catarrhalis	3	3	3	3	2	2	2	2	0	2	2	2	0	0	0	0	0	0	2	2	2	2	2	2
Morganella sp.	2	2	1	1	3	2	2	2	0	2	2	0	0	0	0	0	0	3	2	2	2	2	2	2
P. aeruginosa	2	2	1	1	1	1	0	3	1	3	3	0	0	0	0	0	0	1	2*	2	2	2	0	1
Proteus sp.	2	2	1	1	3	2	2	2	0	3	3	0	0	0	0	0	0	2	2	2	2	2	2	2
Providencia sp.	2	2	1	1	3	2	2	2	0	3	3	0	0	0	0	0	0	2	2	2	2	2	2	2
Salmonella sp.	0	0	0	0	1	2	2	2	3	3	3	2	0	0	0	0	0	0	2	2	2	2	2	2
Serratia marcescens	3	2	3	2	2	2	2	2	0	3	3	2	0	0	0	0	0	3	2	2	2	2	2	2
Shigella sp.	3	3	3	3	2	2	2	2	3	3	3	2	0	0	0	0	0	0	2	2	2	2	2	2
Stenotrophomonas (Xanthomonas) maltophilia	0	0	0	0	3	2	2	3	2	0	1	1	0	0	0	0	0	0	0	2	0	2	0	0
Vibrio vulnificus	0	0	0	0	3	3	3	3	3	0	0	3	0	0	0	0	0	0	0	0	0	0	0	0
Yersinia enterocolitica	2	2	2	0	2	2	2	2	0	2	3	3	0	0	0	0	0	0	0	0	0	0	0	0
Anaerobic Gram Positive Cocci (chains)																								
Peptostreptococcus	0	0	0	0	0	0	3	0	0	0	0	2	3	3	2	0	0	0	2	2	2	2	2	2
Anaerobic Gram Positive Bacilli																								
Actinomyces sp.	0	0	0	0	0	0	3	0	0	0	0	3	0	3	0	0	0	0	2	2	2	2	2	0

1 = Preferred antibiotic—High degree of activity against the isolate and likely to be clinically effective, most strains susceptible, has a favorable PK/PD characteristics, has a good safety profile, and has a "low resistance" potential (see Chapter 11 Drug Summaries for antibiotic dosing details). 2 = Alternate choice—With many attributes of a preferred antibiotic. 3 = Acceptable, but preferably select an alternate antibiotic. 0 = No activity or no data or limited experience. *May be effective initially but as a "high resistance" potential, antibiotic resistance may develop during/after therapy.

Table 3.3 Antibiotic Susceptibility Profiles (Aminoglycosides, Fluoroquinolones, Carbapenems, and Miscellaneous Others) *(contd)*

ORGANISMS	Amino-glycosides				Fluoro-quinolones				Miscellaneous										Carbapenems*					
	Gentamicin (IV)	Tobramycin (IV)	Amikacin (IV)	Plazomycin (IV)	Ciprofloxacin (IV/PO)	Levofloxacin (IV/PO)	Moxifloxacin (IV/PO)	Delafloxacin (IV/PO)	Colistin (IV) Polymyxin B (IV)	Aztreonam (IV)	Aztreonam/ Avibactam (IV)	Tigecycline (IV)	Vancomycin (IV)	Q/D† (IV)	Linezolid (IV/PO)	Daptomycin (IV)	Nitrofurantoin§ (PO)	Fosfomycin (IV/PO)	Imipenem (IV)	Meropenem/ Vaborbactam (IV)	Meropenem (IV)	Imipenem/ Relabactam (IV)	Ertapenem (IV)	Doripenem (IV)
Anaerobic Gram Negative Bacilli																								
Bacteroides fragilis group (*Parabacteroides distasonis, B. ovatus, B. thetaiotaomicron, vulgatus*)	0	0	0	0	0	0	2	2	0	0	0	1	0	3	0	0	0	0	1	2	1	2	1	2
Prevotella sp. B.	0	0	0	0	2	2	2	2	0	0	0	2	0	0	0	0	0	0	2	2	2	2	2	2

1 = Preferred antibiotic—High degree of activity against the isolate and likely to be clinically effective, most strains susceptible, has a favorable PK/PD characteristics, has a good safety profile, and has a "low resistance" potential (see Chapter 11 Drug Summaries for antibiotic dosing details).
2 = Alternate choice—With many attributes of a preferred antibiotic.
3 = Acceptable, but preferably select an alternate antibiotic.
0 = No activity or no data or limited experience.
† Q/D: Quinupristin/Dalfopristin
§ For acute uncomplicated cystitis (AUC) or catheter associated bacteriuria (CAB) only.
* ± β-lactamase inhibitors

Gram Stain of Isolates
(by Morphology, Arrangement, Oxygen Requirements)

AEROBIC ISOLATES*

* Traditional names of most organisms have been retained for clarity in this section.

* Oxidase negative.   (α) = α (alpha) hemolysis on BAP.   (m) = motile.
[t] Catalase positive.   (β) = β (beta) hemolysis on BAP.   (v) = Gram variable bacilli.
§ Non-lactose fermenter.   (γ) = γ (gamma) hemolysis on BAP.

CAPNOPHILIC ISOLATES[+]

+ Capnophilic organisms grow best under increased CO_2 tension.   (m) = motile.

ANAEROBIC ISOLATES

[++] **Microaerophilic organisms. Grow best under decreased O$_2$ concentration.**
* **Oxidase negative.**   (m) = motile.
[†] **Catalase positive.**   (v) = Gram variable bacilli.

YEASTS/FUNGI

Alphabetical Index of Isolates

Table 3.4 Key Factors in Antibiotic Selection

- **Select an antibiotic with a high degree of activity against the known pathogen** (not colonizers).
- **Dose appropriate for the target tissue to assure therapeutic/effective concentrations at site of infection**. If necessary, adjust dose ↑ for tissue targets that require higher doses, e.g., bacterial meningitis, endocarditis, etc., or ↓ dose for sites with antibiotic concentrations that are above serum concentrations, e.g., skin, urine, etc.
- **Select an empiric antibiotic with a "low resistance" potential** avoid, if possible, antibiotics with a "high resistance" potential (also with a high degree of activity against the presumed pathogen). Select a "low resistance" potential antibiotic for the same/different class with a high degree of activity.
- **Select antibiotic with a good safety profile** and minimal potential for drug-drug interactions.
- **Select antibiotic that is relatively cost effective** (first take into account the above principles).

Table 3.5 Clinically Relevant Types of Antibiotic Resistance

High Level/Absolute Resistance (dose independent)

- Resistant isolate MIC beyond achievable serum concentrations
- High level/absolute resistance cannot be overcome using high antibiotic doses

Relative Resistance (dose dependent)

- Relatively resistant = susceptible – dose dependent (S–DD)
- Consider "intermediate" susceptibility as "susceptible" rather than resistant if achievable levels exceed the MIC
- Non-susceptible or relatively resistant can be overcome with high doses
  Examples:
    - PCN with S. pneumoniae
    - Meropenem or cefepime with P. aeruginosa
    - Tigecycline with Acinetobacter baumannii

Cross Resistance between Classes ("MIC drift")

  Example:

  P. aeruginosa treated with gentamicin increases MICs to other aminoglycosides, e.g., tobramycin, amikacin and other *unrelated* antibiotic classes with antipseudomonal activity.

    - ↑ Ciprofloxacin MICs
    - ↑ Levofloxacin MICs
    - ↑ Cefepime MICs
    - ↑ Imipenem MICs

Table 3.6 Clinical Significance of AEROBIC Isolates Pending Susceptibility Testing

	GRAM POSITIVE COCCI (clusters)		
Isolate	Isolate Significance	Therapy	Comments
Staphylococcus aureus (MSSA/MRSA)	• CSF = C*, P (CNS shunts) • Blood = C*, P (from soft tissue/bone infection, abscess, IV line infection, ABE, PVE) • Sputum = C, P (S. aureus pneumonia is rare; only with viral influenza) • Urine = C, P (S. aureus is not a uropathogen and usually due to skin contamination of urine specimen. Rarely, due to overwhelming S. aureus bacteremia) • Stool = C, P (enterocolitis) • Wound = C, P (abscess)	<u>MSSA:</u> Nafcillin (IV), Cefazolin (IV), Clindamycin (IV/PO), a "respiratory quinolone" (IV/PO), Minocycline (IV/PO), Daptomycin (IV), any carbapenem (IV), Linezolid (IV/PO), Tigecycline (IV), Telavancin (IV) <u>Hospital-acquired MRSA (HA-MRSA)/</u> <u>Community-onset MRSA (CO-MRSA):</u> Ceftaroline fosamil (IV), Daptomycin (IV), Linezolid (IV/PO), Tigecycline (IV), Vancomycin (IV), Minocycline (IV/PO), Quinupristin/Dalfopristin (IV), Telavancin (IV) <u>Oral Therapy of Community acquired MRSA (CA-MRSA):</u> Minocycline preferred. Alternately, Doxycycline*, TMP-SMX, Clindamycin <u>VISA/VRSA:</u> Linezolid (IV/PO), Daptomycin (IV), Telavancin (IV)	<u>MSSA:</u> For oral treatment, 1st generation cephalosporins (IV) preferred to oral anti-staphylococcal penicillins (e.g., dicloxacillin) <u>MRSA:</u> *in-vitro susceptibility testing is unreliable; treat MRSA infections empirically.* Most effective drugs for MRSA are vancomycin, linezolid, ceftaroline fosamil, quinupristin/dalfopristin, minocycline, daptomycin, tigecycline. **Preferentially use minocycline instead of doxycycline for MSSA/MRSA.** Community-acquired MRSA (CA-MRSA) SCC mec IV,V CA-MRSA has different susceptibilities than HA-MRSA/CO-MRSA. CA-MRSA strains with Panton-Valentin Leukocidin PVL+ gene cause two distinct clinical syndromes: severe necrotizing pneumonia (with viral influenza) and severe necrotizing fasciitis/pyomyositis. **CA-MRSA is usually susceptible to doxycycline in vitro, but minocycline more effective in vivo than doxycycline.** *Drugs effective against HA-MRSA/CO-MRSA are also effective against CA-MRSA. However, drugs effective against CA-MRSA usually not effective against HA-MRSA/CO-MRSA* MSSA/MRSA: Non-continuous or low-grade blood culture positivity (1/4) usually indicates skin contamination during venipuncture Continuous high-grade blood culture positivity (3/4 or 4/4) usually indicates intra-vascular infection, osteomyelitis, or abscess.

Organism	Susceptibility Profile	Initial Therapy	Comments
Staphylococcus epidermidis (MSSE/MRSE) or coagulase-negative staphylococci (CoNS) Staphylococcus lugdunensis	• CSF = C*, P (CNS shunts) • Blood = C*, P (from IV lines, infected implants, prosthetic valve endocarditis [PVE], rarely from native valve subacute bacterial endocarditis [SBE]) • Sputum = C • Urine = C (may be reported as S. saprophyticus; request novobiocin sensitivity tc differentiate S. epidermidis from other coagulase-negative staphylococci) • Stool = NP • Wound = C, P (infected foreign body drainage)	MSSE: Linezolid (IV/PO), Daptomycin (IV), Vancomycin (IV), Telavancin (IV), any carbapenem (IV), a "respiratory quinolone" (IV/PO), Minocycline (IV/PO) MRSE: Linezolid (IV/PO), Daptomycin (IV), Vancomycin (IV), Quinupristin/Dalfopristin (IV), Minocycline (IV/PO)	VISA/VRSA: MICs for vancomycin sensitive (VSSA), heteroresistant vancomycin intermediate (hVISA), intermediate (VISA), and resistant (VRSA) S. aureus are ≤ 2 mcg/mL, < 4 mcg/mL (with subpopulations > 4 mcg/mL, 2–4 mcg/mL, and ≥ 16 mcg/mL, respectively. *Empiric therapy of selected pathogens (Table 3.11) p. 258* Usually non-pathogenic in absence of prosthetic/implant materials. Common cause of PVE; rare cause of native valve SBE. Treat foreign body-related infection until foreign body is removed. S. lugdunensis is a CoNS but is often misidentified as S. aureus since it produces "clumping factor" which gives a + slide test but – tube coagulase test*. Resembles S. aureus in terms of invasiveness/virulence. Unlike S. aureus, S. lugdensis is pan-sensitive to antibiotics which is another clue the isolate is not S. aureus. S. lugdensis bacteremia associated with community acquired (not nosocomial) SBE. *S. aureus [+ bound coagulase (slide test) + free coagulase (tube test)]

C = colonizer; C* = skin contaminant; NP = non-pathogen at site; P = pathogen at site; (IV/PO) = IV or PO. See p. xi for all other abbreviations.
* Minocycline (IV/PO) preferred.

Table 3.6 Clinical Significance of AEROBIC Isolates Pending Susceptibility Testing *(cont'd)*

Isolate	Isolate Significance	GRAM POSITIVE COCCI (clusters) Preferred Therapy	Alternate Therapy	Comments
Staphylococcus saprophyticus (coagulase negative staphylococci)	• CSF = NP • Blood = NP • Sputum = NP • Urine = P (cystitis) • Stool = NP • Wound = NP	Preferred therapy Amoxicillin (PO) TMP–SMX (PO) Nitrofurantoin (PO) Alternate therapy Any quinolone (PO) Any 1st generation cephalosporin (PO)		S. saprophyticus UTI is associated with a urinary "fishy odor" (like bacterial vaginosis), alkaline urine pH, and microscopic hematuria. Novobiocin sensitivity (only for CoNS urinary isolates) differentiates coagulase negative staphylococci (sensitive) from S. saprophyticus (resistant).

		GRAM POSITIVE COCCI (chains)		
Enterococcus faecalis (VSE)	• CSF = NP (except from S. stercoralis hyperinfection or V-P shunt infection) • Blood = C*, P (from GI/GU source, SBE) • Sputum = NP • Urine = C, P (cystitis, pyelonephritis) • Stool = NP • Wound = C, NP	Non-SBE Ampicillin (IV) Amoxicillin (PO) Meropenem (IV) Piperacillin/ Tazobactam (IV) Linezolid (IV/PO) Tigecycline (IV) Daptomycin (IV) SBE Gentamicin + Ampicillin (IV) **or** Vancomycin (IV) Meropenem (IV) Piperacillin/ Tazobactam (IV) Linezolid (IV/ PO)	Non-SBE Cefoperazone (IV) Chloramphenicol (IV) Levofloxacin (IV/PO) Moxifloxacin (IV/PO) Nitrofurantoin (PO) (UTIs only) SBE Levofloxacin (IV/PO) Moxifloxacin (IV/PO) Cefoperazone (IV) Daptomycin Linezolid	Sensitive to ampicillin, not penicillin. Cause of intermediate (severity between ABE and SBE) endocarditis, hepatobiliary infections, and UTIs. Enterococci (E. faecalis, E. faecium) are the only cause of SBE (below the waist) from GI/GU sources. Permissive pathogen (i.e., usually does not cause infection alone) in the abdomen/pelvis (except in gallbladder or urinary bladder/kidneys). Cefoperazone is the only cephalosporin with anti-E. faecalis (VSE) activity (MIC ~ 32 mcg/mL). Quinupristin/dalfopristin is not active against E. faecalis (VSE). Treat vancomycin resistant E. faecalis as VRE. *Empiric therapy of selected pathogens (Table 3.11) p. 258*

Enterococcus faecium (VRE)	• CSF = NP (except from S. stercoralis hyperinfection or V-P shunt infection) • Blood = C*, P,*from GI/GU source, SBE) • Sputum = C • Urine = C, P (UTIs) • Stool = NP • Wound = C, NP	Non-SBE Linezolid (IV/PO), Quinupristin/Dalfopristin (IV), Doxycycline (IV/PO), Minocycline (IV/PO), Tigecycline (IV), Chloramphenicol (IV/PO), Daptomycin (IV), Nitrofurantoin (PO),* Fosfomycin* SBE Linezolid (IV/PO) Quinupristin/Dalfopristin (IV) Daptomycin (IV)	Same spectrum of infection as E. faecalis (VSE). Colonization common; infection less common. Fecal carriage is intermittent but prolonged. In vitro sensitivity ≠ in vivo efficacy. Increased prevalence of E. faecalis (VRE) related to vancomycin IV (not PO) use. Nitrofurantoin preferred for VRE lower UTIs/catheter-associated bacteriuria (CAB). Empiric therapy of selected problem pathogens (Table 3.11) p. 258
Group A streptococci (GAS)	• CSF = C* • Blood = P (cellulitis) • Sputum = P rare cause of CAP • Urine = NP • Stool = NP • Wound = C, P (cellulitis) • Throat = C, P (pharyngitis) (pharynx is colonized commonly with Group A streptococci in ~ 30% of patients with EBV IM)	Amoxicillin (PO) Any β-lactam (IV/PO)	Penicillin (PO) Clindamycin (IV/PO)	For Group A streptococcal pharyngitis, amoxicillin is preferred over penicillin. Clindamycin is best for elimination of carrier states, and for penicillin-allergic patients with streptococcal pharyngitis. Any β-lactam is equally effective against Group A streptococci. Nafcillin is the most active anti-staphylococcal penicillin against Group A streptococci. Erythromycin is no longer reliable against Group A streptococci due to increasing resistance. Doxycycline has little/no activity against Group A streptococci.
Group B streptococci (S. agalactiae)	• CSF = P • Blood = P (from urine source, Skin)	Non-SBE, non-CNS Clindamycin (IV/PO)	Non-SBE, non-CNS Vancomycin (IV) Amoxicillin (PO)	Cause of UTIs in diabetics and the elderly. Cause of neonatal GBS sepsis and meningitis. Infection is uncommon in the general population. Rarely a cause of SBE

C = colonizer; C* = skin contaminant; NP = non-pathogen at site; P = pathogen at site; (IV/PO) = IV or PO. See p. xi for all other abbreviations.

*For acute uncomplicated cystitis (AUC) or catheter associated bacteriuria (CAB) only.

Table 3.6 Clinical Significance of AEROBIC Isolates Pending Susceptibility Testing *(cont'd)*

		GRAM POSITIVE COCCI (chains)		
Isolate	**Isolate Significance**	**Preferred Therapy**	**Alternate Therapy**	**Comments**
	• Sputum = NP • Urine = P (UTIs, especially in diabetics, elderly) • Stool = C • Wound = C, P (diabetic foot infections)	Any 1st, 2nd, 3rd generation cephalosporin (IV/PO) SBE Ceftriaxone (IV) Penicillin (IV) Vancomycin (IV) CNS Ceftriaxone (IV) Penicillin (IV)	SBE Meropenem (IV) Ertapenem (IV) Linezolid (IV/PO) CNS Chloramphenicol (IV) Linezolid (IV/PO)	Non-pregnant adults. On Gram stain, GBS appear larger/rounder than S. pneumoniae. Colonies of GBS slightly β-hemolytic on BAP have a "sheen" (vs. S. pneumoniae which is α-hemolytic). Aminoglycosides and tetracyclines are ineffective.
Group C, F, G streptococci	• CSF = P (rarely ABM) • Blood = P (from skin/soft tissue infection, SBE) • Sputum = C • Throat = C (especially with viral pharyngitis), P (pharyngitis in medical personnel) • Urine = NP • Stool = NP • Wound = P (rarely cellulitis)	Ceftriaxone (IV) Penicillin (IV) Ampicillin (IV) Clindamycin (IV/PO)	Vancomycin (IV) Amoxicillin (PO) Any 1st, 2nd, 3rd generation cephalosporin (IV) Meropenem (IV) Ertapenem (IV)	Group C, G streptococci may cause pharyngitis, wound infections, and rarely SBE. Group G streptococci associated with malignancies. Common pharyngeal colonizers in medical personnel.

		GRAM POSITIVE COCCI (chains)		
Streptococcus (bovis) gallolyticus	• Blood = P (SB= from GI source) • Urine = NP	Ceftriaxone (IV) Ampicillin (IV) Clindamycin (IV/PO)	Vancomycin (IV) Amoxicillin (PO) Any cephalosporin (IV)	Associated with GI malignancies. Non-enterococcal Group D streptococci (e.g., S. bovis) are sensitive to penicillin.
Viridans streptococci (S. anginosus, S. mitis, S. mutans, S. sanguis, S. salivarius)	• CSF = NP (aseptic meningitis with SBE) • Blood = C*, P (1° bacteremia, SBE) • Sputum = NP • Urine = NP • Stool = NP • Wound = NP	Ceftriaxone (IV) Any cephalosporin (IV/PO)	Amoxicillin (PO) Meropenem (IV) Ertapenem (IV) Vancomycin (IV)	Low-grade blood culture positivity (1/4) indicates contamination during venipuncture. Continuous/high-grade blood culture positivity (3/4 or 4/4) indicates SBE until proven otherwise. S. anginosus, S. constellatus prone to invasive disease, bacteremia and abscess formation.
		GRAM POSITIVE COCCI (pairs)		
Leuconostoc	• CSF = NP • Blood = P (PVE) • Sputum = NF • Urine = P (UTIs) • Stool = NP • Wound = NP	Penicillin (IV) Ampicillin (IV) Clindamycin (IV/PO)	Amoxicillin (PO) Erythromycin (IV) Minocycline (IV/PO) Clarithromycin XL (PO)	Coccobacillary forms resemble streptococci/enterococci. Cause of infection in compromised hosts. Rare cause of IV line infection. Intrinsically vancomycin resistant.
Streptococcus pneumoniae	• CSF = P (ABM) • Blood = P (from respiratory tract source) • Sputum = C, P • Urine = NP • Stool = NP	Multidrug Resistant S. pneumoniae (MDRSP) A "respiratory quinolone" (IV/PO), Telithromycin (PO), Ertapenem (IV), Meropenem (IV), Cefepime (IV), Linezolid (IV/PO), Vancomycin (IV)	Amoxicillin (PO) Erythromycin (IV) Minocycline (IV/PO) Clarithromycin XL (PO)	Penicillin-resistant S. pneumoniae (PRSP) are still sensitive to full-dose/high-dose β-lactams. If possible, avoid macrolides, as > 30% of S. pneumoniae are macrolide resistant (MRSP). (~ 20–25% are naturally resistant and 10–15% acquire macrolide resistance).

C = colonizer; C* = skin contaminant; NP = non-pathogen at site; P = pathogen at site; (IV/PO) = IV or PO. See p. xi for all other abbreviations.

Table 3.6 Clinical Significance of AEROBIC Isolates Pending Susceptibility Testing *(cont'd)*

Isolate	Isolate Significance	Preferred Therapy	Alternate Therapy	Comments
GRAM POSITIVE COCCI (pairs)				
	• Wound = P (cellulitis only in SLE)		Sensitive or relatively PCN-resistant Doxycycline (IV/PO), any cephalosporin (IV/PO), Clindamycin (IV/PO), Amoxicillin/Clavulanic acid (PO)	
GRAM NEGATIVE COCCI (pairs)				
Neisseria gonorrhoeae (GC)	• CSF = NP • Blood = P (from pharyngitis, proctitis, ABE) • Sputum = NP • Urine = P (urethritis) • Stool = NP • Wound = NP • Rectal discharge = P (GC proctitis)	Penicillin-sensitive N. gonorrhoeae (PSNG) Ceftriaxone (IV/IM) Any quinolone (IV/PO) PRNG Ceftriaxone (IV/IM)	Penicillin-sensitive N. gonorrhoeae (PSNG) Penicillin (IV/IM) Amoxicillin (PO) Doxycycline (IV/PO) PPNG Spectinomycin (IM) Any quinolone (PO) Any cephalosporin (IV/PO)	Cause of "culture negative" right-sided ABE. May be cultured from synovial fluid/blood in disseminated GC infection (arthritis-dermatitis syndrome). Spectinomycin is ineffective against pharyngeal GC/incubating syphilis. PRNG are tetracycline-resistant (TRNG). GC strains from Hawaii/California have increased quinolone resistance; use cefixime or ceftriaxone for such strains. Treat possible Chlamydia trachomatis co-infection and sexual partners.
Neisseria meningitidis (MC)	• CSF = P (ABM) • Blood = P (acute/chronic meningococcemia) • Sputum = C, P (only in closed populations, e.g., military recruits)	Penicillin (IV) Ampicillin (IV) Any 3rd generation cephalosporin (IV)	Chloramphenicol (IV/PO) Cefepime (IV) Meropenem (IV)	In ABM, do not decrease meningeal dose of β-lactam antibiotics as patient improves, since CSF penetration/concentration decreases as meningeal inflammation decreases. Chloramphenicol is an excellent choice for penicillin-allergic patients. Preferred meningococcal prophylaxis is an oral quinolone (single dose).

		GRAM POSITIVE BACILLI	
Arcanobacterium (Corynebacterium) haemolyticus	• Urine C, P (urethritis rarely) • Stool = NP • Wound = NP • CSF = NP • Blood = NP • Sputum = P (oropharyngeal secretions) • Urine = NP • Stool/Wound = NP	Doxycycline (PO)	Erythromycin (PO) Azithromycin (PO) Any 1st, 2nd, 3rd generation cephalosporin (PO) Clarithromycin XL (PO)	Causes membranous pharyngitis with scarlet fever-like rash. Differentiate from C. diphtheriae (catalase +) and is not hemolytic on human or horse blood agar. A. hemolyticus (catalase –). β-hemolytic on human or horse blood agar. Penicillin and ampicillin are less effective than erythromycin or doxycycline.
Bacillus anthracis (naturally acquired)	• CSF = P (ABM) • Blood = P (septicemia; isolation required; dangerous) • Sputum = P (mediastinitis; anthrax pneumonia rare) • Urine = NP • Stool = NP • Wound = P (ulcer; isolation required; dangerous)	Penicillin (IV) Doxycycline (IV/PO) Any quinolone (IV/PO)	Amoxicillin (PO) Ampicillin (IV)	Doxycycline may be used for therapy/outbreak prophylaxis. Streptobacillary configuration in blood. Causes hemorrhagic meningitis, wound infections, and bacteremia. Quinolones are effective. Alert microbiology laboratory of potentially biohazardous specimens.
Bacillus cereus, subtilis, megaterium	• CSF = NP • Blood = C*, P (leukopenic compromised hosts)	Vancomycin (IV) Clindamycin (IV/PO)	Meropenem (IV) Any quinolone (IV/PO)	Soil organisms not commonly pathogenic for humans. Suspect pseudoinfection if isolated from clinical specimens. Look for soil/dust contamination of blood culture tube top/

C = colonizer; C* = skin contaminant; NP = non-pathogen at site; P = pathogen at site; (IV/PO) = IV or PO. See p. xi for all other abbreviations.

Table 3.6 Clinical Significance of AEROBIC Isolates Pending Susceptibility Testing *(cont'd)*

Isolate	Isolate Significance	GRAM POSITIVE BACILLI		Comments
		Preferred Therapy	Alternate Therapy	
	• Sputum = NP • Urine = NP • Stool = NP • Wound = NP			apparatus. Rare pathogen in leukopenic compromised hosts.
Corynebacterium diphtheriae	• CSF = NP • Blood = NP • Sputum = P (oropharyngeal secretions) • Urine = NP • Stool = NP • Wound = P (wound diphtheria)	Penicillin (IV) Erythromycin (IV) Clindamycin (IV/PO)	Doxycycline (IV/PO) Clarithromycin XL (PO) Rifampin (PO)	Administer diphtheria antitoxin as soon as possible. Antibiotic therapy is adjunctive, since diphtheria is a toxin-mediated disease. Patients may die unexpectedly from toxin-induced myocarditis during recovery.
Corynebacterium jeikeium (JK)	• CSF = C*, P (CSF shunts) • Blood = C*, P (from IV lines) • Sputum = NP • Urine/Stool = NP • Wound = C	Vancomycin (IV) Linezolid (IV/PO)	Quinupristin/ Dalfopristin (IV)	Cause of IV line/foreign body infections. In-vitro testing is not always reliable. Highly resistant to most anti-gram positive antibiotics.
Erysipelothrix rhusiopathiae	• CSF = NP • Blood = P (from SBE) • Sputum = NP • Urine = NP • Stool = NP • Wound = P (chronic erysipelas-like skin lesions)	Penicillin (IV) Ampicillin (IV) Amoxicillin (PO)	Any 3rd generation cephalosporin (IV) Any quinolone (IV/PO)	Cause of "culture-negative" SBE. Susceptible to clindamycin but resistant to vancomycin.

Listeria monocyto-genes	• CSF = P (ABM) • Blood = P (1° bacteremia, SBE) • Sputum = NP • Urine = NP • Stool = NP • Wound = NP	Ampicillin (IV) Amoxicillin (PO) Chloram-phenicol (IV) CNS Ampicillin (IV) TMP-SMX (IV/PO) Chlorampheni-col (IV/PO) SBE Ampicillin (IV)	Meropenem (IV) Linezolid (IV/PO) CNS Meropenem (IV) (meningeal doses) Linezolid (IV/PO) SBE Meropenem (IV) Linezolid (IV/PO)	Listeria ABM is common in T-cell deficiencies (e.g., lymphoma, steroids, HIV). Causes SBE in normal hosts, and is the commonest cause of ABM in non-neutropenic cancer patients. 3rd generation cephalosporins are ineffective against Listeria. *Empiric therapy of selected problem pathogens (Table 3.11) p. 260*
Nocardia asteroides, brasiliensis	• CSF = P (brain abscess) • Blood = P (from lung/soft tissue source) • Sputum = P (pneumonia, lung abscess) • Urine/Stool = NP • Wound = P (skin lesions from direct inoculation or dissemination)	TMP-SMX (IV/PO) Minocycline (IV/PO) Doxycycline (IV/PO)	Imipenem (IV) Mevopenem (IV) Linezolid (IV/PO) Ceftriaxone (IV)	Branched, filamentous, beady hyphae are typical, but coccobacillary and bacillary forms are also common. Nocardia are Gram-positive, aerobic, and weakly acid fast. Linezolid is active against Nocardia *Empiric therapy of selected problem pathogens (Table 3.11) p. 260*
Rhodococcus equi	• CSF = NP • Blood = P (from pneumonia, lung abscess) • Sputum = F (pneumonia with abscess/cavitation)	Any quinolone (IV/PO) Vancomycin (IV)	Erythromycin (IV) Imipenem (IV) Meropenem (IV) Doxycycline (IV/PO) TMP-SMX (IV/PO)	Causes TB-like community-acquired pneumonia in HIV. Filamentous bacteria break into bacilli/cocci. Aminoglycosides and β-lactams relatively ineffective.

C = colonizer; C* = skin contaminant; NP = non-pathogen at site; P = pathogen at site; (IV/PO) = IV or PO. See p. xi for all other abbreviations.

Table 3.6 Clinical Significance of AEROBIC Isolates Pending Susceptibility Testing *(cont'd)*

Isolate	Isolate Significance	Preferred Therapy	Alternate Therapy	Comments
		GRAM POSITIVE BACILLI		
	• Urine = NP • Stool = NP • Wound = NP			
		GRAM NEGATIVE BACILLI		
Acinetobacter baumannii, lwoffi, calcoaceticus, haemolyticus	• CSF = C* (ABM 2° to EVDs or CNS shunts) • Blood = P (from IV line, lung, or urine source) • Sputum = C, P (only with VAP outbreaks) • Urine = C, P (CAB) • Stool = NP • Wound = P (cellulitis)	Minocycline (IV/PO) Any carbapenem (IV) Ampicillin/ Sulbactam (IV) Tigecycline (IV) Colistin (IV) Polymyxin B (IV) Amikacin (IV)	Any 3rd generation cephalosporin (IV) (except Ceftazidime) Cefepime (IV) Aztreonam (IV) Fosfomycin (PO) (only Cystitis/CAB)	Colonization common; infection uncommon. If possible, avoid treating Acinetobacter common colonizer of respiratory secretions or urine (CAB). Occurs only in outbreaks of ventilator-associated pneumonia. Use meropenem for MDR susceptible isolates. For meropenem resistant isolates, colistin, polymyxin B, tigecycline, minocycline, or doripenem usually effective *Empiric therapy of selected problem pathogens (Table 3.11) p. 259*
Aeromonas hydrophila	• CSF = NP • Blood = P (from wound, urine, or GI source) • Sputum = NP • Urine = C, P (CAB) • Stool = P (diarrhea) • Wound = P (cellulitis)	Gentamicin (IV) TMP-SMX (IV/PO) Any quinolone (IV/PO)	Doxycycline (IV/PO) Any 3rd generation cephalosporin (IV/PO) Any carbapenem (IV) Aztreonam (IV)	Cause of wound infection, septic arthritis, diarrhea, and necrotizing soft tissue infection resembling gas gangrene.
Aggregatibacter (Actinobacillus) actinomycetemcomitans	• CSF = NP • Blood = P (from abscess, SBE) • Sputum = NP • Urine/Stool = NP	Any quinolone (IV/PO) Any 3rd generation cephalosporin (IV/PO)	Penicillin (IV) + Gentamicin (IV) TMP-SMX (IV/PO)	Cause of "culture-negative" SBE. One of the HACEK organisms. Found with Actinomyces in abscesses. Resistant to erythromycin and clindamycin.

Organism	Site	Preferred Therapy	Alternate Therapy	Comments
	· Wound = P (from abscess, draining fistulous tract)			Water-borne pathogen resembling Acinetobacter microbiologically. Resistant to aminoglycosides and 1st, 2nd generation cephalosporins.
Alcaligenes (Achromobacter) xylosoxidans	· CSF = P (rarely ABM) · Blood = P (from urine) · Sputum = NP · Urine = P (CAB) · Stool = NP · Wound = P (cellulitis rare)	Imipenem (IV) Meropenem (IV) Any 3rd generation cephalosporin (IV/PO)	Any quinolone (IV/PO) Cefepime (IV) Aztreonam (IV)	
Bartonella henselae, quintana, bacilliformis	· CSF = NP · Blood = P (from skin source, SBE) · Sputum = NP · Urine = NP · Stool = NP · Wound = P (skin lesions)	Doxycycline (IV/PO) Azithromycin (PO)	Clarithromycin XL (PO) Any quinolone (IV/PO) Any aminoglycoside (IV)	B. henselae (bacteremia, endocarditis, peliosis hepatis, bacillary angiomatosis); B. quintana (relapsing, trench fever, bacillary angiomatosis); B. bacilliformis (Oroyo fever, Carrion's disease). May present as FUO. Titers may cross react with C. burnetii (Q fever). TMP–SMX and cephalosporins are ineffective.
Bordetella pertussis, parapertussis	· CSF = NP · Blood = P (from respiratory tract source) · Sputum = C, P (pertussis) · Urine = NP · Stool = NP · Wound = NP	Erythromycin (IV) Clarithromycin XL (PO) Azithromycin (IV/PO)	Any quinolone (IV/PO) TMP–SMX (IV/PO) Doxycycline (IV/PO)	Causes pertussis in children and incompletely/non-immunized adults. Macrolides remain the preferred therapy. Resistant to penicillins, cephalosporins, and aminoglycosides.
Brucella abortus, canis, suis, melitensis	· CSF = P (meningitis) · Blood = P (from abscess, SBE)	Doxycycline (IV/PO) + Gentamicin (IV)	TMP–SMX (IV/PO) + Gentamicin (IV)	Causes prolonged relapsing infection. Zoonotic cause of brucellosis/Malta fever. Resistant to penicillins.

C = colonizer; C* = skin contaminant, NP = non-pathogen at site; P = pathogen at site; (IV/PO) = IV or PO. See p. xi for all other abbreviations.

Table 3.6 Clinical Significance of AEROBIC Isolates Pending Susceptibility Testing (cont'd)

		GRAM NEGATIVE BACILLI		
Isolate	Isolate Significance	Preferred Therapy	Alternate Therapy	Comments
	• Sputum = NP • Urine = P (pyelonephritis) • Stool/Wound = NP	Doxycycline + Streptomycin (IM)	Doxycycline (IV/PO) + Rifampin (PO) Any quinolone (IV/PO) + Rifampin (PO)	
Burkholderia (Pseudomonas) cepacia (BCC)	• CSF = NP • Blood = P (usually from IV line/urinary tract infection) • Sputum = C (not a cause of VAP) • Urine = C • Stool = NP • Wound = NP	TMP-SMX (IV/PO) Minocycline (IV/PO) Meropenem (IV)	A "respiratory quinolone" (IV/PO) Chloramphenicol (IV/PO) Cefepime (IV)	Common colonizer of ulcers, body fluids, and wounds. Opportunistic pathogen in cystic fibrosis/bronchiectasis. Resistant to aminoglycosides, colistin, and polymyxin B. *Empiric therapy of selected problem pathogens (Table 23.11) p. 260*
Burkholderia (Pseudomonas) pseudomallei	• CSF = NP • Blood = P (from septicemic melioidosis) • Sputum = P (chronic cavitary pneumonia) • Urine = NP • Stool = NP • Wound = NP	Imipenem (IV) Meropenem (IV) Ceftazidime (IV) Doxycycline (IV/PO)	Chloramphenicol (IV) TMP-SMX (IV/PO) Amoxicillin/ Clavulanic acid (PO)	Acute (septicemia)/chronic (cavitary CAP/ abscesses) melioidosis endemic in S.E. Asia. Chronic melioidosis resembles reactivation TB, but has lower lobe distribution. Prolonged latency until reactivation years later. Slow response to effective therapy (1–2 weeks). Prolonged therapy needed to prevent relapse (≥ 3 months). Oxidase positive. Resistant to penicillin, aminoglycosides, colistin.
Campylobacter fetus	• CSF = P (ABM) • Blood = P (from vascular source)	Gentamicin (IV) Imipenem (IV) Meropenem (IV)	Chloramphenicol (IV) Ampicillin (IV)	Causes invasive infection with spread to CNS. CNS infection may be treated with meningeal doses of chloramphenicol, ampicillin,

Subset of pathogens	Specimen	Preferred Therapy	Alternate Therapy	Comments
	• Sputum = NP • Urine = NP • Stool = NP • Wound = NP		Any 3rd generation cephalosporin (IV)	or a 3rd generation cephalosporin. Resistant to erythromycin.
Campylobacter jejuni	• CSF = NP • Blood = P (from GI source) • Sputum = NP • Urine = NP • Stool = P (diarrhea) • Wound = NP	Any quinolone (IV/PO) Erythromycin (PO) Doxycycline (IV/PO)	Azithromycin (PO) Clarithromycin XL (PO)	Commonest cause of acute bacterial diarrhea. Resistant to TMP-SMX.
Cardiobacterium hominis	• CSF = NP • Blood = P (from SBE) • Sputum = NP • Urine = NP • Stool = NP • Wound = NP	Penicillin (IV) + Gentamicin (IV) Ampicillin (IV) + Gentamicin (IV)	Any 3rd generation cephalosporin (IV) + Gentamicin (IV)	Pleomorphic bacillus with bulbous ends. Often appears in clusters resembling rosettes. Indole positive. Cause of "culture-negative" SBE (one of the HACEK organisms). Rare cause of abdominal abscess. Grows best with CO_2 enhancement. Resistant to macrolides and clindamycin.
Chromobacterium violaceum	• CSF = NP • Blood = P (from wound infection) • Sputum = NF • Urine = NP • Stool = NP • Wound = P (drainage from deep soft tissue infection)	Gentamicin (IV) Doxycycline (IV/PO)	Chloramphenicol (IV)	Cause of cutaneous lesions primarily in tropical/subtropical climates. Often mistaken for Vibrio or Alcaligenes. Resistant to β-lactams.
Chryseobacterium (Flavobacterium) meningosepticum	• CSF = P (ABM) • Blood = P (from IV line infection, PVE) • Sputum = NP	CNS TMP-SMX (IV/PO)	CNS Chloramphenicol (IV)	Rare cause of ABM in newborns and PVE in adults. Only unencapsulated Chryseobacterium species. Clindamycin, clarithromycin, and vancomycin are useful only in non-CNS

C = colonizer; C* = skin contaminant; NP = non-pathogen at site; P = pathogen at site; (IV/PO) = IV or PO. See p. xi for all other abbreviations.

Table 3.6 Clinical Significance of AEROBIC Isolates Pending Susceptibility Testing (cont'd)

| | | GRAM NEGATIVE BACILLI | | |
Isolate	Isolate Significance	Preferred Therapy	Alternate Therapy	Comments
	• Urine = C, P (from urologic instrumentation) • Stool = NP • Wound = C, P (cellulitis)	<u>Non-CNS</u> Vancomycin (IV) plus Rifampin (PO) Any quinolone (IV/PO)	<u>Non-CNS</u> Clarithromycin XL (PO) plus Rifampin (PO) Clindamycin (IV/PO)	infections. Resistant to aztreonam and carbapenems.
Citrobacter diversus, freundii, koseri	• CSF = C*, P (from NS procedure) • Blood = C*, P (from IV line/urinary tract infection) • Sputum = C (not pneumonia) • Urine = C, P (from urologic instrumentation) • Stool = NP • Wound = C, P (rarely in compromised hosts)	Any carbapenem (IV) Cefepime (IV) Any quinolone (IV/PO)	Aztreonam (IV) Piperacillin/ Tazobactam (IV) Any 3rd generation cephalosporin (IV)	Common wound/urine colonizer. Rare pathogen in normal hosts. Often aminoglycoside resistant. (C. freundii is usually more resistant than C. koseri).
Edwardsiella tarda	• CSF = NP • Blood = P (from liver abscess) • Sputum/Urine = NP • Stool = P • Wound C, P (wound infection)	Ampicillin (IV) Amoxicillin (PO) Any quinolone (IV/PO)	Doxycycline (IV/PO) Any 3rd generation cephalosporin (IV/PO)	Cause of bacteremia, usually from liver abscess or wound source.

Organism	Site/Specimen	Column 3	Column 4	Comments
Enterobacter agglomerans, cloacae Klebsiella (Enterobacter) aerogenes	• CSF = C* , P (from NS procedure) • Blood = C* , P (from IV line/urinary tract infection) • Sputum = C (not a cause of pneumonia) • Urine = C, P (post-urologic instrumentation) • Stool = NP • Wound = C, P (*rarely in compromised hosts)	Any carbapenem (IV)	Any quinolone (IV/PO) Aztreonam (IV) Piperacillin/ Tazobactam (IV) Cefepime (IV)	Not a cause of community-acquired or nosocomial pneumonia. Common colonizer of respiratory secretions and wound/urine specimens. Antibiotic resistance to E. cloacae > K. aerogenes > E. agglomerans. Treatment of Enterobacter colonizers with ceftazidime or ciprofloxacin may result in MDR Enterobacter sp. Enterobacter CRE usually susceptible to tigecycline, colistin, polymyxin B, ceftazidime/avibactam, fosfomycin. (For CRE see p. 259) *Empiric therapy of selected problem pathogens (Table 3.11) p. 258*
Escherichia coli	• CSF = P (ABM) • Blood = P (from GI/ GU source) • Sputum = P (rarely CAP from urinary source, VAP) • Urine = C, P (CAB, cystitis, pyelonephritis) • Stool = P (diarrhea) • Wound = P (cellulitis)	Any 1st, 2nd, 3rd generation cephalosporin (IV/PO) Amoxicillin (PO) Any quinolone (IV/PO) Ceftriaxone (IV) Nitrofurantoin (PO)*	Aztreonam (IV) Gentamicin (IV) TMP-SMX (IV/PO)	Common pathogen, usually from GI/ GU source. Many strains are resistant to ampicillin and some to 1st generation cephalosporins. MDR/ESBL & E. coli may be treated with a carbapenem. E. coli CRE usually susceptible only to tigecycline, colistin, polymyxin B, ceftazidime/avibactam, nitrofurantoin* fosfomycin.* (For CRE see p. 259)
Francisella tularensis	• CSF = NP • Blood = P (isolation dangerous) • Sputum = P (tularemic pneumonia; isolation dangerous)	Doxycycline (IV/PO) Gentamicin (IV/IM) Streptomycin (IM)	Chloramphenicol (IV/PO) Any quinolone (IV/PO)	Six clinical tularemia syndromes. Alert microbiology laboratory of potentially biohazardous specimens. Do not culture. Resistant to penicillins and cephalosporins. Bioterrorist tularemia is treated the same as naturally-acquired tularemia.

C = colonizer; C* = skin contaminant; NP = non-pathogen at site; P = pathogen at site; (IV/PO) = IV or PO for all other abbreviations.
* For acute uncomplicated cystitis (ALC) or catheter associated bacteriuria (CAB) only.

Table 3.6 Clinical Significance of AEROBIC Isolates Pending Susceptibility Testing (cont'd)

		GRAM NEGATIVE BACILLI		
Isolate	Isolate Significance	Preferred Therapy	Alternate Therapy	Comments
	• Urine/Stool = NP • Wound = P (isolation dangerous)			
Hafnia alvei	• CSF = C, P (from NS procedure) • Blood = C*, P (from IV line/urinary tract infection) • Sputum = C (not pneumonia) • Urine = C, P (post-urologic instrumentation) • Stool = NP • Wound = C, P (rarely in compromised hosts)	Cefepime (IV) Any quinolone (IV/PO) Aztreonam (IV)	Piperacillin/ Tazobactam (IV) Imipenem (IV) Meropenem (IV)	Formerly Enterobacter hafniae. Uncommon nosocomial pathogen. Rarely pathogenic in normal hosts. Cause of UTIs in compromised hosts.
Helicobacter (Campylobacter) pylori	• CSF = NP • Blood = NP • Sputum = NP • Urine = NP • Stool = P (from upper GI tract biopsy specimens, not stool) • Wound = NP	Omeprazole (PO) plus Clarithromycin XL (PO) plus Amoxicillin (PO)	Doxycycline (PO) plus Metronidazole (PO) plus Bismuth subsalicylate (PO)	Optimal therapy awaits definition. Treat until cured. Some strains of resistant H. pylori may respond to treatment with a quinolone. TMP–SMX is ineffective.

		For all Haemophilus species Any 2nd, 3rd generation cephalosporin (IV/PO) Any quinolone (IV/PO) Doxycycline (IV/PO)	For all Haemophilus species Chloramphenicol (IV) TMP-SMX (IV/PO) Azithromycin (PO) Aztreonam (IV) Ampicillin resistant H.influenzae Meropenem (IV) Imipenem (IV) Ertapenem (IV) Cefepime (IV) Aztreonam (IV)	1st generation cephalosporins, erythromycin, and clarithromycin have limited anti-H. influenzae activity; doxycycline and azithromycin are better. Hemophilus species are common colonizers of the respiratory tract. Rarely a cause of "culture-negative" SBE (H. parainfluenzae/aphrophilus are HACEK organisms). H. influenzae (non-hemolytic) and H. parainfluenzae may be differentiated from the throat commensals H. hemolyticus and H. parahemolyticus by hemolysis on sheep agar.
Haemophilus influenzae, parainfluenzae, aphrophilus, paraphrophilus	• CSF = P (ABM) • Blood = P (from respiratory tract or cardiac source) • Sputum = C, P (CAP) • Urine = NP • Stool = NP • Wound = P			
Kingella (Moraxella) kingae	• CSF = NP • Blood = P (from skeletal or cardiac source) • Sputum = C • Urine = NP • Stool/wound = NP	Ampicillin (IV) plus any aminoglycoside (IV)	Any 3rd generation (IV) cephalosporin plus any aminoglycoside (IV) Imipenem (IV) Meropenem (IV) Any quinolone (IV/PO)	Common colonizer of respiratory tract, but rarely a respiratory pathogen. Causes septic arthritis/osteomyelitis in children and endocarditis in adults (one of HACEK organisms). Oxidase positive. Growth enhanced with CO_2.
Klebsiella pneumoniae, oxytoca	• CSF = P (ABM) • Blood = P (from respiratory, GI, GU source)	Tigecycline (IV) Any carbapenem (IV)	Any 3rd generation cephalosporin (IV, PO) except ceftazidime Any quinolone (IV/PO)	TMP-SMX may be ineffective in systemic infection. Anti-pseudomonal penicillins have limited anti-Klebsiella activity. Klebsiella usually susceptible to carbapenems. CRE susceptible to tigecycline, colistin, polymyxin B, ceftazidime/avibactam, fosfomycin. (For CRE see p. 259) *Empiric therapy of selected problem pathogens (Table 3.11) p. 258*

C = colonizer; C* = skin contaminant; NP = non-pathogen at site; P = pathogen at site; (IV/PO) = IV or PO. See p. xi for all other abbreviations.

Table 3.6 Clinical Significance of AEROBIC Isolates Pending Susceptibility Testing *(cont'd)*

		GRAM NEGATIVE BACILLI		
Isolate	Isolate Significance	Preferred Therapy	Alternate Therapy	Comments
Klebsiella ozaenae, rhinoscleromatis	• Sputum = C, P (CAP/VAP) • Urine = C (CAB), P • Stool = NP • Wound = C, P	Any quinolone (PO)	Aztreonam (IV) Cefepime (IV)	NDM-1 metallo β-lactamase strains are carbapenem resistant and usually susceptible only to colistin, tigecycline.
	• CSF = NP • Blood = NP • Sputum = NP • Urine = NP • Stool = NP • Wound = P (rhinoscleromatis lesions)	Any quinolone (PO)	TMP–SMX (PO) + Rifampin (PO)	Skin infection usually requires prolonged treatment for cure (weeks-to-months).
Legionella sp.	• CSF = NP • Blood = NP • Sputum = P (CAP or VAP) • Urine = NP • Stool = NP • Wound = NP	Any quinolone (IV/PO) Doxycycline (IV/PO) Tigecycline (IV) Azithromycin (IV/PO)	Clarithromycin XL (PO) Erythromycin (IV)	Anti-Legionella activity: quinolones > doxycycline > erythromycin. Erythromycin failures are not uncommon. Rarely a cause of culture-negative SBE/PVE.
Leptospira interrogans	• CSF = P (ABM) • Blood = P (1° bacteremia) • Sputum = NP • Urine = P (excreted in urine) • Stool = NP • Wound = NP	Doxycycline (IV/PO) Penicillin G (IV) Any 3rd generation cephalosporin (IV/PO)	Amoxicillin (PO)	Blood/urine cultures may be positive during initial/bacteremic phase, but are negative during immune phase. Relapse is common. Resistant to chloramphenicol.

Moraxella (Branhamella) catarrhalis	• CSF = NP • Blood = P (rarely from CAP) • Sputum = C, P (CAP) • Urine = NP • Stool = NP • Wound = NP	Any 2ⁿᵈ, 3ʳᵈ generation cephalosporin (IV/PO) Any quinolone (IV/PO) Telithromycin (PO) Doxycycline (IV/PO)	Azithromycin (PO) Clarithromycin XL (PO) TMP-SMX (IV/PO) Amoxicillin/ Clavulanic acid (PO)	Almost all strains are β-lactamase positive and resistant to penicillin/ampicillin. β-lactamase-resistant β-lactams are effective. Resembles Acinetobacter on sputum Gram stain.
Morganella morganii	• CSF = NP • Blood = P (from GU source) • Sputum = NP • Urine = P (CAB, cystitis, pyelonephritis) • Stool = NP • Wound = P (cellulitis rare)	Any quinolone (IV/PO) Any 3ʳᵈ generation cephalosporin (IV) Any carbapenem (IV)	Any aminoglycoside (IV) Aztreonam (IV) Cefepime (IV)	Common uropathogen. Causes bacteremia with urosepsis. Rare cause of wound infections.
Ochrobactrum (CDC group Vd) anthropi	• CSF = NP • Blood = P (from IV line infections) • Sputum = C • Urine = C • Stool/Wound = C	Any quinolone (IV/PO) TMP-SMX (IV/PO)	Any aminoglycoside (IV) Imipenem (IV) Meropenem (IV)	Pathogen in compromised hosts. Oxidase and catalase positive. Resistant to β-lactams.
Pasteurella multocida	• CSF = P (ABM) • Blood = P (from respiratory source, bite wound, abscess) • Sputum = C, P (CAP, bronchiectasis)	Amoxicillin (PO) Doxycycline (IV/PO) Penicillin G (IV)	Ampicillin/ Sulbactam (IV) Piperacillin/ Tazobactam (IV) Any quinolone (IV/PO)	Common cause of infection following dog/cat bites. Many antibiotics are effective, but erythromycin is ineffective. Resembles Hemophilus sp. on sputum Gram stain.

C = colonizer; C* = skin contaminant; NP = non-pathogen at site; P = pathogen at site; (IV/PO) = IV or PO. See p. xi for all other abbreviations.

Table 3.6 Clinical Significance of AEROBIC Isolates Pending Susceptibility Testing *(cont'd)*

		GRAM NEGATIVE BACILLI		
Isolate	**Isolate Significance**	**Preferred Therapy**	**Alternate Therapy**	**Comments**
	• Urine = C, P (pyelonephritis) • Stool = NP • Wound = P (human/animal bites)			
Plesiomonas shigelloides	• CSF = NP • Blood = P (from GU source) • Sputum = NP • Urine = NP • Stool = P (diarrhea) • Wound = NP	Any quinolone (PO) TMP–SMX (PO)	Doxycycline (PO) Aztreonam (PO)	Infrequent cause of diarrhea, less commonly dysentery. Oxidase positive. β-lactamase strains are increasing. Resistant to penicillins.
Proteus mirabilis, vulgaris	• CSF = NP • Blood = P (from urinary source) • Sputum = C • Urine = C, P (from urologic instrumentation) • Stool = NP • Wound = C, P (wound infection)	P. mirabilis, (indole –) Ampicillin (IV) Any 1st, 2nd, 3rd. gen. cephalosporin (IV/PO) P. vulgaris, (indole +) Any 3rd generation cephalosporin (IV/PO) Cefepime (IV) Any quinolone (IV/PO)	P. mirabilis, (indole –) TMP–SMX (IV/PO) Amoxicillin (PO) P. vulgaris, (indole +) Aztreonam (IV) Any carbapenem (IV) Any aminoglycoside (IV)	Usually a uropathogen. Most antibiotics are effective against P. mirabilis (indole negative); P. penneri (indole negative P. vulgaris) is resistant to ceftriaxone. Indole positive Proteus sp. require potent antibiotics to treat non-UTIs. P. penneri (indole negative P. vulgaris) resistant to 3rd gen. cephalosporins; use cefepime, a carbapenem, or a quinolone.

Providencia alcalifaciens, rettgeri, stuartii	• CSF = NP • Blood = C*, P (from GU source) • Sputum/Stool = NP • Urine = C, P • Wound = C, P (rare)	Any quinolone (IV/PO) Any 3rd generation cephalosporin (IV/PO) Cefepime (IV) Meropenem (IV) Ertapenem (IV)	Any aminoglycoside (IV) Aztreonam (IV) Piperacillin/ Tazobactam (IV) Imipenem (IV)	Almost always a uropathogen. Formerly classified as indole positive Proteus.
Pseudomonas aeruginosa	• CSF = NP • Blood = P (from respiratory, GU source) • Sputum = C (usually), P (rarely indicates VAP) • Urine = C, P (from urologic instrumentation) • Stool = NP • Wound = C (almost always)	Monotherapy Meropenem (IV) Cefepime (IV) Combination therapy Meropenem (IV) plus either Cefepime (IV) or Amikacin (IV)	Doripenem (IV) Amikacin (IV) Aztreonam (IV) Polymyxin B (IV) Colistin (IV)	Colonization common; infection uncommon. If possible, avoid covering P. aeruginosa in respiratory secretions in ventilated patients (unless tracheobronchitis). For serious systemic P. aeruginosa infection, double drug therapy preferred. All double anti-P. aeruginosa regimens are equally effective. Individual differences in activity (MICs) are unimportant if combination therapy is used. If MDR P. aeruginosa meropenem susceptible, treat with meropenem. If MDR P. aeruginosa meropenem resistant, treat with colistin, polymyxin B, doripenem or ceftazidime/ avibactam usually effective. *Empiric therapy of selected problem pathogens (Table 3.11) p.259*
Pseudomonas (Chryseomonas) luteola (CDC group Ve-1)	• CSF = NP • Blood = P (from IV line infection) • Sputum = NP • Urine = NP • Stool = NP • Wound = NP	Imipenem (IV) Meropenem (IV) Cefepime (IV)	Piperacillin/ Tazobactam (IV) Aztreonam (IV)	Opportunistic pathogen primarily in compromised hosts.

C = colonizer; C* = skin contaminant; NP = non-pathogen at site; P = pathogen at site; (IV/PO) = IV or PO. See p. xi for all other abbreviations.

Table 3.6 Clinical Significance of AEROBIC Isolates Pending Susceptibility Testing (cont'd)

		GRAM NEGATIVE BACILLI		
Isolate	Isolate Significance	Preferred Therapy	Alternate Therapy	Comments
Pseudomonas (Flavimonas) oryzihabitans (CDC group Ve-2)	• CSF = P (NS procedures) • Blood = P (from IV line infection) • Sputum = NP • Urine = NP • Stool = NP • Wound = P (rare)	Imipenem (IV) Meropenem (IV) Cefepime (IV)	Any 3rd generation cephalosporin (IV) Piperacillin/ Tazobactam (IV) Aztreonam (IV)	Rare cause of central IV line infections (usually in febrile neutropenics). Rare cause of peritonitis in CAPD patients. Oxidase negative, unlike other Pseudomonas species.
Salmonella typhi, non-typhi	• CSF = NP • Blood = P (from GI source) • Sputum = NP • Urine = P (only with enteric fever) • Stool = C (carrier), P (gastroenteritis, enteric fever) • Wound = NP	Any quinolone (IV/PO) Any 3rd generation cephalosporin (IV)	Chloramphenicol (IV) TMP–SMX (IV/PO) Doxycycline (IV/PO)	Carrier state is best eliminated by a quinolone or TMP–SMX. If drug therapy fails to eliminate carrier state, look for hepatic/ bladder calculi for persistent focus. Many strains are resistant to ampicillin/amoxicillin.
Serratia marcescens	• CSF = P (from NS procedures) • Blood = P (from IV line or urinary source) • Sputum = C, P (rarely in VAP) • Urine = C, P (post-urologic instrumentation) • Stool = NP • Wound = C, P (rare)	Any 3rd generation cephalosporin (IV/PO) Any quinolone (IV/PO) Cefepime (IV)	Any carbapenem (IV) Gentamicin (IV) Aztreonam (IV) Piperacillin/ Tazobactam (IV)	Enterobacteriaceae. Associated with water sources. Common colonizer of respiratory secretions/urine in ICU. Serratia nosocomial pneumonia and PVE are rare. Cause of septic arthritis, osteomyelitis, and SBE (IV drug abusers). Among the aminoglycosides, gentamicin has the greatest anti-Serratia activity. *Empiric therapy of selected problem pathogens (Table 3.11) p. 259*

Shigella boydii, sonnei, flexneri, dysenteriae	• CSF = NP • Blood = P (from GI source) • Sputum = NP • Urine = NP • Stool = P (Shigella dysentery) • Wound = NP	Any quinolone (IV/PO)	TMP–SMX (IV/PO) Azithromycin (IV/PO)	No carrier state. Severity of dysentery varies with the species: S. dysenteriae (most severe) > S. flexneri > S. sonnei/boydii (least severe).
Steno-trophomonas (Pseudomonas, Xanthomonas) maltophilia	• CSF = C, P (from NS procedures) • Blood = C*, P (from IV line infection; GU source) • Sputum = C (not VAP) • Urine = C, P (from urologic instrumentation) • Stool = NP • Wound = C, P (rarely in compromised hosts)	TMP–SMX (IV/PO) Tigecycline (IV) Minocycline (IV/PO) Ceftazidime/ Avibactam (IV) Ceftolozane/ Tazobactam (IV)	Doxycycline (IV/PO) Any respiratory quinolone (IV/PO)	Common colonizers of wounds, urine, and respiratory secretions. Potential pulmonary pathogen only in bronchiectasis/cystic fibrosis. Although usually carbapenem resistant, ~60% of strains demonstrate synergy with meropenem + levofloxacin. Susceptible to chloramphenicol, rifampin, colistin, polymyxin B. Resistant to aminoglycosides and carbapenems. *Empiric therapy of selected problem pathogens (Table 3.11) p. 259*
Streptobacillus moniliformis	• CSF = P (brain abscess) • Blood = P (from wound) • Sputum = P (lung abscess) • Urine = NP • Stool = NP • Wound = P (from rat bite)	Penicillin (IV) Ampicillin (IV) Amoxicillin (PO)	Doxycycline (IV/PO) Erythromycin (IV) Clindamycin (IV/PO)	Cause of Haverhill fever and rat bite fever, with abrupt onset of fever and severe headache/arthralgias after bite wound has healed. Rat bite site does not ulcerate. No regional adenopathy. Morbilliform/petechial rash. Arthritis in 50%. May cause SBE.

C = colonizer; C* = skin contaminant; NP = non-pathogen at site; P = pathogen at site; (IV/PO) = IV or PO. See p. xi for all other abbreviations.

Table 3.6 Clinical Significance of AEROBIC Isolates Pending Susceptibility Testing *(cont'd)*

		GRAM NEGATIVE BACILLI		
Isolate	Isolate Significance	Preferred Therapy	Alternate Therapy	Comments
Vibrio cholerae	• CSF = NP • Blood = P (from GI source) • Sputum = NP • Urine = NP • Stool = P (cholera) • Wound = NP	Doxycycline (IV/PO) Any quinolone (IV/PO)	TMP–SMX (IV/PO)	No carrier state. Treat for 3 days. Single-dose therapy is often effective. Resistant to ampicillin.
Vibrio parahaemolyticus	• CSF = NP • Blood = P (from GI source) • Sputum = NP • Urine = NP • Stool = P (diarrhea) • Wound = P	Doxycycline (IV/PO)	Any quinolone (IV/PO)	Most cases of gastroenteritis caused by V. parahaemolyticus are self-limited and require no treatment.
Vibrio vulnificus, alginolyticus	• CSF = NP • Blood = P (from GI/wound source) • Sputum = NP • Urine = NP • Stool = P (diarrhea) • Wound = P (water-contaminated wound raw oysters, other shell fish ingestion)	Doxycycline (IV/PO) Any quinolone (IV/PO)	Piperacillin/ Tazobactam (IV) Ampicillin/ Sulbactam (IV)	Causes necrotizing soft tissue infection resembling gas gangrene. Patients are critically ill with fever, bullous lesions, diarrhea, and hypotension. Treat wound infection, bacteremia. Aminoglycoside susceptibilities are unpredictable.
Yersinia enterocolitica	• CSF = NP • Blood = P (from GI source)	Any quinolone (IV/PO)	TMP–SMX (IV/PO) Any 3rd generation cephalosporin (IV/PO)	Cause of diarrhea with abdominal pain. If pain in right lower quadrant, may be mistaken for acute appendicitis.

Organism	Site	Preferred	Alternate	Comments
Yersinia pestis	• Sputum = NP • Urine = NP • Stool = P (diarrhea) • Wound = NP	Gentamicin (IV) Doxycycline (IV/PO)		
	• CSF = NP • Blood = P (septicemic plague; isolation required; dangerous) • Sputum = P (pneumonic plague; isolation required; dangerous) • Urine = NP • Stool = NP • Wound = P (lymph nodes, lymph node drainage; bubonic plague; isolation required; dangerous)	Doxycycline (IV/PO) Streptomycin (IM) Gentamicin (IV/IM) Any quinolone (IV/PO)	Chloramphenicol (IV/PO)	Cause of bubonic, septicemic, and pneumonic plague. Doxycycline or any quinolone may be used for prophylaxis. Alert microbiology laboratory of potentially biohazardous specimens. Do not culture. Bioterrorist plague is treated the same as naturally-acquired plague.

SPIROCHETES

| Borrelia burgdorferi | • CSF = P (neuroborreliosis)
• Blood = P (rarely isolated; requires special media)
• Sputum = NF
• Urine = NP
• Stool = NP
• Wound = P (rarely isolated from erythema migrans lesions) | Doxycycline (PO)
Amoxicillin (PO) | Any cephalosporin (PO)
Azithromycin (PO)
Erythromycin (PO) | Cause of Lyme disease. β-lactams and doxycycline are effective. Erythromycin least effective. Minocycline may be preferred to doxycycline for neuroborreliosis. |

C = colonizer; C* = skin contaminant; NP = non-pathogen at site; P = pathogen at site; (IV/PO) = IV or PO. See p. xi for all other abbreviations.

Table 3.6 Clinical Significance of AEROBIC Isolates Pending Susceptibility Testing (cont'd)

SPIROCHETES

Isolate	Isolate Significance	Preferred Therapy	Alternate Therapy	Comments
Borrelia recurrentis	• CSF = P (ABM) • Blood = P (1° bacteremia) • Sputum = NP • Urine = NP • Stool = NP • Wound = NP	Doxycycline (IV/PO) Azithromycin (IV/PO)	Erythromycin (IV) Penicillin (IV) Ampicillin (IV) Any 1st, 2nd, 3rd generation cephalosporin (IV/PO)	Cause of relapsing fever. May be recovered from septic metastatic foci. Septic emboli may cause sacroiliitis, SBE, myositis, orchitis, or osteomyelitis.
Spirillum minus	• CSF = NP • Blood = P (from wound source, SBE) • Sputum = NP • Urine = NP • Stool = NP • Wound = P (from rat bite)	Penicillin (IV) Amoxicillin (PO)	Doxycycline (IV/PO) Any quinolone (IV/PO)	One cause of rat bite fever. Bite wound heals promptly, but 1–4 weeks later becomes painful, purple and swollen, and progresses to ulceration and eschar formation. Painful regional adenopathy. Central maculopapular rash is common (rarely urticarial). Arthralgias/arthritis rare compared to rat bite fever from Streptobacillus moniliformis.

C = colonizer; C* = skin contaminant; NP = non-pathogen at site; P = pathogen at site; (IV/PO) = IV or PO. See p. xi for all other abbreviations.

Table 3.7 Clinical Significance of CAPNOPHILIC Isolates Pending Susceptibility Testing

		GRAM NEGATIVE BACILLI		
Isolate	Isolate Significance	Preferred Therapy	Alternate Therapy	Comments
Capnocytophaga canimorsus/ cynodegni (DF-2 like)	• CSF = NP • Blood = P (from GI source, bite wound) • Sputum = NP • Urine = NP • Stool = NP • Wound = P (from dog/cat bite)	Ampicillin/ Sulbactam (IV) Piperacillin/ Tazobactam (IV) Imipenem (IV) Meropenem (IV) Ertapenem (IV)	Clindamycin (IV/PO) Any quinolone (IV/PO) Doxycycline (IV/PO)	Associated with animal bites or cancer. May cause fatal septicemia in cirrhotics/asplenics. Resistant to aminoglycosides, metronidazole, TMP–SMX, and aztreonam.
Capnocytophaga ochraceus (DF-1)	• CSF = NP • Blood = P (from GI, wound, abscess source) • Sputum = NP • Urine = NP • Stool = NP • Wound = P	Ampicillin/ Sulbactam (IV) Piperacillin/ Tazobactam (IV) Imipenem (IV) Meropenem (IV) Ertapenem (IV)	Clindamycin (IV/PO) Any quinolone (IV/PO) Doxycycline (IV/PO)	Thin, spindle-shaped bacilli resemble Fusobacteria morphologically. "Gliding motility" seen in hanging drop preparations. Cause of septicemia, abscesses, and wound infections. Resistant to aminoglycosides, metronidazole, TMP–SMX, and aztreonam.
Eikenella corrodens	• CSF = NP • Blood = P (SBE in IV drug abusers) • Sputum = NP • Urine = NP • Stool = NP • Wound = P (IV drug abusers)	Penicillin (IV) Ampicillin (IV) Imipenem (IV) Meropenem (IV) Ertapenem (IV)	Piperacillin (IV) Ampicillin/ Sulbactam (IV) Doxycycline (IV/PO) Amoxicillin (PO)	Cause of "culture-negative" SBE (one of the HACEK organisms). Resistant to clindamycin and metronidazole.

C = colonizer; C* = skin contaminant; NP = non-pathogen at site; P = pathogen at site; (IV/PO) = IV or PO. See p. xi for all other abbreviations.

Table 3.8 Usual Clinical Significance of ANAEROBIC Isolates Pending Susceptibility Testing

Isolate	Isolate Significance	Preferred Therapy	Alternate Therapy	Comments
GRAM POSITIVE COCCI (chains)				
Peptococcus	• CSF = P (brain abscess) • Blood = P (from GI/pelvic source) • Sputum = C, P (aspiration pneumonia, lung abscess) • Urine/Stool = NP • Wound = P (rarely a sole pathogen)	Penicillin (IV) Ampicillin (IV) Amoxicillin (PO) Clindamycin (IV/PO)	Chloramphenicol (IV) Erythromycin (IV) Any carbapenem (IV) Moxifloxacin (IV/PO)	Normal flora of mouth, GI tract, and pelvis. Associated with mixed aerobic/anaerobic dental, abdominal, and pelvic infections, especially abscesses.
Peptostreptococcus	• CSF = P (brain abscess) • Blood = P (GI/pelvic source) • Sputum = C, P (aspiration pneumonia, lung abscess) • Urine/Stool = NP • Wound = P (rarely a sole pathogen)	Penicillin (IV) Ampicillin (IV) Amoxicillin (PO) Clindamycin (IV/PO)	Chloramphenicol (IV) Erythromycin (IV) Any carbapenem (IV) Moxifloxacin (IV/PO)	Normal flora of mouth, GI tract, and pelvis. Associated with mixed aerobic/anaerobic dental, abdominal, and pelvic infections, especially abscesses.
GRAM POSITIVE BACILLI				
Actinomyces israelii, odontolyticus	• CSF = P (brain abscess) • Blood = NP	Amoxicillin (PO) Doxycycline (PO)	Erythromycin (PO) Clindamycin (PO)	Anaerobic and non-acid fast. Usually presents as cervical, facial, thoracic, or abdominal masses/fistulas. Prolonged

	• Sputum = C, P (lung abscess) • Urine = **NP** • Stool = NP • Wound = P (fistulas/ underlying abscess)			(6–12 month) treatment is needed for cure. Unlike Nocardia, Actinomyces rarely causes CNS infections. May be cultured from polymicrobial brain abscess of pulmonary origin. Quinolones, aminoglycosides, metronidazole, and TMP–SMX have little activity.
Arachnia propionica	• CSF = P (brain abscess) • Blood = P (from dental, GI, lung source) • Sputum = C, P (lung abscess) • Urine = **NP** • Stool = NP • Wound = NP	Clindamycin (IV/PO) Ampicillin (IV) **plus** + Gentamicin (IV)	Erythromycin (IV)	Polymicrobial pathogen in dental, lung, and brain abscesses.
Bifidobacterium sp.	• CSF = P, brain abscess, • Blood = NP • Sputum = C, P (lung abscess) • Urine/Stool = NP • Wound = NP	Clindamycin (IV/PO) Ampicillin (IV) **plus** Gentamicin (IV)	Erythromycin (IV)	Usually part of polymicrobial infection.
Clostridium botulinum	• CSF = NP • Blood = NP • Sputum = NP • Urine/Stool = NP • Wound = P (wound botulism)	Penicillin (IV)	Clindamycin (IV/PO) Imipenem (IV) Meropenem (IV)	Give trivalent equine antitoxin as soon as possible. Antibiotic therapy is adjunctive.

C = colonizer; C* = skin contaminant; NP = non-pathogen at site; P = pathogen at site; (IV/PO) = IV or PO. See p. xi for all other abbreviations.

Table 3.8 Usual Clinical Significance of ANAEROBIC Isolates Pending Susceptibility Testing (cont'd)

		GRAM POSITIVE BACILLI		
Isolate	Isolate Significance	Preferred Therapy	Alternate Therapy	Comments
Clostridium difficile	• CSF = NP • Blood = P (rarely from GI source) • Sputum = NP • Urine = NP • Stool = C (normal fecal flora), P (diarrhea/colitis) • Wound = NP	<u>C. difficile diarrhea</u> Vancomycin (PO) Nitazoxanide (PO) <u>C. difficile colitis</u> Metronidazole (IV/PO) Tigecycline (IV)	<u>C. difficile diarrhea</u> Metronidazole (PO) <u>C. difficile colitis</u> Nitazoxanide (PO)	**C. difficile diarrhea** PO vancomycin preferred. PO vancomycin more effective than PO metronidazole. Nitazoxanide also highly effective. PO metronidazole, not PO vancomycin, increases prevalence of VRE. **C. difficile colitis,** use IV or PO metronidazole (IV vancomycin ineffective). Nitazoxanide (PO) or tigecycline (IV) also highly effective. Diagnose C. difficile diarrhea by stool C. difficile toxin assay/PCR. Diagnose C. difficile colitis by C. difficile + toxin assay/PCR plus colitis on abdominal CT scan/colonoscopy.
Clostridium perfringens, septicum, novyi	• CSF = NP • Blood = P (from GI source/malignancy) • Sputum = NP • Urine = NP • Stool = NP • Wound = P (gas gangrene)	Penicillin (IV) Piperacillin/ Tazobactam (IV) Meropenem (IV) Ertapenem (IV)	Clindamycin (IV) Chloramphenicol (IV) Imipenem (IV)	Usual cause of myonecrosis (gas gangrene). Surgical debridement is crucial; antibiotic therapy is adjunctive. Also causes emphysematous cholecystitis/cystitis. Does not form spores in blood cultures as does C. sordelli.
Clostridium tetani	• CSF = NP • Blood = NP	Penicillin (IV) Clindamycin (IV)	Imipenem (IV) Meropenem (IV)	Prompt administration of tetanus immune globulin is crucial. Antibiotic therapy is adjunctive.

	• Sputum = NP • Urine/Stcol = NP • Wound = P (wound tetanus)		
Eubacterium sp.	• CSF = P (brain abscess) • Blood = F (from dental, GI, GU, lung source) • Sputum = P (lung abscess) • Urine/Stool = NP • Wound = NP	Clindamycin (IV/PO) Ampicillin (IV) + Gentamicin (IV)	Erythromycin (IV)	Pathogen in lung/pelvic/brain abscesses, and chronic periodontal disease. Eubacterium bacteremias are associated with malignancies.
Lactobacillus sp.	• CSF = P (ABM) • Blood = P (1° bacteremia, SBE, or from endometritis) • Sputum = NP • Urine = P (rare) • Stool = NP • Wound = NP	Ampicillin (IV) + Gentamicin (IV) Clindamycin (IV/PO)	Erythromycin (IV)	Uncommon pathogen in normal/compromised hosts. Rare cause of SBE. Variably resistant to cephalosporins and quinolones. Some clindamycin-resistant strains. Resistant to metronidazole and vancomycin.
Propionibacterium acnes	• CSF = C*, P (meningitis from NS shunts) • Blood = C*, P (from IV line infection, SBE) • Sputum = NP • Urine = NP • Stool = NP • Wound = C	Penicillin (IV) Clindamycin (IV/PO)	Doxycycline (IV/PO)	Common skin colonizer/blood culture contaminant. Rarely causes prosthetic joint infection, endocarditis, or CNS shunt infection. Resistant to metronidazole.

C = colonizer; C* = skin contaminant; NP = non-pathogen at site; P = pathogen at site; (IV/PO) = IV or PO. See p. xi for all other abbreviations.

Table 3.8 Usual Clinical Significance of ANAEROBIC Isolates Pending Susceptibility Testing *(cont'd)*

			GRAM NEGATIVE BACILLI	
Isolate	Isolate Significance	Preferred Therapy	Alternate Therapy	Comments
Bacteroides fragilis group (*Parabacteroides distasonis, B. ovatus, B. thetaiotaomicron, B. vulgatus*)	• CSF = P (meningitis from *Strongyloides* hyperinfection) • Blood = P (from GI/ pelvic source) • Sputum = NP • Urine = NP, P (only from colonic fistula) • Stool = NP • Wound = NP	Tigecycline (IV) Piperacillin/ Tazobactam (IV) Any carbapenem (IV) Moxifloxacin (IV/PO)	Ampicillin/ Sulbactam (IV) Clindamycin (IV/PO) Metronidazole (IV/PO) plus either Ceftriaxone (IV) *or* Levofloxacin (IV/PO)	Major anaerobe below the diaphragm. Usually part of polymicrobial lower intra-abdominal and pelvic infections. Cefotetan is less effective against B. fragilis DOT strains (B. distasonis, B. ovatus, B. thetaiotaomicron). Resistant to penicillin.
Fusobacterium nucleatum	• CSF = P (brain abscess) • Blood = P (from lung, GI source) • Sputum = P (aspiration pneumonia, lung abscess) • Urine = NP • Stool = NP • Wound = P (rarely)	Clindamycin (IV/PO) Piperacillin/ Tazobactam (IV) Ampicillin/ Sulbactam (IV)	Chloramphenicol (IV) Metronidazole (IV/PO)	Mouth flora associated with dental infections and anaerobic lung infections. F. nucleatum is associated with jugular vein septic phlebitis and GI cancer. Resembles Capnophagia sp. on sputum Gram stain.
Prevotella (*Bacteroides*) *bivia*	• CSF = NP • Blood = P (from dental, lung, pelvic source) • Sputum = P (lung abscess)	Penicillin (IV/ PO) Any β-lactam (IV/PO)	Any quinolone (IV/PO) Doxycycline (IV/PO) Clindamycin (IV/PO)	Cause of dental, oropharyngeal, and female genital tract infections.

	• Urine = NP • Stool = NP • Wound = NP			
Prevotella (Bacteroides) melaninogenicus, intermedius	• CSF = P (brain abscess) • Blood = P (from oral/pulmonary source) • Sputum = P (from aspiration pneumonia, lung abscess) • Urine = NP • Stool = NP • Wound = NP	Aspiration pneumonia/lung abscess Any β-lactam (IV/PO) Any quinolone (IV/PO) Brain abscess Penicillin (IV) Ceftriaxone (IV)	Aspiration pneumonia/lung abscess Doxycycline (IV/PO) Brain abscess Chloramphenicol (IV)	Predominant anaerobic flora of mouth. Known as "oral pigmented" Bacteroides (e.g., B. melanogenicus). Antibiotics used to treat community acquired pneumonia are effective against oral anaerobes (e.g., Prevotella) in aspiration pneumonia; does not require anti-B. fragilis coverage with clindamycin, metronidazole, or moxifloxacin.

C = colonizer; C* = skin contaminant; NP = non-pathogen at site; P = pathogen at site; (IV/PO) = IV or PO. See p. xi for all other abbreviations.

Table 3.9 Clinical Significance of YEAST/FUNGI Pending Susceptibility Testing

| | | | YEAST/FUNGI | |
Isolate	**Usual Isolate Significance	Preferred Therapy	Alternate Therapy	Comments
Aspergillus species	• CSF = P (only from disseminated infection) • Blood = C, P (1° fungemia or from pulmonary source) • Sputum = C, P (pneumonia) • Urine = NP • Stool = NP • Wound = NP, P (rarely, but possible with extensive wounds, e.g., burns)	Isovuconazole (IV/PO) Liposomal amphotericin (IV) Voriconazole (IV/PO)	Posaconazole (IV/PO); Amphotericin B deoxycholate (IV)	A. fumigatus is the usual cause of invasive aspergillosis. Growth of Aspergillus sp. from a specimen can represent airborne contamination. Aspergillus pneumonia and disseminated aspergillosis are not uncommon in patients on chronic steroids or immuno-suppressives (esp. organ transplants). Recovery of Aspergillus from sputum or BAL is not diagnostic of Aspergillus pneumonia. Definitive Dx is by lung biopsy demonstrating vessel/tissue invasion. β 1,3 D-glucan (BG)+, aspergillus galactomannan (GM)+.
Candida albicans	• CSF = P (only from disseminated infection) • Blood = P (1° candidemia or from IV line infection) • Sputum = C	Fluconazole (IV/PO) Micafungin (IV) Caspofungin (IV) Posaconazole (IV/PO) Itraconazole (IV/PO)	Liposomal amphotericin (IV) Isovuconazole (IV/PO) Voriconazole (IV/PO) Anidulafungin (IV)	Common colonizer of GI/GU tracts. Colonization common in diabetics, alcoholics, patients receiving steroids/antibiotics. Commonest cause of fungemia in hospitalized patients. Candidemia secondary to central IV lines should always be treated as possible disseminated disease even though this is not invariably the case. Repeated blood cultures and careful follow-up (including

	• Urine = C, P (from cystitis, pyelonephritis) • Stool = C (source of candiduria) • Wound = NP			ophthalmoscopy) should be undertaken to exclude possible occult dissemination following even a single positive blood culture. Colonization of airways is common, but there is no candidal pneumonia.
Candida non-albicans	• CSF = P (only from disseminated infection) • Blood = P (1° candidemia or from IV line infection) • Sputum = NP • Urine = C (indwelling catheters), P (from cystitis, pyelonephritis) • Stool = C (source of candiduria) • Wound = NF	Micafungin (IV) Isovuconazole (IV/PO) Posaconazole (IV/PO) Voriconazole (IV/PO) Itraconazole (IV/PO) Caspofungin (IV)	Fluconazole (IV/PO) Liposomal amphotericin (IV) Anidulafungin (IV)	Non-albicans Candida cause the same spectrum of invasive disease as C. albicans. Fluconazole susceptibility varies by species. Dose dependent susceptibility with some species eg. C. krusei (almost always) are resistant to fluconazole. C. lusitaniae is often resistant to amphotericin B (deoxycholate and lipid formulations). Other species are generally susceptible to all agents.
Cryptococcus neoformans, gatti	• CSF = P (meningitis, brain abscess) • Blood = P (from pulmonary source) • Sputum = P (pneumonia) • Urine = NP • Stool = NP • Wound = NP*	CNS Liposomal amphotericin (IV) ± Flucytocine (PO) Non-CNS Isovuconazole (IV/PO)	CNS Fluconazole (IV/PO) Non-CNS Itraconazole (IV/PO) Fluconazole (IV/PO)	C. neoformans meningitis may occur with or without dissemination. Cryptococcal pneumonia frequently disseminates to CNS. C. neoformans in blood cultures occurs in compromised hosts (e.g, HIV) and indicates disseminated infection.

C = colonizer; C* = skin contaminant; NP = non-pathogen at site; P = pathogen at site; (IV/PO) = IV or PO. See p. xi for all other abbreviations.
* Cutaneous cryptococcus represents disseminated infection. ** Fungi can produce disseminated infections that involve essentially any organ. Isolation of a fungus from any normal sterile site should be cause for a careful review of the patient's epidemiology, risk factors, and clinical presentation.

Table 3.9 Usual Clinical Significance of YEAST/FUNGI Pending Susceptibility Testing (cont'd)

		YEAST/FUNGI		
Isolate	****Usual Isolate Significance**	**Preferred Therapy**	**Alternate Therapy**	**Comments**
Histoplasma capsulatum	• CSF = P (from disseminated infection, pneumonia) • Blood = P (1° fungemia, rarely SBE) • Sputum = P (pneumonia, mediastinitis) • Urine = P • Stool = P • Wound = P	Isavuconazole (IV/PO) Itraconazole (IV/PO) Liposomal amphotericin (IV)	Fluconazole (IV/PO) Amphotericin B (IV)	Histoplasma recovered from CSF/blood cultures indicates dissemination. Disseminated (reactivated latent) histoplasmosis is most common in compromised hosts (e.g., HIV). Itraconazole is ineffective for meningeal histoplasmosis, but is preferred for chronic suppressive therapy.
Malassezia furfur	• CSF = NP • Blood = P (from IV line infection) • Sputum = NP • Urine = NP • Stool = NP • Wound = P (eosinophilic folliculitis)	Itraconazole (IV/PO) Ketoconazole (PO)	Fluconazole (IV/PO)	M. furfur IV line infections are associated with IV lipid hyperalimentation emulsions. Fungemia usually resolves with IV line removal. Morphology in blood is blunt buds on a broad base yeast. M. furfur requires long chain fatty acids for growth (overlay agar with thin layer of olive oil, Tween 80, or oleic acid).

| Penicillium marneffei | • CSF = NP
• Blood = P (usually from dissemination)
• Sputum = P (pneumonia)
• Urine = NP
• Stool = NP
• Wound = NP* | Liposomal amphotericin (IV)
Itraconazole (IV/PO) | Amphotericin B (IV) | Histoplasma-like yeast forms seen in lymph nodes, liver, skin, bone marrow, blood. Characteristic red pigment diffuses into agar. Closely resembles histoplasmosis yeast forms (H. capsulatum has narrow based budding yeast forms, but P. marneffei has transverse septa). Skin lesions indicate dissemination. May resemble molluscum contagiosum. Hepatosplenomegaly is common. |

C = colonizer; C* = skin contaminant; NP = non-pathogen at site; P = pathogen at site; (IV/PO) = IV or PO. See p. xi for all other abbreviations.

* Cutaneous lesions represents disseminated infection.

** Fungi can produce disseminated infections that involve essentially any organ. Isolation of a fungus from any normal sterile site should be cause for a careful review of the patient's epidemiology, risk factors, and clinical presentation.

Table 3.10 Antibiotic Mechanisms of Action and Resistance

Antibiotic	Mechanism of Action	Mechanism of Resistance
β-lactams (penicillins, cephalosporins, monobactams, carbapenems)	• *Inhibits cell wall synthesis* • Disrupts peptidoglycan cell wall cross-linking	• β-lactam inactivation • Altered PBPs • Reduced porin diffusion
Glycopeptides (teichoplanin, vancomycin, dalbavancin, oritavancin)	• *Inhibits cell wall synthesis* • Blocks glycosyltransferases	• Increased D-Ala-D-Ala target binding
Aminoglycosides (gentamicin, tobramycin, amlkacin)	• *Inhibits protein synthesis* • Binds to 30S ribosomal subunit of the 70S ribosome • Blocks peptide translocation	• Drug modifying (acetylating, adenylating, phosphorylating) enzymes • Efflux pumps
Quinolones (ciprofloxacin, levofloxacin, moxiflocacin)	• *Inhibits DNA synthesis* • Inhibits DNA gyrase and topoisomerase IV	• Altered binding targets • Efflux pumps
Tetracyclines (tetracycline, doxycycline, minocycline)	• *Inhibits protein synthesis* • Binds to 30S ribosomal subunit of the 70S ribosome	• Efflux pumps
Tigecycline	• *Inhibits protein synthesis* • Binds to 30S ribosomal subunit of the 70S ribosome	• Efflux pumps (distinct from tetracyclines)
Macrolides (erythromycin, clarithromycin, azithromycin)	• *Inhibits protein synthesis* • Binds to 50S ribosomal subunit of the 70S ribosome	• Methylation of ribosomal binding sites • Efflux pumps
Streptogramins (quinupristin dalfopristin)	• *Inhibits protein synthesis* • Binds to 50S ribosomal subunit of the 70S ribosome	• Efflux pumps • Methylation of ribosomal binding sites

Table 3.10 Antibiotic Mechanisms of Action and Resistance *(cont'd)*

Antibiotic	Mechanism of Action	Mechanism of Resistance
Oxazolidinones (linezolid, tedizolid)	• *Inhibits protein synthesis* • Binds to 50S ribosomal subunit of the 70S ribosome	• Methylation of ribosomal binding sites
Daptomycin	• *Inhibits cell wall synthesis*	• Reduced drug binding to cell membrane
Sulfonamides (SMX) (sulfamethoxazole)	• *Inhibits dihydropteroate synthesis* • Inhibits dihydrofolate reductase	• Dihydrofolate synthetase resistance
Trimethoprim (TMP)	• *Inhibits folate synthesis* • Inhibits dihydrofolate reductase	• Dihydrofolate reductase resistance
Metronidazole	• *Inhibits nucleic acid synthesis* • Disrupts DNA	• Altered drug activating enzyme • Efflux pumps
Chloramphenicol	• *Inhibits protein synthesis* • Binds to 50S ribosomal subunit of the 70S ribosome	• Drug modifying enzymes (chloramphenicol acetyltransferase)
Polymyxins (polymyxin B, colisin)	• *Disrupts cell membranes*	• Altered cell membrane with reduced drug binding
Nitrofurantoin	• *Inhibits NADH/NADPH reductases* in Kreb's cycle at 3 locations	• Altered drug activating enzymes
Fosfomycin	• *Inhibits cell wall synthesis* • Blocks peptide linkages	• Drug modifying enzymes

Table 3.11 Empiric Antibiotic Therapy of Selected Problem Pathogens
(Preferred and Alternate Therapy choices are NOT listed in any preferential order)

Potential Problem Pathogens	Preferred Therapy	Alternate Therapy

MRSA	Tigecycline
	Minocycline
	Ceftaroline
	Quinupristin/Dalfopristin
	Linezolid
	Daptomycin
	Vancomycin
	Eravacycline
		Clindamycin[mt]
		  (CA-MRSA)
		Doxycycline[mt]
		  (CA-MRSA)
		TMP-SMX[mt]
		  (CA-MRSA)
		Delafloxacin
		Omadacycline

VSE	Ampicillin Piperacillin/Tazobactam Meropenem Tigecycline Linezolid Daptomycin Moxifloxacin Fosfomycin* Nitrofurantoin*	Vancomycin (with gentamicin) Levofloxacin Delafloxacin Eravacycline Omadacycline Fosfomycin* Nitrofurantoin*
VRE	Tigecycline Minocycline Quinupristin/Dalfopristin Daptomycin Linezolid Eravacycline	Chloramphenicol Delafloxacin Fosfomycin Nitrofurantoin*
Klebsiella	Meropenem Cefepime Amikacin Aztreonam Tigecycline Aztreonam/Avibactam Cefiderocol	Levofloxacin Moxifloxacin Delafloxacin Polymyxin B Colistin Fosfomycin Nitrofurantoin*
Enterobacter	3rd generation cephalosporins TMP-SMX Cefepime Meropenem Tigecycline Ceftazidime/Avibactam Ceftolozane/Tazobactam Meropenem/Vaborbactam Aztreonam/Avibactam Fosfomycin Nitrofurantoin* Cefiderocol	Aztreonam 2nd generation cephalosporins[m] Ticarcillin/Clavulanate[m] Piperacillin/Tazobactam[m] Levofloxacin Moxifloxacin Delafloxacin Gentamicin Tobramycin Amikacin Plazomicin Colistin Polymyxin B

Table 3.11 Empiric Antibiotic Therapy of Selected Problem Pathogens *(cont'd)*

Potential Problem Pathogens	Preferred Therapy	Alternate Therapy
Serratia	3rd generation cephalosporins Cefepime TMP-SMX Meropenem Aminoglycosides Aztreonam Polymyxin B Colistin Tigecycline Ceftazidime/Avibactam Ceftolozane/Tazobactam Cefiderocol	2nd generation cephalosporins Piperacillin/Tazobactam[m] Levofloxacin Moxifloxacin Delafloxacin Plazomicin Aztreonam/Avibactam Fosfomycin
P. aeruginosa (meropenem susceptible)	Meropenem Levofloxacin Delafloxacin Polymyxin B Colistin	Gentamicin[m] Tobramycin[m] Amikacin Piperacillin/Tazobactam[m] Cefoperazone Doxycycline* Doripenem Ciprofloxacin Fosfomycin
P. aeruginosa (meropenem resistant)	Fosfomycin Cefiderocol Amikacin Ceftazidime/Avibactam Ceftolozane/Tazobactam Meropenem/Vaborbactam Imipenem/Relebactam	Colistin Doripenem Polymyxin B
CRE*	Tigecycline Cefiderocol Ceftazidime/Avibactam Meropenem/Vaborbactam Imipenem/Relebactam Aztreonam/Avibactam	Polymyxin B, Colistin Aztreonam, Plazomicin Amikacin Minocycline Nitrofurantion* Fosfomycin
Acinetobacter	TMP-SMX Amikacin Minocycline Tigecycline Meropenem[m] Cefiderocol Ceftazidime/Avibactam Ceftolozane/Tazobactam Eravacycline Fosfomycin Meropenem/Vaborbactam Imipenem/Relebactam	Aztreonam[m] Gentamicin[m] Tobramycin[m] Plazomicin Ticarcillin/Clavulanate[m] Piperacillin/Tazobactam[m] Doxycycline Doripenem Omadacycline
S. maltophilia	TMP-SMX Minocycline Doxycycline Tigecycline Polymyxin B Colistin Fosfomycin Aztreonam/Avibactam Cefiderocol	Chloramphenicol Ticarcillin/Clavulanate[m] Piperacillin/Tazobactam[m] Levofloxacin Moxifloxacin Ceftolozane/Tazobactam Meropenem/Vaborbactam Imipenem/Relebactam

* See Table 3.12

Table 3.11 Empiric Antibiotic Therapy of Selected Problem Pathogens *(cont'd)*

Potential Problem Pathogens	Preferred Therapy	Alternate Therapy
B. cepacia[†]	Minocycline TMP-SMX Meropenem Cefepime Ceftazidime/Avibactam Ceftolozane/Tazobactam Meropenem/Vaborbactam Cefiderocol	Doxycycline Chloramphenicol Levofloxacin Ticarcillin/Clavulanate[m] Piperacillin/Tazobactam[m] Imipenem/Relebactam Fosfomycin
Listeria	Ampicillin Chloramphenicol TMP-SMX	Meropenem Linezolid
Nocardia	TMP-SMX Imipenem Doxycycline Minocycline	Meropenem Ceftriaxone Linezolid

* For acute uncomplicated cystitis (AUC) or catheter associated bacteriuria (CAB) only.
† Active against CA-MRSA, but usually ineffective against HA-MRSA or Co-MRSA strain.
m = only moderate activity

Table 3.12 CRE Carbapenemases

Carbapenemase	KPC	MBLs (NDM, VIM, IMP)	OXA-48
Ambler molecular class	A	B	D
Inhibited by classic β-lactamase inhibitors	–	–	–
Inhibited by avibactam	+	–	+
Inhibited by vaborbactam	+	–	–
Inhibited by relebactam	+	–	–

CLINICAL INTERPRETATION OF GRAM STAIN

Table 3.13 Clinical Use of CSF Gram Stain (see Color Atlas of CSF Gram stains)

Gram Stain	Organism	Comments
Gram positive bacilli	Bacillus, Corynebacteria (Pseudomeningitis)	Listeria monocytogenes
Gram negative bacilli	H. influenzae (small, pleomorphic) ± encapsulated	Enteric aerobic bacilli (larger, unencapsulated)

Table 3.13 Clinical Use of CSF Gram Stain *(cont'd)*

Gram Stain	Organism	Comments
Gram positive cocci	Gp B streptococci (pairs/chains) S. pneumoniae (lancet shaped diplococci)	S. aureus (pairs/clusters)* S. epidermidis (pairs/clusters)†
Gram negative diplococci	Neisseria meningitidis	Coffee bean shaped

* Secondary to MSSA/MRSA ABE or CNS shunt infection/EVD.

† Secondary to skin contaminant during LP or CNS shunt infection/EVD.

Table 3.14 Clinical Use of the Sputum Gram Stain (see Color Atlas of Sputum Gram stains)

Gram Stain	Organism	Comments
Gram positive diplococci	S. pneumoniae	Lancet shaped encapsulated diplococci (not streptococci)
Gram positive cocci (grape-like clusters)	S. aureus (MSSA/MRSA)	Clusters predominant. Short chains or pairs may also be present*
Gram positive cocci (short chains or pairs)	Group A streptococci (GAS)	Virulence inversely proportional to length of streptococci. Clusters not present
Gram positive beaded/ filamentous branching organisms	Nocardia	Coccobacillary forms common coccobacilli
Gram negative cocco-bacillary organisms	H. influenzae	Pleomorphic may be encapsulated. Gram negative. Lightly stained
Gram negative bacilli	Klebsiella P. aeruginosa	Plump and encapsulated Thin and unencapsulated. Often arranged in end-to-end pairs
Gram negative diplococci	Moraxella (Branhamella) catarrhalis Neisseria meningitidis	Coffee bean shaped

* Common colonizer of respiratory secretions in ventilated patients. With high spiking fevers, hemoptysis, hypotension, rapid cavitation on CXR represents MSSA/MRSA CAP (not VAP) in adults with simultaneous influenza A CAP.

Table 3.15 Clinical Use of the Urine Gram Stain (see Color Atlas of Urine Gram stains)

Gram Stain	Organism	Comments
Gram positive cocci (clusters)*	S. aureus (MSSA/MRSA)	Skin flora contaminant
	S. epidermidis (CoNS)	Skin flora contaminant
	S. saprophyticus	Uropathogen
Gram positive cocci (chains)	Group B streptococci (GBS)	Uropathogen
	Group D streptococci E. faecalis (VSE) E. faecium (VRE)	Uropathogen; may represent colonization (with minimal pyuria)
Gram negative bacilli*	Coliform bacilli	Uropathogen; may represent colonization (with minimal/moderate pyuria)
Gram negative diplococci*	N. gonorrhoeae	Gonococcal urethritis
	N. meningitidis	Rare cause of urethritis

* Staphylococci (except S. saprophyticus), S. pneumoniae, and B. fragilis are not uropathogens.

REFERENCES

Anaissie EJ, McGinnis MR, Pfaller MA (eds). Clinical Mycology. Churchill Livingstone, New York, 2003.

Bennett JE, Dolin R, Blaser MJ (eds). Mandell, Douglas, and Bennett's Principles and Practice of infectious Diseases (9th Ed), Elsevier Churchill Livingstone, New York, London, 2019.

Bottone EJ (ed). An Atlas of the Clinical Microbiology of Infectious Diseases, Volume 1. Bacterial Agents. The Parthenon Publishing Group, Boca Raton, 2004.

Bottone EJ (ed). An Atlas of the Clinical Microbiology of Infectious Diseases, Volume 2. Viral, fungal, and parasitic agents. Taylor and Francis, New York, London, 2006.

Bowden RA, Ljungman P, Snydman DR (eds). Transplant Infections (3rd Ed), Lippincott Williams & Wilkins, Philadelphia, PA, 2010.

Bryskier A (ed). Antimicrobial Agents. ASM Press, Washington, D.C., 2005.

Cohen J, Powderly WG, Opal S (Eds). Infectious Diseases (4th Ed). Elsevier, Philadelphia, 2016.

de la Maza LM, Pezzlo MT, Shigei JT, et al. (eds). Color Atlas of Medical Bacteriology. ASM Press, Washington, D.C., 2004.

Forbes BA, Sahm DF, Weissfeld AS, et al. (eds). Bailey & Scott's Diagnostic Microbiology (12th Ed), St. Louis, Mosby, 2007.

Gorbach SL, Bartlett JG, Blacklow NR (eds). Infectious Diseases (3rd Ed), Philadelphia, Lippincott, Williams & Wilkins, 2004.

Grayson ML (ed). Kucers' The Use of Antibiotics (6th Ed), ASM Press, Washington, DC, 2010.

Janda JM, Abbott SL (eds). The Enterobacteria (2nd Ed), ASM Press, Washington, D.C., 2006.

Koneman EW, Allen SD, Janda WM, et al. (eds). Color Atlas and Textbook of Diagnostic Microbiology (5th Ed), Lippincott-Raven Publishers, Philadelphia, 1997.

Lorian V (ed). Antibiotics in Laboratory Medicine (5th Ed), Lippincott Williams & Wilkins, Philadelphia, 2005.

Madigan MT, Martinko JM, Parker J (eds). Brock Biology of Microorganisms (10th Ed), Prentice Hall, Upper Saddle River, NJ, 2003.

Scholar EM Pratt WB (eds). The Antimicrobial Drugs (2nd Ed), Oxford University Press, New York, 2000.

Versalovic J, Carroll KC, Funke G, et al. (eds). Manual of Clinical Microbiology (10th Ed), Washington, DC, ASM Press, 2011.

Chapter 4

Parasites, Fungi, Unusual Organisms

Kenneth F. Wagner, DO, James H. McGuire, MD,
Burke A. Cunha, MD, Jean E. Hage, MD,
John H. Rex, MD, Rodger P. Silletti, PhD, Edward J. Bottone, PhD

Parasites, Fungi, Unusual Organisms in Blood

Microfilaria in Blood

Subset	Pathogen	Preferred Therapy	Alternate Therapy
Filariasis	Brugia malayi	Doxycycline 100 mg (PO) of q12h × 6 weeks **plus** Diethylcarbamazine: day 1: 50 mg (PO) day 2: 50 mg (PO) q8h day 3: 100 mg (PO) q8h days 4–14: 2 mg/kg (PO) q8h	Ivermectin 200 mcg/kg (PO) × 1 dose ± Albendazole 400 mg (PO) × 1 dose
	Wuchereria bancrofti	Doxycycline 100 mg (PO) q12h × 6 weeks **plus** Albendazole 400 mg (PO) × 1 dose **plus** Diethylcarbamazine: day 1: 50 mg (PO) day 2: 50 mg (PO) q8h day 3: 100 mg (PO) q8h days 4–14: 2 mg/kg (PO) q8h	Ivermectin 400 mcg/kg (PO) × 1 dose.
Loa Loa (Loiasis)	L. loa	Diethylcarbamazine 2 mg/kg (PO) q8h × 3 weeks	Albendazole 200 mg (PO) q12h × 3 weeks

Brugia malayi

Clinical Presentation: May present as an obscure febrile illness, chronic lymphedema, lymphangitis, or cutaneous abscess. "Filarial fevers" usually last 1 week and spontaneously remit.

Diagnostic Considerations: Diagnosis by demonstrating microfilaria on Giemsa's stained thick blood smear or by using the concentration method; yield is increased by passing blood through a Millipore filter before staining. Several smears should be taken over 24 hours. Adult worms may be detected in scrotal lymphatics by ultrasound. Common infection in Southeast Asia (primarily China, Korea, India, Indonesia, Malaysia, Philippines, Sri Lanka). Most species have nocturnal periodicity (microfilaria in blood at night). Eosinophilia is most common during periods of acute inflammation.

Pitfalls: Genital manifestations—scrotal edema, epididymitis, orchitis, hydrocele—are frequent with W. bancrofti, but rare with B. malayi.

Prognosis: Related to state of health and extent of lymphatic obstruction. No satisfactory treatment is available. Single-dose ivermectin is effective treatment for microfilaremia, but does not kill the adult worm (although diethylcarbamazine kills some). If no microfilaria in blood, full-dose diethylcarbamazine (2 mg/kg q8h) can be started on day one. Antihistamines or corticosteroids may decrease allergic reactions from disintegration of microfilaria.

Wuchereria bancrofti

Clinical Presentation: May present as an obscure febrile illness, chronic lymphedema, lymphangitis, or cutaneous abscess. Genital (scrotal) lymphatic edema, groin lesions, epididymitis, orchitis, hydroceles are characteristic. Chyluria may occur. "Filarial fevers" usually last 1 week and spontaneously remit. Lymphedema worsened by cellulitis associated with Tinea pedis infections.

Diagnostic Considerations: Diagnosis by demonstrating microfilaria on Giemsa's stained thick blood smear or by using the concentration method; yield is increased by passing blood through a Millipore filter before staining. Several smears should to be taken over 24 hours. W. bancrofti is the most common human filarial infection, particularly in Asia (China, India, Indonesia, Japan, Malaysia, Philippines), Southeast Asia, Sri Lanka, Tropical Africa, Central/South America, and Pacific Islands. Most species have nocturnal periodicity (microfilaria in blood at night). Eosinophilia is common.

Pitfalls: Differentiate from "hanging groins" of Loa Loa, which usually do not involve the scrotum.

Prognosis: Related to state of health and extent of lymphatic obstruction. No satisfactory treatment is available. Single-dose ivermectin is effective treatment for microfilaremia, but does not kill the adult worm (although diethylcarbamazine kills some). If no microfilaria in blood, full-dose diethylcarbamazine (2 mg/kg q8h) can be started on day one. Antihistamines or corticosteroids decrease allergic reactions from disintegration of microfilaria. Wolbachia bacteria are endosymbionts in W. bancrofti filariasis. Treatment with doxycycline effective against Wolbachia which are important in microfilarial reproduction.

Loa Loa (Loiasis)

Clinical Presentation: Cutaneous swellings (Calabar swellings) with pruritus. Adults may be visible when migrations under the conjuctiva or under the skin. Disappear in 3 days. Calabar swellings are painless and appear on the extremities. Eosinophilia prominent.

Diagnostic Considerations: Demonstrates of microfilariae in blood (at noon) or by demonstration of L. loa in skin/eye. Immunodiagnosis unhelpful.

Pitfalls: Calabar swellings occur one at time and may last for hours/days.

Prognosis: Poorest with CNS involvement.

Trypanosomes in Blood

Subset	Pathogen	Preferred Therapy	Alternate Therapy
Chagas' disease (American trypanosomiasis)	Trypanosoma cruzi	Nifurtimox 2–3 mg/kg/day (PO) q6h × 30–90 days	Benznidazole 2.5–3.5 mg/kg (PO) q12h × 60 days
Sleeping sickness West African (Gambian) trypanosomiasis	Trypanosoma brucei gambiense	Early disease (hemolymphatic stage) Pentamidine 4 mg/kg (IM) q24h × 7 days	Suramin 1 gm (IV) on days 1, 3, 7, 14 and 21*

Trypanosomes in Blood (cont'd)

Subset	Pathogen	Preferred Therapy	Alternate Therapy
		Late disease (CNS involvement) Eflornithine 400 mg/kg/day (IV) in 4 divided doses × 14 days	Eflornithine 400 mg/kg/day (IV) in 2 divided doses × 7 days *plus* Nifurtimox 15 mg/kg/day (PO) in 3 divided doses × 10 days
Sleeping sickness East African (Rhodesian) trypanosomiasis	Trypanosoma brucei, rhodesiense	Early disease (hemolymphatic stage) Suramin 1 gm on days 1, 3, 7, 14, and 21)*	Pentamidine 4 mg/kg/day (IM/IV) q24h × 7–10 days
		Late disease (CNS involvement) Melarsoprol 2-3-6 mg/kg/day (IV) × 3 days. After 7 days, 3.6 mg/kg/day × 3 days. Repeat 3 series 3.6 mg/kg/day (IV) × 3 days after 7 days.†	

* 100 mg test dose should be given before first dose and monitored for hypotension.

† Steroids may be given to prevent melarsoprol encephalopathy.

Chagas' Disease (Trypanosoma cruzi) American Trypanosomiasis

Clinical Presentation: Presents acutely after bite of infected reduviid (triatoma) bug with unilateral painless periorbital edema (Romaña's sign), or as an indurated area of erythema and swelling with local lymph node involvement (chagoma). Fever, malaise, and edema of the face and lower extremities may follow. Generalized lymphadenopathy and hepatosplenomegaly occur. Patients with chronic disease may develop cardiac involvement (cardiomyopathy with arrhythmias, heart block, heart failure, thromboembolism), GI involvement (megaesophagus, megaduodenum, megacolon) or CNS involvment in HIV/immunosuppressed.

Diagnostic Considerations: Common in Central and South America. Acquired from infected reduviid (triatoma) bug. Transmitted by blood transfusion (~10%), organ transplants, and congenitally. Diagnosis in acute disease by detecting trypanosomes in wet prep of anticoagulated blood or stained buffy coat smears. T. cruzi has largest kinetoplast of all trypanosomes. Resembles histoplasma in bone marrow biopsies, but no kinetoplasts in histoplasma. Amastigote forms present intracellularly in monocytes/histiocytes in Giemsa-stained smears, bone marrow or lymph node aspirates, or xenodiagnosis. Diagnostic tests ELISA, IFA or chemoluminescence immunoassay (CHLIA).

Pitfalls: Do not overlook chronic Chagas' disease in patients from endemic areas with heart block ± apical ventricular aneurysms. May be transmitted by blood transfusion/organ transplantation.

Prognosis: Related to extent of cardiac GI, or CNS involvement.

Sleeping Sickness (T. brucei gambiense/rhodesiense) West African (Gambian)/East African (Rhodesian) Trypanosomiasis

Clinical Presentation: Sleeping sickness from T. brucei gambiense is milder than sleeping sickness from T. brucei rhodesiense, which is usually a fulminant infection. A few days to weeks after bite of tsetse fly, patients progress through several clinical stages:

- *Chancre stage*: Trypanosomal chancre occurs at bite site and lasts several weeks.
- *Hemolymhatic stage (early)*: Blood parasitemia is associated with intermittent high fevers, headaches and insomnia, followed by generalized adenopathy. Posterior cervical lymph node enlargement (Winterbottom's sign) is particularly prominent with T. brucei gambiense. Hepatosplenomegaly and transient edema/pruritus/irregular circinate rash are common. Myocarditis (tachycardia unrelated to fevers) occurs early (before CNS involvement) and is responsible for acute deaths from T. brucei rhodesiense.
- *CNS stage (late)*: Occurs acutely with East African trypanosomiasis or chronically with West African trypanosomiasis after non-specific symptoms, and is characterized by increasing lethargy, somnolence (sleeping sickness), and many subtle CNS findings. Coma and death ensue without treatment. With melarsoprol, use prednisolone 1 mg/kg (PO) q24h (start steroid 1 day prior to first dose and continue to last dose).

Diagnostic Considerations: Diagnosis by demonstrating trypanosomes in blood, chancre, or lymph nodes aspirates by Giemsa stained thin and thick preparations, light microscopy, or buffy coat concentrates with acridine orange. CSF determines early vs. late stage disease (> 20 WBCs/ml).

Pitfalls: Do not overlook other causes of prominent bilateral posterior cervical lymph node enlargement, e.g., lymphoma, EBV. Serum arginase is a biomarker for effective therapy.

Prognosis: Related to extent of cardiac/CNS involvement. Relapse may occur, and may be treated with a 7 day course of eflornithine.

Spirochetes in Blood

Subset	Pathogen	Preferred Therapy	Alternate Therapy
Lyme disease	B. burgdorferi	Ceftriaxone 1 gm (IV) q24h × 2 weeks **or** Doxycycline 200 mg (IV) q12h × 3 days, then 100 mg (IV) q12h × 4 weeks	
Borrelia miyamotoi disease (BMD)	B. miyamotoi	Ceftriaxone 1 gm (IV) q24h × 2 weeks **or** Doxycycline 200 mg (IV) q12h × 3 days, then 100 mg (IV) q12h × 4 weeks	

Spirochetes in Blood *(cont'd)*

Subset	Pathogen	Preferred Therapy	Alternate Therapy
Relapsing fever Louse-borne (LBRF) Tick-borne (TBRF)	Borrelia recurrentis	<u>LBRF</u> Erythromycin 500 mg (PO) × 1 day	<u>LBRF</u> Doxycycline 100 mg (PO) × 1 day
	> 15 Borrelia species (U.S.: B. hermsii; Africa: B. duttonii; Africa/Middle East: B. crocidurae)	<u>TBRF</u> Doxycycline 200 mg (PO) × 3 days, then 100 mg (PO) q12h × 7 days	<u>TBRF with CNS involvement</u> Ceftriaxone 1 gm (IV) q12h × 2 weeks
Rat bite fever	Streptobacillus moniliformis*	Penicillin G 4 mu (IV) q4h × 2 weeks **or** Ceftriaxone 1 g (IV) q24h × 2 weeks	Amoxicillin 1 gm (PO) q8h × 2 weeks **or** Doxycycline 100 mg (PO) q12h × 2 weeks
	Spirillum minus	**or** Doxycycline 200 mg (IV) q12h × 3 days, then 100 mg (IV) q12h × 11 days	

*S. moniliformis SBE treated with penicillin (4 weeks) + gentamicin (2 weeks)

Lyme Disease (Borrelia burgdorferi)

Clinical Presentation: Erythema migrans (EM), annular lesion with central clearing occurs in ~ 75% within 2 weeks of tick bite. Patients appear relatively well with low-grade fevers, headache, arthralgias/myalgias, meningismus. Other manifestations include aseptic meningitis, Bell's palsy, peripheral neuropathy, adenopathy (localized/generalized), or acute heart block, mild ↑ AST/ALT. Lyme disease may present with unilateral large joint arthritis.

Diagnostic Considerations: If present, EM rash is diagnostic and IgM Lyme titers are unnecessary. Serologic diagnosis is by elevated IgM ELISA titers. IgM titers may take 4–6 weeks to become elevated. ↑ IgM titers usually return to normal in 6–9 months, but in some may persist for > 1 year. If IgM ELISA Lyme titer is borderline or suspected as false-positive, obtain an IgM Western Blot (WB). IgM ELISA XR is common with EBV, CMV. If false positive suspected, retest for IgM and IgG ELISA or WB 4 weeks later (false + IgM titers ELISA revert to negative). An equivocal or + ELISA followed by – WB should be considered as –. An equivocal or + ELISA followed by + WB should be considered as +. IgM WB is considered positive if ≥ 2 bands are present (23, 39, 41). An IgM WB is – if < 2 bands listed are present or if other bands are present (not 23, 39, 41). IgG WB is considered as + if any 5 of the following bands are present (18, 23, 28, 30, 39, 41, 45, 58, 66, 93). IgG WB is considered – if no bands are present or if bands other than those listed are present.

Pitfalls: Rash is not always present. Tick bite often goes unnoticed (tick often spontaneously falls off after 1–2 days of feeding). Consider Lyme disease in patients with sudden unexplained acute heart block in areas where Ixodes ticks endemic.

Therapeutic Considerations: B. burgdorferi is highly susceptible to beta-lactams. Highest failure rates with macrolides. For Bell's palsy or neuroborreliosis minocycline may be preferred to doxycycline. Symptoms may persist for 1 year after effective therapy. No rationale to re-treat with antibiotics for post-treatment Lyme disease symptoms (PTLDS). PTLDS patients are not functionally impaired.

Prognosis: Excellent in normal hosts.

Borrelia Miyamotoi Disease (BMD)

Clinical Presentation: B. miyamotoi is transmitted by deer ticks (Ixodes dammini/Ixodes scapularis). Presents acutely with high fevers, chills, severe headache, arthralgias, myalgias, and fatigue. BMD patients appear acutely ill and may appear septic. With BMD, leukopenia, thrombocytopenia, and mild ↑ AST/ALT are usual. Severe headache (no nuchal rigidity) may prompt LP (CSF normal).

Diagnostic Considerations: BMD presents as an ILI or may resemble ehrlichiosis/anaplasmosis. Diagnosis of B. miyamotoi by PCR or elevated IgM titers. Rule out ehrlichiosis/anaplasmosis by IgM titers or PCR. Unlike ehrlichiosis/anaplasmosis with BMD no atypical lymphocytes or morula in neutrophils (HGA). Rash effectively rules out BMD.

Pitfalls: Doesn't resemble Lyme disease even though caused by Borrelia and transmitted by the same tick (Ixodes) vector. Lyme disease co-infection in some. Clinically, most closely resembles ehrlichiosis/anaplasmosis but fevers of shorter duration and unlike ehrlichiosis/anaplasmosis, BMD does not persist beyond the acute presentation. Residual fatigue common.

Therapeutic Considerations: Early empiric doxycycline effective.

Prognosis: Good. A few have recurrent fevers, but no chronic infection.

Relapsing Fever, Louse-borne (LBRF)/Tick-borne (TBRF)

Clinical Presentation: Abrupt onset of "flu-like" illness with high fever, rigors, headache, myalgias, arthralgias, tachycardia, dry cough, abdominal pain after exposure to infected louse or tick. Truncal petechial rash and conjunctival suffusion common. Hepatosplenomegaly (LBRF > TBRF). Bleeding or rash at bite site. ARDS in some with TBRF. Fevers last ~ 1 week, remit for a week, and usually relapse only once in LBRF, but several times in TBRF. Relapses usually last 2–3 days.

Diagnostic Considerations: Borrelia seen in Wright/Giemsa-stained blood smears. LBRF is endemic in South American Andes, Central and East Africa. Soft ticks (Ornithodoros) TBRF main vector. Ticks bite at night, patients do not recall painless tick bite. TBRF is seen throughout the world. With TBRF, meningismus ± facial nerve palsy common with B. duttoni, but rare with B. hermsii.

Pitfalls: Spirochetes are most likely to be seen during febrile periods. Blood smears may be negative if not obtained during fever.

Prognosis: Jarisch-Herxheimer in some LBRF > TBRF within 2 hours after antibiotic therapy. Good if treated early. Usually no permanent sequelae.

Rat Bite Fever (Streptobacillus moniliformis)

Clinical Presentation: Streptobacillus moniliformis is the most common cause of RBF. Abrupt onset of fever, rash and polyarthritis (classic triad), with severe chills. Mono-articular or polyarticular arthritis affects small and large joints (knees). Sore throat, N/V in some. Rat bite site, not indurated, doesn't ulcerate and without regional adenopathy. Hemorrhagic bullae on extremities key diagnostic clue. Extremity rash (MP, petechial or purpuric) involves the palms and soles, but spares face/trunk. Rash desquamates in some.

Diagnostic Considerations: Gram stain of synovial fluid shows few pleomorphic GNB with lateral bulbar swellings in short chains. Blood or synovial fluid cultures diagnostic. Haverhill fever is caused by same organism when ingested (water, milk, meat) often with pharyngitis.

Pitfalls: Blood cultures usually negative in those with arthritis. S. moniliformis inhibited by sodium polyanethol sulfonate (SPS) in aerobic BC bottles. Use only anaerobic bottles for BC. For synovial fluid, culture on TSA enriched with blood/serum. BFP VDRL/RPR in some.

Prognosis: Spontaneous resolution of symptoms < 2 weeks. Serious complications include endocarditis, myocarditis, pericarditis as well as splenic, hepatic, or brain accesses. Some have slowly resolving rash, prolonged migratory arthralgias, and fatigue.

Rat Bite Fever (Spirillum minus)

Clinical Presentation: Infection develops 1–4 weeks following bite of a rat. Rat bite site red, painful, swollen and ulcerated with adenopathy. Fevers and chills, headache, and nausea/vomiting. Recurrent fevers occur in 2–4 days cyctes.

Diagnostic Considerations: Spirochetes are seen in Wright/Giemsa-stained blood smears. Differential diagnosis includes Borrelia recurrentis.

Pitfalls: Macular rash (red/brown) may resemble syphilis, (palms/soles) and BFP VDRL/RPR in 50%. SBE with moniliformis, not S. minus. Bite wound ulcerates with regional adenopathy in S. minus, not Streptobacillus moniliformis.

Prognosis: good.

Intracellular Inclusion Bodies in Blood

Subset	Pathogen	Preferred Therapy	Alternate Therapy
Babesiosis	Babesia microti	Azithromycin 500 mg (PO) × 1, then 250 mg (PO) q24h × 7 days **plus** Atovaquone (suspension) 750 mg (PO) q12h × 7 days	Clindamycin 600 mg (PO) q8h × 7 days **plus** Quinine 650 mg (PO) q8h × 7 days
Ehrlichiosis/ Anaplasmosis	Ehrlichia chaffeensis, ewingii Anaplasma phagocyto- philium	Doxycycline 200 mg (IV/PO) q12h × 3 days, then 100 mg (IV/PO) q12h × 1–2 weeks	Quinolone (IV/PO) q24h × 1–2 weeks **or** Rifampin 300 mg (PO) q12h × 1–2 weeks*

Subset	Therapy
Severe Malaria (Usually P. falciparum)	
	Artesunate 2 mg/kg (IV), then complete 3 days therapy plus **doxycycline** (clindamycin in pregnancy) **or mefloquine or Atovoquone – proguanil** (Malarone) **or** **Artemether-lumefantrine** (80 mg/480 mg) **plus Atovoquone – proguanil** (Malarone) at 0, 8, 24, 36, 48, 60 hours. (6 dose regimen) **or** **Quinine** 20 mg (salt)/kg (IV) over 4 hours (in D_5W), then 10 mg (salt)/kg (IV) over 2 hours q8h until able to take oral meds; complete 7 days total therapy with **doxycycline or oral regimen**.

* Quinidine no longer available in US.

Intracellular Inclusion Bodies in Blood *(cont'd)*

Uncomplicated Malaria (P. falciparum, P. malariae, P. knowlesi or unidentified species)	<u>*Chloroquine sensitive*</u> **Chloroquine phosphate (Aralen)** 600 mg (PO) immediately, followed by 300 mg at 6,24, and 48 hours. <div align="center">***plus***</div>**Tafenoquine** 300 mg (PO) q24h × 3 days <div align="center">**or**</div>**Primaquine phosphate** 30 mg (PO) q24h × 2 weeks. <div align="center">**or**</div>**Hydroxychloroquine (Plaquenil)** 620 mg (PO) then 310 mg (PO) at 6, 24, and 48 hours.
P. vivax and P. ovale	<u>*Chloroquine resistant*</u> **Quinine sulfate** 625 mg (PO) q8h × 7 days ***plus* Doxycycline** 200 mg (PO) q12h × 3 days, then 100 mg (PO) q12h × 4 days. <div align="center">**or**</div>**Atovaquone/proguanil (Malarone)** (250/100 mg tablets) 4 tablets (PO) q12h × 3 days. <div align="center">**or**</div>**Artesunate** 4 mg/kg (PO) × 3 days ***plus* Mefloquine (Larium)** 684 mg (PO) as initial dose followed by 456 mg (PO) given 6–12 hours after initial dose. <div align="center">**or**</div>**Artemether/lumefantrine (Coartem)** 4 tabs = 1 dose (20/120 mg tablets) give initial dose, followed by second dose 8h later, then 1 dose (PO) q12h for 2 days to complete 3 days of therapy. <div align="center">**or**</div>**Pyronaridine/artesunate** (180 mg/60 mg tablets) 1 tablet (PO) q6h × 3 days. <div align="center">**or**</div>**Dihydroartemisinin** 40 mg ***plus* Piperaquine** 320 mg (PO) q24h × 3 days.

For P. vivax single high dose tafenoquine 600 mg (PO) × 6 dose highly effective.

Babesiosis (Babesia microti)
Clinical Presentation: Tickborne "malaria-like illness" with malaise, fever, chills, relative bradycardia, myalgias, arthralgias, headache, abdominal pain, and splenomegaly. Laboratory abnormalities include hemolytic anemia, atypical lymphocytes, relative lymphopenia, thrombocytopenia, ↑ AST/ALT, ↑ AP, elevated ESR, ferritin, and LDH. Incubation periods: naturally acquired = 1–3 weeks; transfusion related = 6–9 weeks.

Diagnostic Considerations: Characteristic four merozoites (often pear shaped) arranged in "Maltese cross" formation (tetrads). Serology diagnostic of acute infection. Hyposplenic patients may have life-threatening infection.

Pitfalls: Co-infection with Lyme disease may occur. No serological cross-reactivity between Babesia and Borrelia (Lyme disease). Merozoites may be confused with P. falciparum malaria. Extracellular ring forms and absence of hemozoin pigment in ring forms distinguish babesiosis from malaria. Highly ↑ ferritin likely due to babesiosis (not HLH which is rare). False + CMV ↑ IgM titer may occur. Doxycycline ineffective.

Prognosis: May be more severe with Lyme disease co-infection. Severe/fatal if ↓/absent splenic function. Exchange transfusions may be life-saving.

Ehrlichiosis (HME)/Anaplasmosis (HGA)

Clinical Presentation: Acute febrile illness with chills, headache, malaise, myalgias, leukopenia, relative lymphopenia, atypical lymphocytes, thrombocytopenia, ↑ LFTs, ↓ ESR, ↑ ferritin. No vasculitis. Resembles Rocky Mountain spotted fever (RMSF), but without rash. HGA vector is Ixodes ticks clinical co-infection with B. burgdorferi (Lyme Disease) is rare, but may occur. Main HME vector Ambylomma americanum (lone star tick).

Diagnostic Considerations: Characteristic "morula" (spherical, basophilic, mulberry-shaped, cytoplasmic inclusion bodies) may be seen (20%) in peripheral blood neutrophils in HGA. Due to false + IgM: confirm with EIA and IFA IgG titers. PCR from blood is sensitive and highly specific for early diagnosis. PCR + early, but rapidly becomes – with treatment.

Pitfalls: No morula with HME. Rash uncommon in HME and rare in HGA. E. chaffeensis (HME) titers will not be elevated with A. phagocytophilium (HGA) and vice versa. Seropositivity increases over time. Blood smears positive early. Unlike BMD, may have prolonged fevers and present as an FUO.

Prognosis: Good if treated early. Delayed response/more severe with Lyme co-infection disease.

Malaria (Plasmodium ovale/vivax/falciparum/malariae/knowlesi)

Clinical Presentation: Presents acutely with fever/chills, severe headaches, cough, nausea/vomiting, diarrhea, abdominal/back pain. Typical "malarial paroxysm" consists of chills, fever and profuse sweating, followed by extreme prostration. There are a paucity of physical findings, but most have tender hepatomegaly/splenomegaly and relative bradycardia. ↑ T. bilirubin, thrombocytopenia, atypical lymphocytes, and mild ↑ AST/ALT common.

Diagnostic Considerations: Diagnosis by visualizing Plasmodium on thick/thin Giemsa or Wright-stained smears.

Pitfalls: Be wary of diagnosing malaria without headache. Dengue most closely resembles malaria. On abdominal US, dengue patients have gallbladder wall thickening/splenomegaly but not hepatomegaly vs. malaria patients which have a normal gallbladder, splenomegaly/heptomegaly. If no atypical lymphocytes on smear (auto cell counters are insensitive to atypical lymphocytes), question the diagnosis of malaria. P. knowlesi (monkey malaria emerging cause of human malaria. Resembles P. malariae (microscopically) but may be severe resembing P. falciparum (clinically). Treat P. knowlesi as chloroquine sensitive (P. vivax, P. ovale, P. malariae) malaria. Avoid monotherapy with artemisinin drugs to prevent MDR malaria.

Prognosis: Related to species degree of parasitemia P. falciparum with high-grade parasitemia is most severe, and may be complicated by coma, hypoglycemia, renal failure, or non-cardiogenic pulmonary edema. If parasitemia exceeds 15%, consider exchange transfusions.

Fungi/Mycobacterium in Blood

See histoplasmosis (treat as pulmonary histoplasmosis), Mycobacterium tuberculosis (treat as pulmonary TB), Mycobacterium avium-intracellulare (treat as pulmonary MAI).

Parasites, Fungi, Unusual Organisms in CSF/Brain

Cysts/Mass Lesions in CSF/Brain

Subset	Pathogens	Preferred Therapy	Alternate Therapy
Cerebral nocardiosis	Nocardia sp.	<u>Preferred IV Therapy:</u> TMP–SMX (TMP 5 mg/kg, SMX 15 mg/kg) (IV) q6h until clinical improvement, then (PO) therapy <u>Alternate IV PO Therapy:</u> Minocycline or Doxycycline 100 mg (IV) q12h until clinical improvement, then (PO) therapy	<u>Preferred PO Therapy</u> TMP–SMX 1 DS tablet (PO) q12h × 6 months <u>Alternate PO Therapy</u> Minocycline 100 mg (PO) q12h × 6 months **or** Doxycycline 100 mg (PO) q12h × 6 months
Cryptococcal meningitis/ cryptococcomas	Cryptococcus neoformans	See p. 22	
Cerebral amebiasis	Entamoeba histolytica	Metronidazole 750 mg (PO) q8h × 10 days **or** Tinidazole 800 mg (PO) q8h × 5 days	
Primary ambic meningo-encephalitis (PAM)	Naegleria fowleri	See p. 21	
Granulomatous ambic encephalitis (GAM)	Acanthamoeba	See p. 21	

Cysts/Mass Lesions in CSF/Brain *(cont'd)*

Subset	Pathogens	Preferred Therapy	Alternate Therapy
Cerebral echinococcosis (hydatid cyst disease)	Echinococcus granulosus or multilocularis	Surgical resection plus Albendazole 400 mg* (PO) q12h until cured	Surgical resection plus Mebendazole 50 mg/kg (PO) q24h until cured
Cerebral gnathostomiasis	Gnathostoma spinigerum	Surgical resection	Albendazole 400 mg (PO) q12h × 3 weeks **or** Ivermectin 200 mcg/kg/d × 2 days
Cerebral coenurosis	Taenia multiceps	Surgical resection	
Neurocysti-cercosis† (NCC)	Taenia solium	Albendazole 400 mg* (PO) q12h (15 mg/kg/day in 2 ÷ doses) × 10 days **plus** Praziquantel 16.7 mg/kg (PO) q8h × (50 mg/kg/day in 3 ÷ doses) × 10 days	Praziquantel 16.7 mg/kg (PO) q8h × (50 mg/kg/day in 3 ÷ doses) × 10 days **or** Albendazole 400 mg* (PO) q12h (15 mg/kg/day in 2 ÷ doses) × 10 days
Cerebral paragonimiasis (lung fluke)	Paragonimus westermani	Praziquantel 25 mg/kg (PO) q8h × 2 days	Bithionol 50 mg/kg (PO) q48h × 2 weeks **or** Tridabendazole 10 mg/kg (PO) q24h × 2 days
Cerebral toxoplasmosis	Toxoplasma gondii	See p. 349	
Chagas' disease (American trypanosomiasis)	Trypanosoma brucei cruzi	Nifurtimox 2 mg/kg (PO) q6h × 4 months	Benznidazole 3.5 mg/kg (PO) q12h × 2 months

*   If < 60 kg, give albendazole 7.5 mg/kg. Maximum daily dose = 800 mg.
†   No need to treat if lesions calcified.
$ If active cysts/inflammation, 1 day before NCC therapy, begin therapy with steroids (prednisone/prednisolone 1 mg/kg/day or 0.1 mg/kg/day × 5–10 days followed by taper).

Cerebral Nocardiosis

Clinical Presentation: CNS mass lesion resembling brain tumor/abscess. 40% of patients with systemic nocardiosis have associated CNS mass lesions.

Diagnostic Considerations: Diagnosis by demonstrating Nocardia (Gram positive, and weakly acid-fast and aerobic. Delicate, beaded, branching filaments) in brain biopsy specimens.

Pitfalls: Usually not limited to brain. Nocardia also in skin, lungs or liver. HIV patients require life-long suppression with TMP–SMX.
Prognosis: Related to immunosuppression, and infection extent.

Cerebral Amebiasis (Entamoeba histolytica)

Clinical Presentation: Rare cause of brain abscess. Onset is frequently abrupt with rapid progression. Suspect in patients with a history of amebiasis and altered mental status/focal neurologic signs. If present, meningeal involvement resembles acute bacterial meningitis. CT/MRI shows focal lesions.

Diagnostic Considerations: Diagnosis by demonstrating E. histolytica trophozoites in wet preps or by trichrome stain from aspirated brain lesions under CT guidance. Worldwide distribution. Mass lesions may be single or multiple, and more commonly involve the left hemisphere. Most patients have concomitant liver ± lung abscesses.

Pitfalls: Trophozoites/cysts in stool are not diagnostic of CNS disease. E. histolytica serology is often positive, but is nonspecific. E. histolytica trophozoites are not present in CSF.

Prognosis: Related to size/location of CNS lesions.

Primary Amebic Meningoencephalitis (Naegleria fowleri) (see p. 23)

Granulomatous Amebic Encephalitis (Acanthamoeba) (see p. 23)

Cerebral Echinococcosis (Echinococcus granulosus) Hydatid Cyst Disease

Clinical Presentation: Most cysts are asymptomatic. Mass lesions may cause seizures, cranial nerve abnormalities, other focal neurologic symptoms.

Diagnostic Considerations: CT/MRI typically shows a single large cyst without edema or enhancement. Multiple cysts are rare. Diagnosis by demonstrating protoscolices in "hydatid sand" in cysts. Usually associated with liver/lung hydatid cysts.

Pitfalls: E. granulosus serology lacks specificity.

Prognosis: Related to size/location of CNS cysts. CSF eosinophilia is not a feature of CNS involvement. Treatment consists of surgical removal of total cyst after instilling cysticidal agent (hypertonic saline, iodophor, ethanol) into cyst plus albendazole.

Cerebral Echinococcosis (Echinococcus multilocularis) Hydatid Cyst Disease

Clinical Presentation: Frequently associated with hydatid bone cysts (may cause spinal cord compression), liver/lung cysts. Peripheral eosinophilia occurs in 50%, but eosinophils are not seen in the CSF.

Diagnostic Considerations: E. multilocularis ELISA is sensitive and specific.

Pitfalls: Praziquantel is ineffective for CNS hydatid cyst disease. Imaging studies suggest carcinoma/sarcoma. Diagnosis is frequently not made until brain biopsy.

Prognosis: If treatment is effective, improvement of CNS lesions is evident in 8 weeks. Brain/bone cysts are difficult to cure.

Cerebral Gnathostomiasis (Gnathostoma spinigerum)

Clinical Presentation: Nausea, vomiting, increased salivation, skin flushing, pruritus, urticaria, and upper abdominal pain 1–6 days after exposure. Cerebral form presents as eosinophilic meningitis with radiculomyeloencephalitis, with headache and severe sharp/shooting pains in extremities often followed by paraplegia and coma. Any cranial nerve may be involved. The most characteristic feature is changing/migratory neurological findings. Intense peripheral eosinophilia occurs in 90% of patients. CSF has eosinophilic pleocytosis and may have RBCs.

Diagnostic Considerations: In cases with ocular involvement, the worm may be seen in the anterior chamber of eye. Specific Gnathostoma serology of CSF is helpful in establishing the diagnosis. Acquired from infected cat/dog feces. Most cases occur in Southeast Asia also Central/South America (Mexico, Peru) and most recently in Africa (Botswana). Few other CNS infections have both RBCs and eosinophils in the CSF.

Pitfalls: Do not miss associated eye involvement or characteristic episodic non-pitting subcutaneous edema.

Prognosis: Related to invasion of medulla/brainstem.

Cerebral Coenurosis (Taenia multiceps)

Clinical Presentation: CNS mass lesion with seizures/cranial nerve abnormalities, often presenting as a posterior-fossa syndrome. Common sites of CNS involvement include paraventricular and basal subarachnoid spaces. Eosinophils not in CSF.

Diagnostic Considerations: Diagnosis by demonstrating protoscolices in brain cyst specimens. Worldwide distribution. Transmitted via dog feces.

Pitfalls: Do not miss associated ocular lesions, which mimic intraocular neoplasms/granulomas.

Prognosis: Related to size/extent of CNS lesions.

Neurocysticercosis (Taenia solium)

Clinical Presentation: Chronic eosinophilic meningitis/mass lesions with onset seizures (late onset). Hydrocephalus is common. Spinal involvement may result in paraplegia. Cerebral cysts are usually multiple.

Diagnostic Considerations: CT/MRI shows enhancing cysts. Diagnosis by specific T. solium serology of serum/CSF. Neurocysticercosis is the most common CNS parasite in Eastern Europe, Asia, Latin America.

Pitfalls: Calcified cysts are not treated. Combined therapy for severe infection (↑ albendazole levels). Cimetidine or ranitidine may be given to ↑ praziquantel levels. Anti-seizure drugs usually given during therapy. Adjunctive therapy includes corticosteroids, anti-epileptics, and or shunt for hydrocephalus.

Prognosis: Related to extent/location of CNS lesions.

Cerebral Paragonimiasis (Paragonimus westermani) Lung Fluke

Clinical Presentation: Can resemble epilepsy, cerebral tumors, or brain embolism. Primary focus of infection is pulmonary, with pleuritic chest pain, cough, and night sweats. CNS findings are a manifestation of extrapulmonary (ectopic) organ involvement.

Diagnostic Considerations: Diagnosis by demonstrating operculated eggs in sputum, pleural fluid, or feces. Multiple sputum samples are needed to demonstrate P. westermani eggs. Charcot-Leyden crystals are seen in sputum. Endemic in Far East, India, Africa, and Central/South America.

Pitfalls: Extrapulmonary (ectopic) organ involvement (cerebral, subcutaneous, abdominal) is common. Up to 20% of patients have normal chest x-rays.

Prognosis: Related to size/location of CNS cysts and extent of lung involvement.

Cerebral Toxoplasmosis (T. gondii) (see p. 349)

Cerebral Cryptococcosis (C. neoformans) (see p. 348)

Chagas' Disease (Trypanosoma cruzi) American Trypanosomiasis

Clinical Presentation: Acute unilateral periorbital cellulitis (Romaña's sign) or regional adenopathy and edema of extremity at site of infected reduviid bug (chagoma). Chronic disease manifests as myocarditis/heart block or megaesophagus, megaduodenum, megacolon. Hepatosplenomegaly is common. Overt CNS signs are frequently absent. CNS Chagas' disease typically have hypodense ring enhancing lesions with surrounding edema on head CT/MRI scans. If meningoencephalitis develops, the prognosis is very poor. In immunosuppressed patients (especially HIV), recrudescence of disease occurs with development of T. cruzi brain abscesses.

Diagnostic Considerations: Diagnosis in acute disease by demonstrating trypanosomes in wet prep of anticoagulated blood or stained buffy coat smears. T. cruzi has the largest kinetoplast of all trypanosomes. Amastigote forms present intracellularly in monocytes/histiocytes in Giemsa-stained smear of bone marrow/lymph node aspirate, or by xenodiagnosis. Serology (mostly used for chronic disease) has limited value in endemic areas due to lack of specificity, but is useful in non-endemic areas. Common in Central/South America. Acquired from infected reduviid (triatoma) bugs, which infest mud/clay/stone parts of primitive dwellings. Infection in humans occurs in areas containing reduviid (triatoma) bugs that defecate during or immediately after a blood meal.

Diagnostic Considerations: Diagnostic tests ELISA, IFA, or chemoluminescence immunoassay (CHLIA).

Pitfalls: Do not overlook diagnosis in persons from endemic areas with unexplained heart block. For children ages 11–16 years, use nifurtimox 3.5 mg/kg (PO) q6h × 3 months. For children < 11 years, use nifurtimox 5 mg/kg (PO) q6h × 3 months.

Prognosis: Related to extent of GI cardiac or CNS involvement. The addition of gamma interferon to nifurtimox × 20 days may shorten the acute phase of the disease.

Parasites, Fungi, Unusual Organisms in Lungs

Pulmonary Cystic Lesions/Masses

Subset	Pathogens	Preferred Therapy	Alternate Therapy
Alveolar echinococcosis	Echinococcus multilocularis	Operable cases Wide surgical resection **plus** Albendazole 400 mg* (PO) q12h **or** Mebendazole 50 mg/kg (PO) q24h until cured	Inoperable cases: Albendazole 400 mg* (PO) q12h × 1 month, then repeat therapy after 2 weeks × 3 cycles (4 total months of albendazole)
Pulmonary amebiasis	Entamoeba histolytica	Metronidazole 750 mg (PO) q8h × 10 days	Tinidazole 800 mg (PO) q8h × 5 days
Pulmonary paragonimiasis (lung fluke)	Paragonimus westermani	Praziquantel 25 mg/kg (PO) q8h × 2 days	Bithionol 50 mg/kg (PO) q48h × 4 weeks **or** Tridabendazole 10 mg/kg (PO) q24h × 2 days

* If < 60 kg, give Albendazole 7.5 mg/kg.

Alveolar Echinococcosis (Echinococcus multilocularis)
Clinical Presentation: Slowly growing cysts remain asymptomatic for 5–20 years, until space-occupying effect elicits symptoms. Rupture/leak into bronchial tree can cause cough, chest pain, and hemoptysis.

Diagnostic Considerations: Diagnosis is suggested by typical "Swiss cheese calcification" findings on chest x-ray, and confirmed by specific E. multilocularis serology (which does not cross react with E. granulosus). Most common in Northern forest areas of Europe, Asia, North America, and Arctic. Acquired by ingestion of viable parasite eggs in food. Tapeworm-infected canines/cats or wild rodents are common vectors. Less common than infection with E. granulosus.

Pitfalls: Do not confuse central cavitary lesions with squamous cell carcinoma.

Prognosis: Related to size/location of cysts.

Pulmonary Amebiasis (Entamoeba histolytica)
Clinical Presentation: Cough, pelvic pain, fever, and right lung/pleural mass mimicking pneumonia or lung abscess. Bronchopleural fistulas may occur. Sputum has "liver-like" taste if cyst ruptures into bronchus. Bacterial co-infection is rare. Amebic lung lesions are associated with hepatic liver abscesses, and invariably involve the right lobe of lung/diaphragm.

Diagnostic Considerations: Diagnosis by aspiration of lungs cysts, which may be massive. Amebic serology is sensitive and specific. Worldwide distribution. Acquired by ingesting amebic cysts. Key to diagnosis is concomitant liver involvement; liver abscess presents years after initial diarrheal episode.

Pitfalls: Lung involvement is rarely the sole manifestation of amebic infection, and is usually due to direct extension of amebic liver abscess (10–20% of amebic liver abscesses penetrate through the diaphragm and into the lungs). Follow metronidazole with paromomycin 500 mg (PO) q8h × 7 days to eliminate intestinal focus.

Prognosis: Related to severity/extent of cysts.

Pulmonary Paragonimiasis (Paragonimus westermani) Lung Fluke

Clinical Presentation: Endemic in Asia, Africa, and Latin America. Mild infection; may be asymptomatic. Acute phase of infection is accompanied by abdominal pain, diarrhea and urticaria, followed by pleuritic chest pain/eosinophilic pleural effusion. Chronic symptoms occur within 6 months after exposure, with dyspnea/dry cough leading to productive cough ± hemoptysis. Complications include lung abscess, bronchiectasis, cough, and night sweats. Eosinophilia may be present acutely.

Diagnostic Considerations: Oriental lung fluke acquired by ingestion of freshwater crayfish/crabs. After penetration of the gut/peritoneal cavity, the fluke migrates through the diaphragm/pleural space and invades lung parenchyma. Incubation period is 2–20 days. Diagnosis by demonstrating operculated eggs not present until 2–3 months after infection in sputum, pleural fluid, or feces. Multiple sputum samples needed to demonstrate P. westermani eggs. Charcot-Leyden crystals are seen in sputum, and characteristic chest x-ray findings of ring-shaped/crescent infiltrates with "thin-walled" cavities are evident in ~ 60%. Chest x-ray findings take months to resolve.

Pitfalls: May have extrapulmonary (ectopic) organ involvement, e.g., cerebral, subcutaneous, abdominal. Up to 20% have normal chest x-rays. Commonest cause of eosinophilic pleural effusions in endemic areas. Diagnosis should be questioned if pleural effusion fluid does not have eosinophils.

Prognosis: Related to degree of lung damage, e.g., bronchiectasis and extrapulmonary organ involvement, especially CNS.

Pulmonary Coin Lesions

Subset	Pathogens	Preferred Therapy	Alternate Therapy
Dog heartworm	Dirofilaria immitis	No therapy necessary	
Aspergilloma	Aspergillus	No therapy if asymptomatic. Surgery for massive hemoptysis	Itraconazole 200 mg (PO) solution q24h × 3–6 months **or** Voriconazole (see "usual dose" in DS,) × 3–6 months

Dog Heartworm (Dirofilaria immitis)

Clinical Presentation: Asymptomatic "coin lesion" after bite of infected mosquito transmits parasite from dogs to humans. Differential diagnosis includes granulomas and malignancy.

Diagnostic Considerations: Diagnosis by specific serology or pathological demonstration of organism in granuloma, usually when a coin lesion is biopsied to rule out malignancy. Worldwide distribution. Acquired from pet dogs. Dirofilariasis causes dog heartworm in carrier, but presents as a solitary lung nodule in humans.

Pitfalls: Coin lesion or CXR often resembling bronchogenic carcinomas.

Prognosis: Excellent.

Pulmonary Aspergilloma

Clinical Presentation: Coin lesion(s) ± productive cough, hemoptysis, wheezing. May be asymptomatic. Usually occurs in pre-existing cavitary lung lesions, especially TB with cavity > 2 cm.

Diagnostic Considerations: Diagnosis by chest x-ray appearance of fungus ball in cavity. ↑ Aspergillus precipitins (PPTNs) best test. Aspergillus hyphae and "fruiting bodies" (conidiophores) in respiratory specimens. May present with "crescent sign" on chest x-ray (white fungus ball silhouetted against black crescent of the cavity).

Pitfalls: Role of itraconazole or voriconazole as therapy is unclear. Surgical resection for severe hemoptysis.

Prognosis: Related to degree of hemoptysis.

Pulmonary Infiltrates/Mass Lesions¶

Subset	Pathogens	Preferred Therapy	Alternate Therapy
Pulmonary blastomycosis	Blastomyces dermatitidis	**Mild illness:** Itraconazole 200 mg (PO) TID × 3 days and then q24h or q12h for 6–12 months. **Moderately severe or severe illness:** Liposomal amphotericin (L-amb) for 1–2 weeks followed by itraconazole as above.	Fluconazole has been disappointing; its use is limited to specialized settings such as CNS blastomycosis. Amphotericin B 0.7–1 mg/kg may be used as initial therapy instead of Liposomal amphotericin (L-amb).

¶ **See Color Atlas** (center of book).

Pulmonary Infiltrates/Mass Lesions *(cont'd)*

Subset	Pathogens	Preferred Therapy	Alternate Therapy
Pulmonary histo-plasmosis	Histoplasma capsulatum	**Mild illness:** Therapy is not always needed, but symptoms lasting more than a month may be treated with Itraconazole 200 mg (PO) q8h × 3 days and then q24h or q12h for a total of 6–12 weeks. **Moderately severe or severe illness:** Isavunconazole 200 mg (IV) q8h × 48 hours then 200 mg (IV/PO) until cured **or** Liposomal amphotericin (L-amb) for 1–2 weeks followed by Itraconazole as above. Chronic cavity histoplasmosis requires at least a year of therapy.	Posaconazole 400 mg (PO) q12h until cured* **or** Itraconazole 200 mg (IV) q12h × 2 days, then 200 mg (IV) q24h × 1–2 weeks, then 200 mg (PO) solution q12h until cured†
Pulmonary para-coccidioido-mycosis (South American blasto-mycosis)	Para-coccidioides brasiliensis	Isavunconazole 200 mg (IV) q8h × 48 hours then 200 mg (IV/PO) until cured **or** Itraconazole 200 mg (PO) q24h × 6 months **or** Ketoconazole 400 mg (PO) q24h × 18 months	Amphotericin B 0.5 mg/kg (IV) q24h until 1.5–2.5 gm given
Pulmonary actino-mycosis	Actinomyces israelii	Amoxicillin 1 gm (PO) q8h × 6 months **or** Doxycycline 100 mg (PO) q12h × 6 months	Clindamycin 300 mg (PO) q8h × 6 months **or** Chloramphenicol 500 mg (PO) q6h × 6 months
Pulmonary aspergillosis	Aspergillus (BPA)	Systemic oral steroids	Itraconazole 200 mg (PO) q12h × 8 months
Acute invasive pneumo-nia/ aspergillus Chronic pneumonia aspergillus	Aspergillus	<u>Preferred Therapy</u> Isavunconazole 200 mg (IV) q8h × 48 hours then 200 mg (IV/PO) until cured **or** Voriconazole*†§ **or** Liposomal amphoterin (L-amb) (IV) q24h until cured§	<u>Alternate Therapy</u> Posaconazole 400 mg (PO) q12h until cured* **or** Itraconazole 200 mg (IV) q12h × 2 days, then 200 mg (IV) q24h × 1–2 weeks, then 200 mg (PO) solution q12h until cured†

*   Initiate therapy with Itraconazole 200 mg (IV) q12h × 7–14 days.
†   Follow with Itraconazole 200 mg (PO) solution q12h until cured.
§   For usual dose, see Chapter 11 (Drug Summaries)

Pulmonary Infiltrates/Mass Lesions (cont'd)

Subset	Pathogens	Preferred Therapy	Alternate Therapy
Pulmonary sporotrichosis	Sporothrix schenckii	Liposomal amphotericin (L-amb) (IV) q24h × 3 weeks **or** Amphotericin B 0.5 mg/kg (IV) q24h until 1–2 gm given	Itraconazole 200 mg (PO)* q12h until cured **or** Liposomal amphotericin (L-amb) (IV) q24h until cured§
Pulmonary coccidioidomycosis	Coccidioides immitis	Isavuconazole 200 mg (IV) q8h × 48 hours, then 200 mg (IV/PO) q24h until cured **or** Itraconazole 200 mg (PO)* q12h until cured **or** Fluconazole 800 mg (IV or PO) × 1 dose, then 400 mg (PO) q24h until cured	Liposomal amphotericin (L-amb) (IV) q24h × 7 days§ **or** Amphotericin B 1 mg/kg (IV) q24h × 7 days†
Pulmonary nocardiosis	Nocardia asteroides	TMP–SMX 5–10 mg/kg/d (TMP) in 2–4 doses (IV) × 3–6 weeks, then 1 DS tablet (PO) q12h until cured	Minocycline 100 mg (PO) q12h until cured
Pulmonary cryptococcosis	Cryptococcus neoformans	Fluconazole 800 mg (IV or PO) × 1 dose, then 400 mg (PO) q24h until cured **or** Isavuconazole 200 mg (IV) q8h × 48 hours, then 200 mg (IV/PO) q24h until cured	Amphotericin B 0.5 mg/kg (IV) q24h until 1–2 grams given **or** Liposomal amphotericin (L-amb) (IV) q24h × 3 weeks§
Pulmonary zygomycosis (mucormycosis)	Rhizopus/ Mucor/ Absidia	Isavuconazole 200 mg (IV) q8h × 48 hours, then 200 mg (IV/PO) q24h until cured **or** Liposomal amphotericin (L-amb) (IV) q24h × 1–2 weeks†§ or × 3 wks	Voriconazole until cured§ **or** Itraconazole 200 mg (PO)* q12h until cured
Pulmonary pseudallescheriasis	Pseudallescheria boydii/ Scedosporium apiospermum	Voriconazole until cured§	Itraconazole 200 mg (PO)* q12h until cured

BPA = bronchopulmonary aspergillosis.

* Initiate therapy with itraconazole 200 mg (IV) q12h × 7–14 days.

† Follow with itraconazole 200 mg (PO) solution q12h until cured.

§ For usual dose see Chapter 11 (Drug Summaries)

Pulmonary Blastomycosis (Blastomyces dermatitidis)

Clinical Presentation: Highly variable. May present as a chronic/non-resolving pneumonia with fever/cough and characteristic "right-sided perihilar infiltrate" ± small pleural effusion.

Diagnostic Considerations: Usual sites of dissemination include skin, bones and prostate, not CNS or adrenals. Blastomyces serology may XR (false +) with Aspergillus, Coccidiodides, Histoplasma, or paracoccidiomycosis. β 1,3 D-glucan (BG) –, aspergillus galactomannan (GM) – .

Pitfalls: Dissemination to extra-pulmonary sites may occur years after pneumonia.

Prognosis: Related to severity/extent of infection. One-third of cases are self-limited and do not require treatment.

Pulmonary Histoplasmosis (Histoplasma capsulatum)

Clinical Presentation: Acute primary infection presents as self-limiting flu-like illness with fever, headache, nonproductive cough, chills, and chest pain. Minority of patients become overtly ill with complicated respiratory or progressive pulmonary infection. Can cause arthralgias, E. nodosum, E. multiforme, or pericarditis. May occur in outbreaks. Chronic infection presents as chronic pneumonia resembling TB or chronic disseminated infection. Eosinophilia common.

Diagnostic Considerations: May be recovered from sputum or demonstrated in lung tissue specimens. Worldwide distribution, but most common in Central/South Central United States. Acute disseminated histoplasmosis suggests HIV. Intracellular (PMNs/monocytes) organisms may be seen in Wright/Giema stained peripheral blood smears/buffy coat smears in disseminated infection. Acute histoplasmosis with immunodiffu-sion (ID) assay M band precipitins; chronic histoplasmosis with ID assay M band precipi-tins or CF ≥ 1:32. Histoplasma urinary antigen useful in diagnosis of acute/disseminated histoplasmosis. Histoplasma serology may XR (false +) with coccidiomycosis, blastomy-cosis, TB or sarcoidosis. Histoplasma urinary antigen may XR with acute/chronic coc-cidiomycosis (false + histoplasma urinary antigen may provide a clue to the presence of coccidiomycosis). β 1,3 D-glucan (BG) +, aspergillus galactomannan (GM) + .

Pitfalls: Pleural effusion is uncommon. Do not treat old/inactive/minimal histoplasmosis, histoplasmosis pulmonary calcification, or histoplasmosis fibrosing mediastinitis. Differentiate from TB and kala-azar. Resembles kala-azar histologically, but rod-shaped kinetoplasts (kala-azar) are absent extracellularly.

Prognosis: Related to severity/extent of infection. No treatment is needed for self-limiting acutehistoplasmosis presenting as flu-like illness. HIV patients should receive life-long suppressive therapy with itraconazole 200 mg (PO) solution q24h.

Pulmonary Paracoccidioidomycosis (South American Blastomycosis)

Clinical Presentation: Typically presents as a chronic pneumonia syndrome with productive cough, blood-tinged sputum, dyspnea, and chest pain. May also develop fever, malaise, weight loss, mucosal ulcerations in/around mouth and nose, dysphagia, changes in voice, cutaneous lesions on face/limbs, or cervical adenopathy. Can disseminate to prostate, epididymis, kidneys, or adrenals.

Diagnostic Considerations: Characteristic "pilot wheel" shaped yeast in sputum. Diagnosis by culture and stain (Gomori) of organism from clinical specimen. Found only in Latin American. One-third of cases have only pulmonary involvement. Skin test is non-specific/non-diagnostic.

Pitfalls: No distinguishing radiologic features. No clinical adrenal insufficiency, in contrast to TB or histoplasmosis. Hilar adenopathy/pleural effusions are uncommon.

Prognosis: Related to severity/extent of infection. HIV requires life-long suppression with TMP-SMX 1 DS tablet (PO) q24h or itraconazole 200 mg (PO) solution q24h.

Pulmonary Actinomycosis (Actinomyces israelii)

Clinical Presentation: Indolent, slowly progressive infiltrates involving the pulmonary parenchyma ± pleural space. Presents with fever, chest pain, weight loss. Cough/hemoptysis are less common. Chest wall sinuses frequently develop. Chest x-ray shows adjacent dense infiltrate. "Sulfur granules" are common in sinus drainage fluid.

Diagnostic Considerations: Diagnosis by stain/culture of drainage from sinuses or lung/bone biopsy specimens. Actinomyces are non-acid fast and anaerobic to micro-aerophilic.

Pitfalls: No CNS lesions, but bone erosion is common with chest lesions. Prior antibiotic therapy may interfere with isolation of organism.

Prognosis: Excellent when treated until lesions resolve. Use IV regimen in critically ill patients, then switch to oral regimen.

Bronchopulmonary Aspergillosis (BPA/ABPA)

Clinical Presentation: Migratory pulmonary infiltrates in chronic asthmatics. Eosinophilia is common, and sputum shows Charcot-Leyden crystals/brown flecks containing Aspergillus.

Diagnostic Considerations: Diagnosis by Aspergillus in sputum and high-titers of Aspergillus precipitins (PPTNs) in serum. BPA is an allergic reaction in chronic asthmatics, not an infectious disease. Pulmonary infiltrates with peripheral eosinophilia in chronic asthmatics suggests the diagnosis.

Pitfalls: Correct diagnosis is important since therapy is steroids, not antifungals.

Prognosis: Related to severity/duration of asthma and promptness of steroid therapy.

Acute Invasive Aspergillus Pneumonia

Chronic Aspergillus Pneumonia

Clinical Presentation: Occurs in patients with AIDS, chronic granulomatous disease, alcoholism, diabetes, and those receiving steroids for chronic pulmonary disease. Usual

features include chronic productive cough ± hemoptysis, low-grade fever, weight loss, and malaise. Chronic Aspergillus pneumonia resembles TB, histoplasmosis, melioidosis.
Diagnostic Considerations: Diagnosis by lung biopsy demonstrating septate hyphae invading lung parenchyma. Aspergillus may be in sputum, but is not diagnostic of aspergillus pneumonia. β 1,3 D-glucan (BG) + , aspergillus galactomannan (GM) + .
Pitfalls: May extend into chest wall, vertebral column, or brachial plexus.
Prognosis: Related to severity/extent of infection. Cavitation is a favorable prognostic sign.

Pulmonary Sporotrichosis (Sporothrix schenckii)
Clinical Presentation: Usually presents as productive cough, low-grade fever, and weight loss. Chest x-ray shows cavitary thin-walled lesions with associated infiltrate. Hemoptysis is unusual. Differential diagnosis includes other thin-walled cavitary lung lesions (e.g., coccidioidomycosis, atypical TB, paragonimiasis).
Diagnostic Considerations: Diagnosis by lung biopsy demonstrating invasive lung disease, not broncho-alveolar lavage. Usually a history of puncture/traumatic wound involving an extremity. May be associated with septic arthritis/osteomyelitis.
Pitfalls: Sporotrichosis in lungs implies disseminated disease. May need repeated attempts at culture.
Prognosis: Related to extent of infection/degree of immunosuppression.

Pulmonary Coccidioidomycosis (Coccidioides immitis)
Clinical Presentation: Usually presents as a solitary, peripheral, thin-walled cavitary lesion in early or later stage of primary infection. May present as a solitary pulmonary nodule. E. nodosum and bilateral hilar adenopathy are common (in contrast to sporotrichosis). Hemoptysis is unusual.
Diagnostic Considerations: Diagnosis by demonstration of spherules with endospores in sputum/BAL or biopsy specimens/Coccidioides serology. Increased incidence of dissemination in Filipinos, Blacks, and American Indians. Eosinophils in CSF in disseminated infection with CNS involvement. May be associated with chronic meningitis/osteomyelitis. CF IgG titer ≥ 1:32 diagnostic of active disease. Coccidioides CF may XR (false +) with Blastomyces, Histoplasma, Cryptococci, Torulopsis, or TB (XR minimal with EIA). (False + histoplasma urinary antigen may provide a clue to the presence of coccidiomycosis).
Pitfalls: Dissemination is preceded by ↓ Coccidioides titers/disappearance of Erythema nodosum.
Prognosis: Related to extent of infection/degree of immunosuppression.

Pulmonary Nocardiosis (Nocardia asteroides)
Clinical Presentation: Usually presents as a dense lower lobe lung mass ± cavitation. May have associated mass lesions in CNS. Chest wall sinuses are more common with Actinomycosis.

Diagnostic Considerations: Diagnosis by demonstrating organisms by stain/culture of lung specimens. Nocardia are weakly acid-fast and aerobic.

Pitfalls: Use IV regimens in critically ill patients. HIV patients require life-long suppressive therapy with TMP–SMX or minocycline.

Prognosis: Related to extent of infection/degree of immunosuppression.

Pulmonary Cryptococcosis (Cryptococcus neoformans)

Clinical Presentation: Individual focus of infection is usually inapparent/minimal when patient presents with disseminated cryptococcal infection. Pneumonia is typically a minor part of disseminated disease; CNS manifestations usually predominate (e.g., headache, subtle cognitive changes, occasional meningeal signs, focal neurological deficits).

Diagnostic Considerations: Diagnosis by serum cryptococcal antigen, by demonstrating encapsulated yeasts in sputum/lung specimens, or by culture of pulmonary specimens. β 1,3 D-glucan (BG) – , aspergillus galactomannan (GM) – .

Pitfalls: Clinical presentation of isolated cryptococcal pneumonia is rare. In HIV, false + cryptococcal antigen may occur with BBL Port-A-Cul transport vials. Patients require life-long suppressive therapy with fluconazole.

Prognosis: Related to extent of dissemination/degree of immunosuppression.

Pulmonary Zygomycosis (Mucormycosis) (Rhizopus/Mucor/Absidia/Cunninghamella)

Clinical Presentation: Progressive pneumonia with fever, dyspnea, hemoptysis and cough unresponsive to antibiotic therapy. Usually seen only in compromised hosts. Chest x-ray is not characteristic, but shows infiltrate with consolidation in > 50% of patients. Cavitation occurs in 40% as neutropenia resolves.

Diagnostic Considerations: Diagnosis by demonstrating branched sparsely septate "ribbon-like" hyphae often with right angle branching in biopsy specimens in lung biopsy. Pleural effusion is not a feature of pulmonary mucormycosis. β 1,3 D-glucan (BG) –, aspergillus galactomannan (GM) – .

Pitfalls: Causes rhinocerebral mucormycosis in diabetics, pneumonia in leukopenic compromised hosts.

Prognosis: Related to degree of immunosuppression and underlying disease. Angioinvasive with a propensity for dissemination.

Pulmonary Pseudallescheriasis (P. boydii/S. apiospermum)

Clinical Presentation: Progressive pulmonary infiltrates indistinguishable from Aspergillosis or Mucor. Usually seen only in compromised hosts (e.g., prolonged neutropenia, high-dose steroids, bone marrow or solid organ transplants, HIV). Manifests as cough, fever, pleuritic pain, and often hemoptysis. No characteristic chest x-ray appearance.

Diagnostic Considerations: Diagnosis by culture of organisms in lung biopsy. Hemoptysis is common in patients with cavitary lesions. CNS involvement is rare.

Pitfalls: One of few invasive fungi unresponsive to amphotericin B deoxycholate. Cause of sinusitis in diabetics, and pneumonia in leukopenic compromised hosts.

Prognosis: Related to severity/extent of infection and degree of immunosuppression. Cavitary lesions causing hemoptysis often require surgical excision. Disseminated infection is often fatal.

Parasites, Fungi, Unusual Organisms in Heart

Chagas' Disease (Trypanosoma cruzi) American Trypanosomiasis

Subset	Pathogens	Preferred Therapy	Alternate Therapy
Chagas' disease (American trypanosomiasis)	Trypanosoma cruzi	Benznidazole 2.5–3.5 mg/kg (PO) q12h × 60 days	Nifurtimox 2–3 mg/kg/day (PO) q6–8h × 90 days

Parasites, Fungi, Unusual Organisms in the Liver

Liver Flukes

Subset	Pathogens	Preferred Therapy	Alternate Therapy
Fascioliasis	Fasciola hepatica Fasciola gigantica	Tridabendazole 600 mg (PO) q12h × 14 days	Bithionol 30–50 mg/kg (PO) q48h × 20–30 days **or** Nitazoxanide 500 mg (PO) q12h × 7 days
Clonorchiasis/ Opisthorchiasis	Clonorchis sinensis Opisthorchis viverrini	Praziquantel 25 mg/kg (PO) q8h × 2 days	<u>C. sinensis/O. viverrini</u> Albendazole 10 mg/kg (PO) q24h × 7 days <u>O. viverrini:</u> Tribendimidine 400 mg (PO) × 1 dose

Hepatic Fascioliasis (F. hepatica/F. gigantica) Liver Fluke

Clinical Presentation: Frequently asymptomatic, but may present acutely with fever, right upper quadrant pain, nausea, diarrhea, wheezing, urticaria, hepatomegaly, eosinophilia, anemia. ELISA, IHA, CF, CIE serology helpful with acute diagnosis. Aspiration of biliary fluid may show flukes/eggs. Chronic disease is associated with gallstones, cholecystitis, cholangitis, liver abscess, generalized adenopathy. Subacute nodules, hydrocele, lung/brain abscess can be seen in ectopic forms.

Diagnostic Consideration: Diagnosis by F. hepatica/F. gigantica eggs in stool. F. hepatica eggs indistinguishable from Fasciolopsis buski (giant intestinal fluke) eggs. Endemic in sheep-raising areas (sheep liver flukes). Acquired from freshwater plants (watercress). Not associated with cholangiocarcinoma.

Pitfalls: May present as Katayama syndrome resembling schistosomiasis, with high fever, eosinophilia, and hepatosplenomegaly. Unlike other trematodes, praziquantel is ineffective. Chronic F. hepatica often asymptomatic, but may present with intermittent biliary colic. No eosinophilia. Abdominal ultrasound/CT shows crescentic/leaf shaped defects in gallbladder/hepatic ducts.

Prognosis: Related to extent/location of liver damage.

Hepatic Clonorchiasis (C. sinensis)/Opisthorchis (O. viverrini) Liver Flukes

Clinical Presentation: Frequently asymptomatic, but may present 2–4 weeks after ingestion of fluke with fever, tender hepatomegaly, rash, and eosinophilia. Chronically presents as recurrent cholangitis, chronic cholecystitis, or pancreatitis. Associated with cholangiocarcinoma (unlike fascioliasis).

Diagnostic Considerations: Diagnosis by visualizing C. sinensis/O. viverrini (operculated lemon-shaped) eggs (morphologically indistinguishable) in stool. Clonorchiasis is acquired from ingesting raw/inadequately cooked infected freshwater (Cyprinoid) fish in Southeast Asia. Opisthorchiasis is acquired from ingesting raw/inadequately cooked infected freshwater fish/crayfish from Laos, Cambodia, or Thailand.

Pitfalls: Cholecystitis with eosinophilia should suggest clonorchiasis or ascariasis.

Prognosis: Related to extent/location of hepatic damage. Associated with cholangiocarcinoma.

Cystic Masses in Liver

Subset	Pathogens	Preferred Therapy	Alternate Therapy
Hepatic amebiasis	Entamoeba histolytica	Metronidazole 750 mg (PO) q8h × 7–10 days	Tinidazole 2 gm/day (PO) in 3 divided doses × 3 days
Hepatic echinococcosis (hydatid cyst disease)	Echinococcus granulosus	Operable Surgical resection **plus** Albendazole 400 mg* (PO) q12h × 1–6 months	Inoperable Albendazole 400 mg* (PO) q12h × 1–6 months

* If < 60 kg, give albendazole 7.5 mg/kg.

Hepatic Amebiasis (Entamoeba histolytica)

Clinical Presentation: Antecedent (years prior) mild amebic dystery. Severe cases of amebic dysentery tend not to develop liver abscesses later. Presents insidiously with weight loss and night sweats to acutely ill with fever, nausea, vomiting, right upper quadrant pain. Typically, amebic liver abscesses are single, affect the right posterior lobe of liver, and do not show air/fluid levels. (In contrast, bacterial liver abscesses are usually multiple, and in all lobes of liver, and often show air/fluid levels.) Amebic liver abscesses do not calcify like hydatid cysts.

Diagnostic Considerations: Diagnosis by E. histolytica ↑ HI or EIA titers. E. histolytica in abscess wall. Worldwide distribution. Acquired by ingesting amebic cysts. Amebic liver abscess usually presents years after initial mild amebic dysenteric episode.t

Pitfalls: Amebic abscess fluid ("anchovy paste") contains no PMNs or amebas; amebas are found only in abscess wall. Eosinophilia is not a feature of amebiasis.

Prognosis: Related to health of host/extrapulmonary spread.

Hepatic Echinococcosis (Echinococcus granulosus) Hydatid Cyst Disease

Clinical Presentation: Right upper quadrant pain/mass when cysts enlarge enough to cause symptoms. Hepatic cysts are unilocular in 70%, multilocular in 30%.

Diagnostic Considerations: Diagnosis by demonstrating E. granulosus scolices/hooklets in cyst/hydatid sand. Serology is unreliable. Worldwide distribution in sheep/cattle raising areas. Acquired by ingestion of eggs from dogs.

Pitfalls: Eosinophilia not a feature of hydatid cyst disease. Hydatid cysts are multifaceted, loculated, and calcified.

Prognosis: Related to location/extent of extrahepatic cysts. Large cysts are best treated by surgical removal after injection with hypertonic saline, alcohol, or iodophor to kill germinal layer/daughter cysts. Percutaneous drainage under ultrasound guidance plus albendazole may be effective.

Hepatomegaly

Subset	Pathogens	Preferred Therapy	Alternate Therapy
Visceral leishmaniasis (Kala-azar)	Leishmania donovani	Antimony stibogluconate 20 mg/kg (IV/IM) q24h × 28 days **or** Liposomal amphotericin (L-amb): **Immunocompetent adults:** 3 mg/kg (IV) q24h on days 1–5,14, and 21 **Immunocompromised adults:** 4 mg/kg (IV) q24h on days 1–5, 10, 17, 24, 31, and 38)*	Miltefosine 2.5 mg/kg* (PO) q24h × 28 days **or** Paromomycin 15 mg/kg (IM) q24h × 21 days
Indian (Bihar state) visceral leishmaniasis (Kala-azar)	L. donovani	Liposomal amphotericin (L-amb)† 5 mg/kg (IV) × 1 dose, then Miltefosine 50 mg (PO with food) q12h × 7–14 days	
Schistoso-miasis	Schistosoma mansoni	Praziquantel 20 mg/kg (PO) q12h × 2 doses	Oxamniquine 15 mg/kg (PO) × 1 dose¶
	Schistosoma japonicum	Praziquantel 20 mg/kg (PO) q8h × 3 doses	None

*   Maximum 150 mg (PO)/day.
†   Ultra short course therapy is 10 mg/kg (IV) × 2 days.
¶   In Africa, give 20 mg/kg (PO) q24h × 3 days.

Visceral Leishmaniasis (Leishmania donovani) Kala-azar

Clinical Presentation: Subacute or chronic systemic cases manifest months to years after initial exposure to Leishmania, most often with fever, weight loss, anemia, hepatosplenomegaly ± generalized adenopathy. Long eyelashes in some. Laboratory abnormalities include leukopenia, anemia, and polyclonal gammopathy on SPEP. Incubation period is usually 3–8 months. May have atypical presentation in HIV (e.g., no splenomegaly). Acutely can mimic malaria with chills/temperature spikes. Post–kala-azar dermatitis may resemble leprosy, and is persistent/common on face.

Diagnostic Considerations: Double quotidian fever (double daily temperature spike) in persons from endemic areas with hepatosplenomegaly suggests the diagnosis. Kala-azar in children may have ↑ triglycerides/↓ HDL. Diagnosis by liver/bone marrow or buffy coat smear. Histologically, Kala-azar resembles histoplasmosis. Key diagnostic finding in tissue biopsy specimens is intracellular amastigotes with adjacent rod-shaped kineto-plasts. L. donovani serology is specific; immunochromatographic Anti-K39 strip test is also useful. Most common in Southern Europe, Middle East, Asia, Africa, South America. Facial lesion is a clue to the diagnosis.

Pitfalls: In acute cases, can mimic malaria with chills and temperature spikes, but no thrombocytopenia or atypical lymphocytes. Antimony resistance is common in India (Bihar state).

Prognosis: Related to degree of liver/spleen involvement.

Hepatic Schistosomiasis (Schistosoma mansoni/japonicum)

Clinical Presentation: May present acutely with Katayama fever (serum sickness-like illness with wheezing and eosinophilia) 4–8 weeks after exposure. May be accompanied or followed by fever/chills, headache, cough, abdominal pain, diarrhea, generalized lymphadenopathy, or hepatosplenomegaly. Laboratory abnormalities include leukocytosis, eosinophilia, and polyclonal gammopathy on SPEP. Resolves spontaneously after 2–4 weeks. After 10–15 years, may present chronically as hepatosplenic schistosomiasis, with pre-sinusoidal portal hypertension, hepatomegaly (L > R lobe enlargement), no jaundice, and intact liver function.

Diagnostic Considerations: Diagnosis by S. mansoni/S. japonicum eggs in stool/liver biopsy. Serology is good for acute (not chronic) schistosomiasis. CT/MRI of liver shows "turtle back" septal calcifications. Rare complications include cor pulmonale and protein-losing enteropathy. Increased incidence of hepatitis B/C and chronic Salmonella infections. Renal complications include glomerulonephritis and nephrotic syndrome.

Pitfalls: Chronic schistosomiasis is not associated with eosinophilia. S. hematobium does not infect the liver/spleen. Oxamniquine is contraindicated in pregnancy.

Prognosis: Related to egg burden.

Parasites, Fungi, Unusual Organisms in Stool/Intestines

Intestinal Protozoa

Subset	Pathogens	Preferred Therapy	Alternate Therapy
Amebiasis	E. histolytica	See p. 94	
Giardiasis	Giardia lamblia	Tinidazole 2 gm (PO) × 1 dose or Metronidazole 250 mg (PO) q8h × 5–7 days	
Cystoisosporiasis (Isospora)	C. (Isospora) belli	TMP–SMX 1 DS tablet (PO) q12h × 10 days **or** Nitazoxanide 500 mg (PO) × 3 days (for HIV, see p. 334)	Ciprofloxacin 500 mg (PO) q12h × 7 days **or** Pyrimethamine 75 mg (PO) q24h + folinic acid 10 mg (PO) q24h × 2 weeks then q12h × 3 weeks
Dientamoebiasis	Dientamoeba fragilis	Iodoquinol 650 mg (PO) q8h × 20 days	Doxycycline 100 mg (PO) q12h × 10 days **or** Metronidazole 500–750 mg (PO) q8h × 10 days
Blastocystis	Blastocystis hominis	Nitazoxanide 500 mg (PO) q12h × 3 days	Iodoquinol 650 mg (PO) q8h × 20 days **or** TMP–SMX 1 DS tablet (PO) q12h × 7 days
Cyclospora	Cyclospora	TMP–SMX 1 DS (PO) q12h × 10 days **or** Nitazoxanide 500 mg (PO) q12h × 3 days	
Cryptosporidiosis	Cryptosporidia	Nitazoxanide 500 mg (PO) q12h × 3 days	
Balantidiasis	Balantidium coli	Doxycycline 100 mg (PO) q12h × 10 days	Iodoquinol 650 mg (PO) q8h × 20 days **or** Metronidazole 750 mg (PO) q8h × 5 days

Amebiasis (Entamoeba histolytica) (see p. 94)

Giardiasis (Giardia lamblia) (see p. 94)

Cystoisosporiasis (C. isospora) belli
Clinical Presentation: Acute/subacute onset of diarrhea. C. (Isospora) belli is the only protozoa with eosinophils in stool.

Diagnostic Considerations: Diagnosis by demonstrating oocysts in stool and organisms in intestinal biopsy specimen. Associated with HIV, immigration from Latin America, daycare centers, and mental institutions. If stool exam is negative, "string test"/ duodenal aspirate and biopsy may be helpful.

Pitfalls: Difficult to eradicate; may last months. Multiple stool samples may be needed for diagnosis. Add folinic acid 10 mg (PO) q24 if pyrimethamine is used.

Prognosis: Related to adequacy of treatment/degree of immunosuppression.

Dientamoebiasis (Dientamoeba fragilis)

Clinical Presentation: Acute/subacute onset of diarrhea. No cyst stage. Lives only as trophozoite. Among intestinal protozoa, only D. fragilis and I. belli are associated with peripheral eosinophilia.

Diagnostic Considerations: Diagnosis by demonstrating trophozoites in stool/intestinal by trichrome stain. Mucus in diarrheal stools, not blood. May have abdominal pain. Diarrhea may last for months/years.

Pitfalls: Frequently associated with pinworm (Enterobius vermicularis) infection. Metronidazole failures common.

Prognosis: Related to adequacy of fluid replacement/underlying health of host.

Blastocystis (Blastocystis hominis)

Clinical Presentation: Acute/subacute onset of diarrhea.

Diagnostic Considerations: Diagnosis by demonstrating cysts which vary greatly in size (6–40 μm). No trophozoites in stools, in stool by trichrome stain. Trichrome stain reveals characteristic "halo" (slime capsule) in stool specimens. No trophozoites in stools.

Pitfalls: Uncommon GI pathogen. Consider as cause of diarrhea only after other pathogens excluded.

Prognosis: Related to adequacy of fluid replacement/underlying health of host.

Cyclospora (see p. 97; for HIV, see Chapter 5)

Cryptosporidiosis (see p. 97; for HIV, see Chapter 5)

Balantidiasis (Balantidium coli)

Clinical Presentation: Acute/subacute onset of diarrhea. Fecal WBCs only with mucosal invasion. Largest intestinal protozoa and only ciliated protozoa to infect humans.

Diagnostic Considerations: Diagnosis by demonstrating trophozoites (cysts rarely seen) in stool/intestinal biopsy specimen. Identifying features include darkly staining "kidney shaped" macronucleus (also has micronucleus) and large size. Fulminant dysentery seen only in debilitated/compromised hosts.

Pitfalls: Stools not bloody. Diarrhea may be intermittent.

Prognosis: Related to adequacy of fluid replacement/underlying health of host.

Intestinal Nematodes (Roundworms)

Subset	Pathogens	Preferred Therapy	Alternate Therapy
Capillariasis	Capillaria (Aonchotheca) philippinensis	Mebendazole 200 mg (PO) q12h × 20 days	Albendazole 400 mg (PO) q24h × 10 days
Angiostrongyliasis (rodent lung/ intestinal worm)	Angiostrongylus cantonensis	Albendazole 400 mg (PO) q12h × 2–3 weeks **plus** corticosteroids	Mebendazole 200–400 mg (PO) q8h × 10 days
Hookworm	Necator americanus/ Ancylostoma duodenale	Albendazole 400 mg (PO) × 1 dose **or** Mebendazole 100 mg (PO) q12h × 3 days or 500 mg (PO) × 1 dose	Pyrantel pamoate 11 mg/kg (PO) q24h × 3 days (max. 1 gm/ day)
Strongyloidiasis	Strongyloides stercoralis	Ivermectin 200 mcg/kg (PO) q24h × 2 days **or** Thiabendazole 25 mg/ kg (PO) q12h × 2 days (max. 3 gm/day)	Albendazole 400 mg (PO) q24h × 3 days
Ascariasis	Ascaris lumbricoides	Albendazole 400 mg (PO) × 1 dose **plus** Pyrantel pamoate 11 mg/kg (PO) q24h × 3 days (max. 1gm/day) **or** Mebendazole 100 mg (PO) q12h × 3 days or 500 mg (PO) × 1 dose	Ivermectin 200 mcg/ kg (PO) × 1 dose*
Trichostrongyliasis	Trichostrongylus orientalis	Pyrantel pamoate 11 mg/kg (PO) × 1 dose (max. 1 gm)	Albendazole 400 mg (PO) × 1 dose **or** Mebendazole 100 mg (PO) q12h × 3 days

* Avoid in young children and pregnant adults.

Intestinal Nematodes (Roundworms) *(cont'd)*

Subset	Pathogens	Preferred Therapy	Alternate Therapy
Pinworm	Enterobius vermicularis	Pyrantel pamoate 11 mg/kg (PO) × 1 dose (max. 1 gm); repeat in 2 weeks **or** Albendazole 400 mg (PO) × 1 dose; repeat in 2 weeks	Ivermectin 200 mcg/kg (PO) × 1 dose **or** Mebendazole 100 mg (PO) × 1 dose; repeat in 2 weeks
Whipworm	Trichuris trichiura	Mebendazole 100 mg (PO) q12h × 3–7 days	Albendazole 400 mg (PO) q24h × 3 days **or** Ivermectin 200 mcg/kg (PO) q24h × 3 days

Capillariasis (Capillaria philippinensis)

Clinical Presentation: Intermittent voluminous watery diarrhea ± malabsorption. Fever is uncommon.

Diagnostic Considerations: Diagnosis by demonstrating ova or parasite in stools. Resembes Trichuris, but C. philippinensis ova have non-protruding polar plugs, are smaller, and have a "pitted shell" (striated) with prominent polar plugs. Peripheral eosinophilia is uncommon until after therapy.

Pitfalls: Serology is positive in 85%, but cross-reacts with other parasites.

Prognosis: Related to severity of malabsorption/extra-intestinal disease.

Angiostrongyliasis (A. cantonensis) Rodent Lung/Intestinal Worm

Clinical Presentation: Presents as appendicitis (worm resides and deposits eggs in arteries/arterioles around ileocecum/appendix).

Diagnostic Considerations: Diagnosis by demonstrating organism in biopsied/excised tissue. May involve proximal small bowel, liver, CNS. When in CNS, a cause of eosinophilic meningitis.

Pitfalls: Can present as RLQ mass/fever resembling regional enteritis (Crohn's disease), but with eosinophilia and leukocytosis.

Prognosis: Related to severity of malabsorption and extra-intestinal disease.

Hookworm (Necator americanus/Ancylostoma duodenale)

Clinical Presentation: Pruritic, vesicular eruptions at site of filariform larval entry ("ground itch"). Pulmonary symptoms and transient eosinophilia may occur during migratory phase to intestines. Later, abdominal pain, diarrhea, weight loss, hypoalbuminemia, and anemia develop.

Diagnostic Considerations: Diagnosis by demonstrating eggs in stools. Hookworm eggs do not have "pointed ends", larvae rare in fresh stool specimens (eggs may hatch if stools allowed to stand too long prior to examination). N. americanus can ingest 0.3 mL of blood/worm/day, much greater than A. duodenale. Anemia may be severe with heavy infestation (up to 100 mL/day).

Pitfalls: Eggs in fresh stool, not rhabditiform larvae vs. S. stercoralis.

Prognosis: Related to severity of anemia/malabsorption.

Strongyloidiasis (Strongyloides stercoralis)

Clinical Presentation: Pruritic, papular, erythematous rash. Pulmonary symptoms (cough, asthma) may occur during lung migration phase. May develop Loeffler's syndrome (pulmonary infiltrates with eosinophilia) or ARDS in heavy infections. Intestinal phase associated with colicky abdominal pain, diarrhea, and malabsorption.

Diagnostic Considerations: Diagnosis by demonstrating larvae in stool specimens/duodenal fluid. Usually asymptomatic in normal hosts, but causes "hyperinfection syndrome" in compromised hosts. CNS strongyloides (part of hyperinfection syndrome) should suggest diagnosis of HIV in non-immunosuppressed patients. Diarrhea/abdominal pain mimics regional enteritis (Crohn's disease) or ulcerative colitis. Malabsorption is common and mimics tropical sprue. Anemia is usually mild.

Pitfalls: Usually rhabditiform larvae (not eggs) in stools.

Prognosis: Related to severity of malabsorption.

Ascariasis (Ascaris lumbricoides)

Clinical Presentation: Pulmonary symptoms (cough, asthma) may occur during larval lung migration phase. May develop Loeffler's syndrome (pulmonary infiltrates with eosinophilia), as with hookworm/Strongyloides. Intestinal symptoms develop late. Usually asymptomatic unless intestinal/biliary obstruction occurs. Can obstruct the appendix/pancreatic duct.

Diagnostic Considerations: Diagnosis by demonstrating eggs in stool specimens. Abdominal ultrasound can detect obstruction from adult worms. Most infections are asymptomatic; symptoms are related to "worm burden"/ectopic migration. Each female worm may produce up to 250,000 eggs/day.

Pitfalls: Lung involvement (bronchospasm, bronchopneumonia, lung abscess) is prominent in HIV.

Prognosis: Related to worm burden/extra-intestinal organ invasion.

Trichostrongyliasis (Trichostrongylus orientalis)

Clinical Presentation: Mild intestinal symptoms with persistent eosinophilia.

Diagnostic Considerations: Diagnosis by demonstrating eggs in stool specimens. Most prevalent in the Middle East and Asia. Mild anemia. Eosinophilia is usually > 10%.

Pitfalls: Must differentiate eggs from hookworm, and rhabditiform larvae from Strongyloides. T. orientalis eggs have one or both "pointed ends."

Prognosis: Related to extent of disease/underlying health of host.

Pinworm (Enterobius vermicularis)

Clinical Presentation: Primarily affects children. Perianal pruritus (ectopic migration) is the main symptom. Worm lives in the cecum, but patients do not have intestinal symptoms.

Diagnostic Considerations: Scotch tape of anus at night can be used to detect eggs left by migrating female worms (Scotch tape test).

Pitfalls: Abdominal pain and diarrhea should prompt search for Dientamoeba fragilis, since co-infection is common.

Prognosis: Excellent.

Whipworm (Trichuris trichiura)

Clinical Presentation: May present as "chronic appendicitis." Severe infestation may cause bloody diarrhea/abdominal pain ("Trichuris dysentery syndrome"), rectal prolapse.

Diagnostic Considerations: Diagnosis by demonstrating large eggs with bile-stained, triple-layered eggshell walls and doubly operculated transparent protruding plugs. Most patients are asymptomatic or mildly anemic.

Pitfalls: Commonly co-exists with Ascaris, hookworm, or E. histolytica.

Prognosis: Related to severity/extent of dysentery. May need retreatment if heavy infection.

Intestinal Cestodes (Tapeworms)

Subset	Pathogens	Preferred Therapy	Alternate Therapy
Beef tapeworm	Taenia saginata	Praziquantel 5–10 mg/kg (PO) × 1 dose	Niclosamide 2 gm (PO) × 1 dose **or** Nitazoxanide 500 mg (PO) q12h × 3 days
Pork tapeworm	Taenia solium	Praziquantel 5–10 mg/kg (PO) × 1 dose	Niclosamide 2 gm (PO) × 1 dose **or** Nitazoxanide 500 mg (PO) q12h × 3 days
Dwarf tapeworm	Hymenolepis nana	Praziquantel 25 mg/kg (PO) × 1 dose	Nitazoxanide 500 mg (PO) q12h × 3 days **or** Niclosamide 2 gm (PO) × 1 dose, then 1.5 gm q24h × 6 days
Fish tapeworm	Diphyllobothrium latum	Praziquantel 10 mg/kg (PO) × 1 dose	Niclosamide 2 gm (PO) × 1 dose **or** Nitazoxanide 500 mg (PO) q12h × 3 days

Beef Tapeworm (Taenia saginata)/Pork Tapeworm (Taenia solium)

Clinical Presentation: Usually mild symptoms (weight loss, anemia), since most infections are caused by a single tapeworm. Worm segments passed between BMs with T. saginata and with BMs with T. solium.

Diagnostic Considerations: Diagnosis by demonstrating proglottids in stool. Taenia eggs in stool cannot be speciated; all are brown and spherical with a radially-striated inner shell. T. saginata may survive for 10 years, T. solium for 25 years.

Pitfalls: Severe cases may cause appendicitis, intestinal obstruction/perforation.

Prognosis: Related to severity of malabsorption/intestinal obstruction.

Dwarf Tapeworm (Hymenolepis nana)/Rat Tapeworm Hymenolepsis diminuta

Clinical Presentation: Usually asymptomatic.

Diagnostic Considerations: Diagnosis by demonstrating typical eggs in stool, with two shells enclosing inner oncosphere with hooklets and polar filaments. ELISA is positive in 85%, but cross-reacts with Taenia/Cysticercosis. GI symptoms develop with stool egg counts > 15,000/gm. H. diminuta is the rat tapeworm.

Pitfalls: Abdominal pain and diarrhea in heavy infestations.

Prognosis: Related to severity of malabsorption/underlying health of host.

Fish Tapeworm (Diphyllobothrium latum)

Clinical Presentation: Symptoms secondary to macrocytic anemia from vitamin B_{12} deficiency. Most infestations are asymptomatic.

Diagnostic Considerations: Diagnosis by demonstrating operculated eggs and proglottids in stool.

Pitfalls: Vitamin B_{12} deficiency anemia requires prolonged infection (> 3 years).

Prognosis: Related to severity of B_{12} deficiency anemia/underlying health of host.

Intestinal Trematodes (Flukes)

Subset	Pathogens	Preferred Therapy
Fasciolopsiasis	Fasciolopsis buski	Praziquantel 25 mg/kg (PO) q8h × 3 doses
Heterophyiasis	Heterophyes heterophyes Metagonimus yokogawai	Praziquantel 25 mg/kg (PO) q8h × 3 doses

Fasciolopsiasis (Fasciolopsis buski) Intestinal Fluke

Clinical Presentation: Diarrhea with copious mucus in stool. Most cases are asymptomatic.

Diagnostic Considerations: Diagnosis by demonstrating eggs in stool. F. buski eggs are indistinguishable from F. hepatica eggs (liver fluke). May have eosinophilia, low-grade fever ± malabsorption. Intestinal obstruction is the most serious complication.

Pitfalls: Mimics peptic ulcer disease with upper abdominal pain relieved by food.

Prognosis: Related to severity/extent of malabsorption/intestinal obstruction.

Heterophyiasis (Heterophyes heterophyes/Metagonimus yokogawai)
Intestinal Fluke

Clinical Presentation: Usually asymptomatic or mild intestinal symptoms. Embolization of eggs may result in myocarditis, myocardial fibrosis, or cerebral hemorrhage. Eosinophilia may be present.

Diagnostic Considerations: Diagnosis by demonstrating large operculated eggs in stool. Eggs resemble Chlonorchis and Opisthirchis. Small intestine fluke.

Pitfalls: Difficult to differentiate from Clonorchis sinensis. Difficult to diagnose when adult worms not present.

Prognosis: Related to extent/severity of extra-intestinal dissemination to heart, lungs, CNS.

Other Intestinal Infections

Subset	Pathogen	Preferred Therapy
Whipple's disease	Tropheryma whippeli	Ceftriaxone 2 gm (IV) q24h × 2 weeks[†] **then** TMP–SMX 1 DS tablet (PO) q12h* **plus** Streptomycin 1 gm (IM) q24h × 2 weeks

† × 4 weeks for CNS involvement
* TMP–SMX 1 DS tablet (PO) q12h × 1 year. Alternately, doxycycline 100 mg (PO) q12h **plus** hydroxychloroquine 200 mg (PO) q8h × 1 year.

Whipple's Disease (Tropheryma whippeli)

Clinical Presentation: Fever, encephalopathy/dementia, weight loss, migratory polyarthritis, myocarditis, pericarditis, endocarditis (CNE) generalized lymphadenopathy, diarrhea ± malabsorption.

Diagnostic Considerations: Diagnosis by demonstrating organism by PAS staining macrophages in small bowel biopsy specimens or by RT PCR.

Pitfalls: May present with dementia, as CNE, or FUO mimicking celiac disease or lymphoma. Optimum length of treatment is unknown. Relapses occur. T. whippeli normal flora in some healthy adults.

Prognosis: Related to severity/extent of extra-intestinal disease.

Parasites, Fungi, Unusual Organisms in Skin/Muscle

Infiltrative Skin/Subcutaneous Lesions

Subset	Pathogens	Preferred Therapy
Cutaneous leishmaniasis Old World	Leishmania major Leishmania tropica	Sodium stibogluconate 20 mg/kg (IV or IM) q24h × 20 days **or** Pentamidine 2–3 mg/kg (IM) q48h × 4–7 days
New World	Leishmania mexicana	**or** Lipid amphotericin 3 mg/kg (IV) q24h on days 1–5, 14, and 21 **or**
	Leishmania braziliensis	Miltefosine 2.5 mg/kg (PO) q24h × 28 days (max. 150 mg/day)
Leprosy Lepromatous	Mycobacterium leprae	Dapsone 100 mg (PO) q24h × 1–2 years **plus** Clofazimine 50 mg (PO) q24h × 1–2 years **plus** Rifampin 600 mg (PO) monthly × 1–2 years
Non-lepromatous (tuberculoid)	Mycobacterium leprae	Dapsone 100 mg (PO) q24h × 6 months **plus** Rifampin 600 mg (PO) monthly × 6 months
Loa Loa (Loiasis)	L. loa	Diethylcarbamazine 2–3 mg/kg (PO) q8h × 2–3 weeks **or** Albendazole 200 mg (PO) q12h × 3 weeks
Erythrasma	Corynebacterium minutissimum	Erythromycin 250 mg (PO) q6h × 2 weeks

Cutaneous Leishmaniasis (Old World/New World)
Clinical Presentation: Variable presentation. Typically, a nodule develops then ulcerates, with a raised/erythematous outer border and a central area of granulation tissue. May be single or multiple. Usually non-pruritic/non-painful. Occurs weeks after travel to endemic areas (New World leishmaniasis: Latin America; Old World leishmaniasis: Central Asia).
Diagnostic Considerations: Diagnosis by demonstrating Leishmania amastigotes in biopsy specimen.
Pitfalls: Most skin lesions undergo spontaneous resolution. However, treatment is advisable for lesions caused by L. braziliensis or related species causing mucosal leishmaniasis.
Prognosis: Excellent.

Lepromatous Leprosy (Mycobacterium leprae)

Clinical Presentation: Diffuse, symmetrical, red or brown skin lesions presenting as macules, papules, plaques, or nodules. May also present as diffuse thickening of skin, especially involving ear lobes, face, and extremities. Loss of eyebrows/body hair may occur.

Diagnostic Considerations: Diagnosis by demonstrating organism in acid fast stain of tissue specimens. Afebrile bacteremia is frequent, and buffy coat smears positive for M. leprae. Erythema nodosum and polyclonal gammopathy on SPEP are common, and lepromin skin test/PPD are negative (anergic). When present, peripheral neuropathy is often symmetrical and acral in distribution.

Pitfalls: Differential diagnosis is large. Consider leprosy in patients with unexplained skin diseases.

Prognosis: Good if treated early.

Non-Lepromatous (Tuberculoid) Leprosy (Mycobacterium leprae)

Clinical Presentation: Small number of asymmetrical, hypopigmented skin lesions, which are often scaly with sharp borders and associated anesthesia. Asymmetric peripheral nerve trunk involvement is common.

Diagnostic Considerations: Diagnosis by demonstrating granulomas with few acid-fast bacilli. Differentiate from cutaneous leishmaniasis by skin biopsy. Lepromin skin test/PPD are positive and SPEP is normal (in contrast to lepromatous leprosy).

Pitfalls: Wide spectrum of presentations depending on immune status and duration of disease. Differential diagnosis is large. Consider leprosy in patients with unexplained skin diseases.

Prognosis: Good if treated early.

Erythrasma (Corynebacterium minutissimum)

Clinical Presentation: Reddened/raised skin lesions on face/trunk. Not hot or pruritic.

Diagnostic Considerations: Differentiated from Tinea versicolor by culture. C. minutissimum skin lesions fluoresce red under UV light (Wood's lamp).

Pitfalls: Resembles Tinea versicolor, but lesions primarily involve the face, not trunk.

Prognosis: Excellent.

Infiltrative Skin Lesions ± Ulcers/Sinus Tracts/Abscesses

Subset	Pathogens	Preferred Therapy
Cutaneous histoplasmosis	Histoplasma capsulatum	Treat as for disseminated histoplasmosis (p. 282) if part of systematic syndrome. If solely involves the skin, Itraconazole 200 mg (PO) q12h until resolution.
Cutaneous blastomycosis	Blastomyces dermatitidis	Treat the same as pulmonary infection (p. 281)

Infiltrative Skin Lesions ± Ulcers/Sinus Tracts/Abscesses *(cont'd)*

Subset	Pathogens	Preferred Therapy
Cutaneous coccidioidomycosis	Coccidioides immitis	Treat same as pulmonary infection (p. 284)
Cutaneous actinomycosis	Actinomyces israelii	Treat same as pulmonary infection (p. 286)
Cutaneous nocardiosis	Nocardia sp.	Treat same as pulmonary infection (p. 283)
Cutaneous amebiasis	Entamoeba histolytica	Treat same as gastrointestinal infection (p. 94)
Cutaneous mycobacteria *Scrofula*	Mycobacterium tuberculosis	Treat same as pulmonary TB. (p. 55)
	M. scrofulaceum	Surgical excision is curative
M. haemophilum	M. haemophilum	Surgical excision/TMP–SMX 1 DS tablet (PO) q12h **or** Minocycline 100 mg (PO) q12h **or** quinolone (PO) until cured
M. chelonae	M. chelonae	Clarithromycin 500 mg (PO) q12h × 6 months
M. abscessus	M. abscessus	Eravacycline, Azithromycin, Amikacin, Tigecycline, Linezolid × 3–6 months (see Chapter 11 Drug Summaries for dosage.)*
M. fortuitum	M. fortuitum	Minocycline 100 mg (PO) q12h × 6–12 months **or** Doxycycline 100 mg (PO) q12h × 6–12 months **plus** TMP–SMX 1 DS tablet (PO) q12h × 6–12 months
Swimming pool granuloma	M. marinum	Clarithromycin XL 1 gm (PO) q24h × 3 months **plus** Rifampin 600 mg (PO) q24h × 3 months **or** TMP–SMX 1 DS tablet (PO) q12h × 3 months **plus** Ethambutol 15 mg/kg (PO) q24h × 3 months **or** Doxycycline 100 mg (PO) q12h × 3 months
Buruli ulcer	M. ulcerans	TMP–SMX 1 DS tablet (PO) q12h **plus** Ethambutol 15 mg/kg (PO) q24h × 6 weeks
Cutaneous MAI/ MAC	Mycobacterium avium-intracellu-lare/complex	Ethambutol 15 mg/kg (PO) q24h **plus** Azithromycin 1200 mg (PO) weekly × 6 months

*   Combination therapy with ≥ 2 drugs preferred.

Cutaneous Histoplasmosis (Histoplasma capsulatum)
Clinical Presentation: Chronic, raised, verrucous lesions.
Diagnostic Considerations: Diagnosis by demonstrating organism by culture/tissue staining.

Pitfalls: Skin nodules represent disseminated histoplasmosis, not isolated skin infection. Look for histoplasmosis elsewhere (e.g., lung, liver, bone marrow). Skin nodules (± chronic pneumonia) with osteolytic bone lesions suggests. African histoplasmosis due to H. capsulation var. duboisii.

Prognosis: Related to extent of infection/degree of immunosuppression.

Cutaneous Blastomyces (Blastomyces dermatitidis)

Clinical Presentation: Painless, erythematous, well-circumscribed, hyperkeratotic, crusted nodules or plaques that enlarge over time. Some may ulcerate and leave an undermined edge.

Diagnostic Considerations: Diagnosis by demonstrating organism by culture/tissue staining. Blastomyces dermatitidis affects many organs.

Pitfalls: When found in skin, look for Blastomyces elsewhere (e.g., lungs, prostate).

Prognosis: Related to extent of infection/degree of immunosuppression.

Cutaneous Coccidioidomycosis (Coccidioides immitis)

Clinical Presentation: Skin lesions take many forms, including raised verrucous lesions, cold subcutaneous abscesses, indolent ulcers, or small papules.

Diagnostic Considerations: Diagnosis by demonstrating organism by culture/tissue staining.

Pitfalls: Skin nodules represent disseminated coccidioidomycosis, not isolated skin infection. Look for Coccidioides elsewhere (e.g., CNS, bone, lungs).

Prognosis: Related to extent of infection/degree of immunosuppression.

Cutaneous Actinomycosis (Actinomyces israelii)

Clinical Presentation: Erythematous, uneven, indurated, woody, hard, cervicofacial tumor. Localized single/multiple sinus tracts in chest wall, abdominal wall, or inguinal/pelvic area may be present.

Diagnostic Considerations: Diagnosis by demonstrating organism by culture/tissue staining.

Pitfalls: Look for underlying bone involvement.

Prognosis: Good with early/prolonged treatment.

Cutaneous Nocardia (Nocardia brasiliensis)

Clinical Presentation: Subcutaneous abscesses may rupture to form chronically draining fistulas.

Diagnostic Considerations: Diagnosis by demonstrating organism by culture/tissue staining. May present as "Madura foot."

Pitfalls: Look for underlying immunosuppressive disorder.

Prognosis: Related to extent of infection/degree of immunosuppression.

Cutaneous Amebiasis (Entamoeba histolytica)

Clinical Presentation: Ulcers with ragged edges, sinus tracts, amebomas, and strictures may develop around the anus/rectum or abdominal wall.

Diagnostic Considerations: Diagnosis by demonstrating organism by tissue staining.
Pitfalls: If abdominal sinus tract is present, look for underlying ameboma.
Prognosis: Related to extent of infection/degree of organ damage.

Scrofula (Mycobacterium tuberculosis) or (Mycobacterium scrofulaceum)

Clinical Presentation: Cold, chronic, anterior cervical adenopathy ± sinus tracts. Usually
M. tuberculosis in children and *M. scrofulaceum* in adults.
Diagnostic Considerations: Diagnosis by acid-fast stain and culture of node/drainage.
Pitfalls: TB cured by antibiotic therapy alone. No need for surgical excision.
Prognosis: *TB*: Excellent with treatment; *M. scrofulaceum* highly resistant to anti-TB
therapy, excellent with surgical excision.

Cutaneous Mycobacterium haemophilum

Clinical presentation: Particularly common in immunosuppressed/HIV patients, presents as multiple, painful cutaneous ulcers/abscesses ± draining fistulas.
Diagnostic Considerations: Diagnose by PCR.
Pitfalls: Suspect M. haemophilum if drainage from ulcer/abscess is AFB smear + but
fails to grow on AFB media. M. haemophilus grows only on AFB media supplemented
with ferric containing compounds. Susceptible to minocycline, TMP–SMX, or quinolones, but most strains resistant to INH, EMB, RIF, PZA.
Prognosis: Good with surgical excision/prolonged treatment.

Cutaneous Mycobacterium chelonae

Clinical presentation: Present as cold abscesses with draining fistulas.
Diagnostic Considerations: AF culture of wound drainage.
Pitfalls: Some strains clarithromycin resistant. May be susceptible to quinolones, doxy-
cycline, or minocycline.
Prognosis: Good with effective therapy.

Cutaneous Mycobacterium abscessus

Clinical Presentation: Traumatic and post-OP wound infections. Lung airway coloniza-
tion with ↓ PFTs and or pneumonia particularly in CF and lung transplants.
Diagnostic Considerations: Culture/PCR of wound drainage or sputum specimens.
Pitfalls: M. abscesses is the most pathogenic NTM and most chemotherapy resistant.
Prognosis: Related to effectiveness of chemotherapy and status of host defenses.

Cutaneous Mycobacterium fortuitum

Clinical Presentation: Usually associated with chronic foreign body infection, especially infected breast implants. Associated with nail salon footbaths. Present as cold abscesses with draining fistulas.

Diagnostic Considerations: Diagnosis by demonstrating organism by acid fast smear are culture of drainage/infected prosthetic material.

Pitfalls: Highly resistant to anti-TB therapy, may be susceptible to quinolones or linezolid.

Prognosis: Good with surgical excision/prolonged treatment.

Swimming Pool Granuloma (Mycobacterium marinum)

Clinical Presentation: Begins as erythema with tenderness at inoculation site, followed by a papule or violaceous nodule that ulcerates and drains pus. May have sporotrichoid spread. Presents as a skin lesion unresponsive to antibiotics after abrasive water exposure (e.g., fish tank, swimming pool/lake).

Diagnostic Considerations: Diagnosis by demonstrating organism by acid-fast smear/culture.

Pitfalls: Resistant to INH/pyrazinamide. Surgical excision of isolated lesions may be needed.

Prognosis: Good with prolonged therapy.

Buruli Ulcer (Mycobacterium ulcerans)

Clinical Presentation: Begin as a firm, painless, movable, subcutaneous nodule. In 1–2 months, nodule becomes fluctuant, ulcerates, and develops an undermined edge. May have edema around lesion and in extremity (if involved).

Diagnostic Considerations: Diagnosis by acid-fast stain and culture of punch biopsy of ulcer rim. Patient is usually from Africa, but M. ulcerans also exists in Asia, Australia, and Central/South America.

Pitfalls: Steroids/skin grafting sometimes needed.

Prognosis: Good with surgical excision.

Cutaneous MAI (Mycobacterium avium-intracellulare)

Clinical Presentation: Nodules, abscesses, ulcers, plaques, ecthyma and draining sinuses can occur, but are uncommon in normal hosts and usually only seen in immunosuppressed patients.

Diagnostic Considerations: Diagnosis by demonstrating organism by acid-fast staining and culture (for species identification) of tissue biopsy specimens.

Pitfalls: Usually represents disseminated infection. Look for non-cutaneous evidence of infection (e.g., lungs, bone marrow, liver/spleen).

Prognosis: Related to extent of organ damage/degree of immunosuppression.

Skin Vesicles/Bullae

Subset	Pathogens	Preferred Therapy
Herpes simplex	Herpes simplex virus (HSV)	See p. 153
Herpes zoster	Varicella zoster virus (VZV)	See p. 153

Subcutaneous Serpiginous Lesions

Subset	Pathogens	Preferred Therapy
Cutaneous larva migrans (creeping eruption)	Ancylostoma braziliense	Ivermectin 200 mcg/kg (PO) × 1 dose **or** Albendazole 400 mg (PO) q24h × 3–7 days. Children may be treated topically with Albendazole ointment (10%) q8h × 10 days
Guinea worm	Dracunculus medinensis	Surgical removal of worm near skin surface. Metronidazole 250 mg (PO) q8h × 10 days facilitates worm removal
Cutaneous gnathostomiasis	Gnathostoma spinigerum	Surgical removal **or** Albendazole 400 mg (PO) q12h × 3 weeks **or** Ivermectin 200 mcg/kg (PO) q24h × 2 days

Cutaneous Larva Migrans (Ancylostoma braziliense) Creeping Eruption
Clinical Presentation: Intensely pruritic, migratory, subcutaneous, raised serpiginous lesions.
Diagnostic Considerations: Diagnosis by clinical appearance.
Pitfalls: Must be differentiated from "swimmer's itch" caused by schistosomal cercariae.
Prognosis: Excellent with treatment.

Guinea Worm (Dracunculus medinensis)
Clinical Presentation: Serpiginous, raised, subcutaneous tract overlying worm.
Diagnostic Considerations: Diagnosis by demonstrating Dracunculus worm when surgically removed.
Pitfalls: Resembles cutaneous larva migrans, but worm is visible below the skin and lesions are serpiginous with Dracunculus. May be complicated by painful arthritis.
Prognosis: Excellent with treatment. Soaking extremity in warm water promotes emergence/removal of worm. Metronidazole can also be used to decrease inflammation and facilitate worm removal. Mebendazole 200–400 mg (PO) q12h × 6 days may kill worms directly.

Cutaneous Gnathostomiasis (Gnathostoma spinigerum)
Clinical Presentation: Painful, intermittent, subcutaneous swelling with local edema, intense pruritus, and leukocytosis with eosinophilia. Acquired by eating undercooked fish, frogs, and other intermediate larvae-containing hosts. May be complicated by eosinophilic meningitis.

Diagnostic Considerations: Diagnosis by demonstrating Gnathostoma in tissue specimens. Relatively common infection in Thailand and parts of Japan, South America, and Southeast Asia.

Prognosis: Good if limited to the skin and surgically removed. Poor with CNS involvement. Albendazole is preferred.

Skin Papules/Nodules/Abscesses

Subset	Pathogens	Preferred Therapy
Bacillary angiomatosis	Bartonella henselae Bartonella quintana	Doxycycline 100 mg (PO) q12h × 8 weeks **or** Azithromycin 250 mg (PO) q24h **or** Any quinolone (PO) × 8 weeks
Cutaneous Alternaria	Alternaria alternata	Amphotericin B 0.7–1 mg/kg (IV) q24h × 2–3 gm‡ <u>Alternate therapy:</u> Voriconazole*, Itraconazole*, Posaconazole*, Caspofungin*. Treat until cured.
Entomophthoromycosis	E. basidiobolus E. conidiobolus	Amphotericin B 0.7–1 mg/kg (IV) q24h × 1–2 gm‡ **or** TMP–SMX 1 DS tablet (PO) q24h until cured
Chromomycosis	Fonsecaea pedrosoi, compactum Phialophora verrucosa, others	<u>Few small lesions:</u> Wide/deep surgical excision or cryosurgery with liquid nitrogen <u>Larger lesions:</u> Itraconazole 200 mg (PO) solution q24h until lesions regress ± cryosurgery
Cutaneous Fusarium	Fusarium solani	Amphotericin B 0.7–1 mg/kg (IV) q24h × 2–3 gm‡ **or** Voriconazole
Cutaneous Penicillium	Penicillium marneffei	Amphotericin B 0.6 mg/kg (IV) q24h × 14 days,‡ then Itraconazole 200 mg (IV) q12 × 2 days followed by 200 mg (PO) q12h × 10 weeks. For HIV, continue with Itraconazole 200 mg (PO) q24h indefinitely
Cutaneous Prototheca	Prototheca wikermanii	Surgical excision. If excision is incomplete, add either Amphotericin B 0.7–1 mg/kg (IV) q24h × 2–3 gm‡ **or** Itraconazole 200 mg (PO)† q12h until cured
Trichosporon	Trichosporon beigelii	Amphotericin B 0.7–1 mg/kg (IV) q24h × 2–3 gm‡

‡   Liposomal amphotericin (L-amb) may be a suitable alternative.
†   Initiate therapy with Itraconazole 200 mg (IV) q12h × 7–14 days.
*   For usual dose, see Chapter 11 (Drug Summaries)

Skin Papules/Nodules/Abscesses *(cont'd)*

Subset	Pathogens	Preferred Therapy
Cutaneous aspergillosis*	Aspergillus sp.	Voriconazole until cured§ **or** Isavuconazole 200 mg (IV) q8h × 48 hours, then 200 mg (IV/PO) q24h until cured **or** Itraconazole 200 mg (IV) q12h × 7–14 days, then 200 mg (PO) solution q12h until cured
Cutaneous zygomycosis (mucormycosis)	Mucor/Rhizopus/Absidia	Treat as for pulmonary zygomycosis (see p. 283)
Cutaneous coccidioido-mycosis	Coccidioides immitis	Fluconazole 800 mg (PO) × 1 dose, then 400 mg (PO) q24h until cured **or** Itraconazole 200 mg (PO)† q12h until cured Alternate therapy Amphotericin B 1 mg/kg (IV) q24h × 7 days, then 0.8 mg/kg (IV) q48h × 2–3 gm total dose‡
Cutaneous histoplasmosis	Histoplasma capsulatum	Treat as for pulmonary histoplasmosis (see p. 284)
Cutaneous cryptococcosis	Cryptococcus neoformans	Amphotericin B 0.5 mg/kg (IV) q24h × 1–2 gm‡ **or** Lipid amphotericin (L-amb) (IV) q24h × 3 weeks§ **then** Fluconazole 800 mg (PO) × 1 dose, then 400 mg (PO) q24h × 8–10 weeks
Cutaneous sporotrichosis	Sporothrix schenckii	Itraconazole 200 mg (PO). If HIV, chronic suppressive therapy may be needed q24h until 2–4 weeks after all lesions have resolved (typically 3–6 months in total).
Nodular/pustular candidiasis	Candida sp.	If occurs in moist skin areas (under breasts, groin, etc.), treat as mucocutaneous candidiasis (see p. 158). Nodular candidiasis occurring in non-moist skin areas in compromised hosts is a manifestation of disseminated disease and should be treated as such (see pp. 159–160)
Cutaneous onchocerciasis	Onchocerca volvulus	Ivermectin 150 mcg/kg (PO) × 1 dose, repeated q 4–6 months until asymptomatic **plus** Doxycycline 100 mg (PO) q12h × 6 weeks

*   Cutaneous aspergillus is a manifestation of disseminated aspergillosis.
†   Initiate therapy with Itraconazole 200 mg (IV) q12h × 7–14 days.
‡   Liposomal amphotericin (L-amb) may be a suitable alternative.
*   For usual dose, see Chapter 11 (Drug Summaries)

Bacillary Angiomatosis (Bartonella henselae/B. quintana) Peliosis Hepatis

Clinical Presentation: Skin lesions resemble Kaposi's sarcoma. Liver lesions resemble CMV hepatitis in HIV patients.

Diagnostic Considerations: Diagnosis by demonstrating organism by stain/culture of skin lesions or by blood culture. Blood cultures (blood or chocolate agar) should be incubated in $\uparrow$ CO_2 for 21 days.

Pitfalls: Requires life-long suppressive therapy.

Prognosis: Related to extent of infection/degree of immunosuppression.

Cutaneous Alternaria (Alternaria alternata)

Clinical Presentation: Bluish/purple papules that are often painful and non-pruritic. Usually seen only in leukopenic compromised hosts.

Diagnostic Considerations: Diagnosis by demonstrating organism by stain/culture in tissue specimen.

Pitfalls: Skin lesions usually represent disseminated disease in compromised hosts, not local infection. Fluconazole and micafungin ineffective.

Prognosis: Poor and related to degree of immunosuppression.

Cutaneous Basidiobolomycosis (B. ranarum)/Conidiobolus (C. coronatus)

Clinical Presentation: Infection presents as swelling of nose, paranasal tissues and mouth, accompanied by nasal stuffiness, drainage, and sinus pain. Begins as swelling of inferior nasal turbinates and extends until generalized facial swelling occurs. Subcutaneous nodules can be palpated in tissue. Basidiobolomycosis infection presents as a non-painful, firm, slowly progressive, subcutaneous nodule of the trunk, arms, legs, or buttocks.

Diagnostic Considerations: Diagnosis by demonstrating organism by stain/culture in tissue specimen. Skin lesions usually represent disseminated disease in compromised hosts, not localized infection.

Pitfalls: Unlike Mucor, Basidiobolomycosis does not usually invade blood vessels, although tissue infarction/necrosis is occasionally seen in diabetics and immunocompromised patients.

Prognosis: May spontaneously resolve. Surgical removal of accessible nodules and reconstructive surgery may be helpful for disfigurement.

Cutaneous Chromomycosis (F. pedrosoi/F. compactum, P. verrucosa, others)

Clinical Presentation: Warty papule/nodule that enlarges slowly to form a scarred, verrucous plaque. May also begin as a pustule, plaque, or ulcer. Over time, typical papule/nodule ulcerates, and the center becomes dry/crusted with raised margins. Lesions can be pedunculated/cauliflower-like.

Diagnostic Considerations: Diagnosis by demonstrating organism by stain/culture in tissue specimen. Chromomycosis remains localized within cutaneous/subcutaneous tissues.

Pitfalls: May resemble other fungal diseases. Sclerotic bodies in tissue and exudate distinguish chromomycosis from other related fugal diseases.

Prognosis: Related to degree of organ damage.

Cutaneous Fusarium (Fusarium solani)

Clinical Presentation: Presents in compromised hosts as multiple papules or painful nodules, initially macular with central pallor, which then become raised, erythematous, and necrotic. Seen mostly in leukopenic compromised hosts (especially acute leukemia and bone marrow transplants). Also a cause of mycetoma/onychomycosis.

Diagnostic Considerations: Diagnosis by demonstrating organism by stain/culture from blood/tissue. β 1,3 D-glucan (BG) + , aspergillus galactomannan (GM) + .

Pitfalls: Skin lesions usually represent disseminated disease, not localized infection.

Prognosis: Poor/fair. Related to degree of immunosuppression. Amphotericin B lipid formulation (L-amb), colony-stimulating granulocyte factor, and granulocyte transfusions may be useful.

Cutaneous Penicillium (Penicillium marneffei)

Clinical Presentation: Papules, pustules, nodules, ulcers, or abscesses. Mostly seen in HIV (requires life-long suppressive therapy with itraconazole).

Diagnostic Considerations: Diagnosis by demonstrating organism by stain/culture in tissue specimen. Affects residents/visitors of Southeast Asia/Southern China.

Pitfalls: Lesions commonly become umbilicated and resemble molluscum contagiosum. May present as disseminated infection.

Prognosis: Poor and related to degree of immunosuppression.

Cutaneous Prototheca (Prototheca wickermanii)

Clinical Presentation: Most common presentation is a single plaque or papulonodular lesion of the skin or subcutaneous tissue. Lesions are usually painless, slowly progressive (enlarge over weeks to months without healing), well-circumscribed, and may become eczematoid/ulcerated.

Diagnostic Considerations: Diagnosis by demonstrating organism by stain/culture in tissue specimen. Skin lesions in HIV are not different from normal hosts.

Pitfalls: Lesions are usually painless and may resemble eczema.

Prognosis: Poor/fair. Related to degree of immunosuppression. Surgical excision has been successful.

Cutaneous Trichosporon (Trichosporon beigelii)

Clinical Presentation: Seen mostly in leukopenic compromised hosts (especially in acute leukemia, but also in HIV, burn wounds, and organ transplants). Usually presents as multiple red-bluish/purple papules, which are often painful and non-pruritic.

Diagnostic Considerations: Diagnosis by demonstrating organism by stain/culture in tissue specimen.

Pitfalls: Skin lesions usually represent disseminated disease, not localized infection.
Prognosis: Related to extent of infection/degree of immunosuppression.

Cutaneous Aspergillosis (Aspergillus fumigatus)

Clinical Presentation: Seen at site of IV catheter insertion or adhesive dressing applied to skin in leukopenic, compromised hosts. Lesion is similar to pyoderma gangrenosum. May also invade burn wounds and cause rapidly progressive necrotic lesions.

Diagnostic Considerations: Diagnosis by demonstrating organism by stain/culture in tissue specimen. β 1,3 D-glucan (BG) +, aspergillus galactomannan (GM) +.

Pitfalls: Infiltrative/ulcerative skin lesions usually represent disseminated disease in compromised hosts, not localized infection. May cause invasive dermatitis/skin lesions in HIV.

Prognosis: Related to extent of infection/degree of immunosuppression.

Cutaneous Mucormycosis/Rhizopus/Absidia

Clinical Presentation: Necrotic skin lesion secondary to vascular invasion. Involves epidermis and dermis. Black eschars are evident.

Diagnostic Considerations: Diagnosis by demonstrating broad, sparsely septate hyphae often with branches at right angles by stain/culture in tissue specimen.

Pitfalls: Skin lesions usually represent disseminated disease in compromised hosts, not localized infection. Contaminated elastic bandages have been associated with cutaneous Mucor.

Prognosis: Related to extent of infection/degree of immunosuppression.

Cutaneous Coccidioidomycosis (Coccidioides immitis)

Clinical Presentation: Skin lesions may take many forms, including verrucous granulomas, cold subcutaneous abscesses, indolent ulcers, or small papules.

Diagnostic Considerations: Diagnosis by demonstrating organism by stain/culture in tissue specimen.

Pitfalls: Skin lesions usually represent disseminated disease in compromised hosts, not local infection.

Prognosis: Related to extent of infection/degree of immunosuppression.

Cutaneous Histoplasmosis (Histoplasma capsulatum)

Clinical Presentation: Common cutaneous findings include maculopapular eruption, petechiae, and ecchymosis. Histopathology reveals necrosis around superficial dermal vessels.

Diagnostic Considerations: Diagnosis by demonstrating organism by stain/culture in tissue specimen. β 1,3 D-glucan (BG) +, aspergillus galactomannan (GM) +.

Pitfalls: Skin lesions usually represent disseminated disease in compromised hosts, not local infection.

Prognosis: Related to extent of infection/degree of immunosuppression.

Cutaneous Cryptococcosis (Cryptococcus neoformans) Encapsulated Yeast

Clinical Presentation: May present as single or multiple papules, pustules, erythematous indurated plaques, soft subcutaneous masses, draining sinus tracts, or ulcers with undermined edges.

Diagnostic Considerations: Diagnosis by demonstrating encapsulated yeasts in stain/culture in tissue specimen. Cryptococcus Ag ↑ disseminated infection with skin involvement. β 1,3 D-glucan (BG) – , aspergillus galactomannan (GM) – .

Pitfalls: Skin lesions usually represent disseminated disease in compromised hosts, not localized infection. In HIV patients, umbilicated papules resemble molluscum contagiosum. In organ transplants, cellulitis with necrotizing vasculitis may occur.

Prognosis: Related to extent of infection/degree of immunosuppression.

Cutaneous Sporotrichosis (Sporothrix schenckii)

Clinical Presentation: Primary cutaneous lymphatic sporotrichosis starts as a small, firm, movable, subcutaneous nodule, which then becomes soft and breaks down to form a persistent, friable ulcer. Secondary lesions usually develop proximally along lymphatic channels, but do not involve lymph nodes. Plaque form does not spread locally.

Diagnostic Considerations: Diagnosis by demonstrating organism by stain/culture in tissue specimen. Cutaneous disease arises at sites of minor trauma with inoculation of fungus into skin. Skin lesions usually represent disseminated disease in compromised hosts, not localized infection.

Pitfalls: HIV patients with CD₄ < 200 may have widespread lymphocutaneous disease that ulcerates and is associated with arthritis. Unusual in axilla due to increased temperature.

Prognosis: Related to extent of infection/degree of immunosuppression.

Nodular/Pustular Candidiasis (sepsis in chronic steroids, see p. 158)

Cutaneous Onchocerciasis (Onchocerca volvulus)

Clinical Presentation: Early manifestation is pruritic, papular rash with altered pigmentation. Later, papules, scaling, edema, and depigmentation may develop. Nodules develop in deep dermis/subcutaneous tissue (especially over bony prominences) or in deeper sites near joints, muscles, bones. Endemic in Middle East, Central Africa, Central America.

Diagnostic Considerations: Diagnosis by serology/demonstration of microfilaria in thin snips of involved skin or in anterior chamber (by slit lamp) if eye involvement. Intradermal edema produces "peau d'orange" effect with pitting around hair follicles/sebaceous glands.

Pitfalls: Ivermectin is effective against microfilaria, not adult worms. Adults live ~ 18 years.

Prognosis: Related to location/extent of organ damage.

Rickettsia (Typhus and Spotted Fevers)

Subset	Pathogens	Preferred Therapy	Alternate Therapy
Rocky Mountain spotted fever (RMSF) (tick borne)	Rickettsia rickettsii	Doxycycline 200 mg (IV or PO) q12h × 3 days, then 100 mg (IV or PO) × 4 days	Any quinolone (IV **or** PO) × 7 days **or** Chloramphenicol 500 mg (IV or PO) q6h × 7 days
Epidemic (louse-borne) typhus, flying squirrel typhus	Rickettsia prowazekii	Same as RMSF	Same as RMSF
Murine (flea-borne) typhus	Rickettsia typhi	Same as RMSF	Same as RMSF
Scrub (chigger/mite-borne) typhus (Tsutsugamushi fever)	Rickettsia (Orientia) tsutsugamushi	Same as RMSF **or** Azithromycin 500 mg (PO) × 1 dose	Rifampin 600–900 mg (PO) q24h × 7 days
Rickettsialpox	Rickettsia akari	Same as RMSF	Same as RMSF
Tick typhus spotted fevers (Mediterranean spotted fever, Boutonneuse fever, Israeli spotted fever) (tick borne)	Rickettsia conorii Rickettsia parkeri Rickettsia phillipi	Same as RMSF	Same as RMSF
African tick bite fever (tick borne)	Rickettsia africae	Same as RMSF	Same as RMSF

Rocky Mountain Spotted Fever (Rickettsia rickettsii) RMSF

Clinical Presentation: Primary vector in United States is the Dermacentor (dog) tick. Fever with relative bradycardia, severe frontal headache, severe myalgias of abdomen/back/legs 3–12 days after tick bite. Rash begins as erythematous macules on wrists and ankles (3–5 days after tick bite), and progresses to petechiae/palpable purpura with confluent areas of ecchymosis. Periorbital edema, conjunctival suffusion, acute deafness, and edema of the dorsum of the hands/feet are important early signs. Abdominal pain can mimic acute abdomen, and meningismus and headache can mimic meningitis/encephalitis. Hepatosplenomegaly in some. Laboratory findings include normal leukocyte count, thrombocytopenia, ↑ AST/ALT and pre-renal azotemia. Hypotension/shock may occur secondary to myocarditis, which is the most common causes of death.

Diagnosis: Primarily a clinical diagnosis. Diagnosis by (Weil-Felix reactions: OX-19: + + +, OX-2: +, OX-K: −), specific R. rickettsii IFA, complement fixation, ELISA titers or RT-PCR. If RMSF (R. rickettsii) IgM titer ↑ (usually minimally elevated) but IgG titer is negative, ↑ IgM may be false positive. Repeat IgM and IgG titers which should both be ↑ in RMSF. R. parkeri may present as a RMSF-like illness. Unlike RMSF, R. parkeri rash (usually MP, but may be vesiculopapular) is primarily trucal and is accompanied by an eschar at the tick bite site. Like RMSF, the rash of R. parkeri may involve the palms/soles.

Pitfalls: Most cases occur in eastern and southeastern United States, not Rocky Mountain area. Many cases go unrecognized due to nonspecific early findings. Early antibiotic therapy may blunt/eliminate serologic response. Patients with signs/symptoms of RMSF but without a rash should be considered as having ehrlichiosis/anaplasmosis ("spotless RMSF") or BMD until proven otherwise.

Prognosis: Delayed treatment increases the risk of death. Adverse prognostic signs include myocarditis or encephalitis.

Epidemic (Louse-Borne) Typhus (Rickettsia prowazekii)

Clinical Presentation: High fever with relative bradycardia, chills, headache, conjunctival suffusion, and myalgias. A macular, rubella-like, truncal rash develops in most on the fifth febrile day, which may become petechial and involve the extremities, but spares the palms/soles. Facial swelling/flushing occurs at end of first week, along with CNS symptoms (e.g., tinnitus, vertigo, delirium) and GI complaints (diarrhea, constipation, nausea, vomiting, abdominal pain). Hypotension, pneumonia, renal failure, gangrene, cerebral infarction may develop late. Laboratory findings include normal leukocyte count, thrombocytopenia, and ↑ serum creatinine/LFTs. Primary vector is the human body louse; primary reservoir is humans.

Diagnosis: Primarily a clinical diagnosis requiring a high index of suspicion and early empiric therapy (Weil-Felix reactions: OX-19: + + +, OX-2: +, OX-K: −). Specific R. prowazekii antibody titers are confirmatory. Consider epidemic (louse-borne) typhus in febrile impoverished persons infested with lice, especially in Africa and parts of Latin America. Rarely seen in the United States. Milder recrudescent form (Brill-Zinsser disease) is also rare.

Pitfalls: Many cases go unrecognized due to nonspecific early findings. Early therapy is essential.

Prognosis: Gangrene of nose, ear lobes, genitalia, toes, and fingers may develop in severe cases. Death occurs in 10–50% of untreated patients.

Murine (Flea-Borne) Typhus (Rickettsia typhi)

Clinical Presentation: Similar to epidemic typhus but less severe, with fever in most, and headache, myalgias, and a macular rash in half. Laboratory findings include a normal leukocyte count, mild thrombocytopenia, and mildly ↑ AST/ALT. Primary vector is the Asian rat flea (Xenopsylla cheopis); primary reservoir is the commensal rat (Rattus genus). Uncommon in United States; most cases from Texas, California, Florida, Hawaii.

Diagnosis: Primarily a clinical diagnosis requiring a high index of suspicion. More common during summer and fall (Weil-Felix reactions: OX-19: + + +, OX-2: +, OX-K: −). Specific R. typhi antibody titers are confirmatory.

Pitfalls: Rash becomes maculopapular, compared to epidemic typhus, which remains macular. A similar illness is caused by R. felis.

Prognosis: Good if treated early. Death occurs in < 1%.

Scrub Typhus Orientia (Rickettsia) tsutsugamushi: Tsutsugamushi Fever

Clinical Presentation: Fever, chills, headache, myalgias, arthralgias, GI symptoms, other nonspecific complaints. Eschar at mite bite site (tache noire) ± regional adenopathy. A macular, truncal rash develops in most, usually in the first week, and may progress to involve the extremities and face, but spares the palms/soles. Vasculitis may lead to cardiopulmonary (ARDS) CNS (encephalitis) hematologic abnormalities during the second week. Hepatosplenomegaly is common. Laboratory abnormalities include normal/decreased WBC, relative lymphopenia, thrombocytopenia, ↑ CRP, ↑ T. bilirubin, ↑ AST/ALT. Primary vector/reservoir is the larval (chigger) trombiculid mite. Endemic areas include northern Australia, southeastern Asia, Indian subcontinent.

Diagnosis: Presumptive diagnosis is clinical (Weil-Felix reactions: OX-19: –, OX-2: –, OX-K: + + +). Specific R. tsutsugamushi serology is confirmatory.

Pitfalls: DDx includes SFTS (with AMS, diarrhea, leukopenia, N CRP vs. scrub typhus).

Prognosis: Excellent if treated early.

Rickettsialpox (Rickettsia akari)

Clinical Presentation: Milder illness than other rickettsioses, with initial eschar at bite site, high fever, and generalized rash (usually erythematous papules which become vesicular and spares the palms/soles). Fever peak is usually < 104°F, occurs 1–3 weeks after mite bite, and lasts ~ 1 week without therapy. Headache, photophobia, marked diaphoresis, sore throat, GI complaints (nausea/vomiting following initial headache) may occur. Leukopenia may be present. Primary vector is the mouse mite; primary animal reservoir is the house mouse. Rare in the United States.

Diagnosis: Presumptive diagnosis by clinical presentation (Weil-Felix reactions: OX-19: –, OX-2: –, OX-K: ±). Specific R. akari serology is confirmatory.

Pitfalls: Do not confuse with African tick-bite fever, which may also have a vesicular rash.

Prognosis: Excellent even without therapy.

Tick Spotted Fevers (Rickettsia conorii, Rickettsia parkeri) Mediterranean Spotted Fever, Boutonneuse Fever, Israeli Spotted Fever

Clinical Presentation: Similar to RMSF with fever, chills, myalgias, but less severe. Unlike RMSF, an eschar is usually present at the site of the tick bite ± regional adenopathy. Leukocyte count is normal and thrombocytopenia is common. Transmitted by the brown dog tick, Rhipicephalus sanguineus.

Diagnosis: Presumptive diagnosis by clinical presentation (Weil Felix reactions: OX-19: +, OX-2: +, OX-K: +). Specific R. conorii serology is confirmatory.

Pitfalls: Suspect in travelers from endemic areas with a RMSF-like illness. Consider different diagnosis in absence of an eschar.

Prognosis: Good with early treatment. Prostration may be prolonged even with proper therapy.

African Tick Bite Fever (Rickettsia africae)

Clinical Presentation: Similar to murine typhus with fever, chills, myalgias, but regional adenopathy and multiple eschars are common. Incubation period ~ 6 days. Amblyomma hebreum/variegatum tick vectors frequently bite humans multiple times.

Diagnosis: Presumptive diagnosis by clinical presentation (Weil-Felix reactions: OX-19: +, OX-2: +, OX-K: +). Specific R. africae serology is confirmatory.

Pitfalls: Rash is transient and may be vesicular or absent. If unable to take doxycycline, rifampin also effective (300 mg (PO) q8h).

Prognosis: Good even without therapy; excellent with therapy.

Other Skin Lesions

Subset	Pathogens	Topical Therapy	PO Therapy
Tinea versicolor (pityriasis)	Malassezia furfur (Pityrosporum orbiculare)	Clotrimazole cream (1%) or miconazole cream (2%) **or** Ketoconazole cream (2%) daily × 7 days	Ketoconazole 200 mg (PO) q24h × 7 days **or** Itraconazole 200 mg (PO) q24h × 7 days
Eosinophilic folliculitis	Malassezia furfur (Pityrosporum orbiculare)	<u>Preferred Therapy</u> Ketoconazole cream (2%) topically × 2–3 weeks ± Ketoconazole 200 mg (PO) q24h × 2–3 weeks	

Tinea Versicolor/Pityriasis (Malassezia furfur)

Clinical Presentation: Hyper- or hypopigmented scaling papules (0.5–1 cm), which may coalesce into larger plaques. Most commonly affects the upper trunk and arms. May be asymptomatic or pruritic.

Diagnostic Considerations: M. furfur also causes eosinophilic folliculitis in HIV, and catheter-acquired sepsis mostly in neonates or immunosuppressed patients. Diagnosis is clinical.

Pitfalls: Skin pigmentation may take months to return to normal after adequate therapy.

Prognosis: Excellent.

Eosinophilic Folliculitis (Malassezia furfur)

Clinical Presentation: Intensely pruritic folliculitis, usually on lower extremities.

Diagnostic Considerations: Tissue biopsy shows eosinophilic folliculitis. Diagnosis by demonstrating organism by culture on Sabouraud's agar overlaid with olive oil.

Pitfalls: Resembles folliculitis, but lesions are concentrated on lower extremities (not on trunk as with cutaneous candidiasis).

Prognosis: Related to degree of immunosuppression. Use oral therapy if topical therapy fails.

Myositis

Subset	Pathogens	Preferred Therapy
Chromomycosis	Cladosporium/ Fonsecaea	Itraconazole 200 mg (PO) q24h until cured **or** Terbinafine 250 mg (PO) q24h until cured
Trichinosis	Trichinella spiralis	Albendazole 400 mg (PO) q12h × 8–14 days **or** Mebendazole 200–400 mg (PO) q8h × 3 days, then 400–500 mg q8h × 10 days

Chromomycosis (Cladosporium/Fonsecaea)
Clinical Presentation: Subcutaneous/soft tissue nodules or verrucous lesions.
Diagnostic Considerations: Diagnosis by demonstrating organism by culture/tissue biopsy specimen.
Pitfalls: May resemble Madura foot or cause ulcerative lesions in muscle.
Prognosis: Related to degree of immunosuppression.

Trichinosis (Trichinella spiralis)
Clinical Presentation: Muscle tenderness, low-grade fevers, peripheral eosinophilia, conjunctival suffusion.
Diagnostic Considerations: Diagnosis by Trichinella serology or by demonstrating larvae in muscle biopsy.
Pitfalls: ESR is very low (approaching zero), unlike other causes of myositis, which have elevated ESRs.
Prognosis: Excellent with early treatment. Short-term steroids may be useful during acute phase. Therapy is ineffective against calcified larvae in muscle.

REFERENCES

TEXTBOOKS

Anaissie EJ, McGinnis MR. Pfaller MA (eds). Clinical Mycology (2nd Ed), Churchill Livingston, New York, 2009.

Arikan S Rex JH. Antifungal Drugs. In: Manual of Clinical Microbiology (8th Ed), ASM Press, Washington, D.C., 2003.

Bennett JE, Dolin R, Blaser MJ (eds). Mandell, Douglas, and Bennett's Principles and Practice of infectious Diseases (9th Ed), Philadelphia, Elsevier, 2019.

Bope ET, Kellerman RD (eds). Conn's Current Therapy. Elsevier, Philadelphia, PA, 2019.

Bottone EJ (ed). An Atlas of the Clinical Microbiology of Infectious Diseases, Volume 1. Bacterial Agents. The Parthenon Publishing Group, Boca Raton, 2004.

Bottone EJ (ed). An Atlas of the Clinical Microbiology of Infectious Diseases, Volume 2. Viral, fungal, and parasitic agents. Taylor and Francis, 2006.

Bryskier A (ed). Antimicrobial Agents. ASM Press, Washington, D.C., 2005.

Calderone RA (ed). Candida and Candidiasis. ASM Press, Washington D.C., 2002.

Cohen J, Powderly WG, Oral S. (eds). Infectious Diseases (4th Ed), Philadelphia: Elsevier, 2016.

Cook GC (ed). Manson's Tropical Diseases (24th Ed), WB Saunders Company, Ltd., London, 2014.

Cunha BA (ed). Tick-Borne Infectious Diseases. Marcel Dekker, New York, 2000.

Cunha CB, Scholssberg D (eds). Clinical Infectious Disease (3rd Ed), Cambridge University Press, Cambridge, 2020.

Despommier DD, Gwadz RW, Hotez PJ, Knirsch CA (eds). Parasitic Diseases (4th Ed), Apple Trees Productions, LLC, New York, 2000.

Garcia LS (ed). Practical guide to Diagnostic Medical Para-sitology. (5th Ed), ASM Press, Washington, DC, 2007.

Gorbach SL, Bartlett JG, Blacklow NR (eds). Infectious Diseases (3rd Ed), Philadelphia, Lippincott, Williams & Wilkins, 2004.

Guerrant RL, Walker DH, Weller PF (eds). Tropical Infectious Disease: Principles, Pathogens & Practice (3rd Ed), Elsevier, Philadelphia, 2011.

Gutierrez Y (ed). Diagnostic Pathology of Parasitic Infections with Clinical Correlations (2nd Ed), Oxford University Press, New York, 2000.

Howard DH (ed). Pathogenic Fungi in Humans and Animals (2nd Ed), New York, Marcel Dekker, 2003.

Jong E, Sanford C (eds). The Travel and Tropical Medicine Manual (4th Ed), Philadelphia: Saunders Elsevier, 2008.

Keystone JS, Kozarsky PE, Freedman DO, Nothdurft HO, Connor B. Travel Medicine (2nd Ed), Philadelphia: Mosby Elsevier, 2008.

Knipe DM, Howley PM (eds). Fields, Virology (5th Ed), Lippincott Williams & Wilkins, Philadelphia, 2008.

Krauss H, Weber A, Appel M (eds). Zoonoses. Infectious Diseases Transmissible from Animals to Humans (3rd Ed), ASM Press, Washington, D.C. 2003.

Maertens JA, Marr KA (eds). Diagnosis of Fungal Infections. Informa Healthcare, New York, 2007.

Porterfield JS (ed). Exotic Viral Infections. Chapman & Hall Medical, London, 1995.

Raoult D, Parola P. Rickettsial Diseases. Informa Healthcare, New York, 2007.

Richman DD, Whitley RJ, Hayden FG (eds). Clinical Virology (2nd Ed), ASM Press, Washington, DC, 2002.

Scholssberg DM (ed). Current Therapy of Infectious Diseases (3rd Ed), Mosby St. Louis, 2008.

Strickland GT (ed). Hunter's Tropical Medicine and Emerging Infectious Diseases (8th Ed), W.B. Saunders Company, Philadelphia, 2000.

Sun T (ed). Parasitic Disorders: Pathology, Diagnosis, and Management (2nd Ed), Williams & Wilkins, Baltimore, 1999.

Walker DH (ed). Biology of Rickettsial Diseases. CRC Press, Boca Raton, 2000.

Warrell DA, Gilles HM. Essential Malariology (4th Ed), Oxford University Press, New York, 2002.

Yu VL, Jr., Merigan TC, Jr., and Barriere SL (eds.). Antimicrobial Therapy & Vaccines (2nd Ed), Williams & Wilkins, Baltimore, MD, 2005.

Chapter 5

HIV Infection

Paul E. Sax, MD,
Jean E. Hage, MD,
Arthur Gran, MD,
Gina L. Wu, MD,
John Gian, MD,
Jeffrey Baron, PharmD
Amy Brotherton, PharmD

HIV OVERVIEW

Infection with Human Immunodeficiency Virus (HIV-1) leads to a chronic and without treatment usually fatal infection characterized by progressive immunodeficiency, a long clinical latency period, and opportunistic infections. The hallmark of HIV disease is infection and viral replication within T-lymphocytes expressing the CD_4 antigen (helper-inducer lymphocytes), a critical component of normal cell-mediated immunity. Qualitative defects in CD_4 responsiveness and progressive depletion in CD_4 cell counts increase the risk for opportunistic infections such as Pneumocystis (carinii) jiroveci pneumonia, and neoplasms such as lymphoma and Kaposi's sarcoma. HIV infection can also disrupt blood monocyte, tissue macrophage, and B-lymphocyte (humoral immunity) function, predisposing to infection with encapsulated bacteria. Direct attack of CD_4-positive cells in the central and peripheral nervous system can cause HIV meningitis, peripheral neuropathy, and dementia. More than 1 million people in the United States and 30 million people worldwide are infected with HIV. Without treatment, the average time from acquisition of HIV to an AIDS-defining opportunistic infection is about 10 years; survival then averages 1–2 years. There is tremendous individual variability in these time intervals, with some patients progressing from acute HIV infection to death within 1–2 years, and others not manifesting HIV-related immunosuppression for > 20 years after HIV acquisition. Antiretroviral therapy and prophylaxis against opportunistic infections have markedly improved the overall prognosis of HIV disease.

Figure 5.1 Diagnosis, Evaluation, and Treatment of HIV Infection

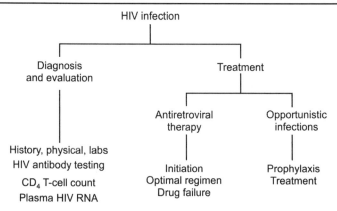

STAGES OF HIV INFECTION

A. **Viral Transmission.** HIV infection is acquired primarily by sexual intercourse (anal, vaginal, infrequently oral), exposure to contaminated blood (primarily needle transmission), or maternal-fetus (perinatal) transmission. Sexual practices with the highest risk of transmission include unprotected receptive anal intercourse (especially with mucosal tearing), unprotected receptive vaginal intercourse (especially during menses), and unprotected rectal/vaginal intercourse in the presence of genital ulcers (e.g., primary syphilis, genital herpes, chancroid). Lower risk sexual practices include insertive anal/vaginal intercourse and oral-genital contact. The risk of transmission after a single encounter with an HIV source has been estimated to be 1 in 150 with needle sharing, 1 in 300 with occupational percutaneous exposure, 1 in 300–1000 with receptive anal intercourse, 1 in 500–1250 with receptive vaginal intercourse, 1 in 1000–3000 with insertive vaginal intercourse, and 1 in 3000 with insertive anal intercourse. Transmission risk increases with the number of encounters and with higher HIV RNA plasma levels. The mode of transmission does not affect the natural history of HIV disease.

B. **Acute (Primary) HIV Infection.** Acute HIV occurs 1–4 weeks after transmission, and is accompanied by a burst of viral replication with a decline in CD_4 cell count. Most patients manifest a symptomatic mononucleosis-like syndrome, which is often overlooked. Acute HIV infection is confirmed by a high HIV RNA in the absence of HIV antibody.

C. **Seroconversion.** Development of a positive HIV antibody test usually occurs within 4 weeks of acute infection, and invariably (with few exceptions) by 6 months.

D. **Asymptomatic HIV Infection** lasts a variable amount of time (average 8–10 years), and is accompanied by a gradual decline in CD_4 cell counts and a relatively stable HIV RNA level (sometimes referred to as the viral "set point").

E. **Symptomatic HIV Infection.** Previously referred to as "AIDS Related Complex (ARC)," findings include thrush or vaginal candidiasis (persistent, frequent, or poorly responsive to treatment), cervical dysplasia/carcinoma in-situ, herpes zoster (recurrent episodes or involving multiple dermatomes), oral hairy leukoplakia, peripheral neuropathy, diarrhea, or constitutional symptoms (e.g., low-grade fevers, weight loss).

F. **AIDS** is defined by a CD_4 cell count < 200/mm³, a CD_4 cell percentage of total lymphocytes <14%, or one of several AIDS-related opportunistic infections. Common opportunistic infections include Pneumocystis (carinii) jiroveci pneumonia, cryptococcal meningitis, recurrent bacterial pneumonia, Candida esophagitis, CNS toxoplasmosis, tuberculosis, and non-Hodgkin's lymphoma. Other AIDS indicators in HIV-infected patients include candidiasis of the bronchi, trachea, or lungs; disseminated/extrapulmonary coccidiomycosis, cryptococcosis, or histoplasmosis; chronic (>1 month) intestinal cryptosporidiosis or isosporiasis; Kaposi's sarcoma;

lymphoid interstitial pneumonia/pulmonary lymphoid hyperplasia; disseminated/ extrapulmonary Mycobacterium (avium-intracellulare, kansasii, other species) infection; progressive multifocal leukoencephalopathy (PML); recurrent Salmonella septicemia; or HIV wasting syndrome.

G. Advanced HIV Disease is diagnosed when the CD_4 cell count is < 50/mm³. Most AIDS-related deaths occur at this point. Common late stage opportunistic infections are caused by CMV disease (retinitis, colitis) or disseminated Mycobacterium avium-intracellulare (MAI).

ACUTE (PRIMARY) HIV INFECTION

A. Description. Acute clinical illness associated with primary acquisition of HIV, occurring 1–4 weeks after viral transmission (range: 6 days to 6 weeks). Symptoms develop in 50–90%, but are often mistaken for the flu, mononucleosis, or other nonspecific viral syndrome. More severe symptoms may correlate with a higher viral set point and more rapid HIV disease progression. Even without therapy, most patients recover, reflecting development of a partially effective immune response and depletion of susceptible CD_4 cells.

B. Differential Diagnosis includes **EBV**, **CMV**, viral hepatitis, enteroviral infection, 2° syphilis, toxoplasmosis, HSV with erythema multiforme, drug reaction, Behcet's disease, acute lupus.

C. Signs and Symptoms usually reflect hematogenous dissemination of virus to lymphoreticular and neurologic sites:
- Fever (97%).
- Pharyngitis (73%). Typically non-exudative (unlike EBV, which is usually exudative).
- Rash (77%). Maculopapular viral exanthem of the face and trunk is most common, but can involve the extremities, palms and soles.
- Arthralgia/myalgia (58%).
- Neurologic symptoms (12%). Headache is most common. Neuropathy, Bell's palsy, and meningoencephalitis are rare, but may predict worse outcome.
- Oral/genital ulcerations, thrush, nausea, vomiting, diarrhea, weight loss.

D. Laboratory Findings
1. **CBC.** Lymphopenia followed by lymphocytosis (common). Atypical lymphocytosis is variable, but usually low level (unlike EBV, where atypical lymphocytosis may be 20–30% or higher). Thrombocytopenia occurs in some.
2. **Elevated transaminases** in some but not all patients.
3. **Depressed CD_4 cell count.** Can rarely be low enough to induce opportunistic infections.

4. **HIV antibody.** Usually negative, although persons with prolonged symptoms of acute HIV may have positive antibody tests if diagnosed late during the course of illness.

E. **Confirming the Diagnosis of Acute HIV Infection**
   1. **Obtain HIV antibody** after informed consent (if required by state law) to exclude prior disease.
   2. **Order viral load test (HIV RNA PCR),** preferably RT-PCR. HIV RNA confirms acute HIV infection prior to seroconversion. Most individuals will have very high HIV RNA (>100,000 copies/mL). Be suspicious of a false-positive test if the HIV RNA is low (< 20,000 copies/mL). For any positive test, it is important to repeat HIV RNA and HIV antibody testing. p24 antigen can also be used to establish the diagnosis, but is less sensitive than HIV RNA PCR.
   3. **Order other tests/serologies if HIV RNA test is negative.** Order throat cultures for bacterial/viral respiratory pathogens, EBV VCA IgM/IgG, CMV IgM/IgG, HHV-6 IgM/IgG, and hepatitis serologies as appropriate to establish a diagnosis for patient's symptoms.

F. **Management of Acute HIV Infection**
   1. **Initiate antiretroviral therapy.** The rationale behind this change is to treat a greater proportion of people with HIV, regardless of disease stage, is based on accumulating evidence of the benefits of earlier initiation of HIV treatment and, conversely, the potential for uncontrolled viral replication and CD_4 depletion.
   2. **Obtain HIV resistance genotype** because of a rising background prevalence of transmission of antiretroviral therapy-resistant virus. A genotype resistance test is preferred; therapy can be started pending results of the test.
   3. **Possible benefits for treatment of acute HIV infection.** Possible (but unproven) benefits include hastening symptom resolution, reducing viral transmission, lowering virologic "set point", and preserving virus-specific CD_4 responses.

APPROACH TO HIV TESTING

A. **Standard HIV Antibody Tests.** Most patients produce antibody to HIV within 6–8 weeks of exposure; half will have a positive antibody test in 3–4 weeks, and nearly 100% will have detectable antibody by 6 months.
   1. **ELISA.** Usual screening test. All positives must be confirmed with Western blot or other more specific tests.
   2. **Western blot.** CDC criteria for interpretation: **positive:** at least two of the following bands: p24, gp41, gp160/120; **negative:** no bands; **indeterminate:** any HIV band, but does not meet criteria for positivity.
   3. **Test performance.** Standard method is ELISA screen with Western blot confirmation.

    a. ELISA negative: Western blot is not required (ELISA sensitivity 99.7%, specificity 98.5%). Obtain HIV RNA if acute HIV infection is suspected.

    b. ELISA positive: Confirm with Western blot. Probability that ELISA and Western blot are both false-positives is extremely low (< 1 per 140,000). Absence of p31 band could be a clue to a false positive Western blot.

    c. Unexpected ELISA/Western blot: Repeat test to exclude clerical/computer error.

4. Indeterminate Western Blot. Common clinical problem, affecting 4–20% of reactive ELISAs. Usually due to a single p24 band or other weak bands. Causes include seroconversion in progress, advanced HIV disease with loss of antibody response, cross-reacting antibody from pregnancy, blood transfusions, organ

Figure 5.2 Laboratory Markers for HIV-1 Infection

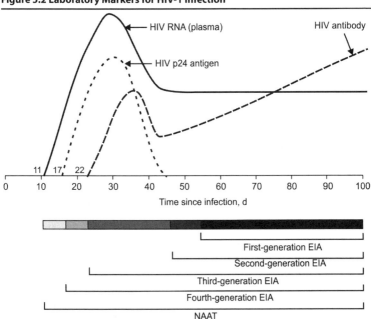

Adapted from: New York State Department of Health AIDS Institute www.hivguidelines.org and
Laboratory Testing for the Diagnosis of HIV Infection Updated Recommendations http://stacks.cdc.gov/view/cdc/23447

Earliest plasma markers for HIV-1 infection are HIV-1 RNA (ribonucleic acid) and HIV-1 p24 antigen. HV-1 RNA can be detected by nucleic acid amplification (NAAT) on day 10 post-infection while HIV-1 p24 antigen can be detected by 4th generation immunoassay on day 15 post-infection. IgM antibodies against HIV-1 can be detected by 4th generation and 3rd generation immunoassays on day 22 post-infection. The IgG antibodies that occur later can be detected by 2nd generation immunoassay (day 38 post-infection) and by 1st generation immunoassay (day 45–50 post-infection).

transplantation, autoantibodies from collagen vascular disease, infection with HIV-2, influenza vaccination, or recipient of HIV vaccine. In low-risk patients, an indeterminate result almost never represents true HIV infection. Since seroconversion in progress is generally associated with high HIV RNA levels, the recommended approach is to order an HIV RNA test.

B. Quantitative Plasma HIV RNA (HIV Viral Load Assays)

1. **Description.** Measures amount of HIV RNA in plasma. High sensitivity of assays allows detection of virus in most patients not on antiviral therapy. Used to diagnose acute HIV infection and more commonly to monitor the response to antiretroviral therapy.

2. **Uses of HIV RNA Assay**

   a. **Confirms diagnosis of acute HIV infection.** A high HIV RNA with a negative HIV antibody test confirms acute HIV infection prior to seroconversion.

   b. **Helpful in initial evaluation of HIV infection.** Establishes baseline HIV RNA and helps (along with CD_4 cell count) determine whether to initiate or defer therapy, as HIV RNA correlates with rate of CD_4 decline.

   c. **Monitors response to antiviral therapy.** HIV RNA changes rapidly decline 2–4 weeks after starting or changing effective antiretroviral therapy, with slower decline thereafter. Patients with the greatest HIV RNA response have the best clinical outcome. No change in HIV RNA suggests therapy will be ineffective.

   d. **Estimates risk for opportunistic infection.** For patients with similar CD_4 cell counts, the risk of opportunistic infections is higher with higher HIV RNAs.

   e. **Correlation between HIV RNA and CD_4.** HIV RNA assays correlate inversely with CD_4 cell counts, but do so imperfectly (e.g., some patients with high CD_4 counts have relatively high HIV RNA levels, and vice versa.) For any given CD_4, higher HIV RNA levels correlate with more rapid CD_4 decline. In response to antiretroviral therapy, changes in HIV RNA generally precede changes in CD_4 cell count.

   f. **Significant change in HIV RNA assay** is defined by at least a 2-fold (0.3 log) change in viral RNA (accounts for normal variation in clinically stable patients), or a 3-fold (0.5 log) change in response to new antiretroviral therapy (accounts for intra-laboratory and patient variability). For example, if an HIV RNA result = 50,000 copies/mL, then the range of possible actual values = 25,000–100,000 copies/mL, and the value needed to demonstrate antiretroviral activity is ≤ 17,000 copies/mL.

3. **Indications for HIV RNA Testing.** Usually performed in conjunction with CD_4 cell counts. Indicated for the diagnosis of acute HIV infection, and for initial evaluation of newly diagnosed HIV. Also recommended 2–8 weeks after initiation of antiretroviral therapy and every 3–4 months in all HIV patients.

4. When to Avoid HIV RNA Testing

a. **During acute illnesses and immunizations.** Patients with acute infections (opportunistic infection, bacterial pneumonia, even HSV recurrences) may experience significant (> 5-fold) rises in HIV RNA, which return to baseline 1–2 months after recovery. Although data are conflicting, many studies show at least a transient increase in HIV RNA levels following influenza and other immunizations, which return to baseline after 1–2 months.

b. **When results of test would not influence therapy.** Frequent scenario in patients with advanced disease who have no antiretroviral options or cannot tolerate therapy.

c. **As a screening test for HIV infection,** except if acute (primary) HIV disease is suspected during the HIV antibody window (i.e., first 3–6 weeks after viral transmission).

INITIAL ASSESSMENT OF HIV INFECTION

A. Clinical Evaluation. History and physical exam should focus on diagnoses associated with HIV infection. Compared to patients without HIV, the severity, frequency, and duration of these conditions are usually increased in HIV disease.

1. **Dermatologic:** Severe herpes simplex (oral/anogenital); herpes zoster (especially recurrent, cranial nerve, or disseminated); molluscum contagiosum; staphylococcal abscesses; tinea nail infections; Kaposi's sarcoma (from HHV-8 infection); petechiae (from ITP); seborrheic dermatitis; new or worsening psoriasis; eosinophilic pustular folliculitis; severe cutaneous drug eruptions (especially sulfonamides).

2. **Oropharyngeal:** Oral candidiasis; oral hairy leukoplakia (from EBV); Kaposi's sarcoma (most commonly on palate or gums); gingivitis/periodontitis; warts; aphthous ulcers (especially esophageal/perianal).

3. **Constitutional symptoms:** Fatigue, fevers, chronic diarrhea, weight loss.

4. **Lymphatic:** Persistent, generalized lymphadenopathy.

5. **Others:** Active TB (especially extrapulmonary); non-Hodgkin's lymphoma (especially CNS); unexplained leukopenia, anemia, thrombocytopenia (especially ITP); myopathy; miscellaneous neurologic conditions (cranial peripheral neuropathies, Guillain-Barre syndrome, mononeuritis multiplex, aseptic meningitis, cognitive impairment).

B. Baseline Laboratory Testing (Table 5.1)

C. CD_4 Cell Count (lymphocyte subset analysis)

1. **Overview.** Acute HIV infection is characterized by a decline in CD_4 cell count, followed by a gradual rise associated with clinical recovery. Chronic HIV infection shows progressive declines (~ 50–80 cells/year) in CD_4 cell count without treatment, followed by more rapid decline 1–2 years prior to opportunistic infection (AIDS-defining diagnosis). Cell counts remain stable

over 5–10 years in 5% of patients, while others may show rapid declines (> 300 cells/year). Since variability exists within individual patients and between laboratories, it is useful to *repeat any value before making management decisions.*

2. **Uses of CD$_4$ Cell Count**
   a. **Gives context of degree of immunosuppression** for interpretation of symptoms/signs (Table 5.2).
   b. **Used to guide therapy.** Guidelines support CD$_4$ < 500/mm^3 as the threshold for initiating treatment, regardless of HIV RNA or symptoms. For prophylaxis against PCP, toxoplasmosis, and MAI/CMV infection, CD$_4$ cell counts of 200/mm^3, < 100/mm^3, and < 50/mm^3 are used as threshold levels, respectively.
   c. **Provides estimate of risk of opportunistic infection or death.** CD$_4$ cell counts < 50/mm^3 are associated with a markedly increased risk of death (median survival 1 year), although some patients with low counts survive > 3 years even without antiretroviral therapy. Prognosis is heavily influenced by HIV RNA, presence/history of opportunistic infections or neoplasms, performance status, and the immune reconstitution response to antiretroviral therapy.

D. HIV RNA Assay (HIV RNA PCR)

Table 5.1 Baseline Laboratory Testing for HIV infected Patients

Test	Rationale
Repeat HIV serology (ELISA/confirmatory Western blot)	Indicated for patients unable to document a prior positive test, and for "low risk" individuals with a positive test (to detect computer/clerical error). Repeat serology is now less important since HIV RNA testing provides an additional means of confirming HIV infection.
CBC with differential, platelets	Detects cytopenias (e.g., ITP) seen in HIV. Needed to calculate CD$_4$ cell count.
Chemistry panel ("SMA 20") and fasting lipid panel	Detects renal dysfunction and electrolyte/LFT abnormalities, which may accompany HIV and associated infections (e.g., HIV nephropathy, HCV). Provides baseline lipid profile (many antiretroviral drugs can affect lipids).
CD$_4$ cell count	Determines the need for antiretroviral therapy and opportunistic infection (OI) prophylaxis. Best test for defining risk of OIs and prognosis.
HIV RNA assay ("viral load")	Provides a marker for the pace of HIV disease progression. Determines indication for and response to antiretroviral therapy.

Table 5.1 Baseline Laboratory Testing for HIV-infected Patients *(cont'd)*

Test	Rationale
Tuberculin skin test (standard 5 TU of PPD)	Detects latent TB infection and targets patients for preventive therapy. Anergy skin tests are no longer indicated due to poor predictive value. HIV is the most powerful co-factor for the development of active TB.
PAP smear	Risk of cervical cancer is nearly twice as high in HIV-positive women compared to uninfected controls.
HLA-B*5701	Needed if Abacavir therapy is planned, to assess risk for severe Abacavir hypersensitivity reactions.
Toxoplasmosis serology (IgG)	Identifies patients at risk for subsequent cerebral/systemic toxoplasmosis and the need for prophylaxis. Those with negative tests should be counseled on how to avoid infection.
Syphilis serology (VDRL or RPR)	Identifies co-infection with syphilis, which is epidemiologically-linked to HIV. Disease may have accelerated course in HIV patients.
Hepatitis C serology (anti-HCV)	Identifies HCV infection and usually chronic carriage. If positive, follow with HCV genotype and HCV viral load assay. If the patient is antibody-negative and at high risk for hepatitis, order HCV RNA to exclude a false-negative result.
Hepatitis B serologies (HBsAb, HBcAb, HBsAg)	Identifies patients who are immune to hepatitis B (HBsAb) or chronic carriers (HBsAg). If all three are negative, hepatitis B vaccine is indicated.
G6PD screen	Identifies patients at risk for dapsone or primaquine associated hemolysis.
CMV serology (IgG)	Identifies patients who should receive CMV negative or leukocyte-depleted blood if transfused.
VZV serology (IgG)	Identifies patients at risk for varicella (chickenpox), and those who should avoid contact with active varicella or herpes zoster patients. Serology-negative patients exposed to chickenpox should receive varicella-zoster immune globulin (VZIG).
Chest X-ray	Sometimes ordered as a baseline test for future comparisons. May detect healed granulomatous diseases/other processes. Indicated in all tuberculin skin test positive patients.

Table 5.2 Use of CD$_4$ Cell Count for Interpretation of Patient Signs/Symptoms

CD$_4$ Cell Count (cells/mm³)	Associated Conditions
> 500	Most illnesses are similar to those in HIV negative patients. Some increased risk of bacterial infections (pneumococcal pneumonia, sinusitis), herpes zoster, tuberculosis, skin conditions.
200–500*	Bacterial infections (especially pneumococcal pneumonia, sinusitis), cutaneous Kaposi's sarcoma, vaginal candidiasis, ITP.
50–200*	Thrush, oral hairy leukoplakia, classic HIV-associated opportunistic infections (e.g., PCP, cryptococcal meningitis, toxoplasmosis). For patients receiving prophylaxis, most opportunistic infection do not occur until CD$_4$ cell counts fall significantly below 100/mm³.
< 50*	"Final common pathway" opportunistic infections (disseminated M. avium complex, CMV retinitis), HIV associated wasting, neurologic disease (neuropathy, encephalopathy).

* Patients remain at risk for all processes noted in earlier stages.

INDICATIONS FOR TREATMENT OF HIV INFECTION

Table 5.3 Initiation of Antiretroviral Therapy in HIV-1 Infected Patients

Clinical Condition and/or CD$_4$ count	Recommendation
Symptomatic HIV disease	ART strongly recommended regardless of CD$_4$ cell count
Pregnant women	
HIV-1 RNA > 100,000 copies/mm³	
Rapid decline in CD$_4$ cell count, >100 cells/mm³ per year	
Acute hepatitis B coinfection	
Acute hepatitis C coinfection	
Active or high risk for cardiovascular disease	
HIV-associated neuropathy	
Symptomatic primary HIV infection	
High risk for secondary HIV transmission (e.g., serodiscordant couples)	
Asymptomatic (any CD$_4$ cell count)	ART is recommended

ART = antiretroviral therapy.

ANTIRETROVIRAL TREATMENT

Table 5.4 ART for Treatment-Naïve Individuals (DHHS Guidelines)

Regimen	Recommended Regimens for Most Patients	Recommended Regimens in Certain Clinical Situations
INSTI based (1 INSTI + 2 NRTIs)	Bictegravir/tenofovir alafenamide[a]/emtricitabine[b]: (BIC/TAF/FTC) **(Biktarvy)**[c] Dolutegravir[d]/abacavir[e]/lamivudine[b]: (DTG/ABC/3TC) **(Triumeq)**[c] Dolutegravir[d] (DTG) **(Tivicay)** *plus* tenofovir alafenamide[a]/emtricitabine[b] (TAF/FTC) **(Descovy)** *or* tenofovir disoproxil fumarate[a]/emtricitabine[b] (TDF/FTC) **(Truvada)** *or* tenofovir disoproxil fumarate[a]/lamivudine[b] (TDF/3TC) **(Cimduo)** Raltegravir[f] (RAL) **(Isentress)** *plus* tenofovir alafenamide[a]/emtricitabine[b] (TAF/FTC) **(Descovy)** *or* tenofovir disoproxil fumarate[a]/emtricitabine[b] (TDF/FTC) **(Truvada)** *or* tenofovir disoproxil fumarate[a]/lamivudine[b] (TDF/3TC) **(Cimduo)**	Elvitegravir/cobicistat[h]/tenofovir alafenamide[a]/emtricitabine[b]: (EVG/c/TAF/FTC) **(Genvoya)**[c,j] Elvitegravir/cobicistat[h]/tenofovir disoproxil fumarate[a]/emtricitabine[b]: (EVG/c/TDF/FTC) **(Stribild)**[c,i,j]
PI based (1 PI + 2 NRTIs)	None	Darunavir/cobicistat[h]/tenofovir alafenamide[a]/emtricitabine[b]: (DRV/c/TAF/FTC) **(Symtuza)**[c,j] Darunavir/ritonavir[h] (DRV/r) **(Prezista, Norvir)**[i] *or* darunavir/cobicistat[h] (DRV/c) **(Prezcobix)**[i] *plus* tenofovir alafenamide[a]/emtricitabine[b] (TAF/FTC) **(Descovy)** *or* tenofovir disoproxil fumarate[a]/emtricitabine[b] (TDF/FTC) **(Truvada)** *or* tenofovir disoproxil fumarate[a]/lamivudine[b] (TDF/3TC) **(Cimduo)** Atazanavir/ritonavir[h] (ATV/r) **(Reyataz, Norvir)**[i] *or* atazanavir/cobicistat[h] (ATV/c) **(Evotaz)**[i] *plus* tenofovir alafenamide[a]/emtricitabine[b] (TAF/FTC) **(Descovy)** *or* tenofovir disoproxil fumarate[a]/emtricitabine[b] (TDF/FTC) **(Truvada)** *or* tenofovir disoproxil fumarate[a]/lamivudine[b] (TDF/3TC) **(Cimduo)** Darunavir/ritonavir[h] (DRV/r) **(Prezista, Norvir)**[i] *or* darunavir/cobicistat[h] (DRV/c) **(Prezcobix)**[i] *plus* abacavir[e]/lamivudine[b] (ABC/3TC) **(Epzicom)**

Table 5.4 ART for Treatment-Naïve Individuals (DHHS Guidelines) *(cont'd)*

Regimen	Recommended Regimens for Most Patients	Recommended Regimens in Certain Clinical Situations
NNRTI based (1 NNRTI + 2 NRTIs)	None	Doravirine/tenofovir disoproxil fumarate[a]/lamivudine[b]: (DOR/TDF/3TC) **(Delstrigo)**[c]
		Doravirine (DOR) **(Pifeltro)** *plus* tenofovir alafenamide[a]/emtricitabine[b] (TAF/FTC) **(Descovy)**
		Efavirenz[k]/tenofovir disoproxil fumarate[a]/emtricitabine[b]: (EFV/TDF/FTC) **(Atripla)**
		Efavirenz[k]/tenofovir disoproxil fumarate[a]/lamivudine[b]: (EFV/TDF/3TC) **(Symfi, Symfi Lo)**
		Efavirenz[k] (EFV) **(Sustiva)** *plus* tenofovir alafenamide[a]/emtricitabine[b] (TAF/FTC) **(Descovy)**
		Rilpivirine[l]/tenofovir alafenamide[a]/emtricitabine[b]: (RPV/TAF/FTC) **(Odefsey)**[c,j]
		Rilpivirine[l]/tenofovir disoproxil fumarate[a]/emtricitabine[b]: (RPV/TDF/FTC) **(Complera)**[c,j]
Two-drug NRTI-sparing regimens[m]	Dolutegravir[d]/lamivudine[b]: (DTG/3TC) **(Dovato)**[c,g]	Dolutegravir[d]/lamivudine[b]: (DTG/3TC) **(Dovato)**[c,g]
		Darunavir/ritonavir[h] (DRV/r) **(Prezista, Norvir)**[i] *plus* lamivudine (3TC) **(Epivir)**
		Darunavir/ritonavir[h] (DRV/r) **(Prezista, Norvir)**[i] *plus* raltegravir (RAL) **(Isentress)**[n]

3TC, lamivudine; ABC, abacavir; ATV/c, atazanavir/cobicistat; ATV/r, atazanavir/ritonavir; BIC, bictegravir; DOR, doravirine; DRV, darunavir; DRV/c, darunavir/cobicistat; DRV/r, darunavir/ritonavir; DTG, dolutegravir; EFV, efavirenz; EVG, elvitegravir; EVG/c, elvitegravir/cobicistat; FTC, emtricitabine; INSTI, integrase strand transfer inhibitor; NNRTI, nonnucleoside reverse transcriptase inhibitor; NRTI, nucleoside analog reverse transcriptase inhibitor; PI, protease inhibitor; RAL, raltegravir; RPV, rilpivirine; TAF, tenofovir alafenamide; TDF, tenofovir disoproxil fumarate.

[a] TAF and TDF are two different forms of tenofovir; TAF is associated with fewer kidney and bone toxicities; TDF is not recommended in patients with or at risk for kidney or bone disease (osteoporosis or osteopenia).

[b] 3TC may substitute for FTC or vice versa.

[c] Available as a single-tablet regimen.

[d] DTG-based regimens are considered an alternative option in those who are trying to conceive, or those of childbearing potential not using effective contraception, due to low but significant risk of neural tube defects if taken during conception.

[e] ABC use is contraindicated in patients who test positive for HLA-B*5701 allele and should be avoided or used with caution in patients with high cardiovascular risk.

[f] RAL can be given as RAL 400 mg twice daily or RAL 1200 mg (two, 600-mg tablets) once daily.

[g] Not for use in individuals with HIV RNA >500,000 copies/mL, HBV co-infection, or in whom ART must be started prior to the results of HIV genotypic resistance testing or HBV testing.

[h] Cobicistat and ritonavir are potent cytochrome P450 3A4 inhibitors and can increase the concentration of other drugs metabolized by this pathway.

[i] Administer with food.

[j] EVG/c/TDF/FTC should not be started in patients with an estimated CrCl <70 mL/min and should be changed to an alternative regimen if the patient's CrCl falls below 50 mL/min.

[k] EFV should be administered at bedtime on an empty stomach; EFV is a potent cytochrome P450 3A4 inducer and can decrease the concentration of other drugs metabolized by this pathway.

[l] RPV requires acid for absorption and is contraindicated with proton pump inhibitors; RPV is not recommended in patients with pretreatment HIV RNA >100,000 copies/mL or pretreatment CD4 counts of <200 cells/mm³

[m] Consider when ABC, TAF, and TDF cannot be used.

[n] DRV/r plus RAL is not recommended in patients with pretreatment HIV RNA >100,000 copies/mL

https://aidsinfo.nih.gov/guidelines.

Table 5.4 ART for Treatment-Naïve Individuals (DHHS Guidelines) *(cont'd)*

<u>**Preferred ART Regimens for Pregnant Women**</u>
Two-NRTI Backbone:
    Abacavir (ABC)/lamivudine (3TC) **(Epzicom)**
    Tenofovir disoproxil fumarate (TDF)/emtricitabine (FTC) **(Truvada)**
    Tenofovir disoproxil fumarate (TDF)/lamivudine (3TC) **(Cimduo)**
INSTI-based Regimens:
    Raltegravir (RAL) **(Isentress)** *plus* Preferred 2-NRTI Backbone
        Note: <u>**Twice-daily dosing**</u> of RAL is required in pregnancy
    Dolutegravir (DTG) **(Tivicay)** *plus* Preferred 2-NRTI Backbone
        Note: DTG use at conception and in early pregnancy has been associated with a small but
        potential increased risk of neural tube defects; this should be discussed with patients to
        ensure informed decision making
PI-based regimens:
    Atazanavir (ATV)/r **(Reyataz/Norvir)** *plus* Preferred 2-NRTI Backbone
    Darunavir (DRV)/r **(Prezista/Norvir)** *plus* Preferred 2-NRTI Backbone
        Note: <u>**Twice-daily dosing**</u> of DRV is required in pregnancy
<u>**Alternate Regimens**</u>
PI-based:
    Lopinavir (LPV)/r **(Kaletra)** *plus* Preferred 2-NRTI Backbone
        Note: <u>**Twice-daily dosing**</u> of LPV/r is required in pregnancy
NNRTI-based:
    Efavirenz (EFV)/tenofovir disoproxil fumarate (TDF)/emtricitabine (FTC) **(Atripla)**
    Efavirenz (EFV)/tenofovir disoproxil fumarate (TDF)/lamivudine (3TC) **(Symfi)**
    Efavirenz (EFV) **(Sustiva)** *plus* Preferred 2-NRTI Backbone
    Rilpivirine (RPV)/tenofovir disoproxil fumarate (TDF)/emtricitabine (FTC) **(Complera)**
    Rilpivirine (RPV) **(Edurant)** *plus* Preferred 2-NRTI Backbone

Selected Recommendations for Initial ART Regimens (IAS-USA Guidelines)

Regimen	Generally Recommended Initial Regimens	Regimens for those Who are Unable to Take Recommended Regimens
INSTI based (1 INSTI + 2 NRTIs)	Bictegravir/tenofovir alafenamide/emtricitabine: (BIC/TAF/FTC) **(Biktarvy)** Dolutegravir/abacavir/ lamivudine: (DTG/ABC/3TC) **(Triumeq)** Dolutegravir (DTG) **(Tivicay)** plus tenofovir alafenamide/emtricitabine (TAF/FTC) **(Descovy)**	Elvitegravir/cobicistat/tenofovir alafenamide/emtricitabine: (EVG/c/TAF/FTC) **(Genvoya)** Elvitegravir/cobicistat/tenofovir disoproxil fumarate/emtricitabine: (EVG/c/TDF/FTC) **(Stribild)** Raltegravir (RAL) **(Isentress)** plus tenofovir alafenamide/emtricitabine (TAF/FTC) **(Descovy)** or tenofovir disoproxil fumarate/ emtricitabine (TDF/FTC) **(Truvada)**
PI-based (1 PI + 2 NRTIs)		Darunavir/cobicistat/tenofovir alafenamide/ emtricitabine: (DRV/c/TAF/FTC) **(Symtuza)** Darunavir/ritonavir (DRV/r) **(Prezista, Norvir)** or darunavir/cobicistat (DRV/c) **(Prezcobix)** plus tenofovir alafenamide/emtricitabine (TAF/FTC) **(Descovy)** or tenofovir disoproxil fumarate/emtricitabine (TDF/FTC) **(Truvada)**
NNRTI based (1 NNRTI + 2 NRTIs)		Efavirenz/tenofovir disoproxil fumarate/ emtricitabine: (EFV/TDF/FTC) **(Atripla)** Rilpivirine/tenofovir alafenamide/ emtricitabine: (RPV/TAF/FTC) **(Odefsey)** Rilpivirine/tenofovir disoproxil fumarate/ emtricitabine: (RPV/TDF/FTC) **(Complera)**

https://www.iasusa.org/guidelines

ANTIRETROVIRAL TREATMENT FAILURE

Antiretroviral treatment failure can be defined in various ways, as described herewith. Causes of treatment failure include inadequate adherence, pre-existing drug resistance, regimen complexity, side effects, and suboptimal pharmacokinetics. All of these factors can lead to persistent viral replication and evolution of drug resistance. Poor medication adherence is the most common cause of treatment failure.

A. Types of Treatment Failure

1. **Virologic Failure** is most strictly defined as the inability to achieve or maintain virologic suppression. In a treatment-naïve patient, the HIV RNA level should be < 400 copies/mL after 24 weeks or < 50 copies/mL by 48 weeks after starting therapy. Virologic rebound is seen when there is repeated detection of HIV RNA after virologic suppression in either treatment-naïve or treatment-experienced patients.

2. **Immunologic Failure** can occur in the presence or absence of virologic failure and is defined as a failure to increase the CD_4 cell count by 25–50 cells/mm^3 above baseline during the first year of therapy, or as a decrease in CD_4 cell count to below baseline count while on therapy.

3. **Clinical Failure** is the occurrence or recurrence of HIV-related events after at least 3 months on potent antiretroviral therapy, excluding events related to an immune reconstitution syndrome.

4. **Usual Sequence of Treatment Failure.** Virologic failure usually occurs first, followed by immunologic failure, and finally by clinical progression. These events may be separated by months or years and may not occur in this order in all patients.

B. Goals After Virologic Failure. When patients have detectable HIV RNA on treatment, clinicians should attempt to identify the cause of their lack of response and set a treatment goal of achieving full virologic suppression (HIV RNA < 50 copies/mL). In addition to improving clinical and immunologic outcomes, this strategy will also prevent the selection of additional resistance mutations. Provided that medication adherence issues and regimen tolerability have been addressed, the regimen should be changed sooner than later. On the other hand, achieving an undetectable HIV RNA level in patients with an extensive prior treatment history may not be possible. The main goals in these patients should be partial suppression of HIV RNA below the pretreatment level to preserve immune function and prevent clinical progression.

C. Resistance Testing and Selection of New Antiretroviral Therapy. Genotypic assays characterize nucleotide sequences of the reverse transcriptase/protease portions of the virus, and identify resistance mutations associated with various drugs. Phenotypic assays attempt to grow the virus in the presence of drugs, providing a more intuitively applicable measurement of resistance (similar to that done with bacteria). Compared to phenotypic assays, genotypic assays are faster (1–2 weeks vs. 2–4 weeks for results), less expensive ($400 vs. $1000), and have less inter-laboratory variability; however, mutations do not always correlate with resistance and results are difficult to interpret.

Table 5.5 Management of Antiretroviral Treatment Failure

Type of Failure	Recommended Approach	Comments
Limited or intermediate prior treatment	Assess for adherence and regimen tolerability. Obtain genotype resistance test. Select new regimen based on resistance test results and tolerability.	Usually associated with limited or no detectable resistance. If no resistance is found, consider re-testing for resistance 2–4 weeks after resuming antivirals. Stop NNRTIs if resistance is detected. Virologic suppression is likely if adherence is good.
Extensive prior treatment	Assess for adherence and regimen tolerability. Obtain resistance test – consider phenotype, "virtual phenotype," or phenotype-genotype combination if level of resistance is likely to be high. Obtain viral tropism assay to assess possible use of CCR5 antagonist. Select new regimen using at least 2 new active agents; if 2 new active agents not available, continue a "holding" regimen.	In patients with resistance to NRTIs, NNRTIs and PIs, the new regimen should generally contain at least: (1) at least one drug from a new drug class (integrase inhibitor, CCR5 antagonist, or fusion inhibitor); (2) a boosted PI with activity against resistant viruses (tipranavir or darunavir); and (3) one or two NRTIs, one of them 3TC or FTC. A holding regimen should always contain 3TC or FTC plus a boosted PI; NNRTIs should never be used.
Low-level HIV RNA (50–1000 copies)	Assess for adherence, drug-drug interactions, intercurrent illness, recent immunizations. Repeat test in 3–4 weeks.	For low-level viremia followed by undetectable HIV RNA ("blip"), no treatment change is necessary. If HIV RNA is persistently detectable at > 500 copies/mL, obtain resistance test as described above, and treat accordingly. If HIV RNA is persistently detectable at 50–500 copies/mL, consider regimen "intensification" with use of an additional agent.

Table 5.5 Management of Antiretroviral Treatment Failure *(cont'd)*

Type of Failure	Recommended Approach	Comments
<u>Immunologic failure</u> *Detectable HIV RNA*	Assess for adherence and tolerability. If non-adherent, resume treatment after barriers to adherence are addressed. If adherent, obtain resistance testing and alter therapy as described above.	If HIV RNA is back to pretreatment baseline, nonadherence is the most likely explanation.
Suppressed HIV RNA	Investigate for modifiable conditions that may be associated with impaired CD_4 response (chronic HCV, treatment with ZDV, TDF + ddI). If no modifiable conditions found, continue current regimen.	Prognosis for patients with suppressed HIV RNA and immunologic failure better than for those with comparable CD_4 cell counts and detectable viremia.
<u>Clinical failure</u> *Detectable HIV RNA*	Treat OI with appropriate anti-infective therapy. Assess for antiretroviral adherence and tolerability. Send resistance test and choose new regimen based on results of test and other treatment options.	OIs (IRIS excluded) most commonly occur in those not on antiretroviral therapy due to poor compliance and/or regimen tolerability.
Suppressed HIV RNA	Continue current antiretrovirals. Treat OI with appropriate anti-infective therapy. If symptoms persist and IRIS is likely, use adjunctive corticosteroids.	IRIS most likely when baseline CD_4 cell count is low (< 200/mm³); onset usually weeks-to-months after starting a potent regimen. IRIS been reported with virtually all OIs. True clinical progression with suppressed HIV RNA is unusual; IRIS should not be considered a sign of treatment failure.

IRIS = immune reconstitution inflammatory syndrome, OI = opportunistic infection.

PROPHYLAXIS OF OPPORTUNISTIC INFECTIONS IN HIV

Patients with HIV disease are at risk for infectious complications not otherwise seen in immunocompetent patients. Such opportunistic infections occur in proportion to the severity of immune system dysfunction (reflected by CD_4 cell count depletion). While community acquired infections (e.g., pneumococcal pneumonia) can occur at any CD_4 cell count, "classic" HIV-related opportunistic infections (PCP, toxoplasmosis, cryptococcus, disseminated M. avium-intracellulare, CMV) do not occur until CD_4 cell counts are dramatically reduced. Specifically, it is rare to encounter PCP in HIV patients with $CD_4 > 200/mm^3$, and CMV and disseminated MAI occur at median CD_4 cell counts $< 50/mm^3$.

Table 5.6 Overview of Prophylaxis

Infection	Indication	Intervention
PCP	$CD_4 < 200$ cells/mm^3	TMP–SMX
TB (M. tuberculosis)	PPD > 5 mm (current or past) or contact with active case	INH
Toxoplasma	IgG Ab (+) and $CD_4 < 100$ cells/mm^3	TMP–SMX
MAI	$CD_4 < 50/mm^3$	Azithromycin or Clarithromycin
S. pneumoniae	$CD_4 > 200/mm^3$	Pneumococcal vaccine
Hepatitis B (HBV)	Susceptible patients	Hepatitis B vaccine
Hepatitis A (HAV)	HCV (+) and HA Ab (–); HCV (–) and HA Ab (–) gay men and travelers to endemic areas, chronic liver disease	Hepatitis A vaccine
Influenza	All patients	Annual flu vaccine Swine influenza (H_1N_1) vaccine
VZV	Exposure to chickenpox or shingles; no prior history	VZIG

Abbreviations: Ab = antibody; HAV = Hepatitis A virus; HCV = Hepatitis C virus; VZIG = varicella-zoster immune globulin; VZV = varicella- zoster virus; other abbreviations (p. xi).

Table 5.7 Prophylaxis of Opportunistic Infections in HIV

Opportunistic infections	Indication	Preferred	Alternative
Pneumocystis (carinii) jiroveci pneumonia (PCP)	**Start:** CD4 < 200 cells/mm^3 **or** History of AIDS defining illness **Stop:** CD_4 > 200 cell/mm^3 after > 3 months on ART	TMP-SMX 1 DS (PO) q24h	TMP-SMX 1 DS (PO) three times weekly **or** Dapsone 100 mg (PO) q24h or 50 mg (PO) q12h **or** Atovaquone 1500 mg (PO) q24h
Disseminated Myobacterium avium complex (MAC)	**Start:** CD4 cells < 50 cells/mm^3 after ruling out active disseminated MAC disease **or** **Stop:** CD4 cells > 100 cell/mm^3 after > 3 months on ART	Azithromycin 1200 mg (PO) once weekly **or** Clarithromycin 500 mg (PO) q12h **or** Azithromycin 600 mg (PO) twice weekly	Rifabutin (dose adjusted based on concomitant ART); rule out active TB before starting rifabutin
Mycobacterium tuberculosis (TB)	**Start:** Positive screening test for LTB with no evidence of active TB and no prior treatment for active TB or LTB Close contact with a person with infectious TB, with no evidence of active TB, regardless of screening test results **Stop:** after completion of TB treatment course	Isoniazid (NH) 300 mg (PO) q24h + Pyridoxine 25 mg (PO) q24h × 9 months **or** Isoniazid (INH) 900 mg (PO) twice weekly (by DOT) + Pyridoxine 25 mg (PO) q24h × 9 months	Rifampin 600 mg (PO) q24h × 4 months **or** Rifabutin (dose adjusted based on concomitant ART) × 4 months

Table 5.7 Prophylaxis of Opportunistic Infections *(cont'd)*

Opportunistic infections	Indication	Preferred	Alternative
Toxoplasma gondii encephalitis	**Start:** Toxoplasma IgG positive with CD_4 < 100 cells/mm^3 **Stop:** CD_4 > 200 cell/mm^3 after >3 months on ART	TMP-SMX 1 DS (PO) q24h	TMP-SMX 1 DS (PO) three times weekly **or** Dapsone 50 mg (PO) q24h + Pyrimethamine 50 mg + leucovorin 25 mg) PO weekly **or** Dapsone 200 mg (PO) q24h + Pyrimethamine 75 mg + Leucovorin 25 mg) PO weekly **or** Atovaquone 1500 mg (PO) q24h

LTB, latent tuberculosis; TB, tuberculosis.

Infection	Indications and Prophylaxis	Comments
Pneumococcus (S. pneumoniae)	<u>Indications:</u> CD_4 > 200/mm^3 <u>Preferred prophylaxis:</u> Pneumococcal polysaccharide (23 valent) vaccine.* Re-vaccinate × 1 at 5 years	Incidence of invasive pneumococcal disease is > 100-fold higher in HIV patients. Efficacy of vaccine is variable in clinical studies.
Influenza (human seasonal)	<u>Indications:</u> Generally recommended for all patients <u>Preferred prophylaxis:</u> Influenza vaccine (inactivated whole virus and split virus vaccine)*	Give annually (optimally October–January). Some experts do not give vaccine if CD_4 is < 100/mm^3 (antibody response is poor). New intranasal live virus vaccine is contraindicated in immunosuppressed patients.
Hepatitis B (HBV)	<u>Indications:</u> All susceptible (anti-HBcAb negative and anti-HBsAg negative) patients <u>Preferred prophylaxis:</u> Hepatitis B recombinant DNA vaccine*	Response rate is lower than in HIV-negative controls. Repeat series if no response, especially if CD_4 was low during initial series and is now increased.
Hepatitis A (HAV)	<u>Indications:</u> All susceptible patients who are also infected with hepatitis C; HAV-susceptible seronegative gay men or travelers to endemic areas; chronic liver disease; illegal drug users <u>Preferred prophylaxis:</u> Hepatitis A vaccine*	Response rate is lower than in HIV-negative controls.

Table 5.7 Prophylaxis of Opportunistic Infections *(cont'd)*

Infection	Indications and Prophylaxis	Comments
Measles, mumps, rubella	<u>Indications:</u> Patients born after 1957 and never vaccinated; patients vaccinated between 1963–1967 <u>Preferred prophylaxis:</u> MMR (measles, mumps, rubella) vaccine*	Single case of vaccine-strain measles pneumonia in severely immuno-compromised adult who received MMR; vaccine is therefore contraindicated in patients with severe immunodeficiency (CD$_4$ < 200).
H. influenzae	<u>Indications:</u> Not generally recommended for adults <u>Preferred prophylaxis:</u> H. influenzae type B polysaccharide vaccine*	Incidence of H. influenzae disease is increased in HIV patients, but 65% are caused by non-type B strains. Unclear whether vaccine offers protection.
Travel vaccines*	<u>Indications:</u> Travel to endemic areas	All considered safe except oral polio, yellow fever, and live oral typhoid—each a live virus vaccine.

* Same dose as for normal hosts (see p. 372–375). If possible, give vaccines early in course of HIV infection, while immune system may still respond. Alternatively, to increase the likelihood of response in patients with advanced HIV disease, vaccines may be administered after 6–12 months of effective antiretroviral therapy. Vaccines should be given when patients are clinically stable, not acutely ill (e.g., give during a routine office visit, rather than during hospitalization for an opportunistic infection). Live vaccines (e.g., oral polio, oral typhoid, Yellow fever) are generally contraindicated, but measles vaccine is well-tolerated in children, and MMR vaccine is recommended for adults as described above.

TREATMENT OF OPPORTUNISTIC INFECTIONS

Antiretroviral therapy (ART) and specific antimicrobial prophylaxis regimens have led to a dramatic decline in HIV-related opportunistic infections. Today, opportunistic infections occur predominantly in patients not receiving ART (due to undiagnosed HIV infection or nonacceptance of therapy), or in the period after starting ART (due to lack of immune reconstitution or from eliciting a previously absent inflammatory host response). Despite high rates of virologic failure in clinical practice, the rate of opportunistic infections in patients compliant with ART remains low, presumably due to continued immunologic response despite virologic failure, a phenomenon that may be linked to impaired "fitness" (virulence) of resistant HIV strains. For patients on or off ART, the absolute CD$_4$ cell count provides the best marker of risk for opportunistic infections.

Respiratory Tract Opportunistic Infections

Aspergillosis, Invasive Pulmonary

Pathogen	Preferred Therapy	Alternate Therapy
Aspergillus fumigatus (rarely other species)	Voriconazole 400 mg (IV or PO) q12h × 2 days, then 200 mg (IV or PO) q12h until cured (typically 6–18 months)	Amphotericin B 1 mg/kg (IV) q24h until 2–3 gm total dose given (optimal duration of therapy poorly defined) **or** Lipid amphotericin (Abelcet or Ambisome) 5 mg/kg/day (IV) until cured

Clinical Presentation: Pleuritic chest pain, hemoptysis, cough in a patient with advanced HIV disease. Additional risk factors include neutropenia and use of cortico-steroids.

Diagnostic Considerations: Diagnosis by bronchoscopy with biopsy/culture. Open lung biopsy (usually video-assisted thorascopic surgery) is sometimes required. Radio-graphic appearance includes cavitation, nodules, sometimes focal consolidation. Dis-semination to CNS may occur, and manifests as focal neurological deficits.

Pitfalls: Positive sputum culture for Aspergillus in advanced HIV disease should heighten awareness of possible infection.

Therapeutic Considerations: Decrease/discontinue corticosteroids, if possible. If pres-ent, treat neutropenia with granulocyte-colony stimulating factor (G-CSF) to achieve absolute neutrophil count > 1000/mm^3. There are insufficient data to recommend chronic suppressive or maintenance therapy.

Prognosis: Poor unless immune deficits can be corrected.

Bacterial Pneumonia

Usual Pathogens	Preferred Therapy	Comments
Streptococcus pneumoniae (most common) Haemophilus influenzae Pseudomonas aeruginosa	**Monotherapy with** Levofloxacin 750 mg (PO/IV) q24h or Moxifloxacin 400 mg (PO/IV) q24h × 7–14 days **or combination therapy with** Ceftriaxone 1–2 gm (IV) q24h (or Cefotaxime 1 gm [IV] q8h) **plus** Azithromycin 500 gm q24h × 7–14 days	For severe immunodeficiency (CD$_4$ < 100/mm^3), neutropenia, or a prior history of pseudomonas infection, broaden coverage to include *P. aeruginosa* and other Gram-negative bacilli by adding **either** Cefepime 1 gm (IV) q12h **or** Ciprofloxacin 750 mg (PO) q12h or 400 mg (IV) q8h.

Clinical Presentation: HIV-infected patients with bacterial pneumonia present similar to those without HIV, with a relatively acute illness (over days) that is often associated with chills, rigors, pleuritic chest pain, and purulent sputum. Patients who have been ill over weeks to months are more likely have PCP, tuberculosis, or a fungal infection. Since bacterial pneumonia can occur at any CD_4 cell count, this infection is frequently the presenting symptom of HIV disease, prompting initial HIV testing and diagnosis.

Diagnostic Considerations: The most common pathogens are Streptococcus pneumoniae, followed by Haemophilus influenzae. The pathogens of atypical pneumonia (Legionella pneumophila, Mycoplasma pneumoniae, and Chlamydia pneumoniae) are rarely encountered, even with extensive laboratory investigation. A lobar infiltrate on chest radiography is a further predictor of bacterial pneumonia. Blood cultures should be obtained, as HIV patients have an increased rate of bacteremia compared to those without HIV.

Pitfalls: Sputum gram stain and culture are generally only helpful if collected prior to starting antibiotics, and only if a single organism predominates. HIV patients with bacterial pneumonia may rarely have a more subacute opportunistic infection concurrently, such as PCP or TB.

Therapeutic Considerations: Once improvement has occurred, a switch to oral therapy is generally safe. Patients with advanced HIV disease are at greater risk of bacteremic pneumonia due to gram-negative bacilli, and should be covered empirically for this condition.

Prognosis: Response to therapy is generally prompt and overall prognosis is good.

Pneumocystis (carinii) jiroveci Pneumonia (PCP)

Subset	Preferred Therapy	Alternate Therapy
Severe disease ($pO_2 < 70$ mm Hg, A-a gradient > 35)	TMP–SMX (5 mg/kg TMP) (IV) q6h × 21 days **plus** Prednisone 40 mg (PO) q12h on days 1–5, then 40 mg (PO) q24h on days 6–10, then 20 mg (PO) q24h on days 11–21. Methylprednisolone (IV) can be substituted at 75% of prednisone dose	Pentamidine 4 mg/kg (IV) q24h (infused over ≥ 60 minutes) × 21 days plus prednisone × 21 days **or** Primaquine 30 mg (PO) q24h × 21 days plus Clindamycin 600 mg (PO) q8h × 21 days
Mild or moderate disease ($pO_2 > 70$ mm Hg, A-a gradient < 35)	TMP–SMX 2 DS tablets (PO) q6h × 21 days	Dapsone 100 mg (PO) q24h × 21 days plus TMP 5 mg/kg (PO) q8h × 21 days **or** Primaquine 30 mg (PO) q24h × 21 days *plus* Clindamycin 600 mg (PO) q8h × 21 days **or** Atovaquone 750 mg (PO) q12h (with food) × 21 days

Clinical Presentation: Fever, cough, dyspnea; often indolent presentation. Progressive SOB usually over a week. Physical exam is usually normal. Chest x-ray is variable, but commonly shows a diffuse interstitial pattern. High A-a gradient with exercise desaturation.

Diagnostic Considerations: Diagnosis by immunofluorescent stain of induced sputum or bronchoscopy specimen. Highly elevated LDH. β 1,3 D-glucan (BG) + , aspergillus galactomannan (GM) – .

Pitfalls: Slight worsening of symptoms is common after starting therapy, especially if not treated with steroids. Do not overlook superimposed bacterial pneumonia or other secondary infections, especially while on pentamidine. Patients receiving second-line agents for PCP prophylaxis—in particular aerosolized pentamidine— may present with atypical radiographic findings, including apical infiltrates, multiple small-walled cysts, pleural effusions, pneumothorax, or single/multiple nodules.

Therapeutic Considerations: Outpatient therapy is possible for mild disease, but only when close follow-up is assured. Adverse reactions to TMP–SMX (rash, fever, GI symptoms, hepatitis, hyperkalemia, leukopenia, hemolytic anemia) occur in 25–50% of patients, many of whom will need a second-line regimen to complete therapy (e.g., trimethoprim-dapsone or atovaquone). Unless an adverse reaction to TMP–SMX is particularly severe (e.g., Stevens-Johnson syndrome or other life-threatening problem), TMP–SMX may be considered for PCP prophylaxis, since prophylaxis requires a much lower dose (only 10–15% of treatment dose). Patients being treated for severe PCP with TMP–SMX who do not improve after one week may be switched to pentamidine, although there are no prospective data to confirm this approach. In general, patients receiving antiretroviral therapy when PCP develops should have their treatment continued, since intermittent antiretroviral therapy can lead to drug resistance. For newly-diagnosed or antiretroviral-naive HIV patients, treatment of PCP may be completed before starting antiretroviral therapy. Steroids should be tapered, not discontinued abruptly. Adjunctive steroids increase the risk of thrush/herpes simplex infection, but probably not CMV, TB, or disseminated fungal infection.

Prognosis: Usually responds to treatment. Adverse prognostic factors include ↑ A-a gradient, hypoxemia, ↑ LDH.

Pulmonary Tuberculosis (isolates sensitive to INH and Rifampin)

Pathogen	Patients NOT Receiving PIs or NNRTIs	Patients Receiving PIs or NNRTIs*
Mycobacterium tuberculosis (TB)	<u>Initial phase (8 weeks)</u> INH 300 mg (PO) q24h **plus** Rifampin† 600 mg (PO) q24h **plus** Pyrazinamide (PZA) 25 mg/kg (PO) q24h **plus** Ethambutol (EMB) 15–20 mg/kg (PO) q24h <u>Continuation phase (18 weeks)</u> INH 300 mg (PO) q24h **plus** Rifampin† 600 mg (PO) q24h	<u>Initial phase (8 weeks)</u> INH 300 mg (PO) q24h **plus** Rifabutin* **plus** PZA 25 mg/kg (PO) q24h **plus** EMB 15 mg/kg (PO) q24h × 8 weeks. <u>Continuation phase (18 weeks)</u> INH 300 mg (PO) q24h **plus** Rifabutin*

*   Rifabutin dose: If PI is nelfinavir, indinavir, amprenavir or fosamprenavir, then rifabutin dose is 150 mg (PO) q24h. If PI is ritonavir, lopinavir/ritonavir or atazanavir, then rifabutin dose is 150 mg (PO) 2–3 times weekly. If NNRTI is efavirenz, then rifabutin dose is 450 mg (PO) q24h or 600 mg (PO) 2–3 times weekly. If NNRTI is nevirapine, then rifabutin dose is 300 mg (PO) q24h. Rifabutin is **contraindicated** in patients receiving delavirdine rilpivirine, etravirine + ritonavir boosted PI or hard-gel saquinavir. <u>Patients receiving PIs AND NNRTIs</u>: as above, except adjust rifabutin to 300 mg (PO) q24h.

†   For patients receiving triple NRTI regimens, substitute rifabutin 300 mg (PO) q24h for rifampin.

Clinical Presentation: HIV patients with high (> 500/mm³) CD_4 cell counts are more likely to have a typical pulmonary presentation, but patients with advanced HIV disease may have a diffuse interstitial pattern, hilar adenopathy, or a normal chest x-ray. Tuberculin skin testing (TST) is helpful if positive, but unreliable if negative due to anergy.

Diagnostic Considerations: In many urban areas, TB is one of the most common HIV-related respiratory illnesses. In other areas, HIV-related TB occurs infrequently. Maintain a high Index of suspicion for TB in HIV patients with unexplained fevers/pulmonary infiltrates. Urinary lipoarabinomannan glycan (LAM) test useful in smear negative HIV patients.

Pitfalls: Extrapulmonary and pulmonary TB often coexist, especially in advanced HIV disease.

Therapeutic Considerations: Treatment by directly observed therapy (DOT) is strongly recommended for all HIV patients. If patients have cavitary disease or either positive sputum cultures or lack of clinical response at 2 months, total duration of therapy should be increased up to 9 months. If hepatic transaminases are elevated (AST > 3 times normal) before treatment initiation, treatment options include: (1) standard therapy with frequent monitoring; (2) rifamycin (rifampin or rifabutin) + EMB + PZA for 6 months; or (3) INH + rifamycin + EMB for 2 months, then INH + rifamycin for 7 months. Once-weekly rifapentine is not recommended for HIV patients. Non-severe immune reconstitution inflammatory syndrome (IRIS) may be treated with nonsteroidal anti-inflammatory drugs (NSAIDs); severe cases should be treated with corticosteroids. In all cases of IRIS, antiretroviral therapy should be continued if possible. Monitor carefully for signs of rifabutin drug toxicity (arthralgias, uveitis, leukopenia).

Prognosis: Usually responds to treatment. Relapse rates are related to the degree of immunosuppression and local risk of re-exposure to TB.

CNS Opportunistic Infections

CMV Retinitis

Preferred Therapy, Duration of Therapy, Chronic Maintenance	Alternate Therapy	Other Options/Issues
Preferred therapy for CMV retinitis *For immediate sight-threatening lesions* Ganciclovir intraocular implant + valganciclovir 900 mg (PO) q12h for 14–21 days, then q24h daily) One dose of intravitreal ganciclovir may be administered immediately after diagnosis until ganciclovir implant can be placed *For small peripheral lesions* Valganciclovir 900 mg (PO) q12h × 14–21 days, then 900 mg (PO) q24h	Alternative therapy for CMV retinitis Ganciclovir 5 mg/kg (IV) q12h × 14–21 days, then 5 mg/kg (IV) q24h; **or** Ganciclovir 5 mg/kg (IV) q12h × 14–21 days, then Valganciclovir 900 mg (PO) q24h **or** Foscarnet 60 mg/kg (IV) q8h or 90 mg/kg (IV) q12h × 14–21 days, then 90–120 mg/kg (IV) q24h; **or** Cidofovir 5 mg/kg (IV) q week × 2 weeks, then 5 mg/kg (IV) every other week with saline hydration before and after therapy plus probenecid 2 g (PO) 3 hours before the dose followed by 1 g (PO) 2 hours after the dose, and 1 g (PO) 8 hours after the dose (total of 4 g) **Note:** This regimen should be avoided in patients with sulfa allergy because of cross hypersensitivity with probenecid	The choice of initial therapy for CMV retinitis should be individualized, based on location and severity of the lesion(s), level of immunosuppression, and other factors such as concomitant medications and ability to adhere to treatment Initial therapy in patients with CMV retinitis, esophagitis, colitis, and pneumonitis should include initiation or optimization of ART In patients with CMV neurological disease, localized morbidity might occur because of IRIS, a brief delay in initiation of ART until clinical improvement might be prudent Maintenance therapy for CMV retinitis can be safely discontinued in patients with inactive disease and sustained CD_4+ count

CMV Retinitis *(cont'd)*

Preferred Therapy, Duration of Therapy, Chronic Maintenance	Alternate Therapy	Other Options/Issues
<u>Preferred chronic maintenance therapy (secondary prophylaxis) for CMV retinitis</u> Valganciclovir 900 mg (PO) daily **or** Ganciclovir implant (may be replaced every 6–8 months if CD$_4$+ count remains < 100 cells/μL) + Valganciclovir 900 mg (PO) q24h until immune recovery	<u>Alternative chronic maintenance (secondary prophylaxis) for CMV retinitis</u> Ganciclovir 5 mg/kg IV 5–7 times weekly **or** Foscarnet 90–120 mg/kg (IV) q24h **or** Cidofovir 5 mg/kg (IV) of other week with saline hydration and probenecid (as above)	(> 100 cells/mm^3 for ≥ 3–6 months); consultation with ophthalmologist is advised Patients with CMV retinitis who discontinued maintenance therapy should undergo regular eye examination, optimally every 3 months, for early detection of relapse or immune recovery uveitis (IRU) IRU might develop in the setting of immune reconstitution. <u>Treatment of IRU:</u> periocular corticosteroid or short courses of systemic steroid

CMV Encephalitis

Pathogen	Preferred Therapy	Alternate Therapy
Cytomegalovirus (CMV)	<u>Acute therapy</u> Ganciclovir (GCV) 5 mg/kg (IV) q12h until symptomatic improvement (typically > 3 weeks). *For severe cases,* consider acute therapy with Ganciclovir 5 mg/kg (IV) q12h plus Foscarnet 90 mg/kg (IV) q24h until improvement <u>Follow with lifelong suppressive therapy</u> Valganciclovir 900 mg (PO) q24h	<u>Acute therapy</u> Foscarnet 60 mg/kg (IV) q8h or 90 mg/kg (IV) q12h × 3 weeks <u>Follow with lifelong suppressive therapy</u> Valganciclovir 900 mg (PO) q24h

CMV Retinitis
Clinical Presentation: Blurred vision, scotomata, field cuts common. Often bilateral, even when initial symptoms are unilateral.

Diagnostic Considerations: Diagnosis by characteristic hemorrhagic ("tomato soup and milk") retinitis on funduscopic exam. Consult ophthalmology in suspected cases.

Pitfalls: May develop immune reconstitution vitreitis after starting antiretroviral therapy.

Therapeutic Considerations: Oral valganciclovir is the preferred option for initial and maintenance therapy. Lifelong maintenance therapy for CMV retinitis is required for CD_4 counts < 100/mm^3, but may be discontinued if CD_4 counts increase to > 100–150/mm^3 for 6 or more months in response to antiretroviral therapy (in consultation with ophthalmologist). Patients with CMV retinitis who discontinue therapy should undergo regular eye exams to monitor for relapse. Ganciclovir intraocular implants might need to be replaced every 6–8 months for patients who remain immunosuppressed with CD_4 < 100–150/mm^3. Immune recovery uveitis (IRU) may develop in the setting of immune reconstitution due to ART and be treated by ophthalmologist with periocular corticosteroid, sometimes systemic corticosteroid.

Prognosis: Good initial response to therapy. High relapse rate unless CD_4 improves with antiretroviral therapy.

CMV Encephalitis

Clinical Presentation: Encephalitis presents as fever, mental status changes, and headache evolving over 1–2 weeks. True meningismus is rare. CMV encephalitis occurs in advanced HIV disease (CD_4 < 50/mm^3), often in patients with prior CMV retinitis. Polyradiculitis presents as rapidly evolving weakness/sensory disturbances in the lower extremities, often with bladder/bowel incontinence. Anesthesia in "saddle distribution" with ↓ sphincter tone possible.

Diagnostic Considerations: CSF may show lymphocytic or neutrophilic pleocytosis; glucose is often decreased. For CMV encephalitis, characteristic findings on brain MRI include confluent periventricular abnormalities with variable degrees of enhancement. Diagnosis is confirmed by CSF CMV PCR (preferred), CMV culture, or brain biopsy.

Pitfalls: For CMV encephalitis, a wide spectrum of radiographic findings are possible, including mass lesions (rare). Obtain ophthalmologic evaluation to exclude active retinitis. For polyradiculitis, obtain sagittal MRI of the spinal cord to exclude mass lesions, and CSF cytology to exclude lymphomatous involvement (can cause similar symptoms).

Therapeutic Considerations: For any established CMV disease, optimization of antiretroviral therapy is important along with initiating anti-CMV therapy. Ganciclovir plus foscarnet may be beneficial as initial therapy for severe cases. Consider discontinuation of valganciclovir maintenance therapy if CD_4 increases to > 100–150/mm^3 × 6 months or longer in response to antiretroviral therapy.

Prognosis: Unless CD_4 cell count increases in response to antiretroviral therapy, response to anti-CMV treatment is usually transient, followed by progression of symptoms.

Cryptococcal Meningitis

Pathogen	Preferred Therapy	Alternate Therapy
Cryptococcus neoformans	Acute infection (induction therapy) Amphotericin B 0.7 mg/kg (IV) q24h × 2 weeks ± flucytosine (5-FC) 25 mg/kg (PO) q6h × 2 weeks **or** Lipid amphotericin 4 mg/kg (IV) q24h × 2 weeks ± flucytosine (5-FC) 25 mg/kg (PO) q6h × 2 weeks Consolidation therapy Fluconazole 400 mg (PO) q24h × 8 weeks or until CSF cultures are sterile Chronic maintenance therapy (secondary prophylaxis) Fluconazole 200 mg (PO) q24h	Acute infection (induction therapy) Amphotericin B 0.7 mg/kg/day (IV) × 2 weeks **or** Fluconazole 400–800 mg (IV or PO) q24h × 6 weeks (less severe disease) **or** Fluconazole 400–800 mg (IV or PO) q24h *plus* Flucytosine (5-FC) 25 mg/kg (PO) q6h × 4–6 weeks Consolidation therapy Itraconazole 200 mg (PO) q12h × 8 weeks or until CSF cultures are sterile Chronic maintenance therapy Itraconazole 200 mg (PO) q24h for intolerance to Fluconazole or failed Fluconazole therapy

Clinical Presentation: Often indolent onset of fever, headache, subtle cognitive deficits. Occasional meningeal signs and focal neurologic findings, though non-specific presentation is most common.

Diagnostic Considerations: Diagnosis usually by cryptococcal antigen; India ink stain of CSF is less sensitive. Diagnosis is essentially excluded with a negative serum cryptococcal antigen (sensitivity of test in AIDS patients approaches 100%). If serum cryptococcal antigen is positive, CSF antigen may be negative in disseminated disease without spread to CNS/meninges. Brain imaging is often normal, but CSF analysis is usually abnormal with a markedly elevated opening pressure.

Pitfalls: Be sure to obtain a CSF opening pressure, since reduction of increased intracranial pressure is critical for successful treatment. Remove sufficient CSF during the initial lumbar puncture (LP) to reduce closing pressure to < 200 mm H_2O or 50% of opening pressure. Increased intracranial pressure requires repeat daily lumbar punctures until CSF pressure stabilizes; persistently elevated pressure should prompt placement of a lumbar drain or ventriculo-peritoneal shunting. Adjunctive corticosteroids are not recommended.

Therapeutic Considerations: Optimal total dose/duration of amphotericin B prior to fluconazole switch is unknown (2–3 weeks is reasonable if patient is doing well). Treatment with 5-FC is optional; however, since 5-FC is associated with more rapid sterilization of CSF, it is reasonable to start 5-FC and then discontinue it for toxicity (neutropenia, nausea). Fluconazole is preferred over itraconazole for lifelong maintenance therapy. Consider discontinuation of chronic maintenance therapy in patients who remain asymptomatic with CD_4 >100–200/mm³ for > 6 months due to ART.

Prognosis: Variable. Mortality up to 40%. Adverse prognostic factors include increased intracranial pressure, abnormal mental status.

Progressive Multifocal Encephalopathy (PML)

Pathogen	Therapy
Reactivation of latent papovavirus (JC strain most common)	Effective antiretroviral therapy with immune reconstitution

Clinical Presentation: Hemiparesis, ataxia, aphasia, other focal neurologic defects, which may progress over weeks to months. Usually alert without headache or seizures on presentation.

Diagnostic Considerations: Demyelinating disease caused by reactivation of latent papovavirus (JC strain most common). Diagnosis by clinical presentation and MRI showing patchy demyelination of white matter ± cerebellum≠brainstem. JC virus PCR of CSF is useful for noninvasive diagnosis. In confusing or atypical presentation, biopsy may be needed to distinguish PML from other opportunistic infections, CNS lymphoma, or HIV encephalitis/encephalopathy.

Pitfalls: Primary HIV-related encephalopathy has a similar appearance on MRI.

Therapeutic Considerations: Most effective therapy is antiretroviral therapy with immune reconstitution. Some patients experience worsening neurologic symptoms once ART is initiated due to immune reconstitution induced inflammation. ART should be continued, with consideration of adjunctive steroids. Randomized controlled trials have evaluated cidofovir and vidarabine—neither is effective nor recommended.

Prognosis: Rapid progression of neurologic deficits over weeks to months is common. Best chance for survival is immune reconstitution in response to antiretroviral therapy, although some patients will have progressive disease despite immune recovery.

Toxoplasma Encephalitis

Pathogen	Preferred Therapy	Alternate Therapy
Toxoplasma gondii	<u>Acute therapy (× 6–8 weeks until good clinical response)</u> Pyrimethamine 200 mg (PO) × 1 dose, then 50 mg (< 60 kg body weight) or 75 mg (> 60 kg) (PO) q24h	<u>Acute therapy (× 6–8 weeks until good clinical response)</u> Pyrimethamine 200 mg (PO) × 1 dose, then 50 mg (< 60 kg body weight) or 75 mg (> 60 kg) (PO) q24h **plus** Clindamycin 600 mg (IV or PO) q6h plus Leucovorin 10 mg (PO) q24h

Toxoplasma Encephalitis *(cont'd)*

Pathogen	Preferred Therapy	Alternate Therapy
	plus Sulfadiazine 1000 mg (< 60 kg) or 1500 mg (> 60 kg) (PO) q6h **plus** Leucovorin 10–25 mg (PO) q24h *For severely ill patients who cannot take oral medications* TMP–SMX (5 mg/kg TMP and 25 mg/kg SMX) (IV) q12h	**or** TMP–SMX (5 mg/kg) (IV/PO) q12h **or** Atovaquone 1500 mg (PO) q12h (with meals or nutritional supplement) plus Pyrimethamine (as above) **or** Atovaquone 1500 mg (PO) q12h (with meals or nutritional supplement) plus Sulfadiazine 1000–1500 mg (PO) q6h **or** Atovaquone 1500 mg (PO) q12h (with meals) **or** Pyrimethamine (see above) **plus** leucovorin 10 mg (PO) q24h plus Azithromycin 900–1200 mg (PO) q24h
	<u>Follow with lifelong suppressive therapy</u> Sulfadiazine 500–1000 mg (PO) q6h **plus** Pyrimethamine 50 mg (PO) q24h **plus** Leucovorin 10–25 mg (PO) q24h	<u>Lifelong suppressive therapy</u> Clindamycin 600 mg (PO) q8h **plus** Pyrimethamine 50 mg (PO) q24h **plus** Leucovorin 10–25 mg (PO) q24h (2nd choice regimen) **or** Atovaquone 750 mg (PO) q12h ± Pyrimethamine 25 mg (PO) q24h **plus** Leucovorin 10 mg (PO) q24h (3rd choice regimen)

Clinical Presentation: Wide spectrum of neurologic symptoms, including sensorimotor deficits, seizures, confusion, ataxia. Fever/headache are common.

Diagnostic Considerations: Diagnosis by characteristic radiographic appearance and response to empiric therapy in a for T. gondii seropositive patient.

Pitfalls: Use leucovorin (folinic acid) 10 mg (PO) daily with pyrimethamine-containing regimens, not folate/folic acid. Radiographic improvement may lag behind clinical response.

Therapeutic Considerations: Alternate agents include atovaquone, azithromycin, clarithromycin, minocycline (all with pyrimethamine if possible). Decadron 4 mg (PO or IV) q6h is useful for edema/mass effect. Chronic suppressive therapy can be discontinued if patients are free from signs and symptoms of disease and have a CD_4 cell count > 200/mm³ for > 6 months due to ART.

Prognosis: Usually responds to treatment if able to tolerate drugs. Clinical response is evident by 1 week in 70%, by 2 weeks in 90%. Radiographic improvement is usually apparent by 2 weeks. Neurologic recovery is variable.

Gastrointestinal Tract Opportunistic Infections

Campylobacter (C. jejuni) Enteritis

Subset	Preferred Therapy
Mild disease	Might withhold therapy unless symptoms persist for several days
Moderate disease	Ciprofloxacin 500 mg (PO) q12h × 1 week **or** Azithromycin 500 mg (PO) q24h × 1 week
Bacteremia	Ciprofloxacin 500 mg (PO) q12h × 2 weeks* **or** Azithromycin 500 mg (PO) q24h × 2 weeks*

*   Consider addition of aminoglycoside in bacteremic patients.

Clinical Presentation: Acute onset of diarrhea, sometimes bloody; constitutional symptoms may be prominent.

Diagnostic Considerations: Diagnosis by stool culture; bacteremia may rarely occur, so blood cultures also indicated. Suspect campylobacter in AIDS patient with diarrhea and curved gram-negative rods in blood culture. Non-jejuni species may be more strongly correlated with bacteremia.

Therapeutic Considerations: Optimal therapy not well defined. Treat with quinolone or azithromycin; modify therapy based on susceptibility testing. Quinolone resistance can occur and correlates with treatment failure. Role of aminoglycoside is unclear.

Prognosis: Depends on underlying immune status; prognosis is generally good.

Clostridium difficile Diarrhea/Colitis

Pathogen	Preferred Therapy	Alternate Therapy
C. difficile	Metronidazole 500 mg (PO) q8h × 10–14 days. Avoid use of C. difficile associated antibiotics if possible.	Vancomycin 250 mg (PO) q6h × 10–14 days. Avoid use of C. difficile associated antibiotics if possible.

Clinical Presentation: Diarrhea and abdominal pain following antibiotic therapy. Diarrhea may be watery or bloody. Proton pump inhibitors increase the risk. Among antibiotics, clindamycin and beta-lactams are most frequent. Rarely due to aminoglycosides, linezolid, doxycycline, TMP–SMX, carbapenems, daptomycin, vancomycin.

Diagnostic Considerations: Most common cause of bacterial diarrhea in the U.S. among HIV patients. Watery diarrhea with positive C. difficile toxin in stool specimen. C. difficile stool toxin test is sufficiently sensitive/specific. If positive, no need to retest until negative (endpoint is end of diarrhea); if negative, no need to retest (repeat tests will be negative). C. difficile colitis may be distinguished clinically from C. difficile diarrhea by temperature > 102°F, ↑ WBC, ↑ ESR, and/or abdominal pain. C. difficile virulent epidemic strain is type B1 (toxinotype III), which produces 20 times the amount of toxin A/B compared to less virulent strains.

Pitfalls: In a patient with C. difficile diarrhea, C. difficile colitis is suggested by the presence of ↑ WBC, ↑ ESR, abdominal pain and temperature > 102°F; confirm diagnosis with CT of abdomen, which will show colonic wall thickening. New virulent strain of C. difficile may present with colitis with temperature ≤ 102°F, little/no ↑ WBC, and little/no abdominal pain; confirm diagnosis with CT/MRI of abdomen. C. difficile toxin may remain positive in stools for weeks following treatment; do not treat positive stool toxin unless patient has symptoms.

Therapeutic Considerations: Initiate therapy for mild disease with metronidazole; symptoms usually begin to improve within 2–3 days. For moderate or severe disease, or with evidence of colitis clinically (leukocytosis, fever, colonic thickening on CT scan), vancomycin has become the preferred agent in many centers due to concern for the more virulent strain, and based on the results of some observational studies suggesting vancomycin is more effective. The duration of therapy should be extended beyond 14 days if other systemic antibiotics must be continued. Relapse occurs in 10–25% of patients, and rates may be higher in patients with HIV due to the frequent need for other antimicrobial therapy. First relapses can be treated with a repeat of the initial regimen of metronidazole or vancomycin. For multiple relapses, a long-term taper is appropriate: week 1–125 mg 4x/day; week 2–125 mg 2x/day; week 3–125 mg once daily; week 4–125 mg every other day; weeks 5 and 6–125 mg every three days. Every effort should be made to resume a normal diet and to avoid other antibacterial therapies. Probiotic treatments (such as lactobacillus or Saccharomyces boulardii) have not yet been shown to reduce the risk of relapse in controlled clinical trials.

Prognosis: Prognosis with C. difficile colitis is related to severity of the colitis.

CMV Esophagitis/Colitis

Infection	Preferred Therapy	Alternate Therapy
Initial infection	Ganciclovir 5 mg/kg (IV) q12h × 3–4 weeks or until signs and symptoms have resolved. **or** Valganciclovir 900 mg (PO) q12h can be used if able to tolerate oral intake. Maintenance therapy is generally not necessary but should be considered after relapses	Foscarnet 90 mg/kg (IV) q12h × 3–4 weeks or until signs and symptoms have resolved **or** Cidofovir 5 mg/kg (IV) q every other week with saline hydration and probenecid (see CMV retinitis)
Relapses	Valganciclovir 900 mg (PO) q24h indefinitely; consider discontinuation if $CD_4 > 200/mm^3$ for ≥ 6 months on ART	

Clinical Presentation: Localizing symptoms, including odynophagia, abdominal pain, diarrhea, sometimes bloody stools.

Diagnostic Considerations: Diagnosis by finding CMV inclusions on biopsy. CMV can affect the entire GI tract, resulting in oral/esophageal ulcers, gastritis, and colitis (most common). CMV colitis varies greatly in severity, but typically causes fever, abdominal cramping, and sometimes bloody stools.

Pitfalls: CMV colitis may cause colonic perforation and should be considered in any AIDS patient presenting with an acute abdomen, especially if radiography demonstrates free intraperitoneal air.

Therapeutic Considerations: Duration of therapy is dependent on clinical response, typically 3–4 weeks. Consider chronic suppressive therapy for recurrent disease. Screen for CMV retinitis.

Prognosis: Relapse rate is greatly reduced with immune reconstitution due to antiretroviral therapy.

Cryptosporidia Enteritis

Pathogen	Preferred Therapy	Alternate Therapy
Cryptosporidium sp.	Effective ART with immune reconstitution to CD$_4$ > 100/mm^3 can result in complete resolution of symptoms and clearance of infection	Nitazoxanide 500 mg (PO) q12h × 4–6 weeks **or** Paromomycin 1 gm (PO) q12h × 2–4 weeks

Clinical Presentation: High-volume watery diarrhea with weight loss and electrolyte disturbances, especially in advanced HIV disease.

Diagnostic Considerations: Spore-forming protozoa. Diagnosis by AFB smear of stool demonstrating characteristic oocyte. Malabsorption may occur.

Pitfalls: No fecal leukocytes; organisms are not visualized on standard ova and parasite exams (need to request special stains).

Therapeutic Considerations: Anecdotal reports of antimicrobial success. Newest agent nitazoxanide may be effective in some settings, but no increase in cure rate for nitazoxanide if CD$_4$ < 50/mm^3. Immune reconstitution in response to antiretroviral therapy is the most effective therapy, and may induce prolonged remissions and cure. Anti-diarrheal agents (Lomotil, Pepto-Bismol) are useful to control symptoms. Hyperalimentation may be required for severe cases.

Prognosis: Related to degree of immunosuppression/response to antiretroviral therapy.

Cystoisospora (Isospora) belli Enteritis

Subset	Preferred Therapy	Alternate Therapy
Acute infection	TMP 160 mg and SMX 800 mg (IV or PO) q6h × 10 days **or** TMP 320 mg and SMX 1600 mg (IV or PO) q12h × 10–14 days	Pyrimethamine 50–75 mg (PO) q24h **plus** Leucovorin 5–10 mg (PO) q24h **or** Ciprofloxacin 500 mg (PO) q12h or other fluoroquinolones

Cystoisospora (Isospora) belli Enteritis (cont'd)

Subset	Preferred Therapy	Alternate Therapy
Chronic maintenance therapy for CD$_4$ < 200 (secondary prophylaxis)	TMP 320 mg *plus* SMX 1600 mg (PO) q24h*	Pyrimethamine 25 mg (PO) q24h *plus* Leucovorin 5–10 mg (PO) q24h*

* Discontinuation of secondary prophylaxis may be considered if CD$_4$ > 200/mm³ for > 3 months.

Clinical Presentation: Severe chronic diarrhea without fever/fecal leukocytes.

Diagnostic Considerations: Spore-forming protozoa (Isospora belli). Oocyst on AFB smear of stool larger that cryptosporidium (20–30 microns vs. 4–6 microns). More common in HIV patients from the tropics (e.g., Haiti). Less common than cryptosporidium or microsporidia. Malabsorption may occur.

Pitfalls: Multiple relapses are possible.

Therapeutic Considerations: Chronic suppressive therapy may be required if CD$_4$ does not increase.

Prognosis: Related to degree of immunosuppression/response to antiretroviral therapy.

Comments: Immune reconstitution with ART results in fewer relapses.

Microsporidia Enteritis

Pathogen	Therapy*
Microsporidia other than Enterocytozoon bienuesi	Albendazole 400 mg (PO) q12h (continue until CD$_4$ > 200/mm³)
Enterocytozoon bienuesi	Nitazoxanide 1 gm (PO) q12h × 60 days **or** Fumagillin 60 mg (PO) q24h (not available in the U.S.)
Trachipleistophora or Brachiola	Itraconazole 400 mg (PO) q24h plus Albendazole 400 mg (PO) q12h

* Regardless of species, ART with immune reconstitution is a critical component of treatment.

Clinical Presentation: Intermittent chronic diarrhea without fever/fecal leukocytes.

Diagnostic Considerations: Spore-forming protozoa (S. intestinalis, E. bieneusi). Diagnosis by modified trichrome or fluorescent antibody stain of stool. Microsporidia can rarely disseminate to sinuses/cornea. Severe malabsorption may occur.

Pitfalls: Microsporidia is too small for detection by routine microscopic examination of stool.

Therapeutic Considerations: Albendazole is less effective for E. bieneusi than S. intestinalis, but speciation is usually not possible. May consider treatment discontinuation for $CD_4 < 200/mm^3$ if patient remains asymptomatic (no signs or symptoms of microsporidiosis). If ocular infection is present, continue treatment indefinitely.

Prognosis: Related to degree of immunosuppression/response to antiretroviral therapy.

Oropharyngeal/Esophageal Candidiasis

Infection	Therapy	Fluconazole Resistant
Oropharyngeal candidiasis (thrush)	<u>Preferred therapy</u> Fluconazole 100 mg (PO) q24h × 1–2 weeks <u>Alternate therapy</u> Itraconazole oral solution 200 mg (PO) q24h × 1–2 weeks **or** Clotrimazole troches 10 mg (PO) 5x/day × 1–2 weeks or nystatin suspension 4–6 mL q6h **or** 1–2 flavored pastilles 4–5x/day × 1–2 weeks	Fluconazole at doses up to 800 mg (PO) q24h × 1–2 weeks **or** Caspofungin 70 mg (IV) on day 1, then 50 mg (IV) q24h × 1–2 weeks **or** Micafugin 150 mg (IV) q24h × 1–2 weeks
Esophageal candidiasis	<u>Preferred therapy</u> Fluconazole 100 mg (up to 400 mg) (IV or PO) q24h × 1–2 weeks <u>Alternate therapy</u> Itraconazole oral solution 200 mg (PO) q24h × 2–3 weeks **or** Voriconazole 200 mg (PO) q24h × 2–3 weeks **or** Caspofungin 50 mg (IV) q24h × 2–3 weeks	Amphotericin B 0.3 mg/kg (IV) q24h × 1–2 weeks **or** Lipid amphotericin 3–5 mg/kg (IV) q24h × 1–2 weeks

Oral Thrush (Candida)

Clinical Presentation: Dysphagia/odynophagia. More common/severe in advanced HIV disease.

Diagnostic Considerations: Pseudomembranous (most common), erythematous, and hyperplastic (leukoplakia) forms. Pseudomembranes (white plaques on inflamed base) on buccal muscosa/tongue/gingiva/palate scrape off easily, hyperplastic lesions do not. Diagnosis by clinical appearance ± KOH/gram stain of scraping showing yeast/pseudomycelia. Other oral lesions in AIDS patients include herpes simplex, aphthous ulcers, Kaposi's sarcoma, oral hairy leukoplakia.

Pitfalls: Patients may be asymptomatic.

Therapeutic Considerations: Fluconazole is superior to topical therapy in preventing relapses of thrush and treating Candida esophagitis. Continuous treatment with fluconazole may lead to fluconazole-resistance, which is best treated initially with itraconazole suspension and, if no response, with IV caspofungin or amphotericin. Chronic suppressive therapy is usually only considered for severely immunosuppressed patients.

Prognosis: Improvement in symptoms are often seen within 24–48 hours.

Candida Esophagitis

Clinical Presentation: Dysphagia/odynophagia, almost always in the setting of oropharyngeal thrush. Fever is uncommon.

Diagnostic Considerations: Most common cause of esophagitis in HIV disease. For persistent symptoms despite therapy, endoscopy with biopsy/culture is recommended to confirm diagnosis and assess azole-resistance.

Pitfalls: May extend into stomach. Other common causes of esophagitis include CMV, herpes simplex, and aphthous ulcers. Rarely, Kaposi's sarcoma, non-Hodgkin's lymphoma, zidovudine, dideoxycytidine, and other infections may cause esophageal symptoms.

Therapeutic Considerations: Systemic therapy is preferred over topical therapy. Failure to improve on empiric therapy mandates endoscopy to look for other causes, especially herpes viruses/aphthous ulcers. Consider maintenance therapy with fluconazole for frequent relapses, although the risk of fluconazole resistance is increased. Fluconazole-resistance is best treated initially with itraconazole suspension and, if no response, with IV caspofungin, micafungin, or amphotericin.

Prognosis: Relapse rate related to degree of immunosuppression.

Salmonella Gastroenteritis (non-S. typhi)

Subset	Preferred Therapy	Alternate Therapy
Mild disease	Ciprofloxacin 750 mg (PO) q12h × 1–2 weeks	TMP–SMX 1 DS (PO) q12h × 2 weeks **or**
$CD_4 < 200$	Ciprofloxacin 750 mg (PO) q12h × 4–6 weeks	Ceftriaxone 2 gm (IV) q24h × 2 weeks **or**
Bacteremia	Ciprofloxacin 750 mg (PO) q12h × 4–6 weeks, then 500 mg (PO) q12h indefinitely	Cefotaxime 1 gm (IV) q8h × 2 weeks

Clinical Presentation: Patients with HIV are at markedly increased risk of developing salmonellosis. Three different presentations may be seen: (1) self-limited gastroenteritis, as typically seen in immunocompetent hosts; (2) a more severe and prolonged diarrheal disease, associated with fever, bloody diarrhea, and weight loss; or (3) Salmonella septicemia, which may present with or without gastrointestinal symptoms.

Diagnostic Considerations: The diagnosis is established through cultures of stool and blood. Given the high rate of bacteremia associated with Salmonella gastroenteritis—especially in advanced HIV disease—blood cultures should be obtained in any HIV patient presenting with diarrhea and fever.

Pitfalls: A distinctive feature of salmonella bacteremia in patients with AIDS is its propensity for relapse (rate > 20%).

Therapeutic Considerations: The mainstay of treatment is a fluoroquinolone; greatest experience is with ciprofloxacin, but newer quinolones (moxifloxacin, levofloxacin) may also be effective. For uncomplicated salmonellosis in an HIV patient with $CD_4 > 200/mm^3$, 1–2 weeks of treatment is reasonable to reduce the risk of extraintestinal spread. For patients with advanced HIV disease ($CD_4 < 200/mm^3$) or who have salmonella bacteremia, at least 4–6 weeks of treatment is required. Chronic suppressive therapy, given for several months or until antiretroviral therapy-induced immune reconstitution ensues, is indicated for patients who relapse after cessation of therapy. Consider using ZDV as part of the antiretroviral regimen (ZDV is active against Salmonella).

Prognosis: Usually responds well to treatment. Relapse rate in AIDS patients with bacteremia is > 20%.

Shigella (Shigella sp.) Enteritis

Subset	Preferred Therapy	Alternate Therapy
No bacteremia	Fluoroquinolone (IV or PO) × 3–7 days	TMP–SMX 1 DS tablet (PO) q12h × 3–7 days **or** Azithromycin 500 mg (PO) on day 1, then 250 mg (PO) q24h × 4 days
Bacteremia	Extend treatment duration to 14 days	Extend treatment duration to 14 days

Clinical Presentation: Acute onset of bloody diarrhea/mucus.

Diagnostic Considerations: Diagnosis by demonstrating organism in stool specimens. Shigella ulcers in colon are linear, serpiginous, and rarely lead to perforation. More common in gay men.

Therapeutic Considerations: Shigella dysentery is more acute/fulminating than amebic dysentery. Shigella has no carrier state, unlike Entamoeba. Shigella infections acquired outside of United States have high rates of TMP–SMX resistance. Therapy is indicated to shorten the duration of illness and to prevent spread of infection. Shigella has no carrier state.

Prognosis: Good if treated early. Severity of illness related to Shigella species: S. dysenteriae (most severe) > S. flexneri > S. boydii/S. sonnei (mildest).

TREATMENT OF OTHER OPPORTUNISTIC INFECTIONS IN HIV

Candida Vaginitis

Pathogen	Therapy
Candida albicans	Intravaginal miconazole suppository 200 mg q24h × 3 days or miconazole 3% × 7 days **or** Nystatin vaginal tablet 100,000U q24h × 14 days **or** Itraconazole 200 mg (PO) q12h × 1 day (or 200 mg q24h × 3 days) **or** Fluconazole 150 mg (PO) × 1 dose

Clinical Presentation: White, cheesy, vaginal discharge or vulvar rash ± itching/pain. Local infection not a sign of disseminated disease.
Diagnostic Considerations: Local infection. Not a manifestation of disseminated disease.
Pitfalls: Women with advanced AIDS receiving fluconazole may develop fluconazole-resistant Candida.
Therapeutic Considerations: For recurrence, consider maintenance with fluconazole 100–200 mg (PO) weekly.
Prognosis: Good response to therapy. Relapses are common.

Coccidioidomycosis (C. immitis)

Infection	Therapy*
Non-meningeal infection	<u>Acute therapy (diffuse pulmonary or disseminated disease)</u> Amphotericin B 0.5–1.0 mg/kg (IV) q24h until clinical improvement (usually 500–1000 mg total dose). Some specialists add an azole to amphotericin B therapy <u>Acute therapy (milder disease)</u> Fluconazole 400–800 mg (PO) q24h or Itraconazole 200 mg (PO) q12h <u>Chronic maintenance therapy (secondary prophylaxis)</u> <u>Preferred</u>: Fluconazole 400 mg (PO) q24h indefinitely; <u>alternative</u>: or Itraconazole 200 mg capsule (PO) q12h indefinitely
Meningeal infection*	<u>Acute therapy</u> Fluconazole 400–800 mg (IV) or (PO) q24h. Intrathecal amphotericin B if no response to azole therapy <u>Chronic maintenance therapy (secondary prophylaxis)</u> Fluconazole 400 mg (PO) q24h or Itraconazole 200 mg capsule (PO) q12h indefinitely

* Therapy for meningeal infection should be lifelong with fluconazole 400–800 mg q24h. There are insufficient data to recommend discontinuation of chronic maintenance therapy in other settings.

Clinical Presentation: Typically a complication of advanced HIV infection (CD_4 cell count < 200/mm³). Most patients present with disseminated disease, which can manifest as fever, diffuse pulmonary infiltrates, adenopathy, skin lesions (multiple forms – verrucous, cold abscesses, ulcers, nodules), and/or bone lesions. Approximately 10% will have spread to the CNS in the form of meningitis (fever, headache, altered mental status).

Diagnostic Considerations: Consider the diagnosis in any patient with advanced HIV-related immunosuppression who has been in a C. immitis endemic area (southwestern US, northern Mexico) and presents with a systemic febrile syndrome. Diagnosis can be made by culture of the organism, visualization of characteristic spherules on histopathology, or a positive complement-fixation antibody (≥ 1:16). In meningeal cases, CSF profile shows low glucose, high protein, and lymphocytic pleocytosis.

Pitfalls: Antibody titers often negative on presentation. CSF profile of meningitis can be similar to TB.

Prognosis: Related to extent of infection and degree of immunosuppression. Clinical response tends to be slow, especially with a high disease burden and advanced HIV disease. Meningeal disease is treated lifelong regardless of CD_4 recovery.

Extrapulmonary Tuberculosis

Pathogen	Therapy
Mycobacterium tuberculosis	Treat the same as pulmonary TB (see p. 326). May require longer duration of therapy based on clinical response

Clinical Presentation: Multiple presentations possible (e.g., lymphadenitis, osteomyelitis, meningitis, hepatitis). Dissemination is more common in patients with low CD_4 cell counts (< 100/mm³).

Diagnostic Considerations: Diagnosis by isolator blood cultures or tissue biopsy.

Pitfalls: Patients with disseminated disease frequently have pulmonary disease, which has implications for infection control.

Therapeutic Considerations: Response to therapy may be slower than in normal hosts.

Prognosis: Usually responsive to therapy.

Herpes Simplex Virus (HSV) Disease

Infection	Preferred Therapy	Alternate Therapy
Orolabial lesions or initial/recurrent genital HSV	Famciclovir 500 mg (PO) q12h × 1–2 weeks **or** Valacyclovir 1 gm (PO) q12h × 1–2 weeks **or** Acyclovir 400 mg (PO) q8h × 1–2 weeks	Acyclovir-resistant HSV Foscarnet 60–100 mg/kg (IV) q12h until clinical response **or** Cidofovir 5 mg/kg (IV) weekly until clinical response

Herpes Simplex Virus (HSV) *(cont'd)*

Infection	Preferred Therapy	Alternate Therapy
Moderate-to-severe mucocutaneous HSV	Initial therapy: Acyclovir 5 mg/kg (IV) q8h × 2–7 days. If improvement, switch to Famciclovir 500 mg (PO) q12h **or** valacyclovir 1 gm (PO) q12h **or** acyclovir 400 mg (PO) q8h to complete 7–10 days	<u>Acyclovir-resistant HSV</u> Foscarnet 60–100 mg/kg (IV) q12h until clinical response **or** Cidofovir 5 mg/kg (IV) weekly until clinical response
HSV keratitis	Trifluridine 1% ophthalmic solution, one drop onto cornea q2h, not to exceed 9 drops per day and no longer than 21 days. Treatment in conjunction with ophthalmology consultation	<u>Acyclovir-resistant HSV</u> Foscarnet 60–100 mg/kg (IV) q12h until clinical response **or** Cidofovir 5 mg/kg (IV) weekly until clinical response
HSV encephalitis	Acyclovir 10 mg/kg (IV) q8h × 2–3 weeks **or** Valacyclovir 1 gm (PO) q6h × 2–3 weeks	<u>Acyclovir-resistant HSV</u> Foscarnet 60–100 mg/kg (IV) q12h until clinical response **or** Cidofovir 5 mg/kg (IV) weekly until response
Multiple mucocutaneous (oral or anogenital) relapses (chronic suppressive therapy)	Acyclovir 400 mg (PO) q12h **or** Famciclovir 250 mg (PO) q12h **or** Valacyclovir 500 mg (PO) q12h	Patients may be able to titrate dose downward to maintain response

Herpes Simplex (genital/oral)

Clinical Presentation: Painful, grouped vesicles on an erythematous base that rupture, crust, and heal within 2 weeks. Lesions may be chronic, severe, ulcerative with advanced immunosuppression.

Diagnostic Considerations: Diagnosis by viral culture of swab from lesion base/roof of blister; alternative diagnostic techniques include Tzanck prep or immunofluorescence staining.

Pitfalls: Acyclovir prophylaxis is not required in patients receiving ganciclovir or foscarnet.

Therapeutic Considerations: In refractory cases, consider acyclovir resistance and treat with foscarnet. Topical trifluridine ophthalmic solution (Viroptic 1%) may be considered for direct application to small, localized areas of refractory disease; clean with hydrogen peroxide, then debride lightly with gauze, apply trifluridine, and cover with bacitracin/polymyxin ointment and nonadsorbent gauze; topical cidofovir (requires compounding) also may be tried. Chronic suppressive therapy with oral acyclovir, famciclovir, or valacyclovir may be indicated for patients with frequent recurrences, dosing similar to HIV-negative patients.

Prognosis: Responds well to treatment except in severely immunocompromised patients, in whom acyclovir resistance may develop. Prognosis for HSV meningitis is excellent.

Herpes Encephalitis (HSV-1)

Clinical Presentation: Acute onset of fever and change in mental status.

Diagnostic Considerations: EEG is abnormal early (< 72 hours), showing unilateral temporal lobe abnormalities. Brain MRI is abnormal before CT scan, which may require several days before a temporal lobe focus is seen. Definitive diagnosis is by CSF PCR for HSV-1 DNA. Profound decrease in sensorium is characteristic of HSV meningoencephalitis. CSF may have PMN predominance and low glucose levels, unlike other viral causes of meningitis. A different clinical entity is HSV meningitis, which is usually associated with HSV-2 and can recur with lymphocytic meningitis.

Pitfalls: Rule out noninfectious causes of encephalopathy. Surprisingly, HIV encephalitis is a relatively rare cause of encephalitis in patients with HIV.

Therapeutic Considerations: Treat as soon as possible since neurological deficits may be mild and reversible early on, but severe and irreversible later.

Prognosis: Related to extent of brain injury and early antiviral therapy. Prognosis for HSV meningitis is excellent.

Histoplasmosis (H. capsulatum), Disseminated

Subset	Preferred Therapy	Alternate Therapy
Acute phase (3–10 days or until clinically improved)	Liposomal amphotericin (L-amb) 3 mg/kg × 1–2 weeks or other lipid associated formulations at 5 mg/kg	Amphotericin B doxycholate 0.7–1 mg/kg **or** Intravenous Itraconazole (200 mg q12 × 4 doses then 200 mg q24)
Continuation phase	Itraconazole 200 (PO) TID × 3 days and then QD or BID for atleast 12 months (adequate serum levels should be confirmed). Immunosuppressed patients may require lifelong suppressive therapy.	Itraconazole oral solution 200 mg (PO) q12h × 12 weeks **or** Fluconazole 800 mg (PO) q24h × 12 weeks
Meningitis	Amphotericin B deoxycholate 0.7 mg/kg (IV) q24h × 12–16 weeks **or** Liposomal amphotericin (L-amb) 4 mg/kg (IV) q24h × 12–16 weeks	Fluconazole 800 mg (PO) q24h × 12 weeks

* Duration of therapy dependent on response to therapy.

Clinical Presentation: Two general forms: Mild disease with fever/lymph node enlargement (e.g., cervical adenitis), or severe disease with fever, wasting ± diarrhea/ meningitis/GI ulcerations.

Diagnostic Considerations: Diagnosis by urine/serum histoplasmosis antigen, sometimes by culture of bone marrow/liver or isolator blood cultures. May occur in patients months to years after having lived/moved from an endemic area.

Pitfalls: Relapse is common after discontinuation of therapy. Cultures may take 7–21 days to turn positive.

Therapeutic Considerations: Initial therapy depends on severity of illness on presentation. Extremely sick patients should be started on amphotericin B deoxycholate, with duration of IV therapy dependent on response to treatment. Mildly ill patients can be started on itraconazole. All patients require chronic suppressive therapy, with possible discontinuation for immune reconstitution with CD_4 counts > 100/mm³ for at least 6 months. HIV patients with CD_4 > 500/mm³ and acute pulmonary histoplasmosis might not require therapy, but a short course of itraconazole (4–8 weeks) is reasonable to prevent systemic spread.

Prognosis: Usually responds to treatment, except in fulminant cases.

Mycobacterium avium-complex (MAC)

Pathogen	Preferred Therapy	Alternate Therapy
Mycobacterium avium-complex (MAC)	At least 2 drugs as initial therapy Clarithromycin 500 mg (PO) q12h plus ethambutol 15 mg/kg (PO) q24h (usually 800 mg or 1200 mg daily). Consider adding third drug, rifabutin 300 mg (PO) q24h, for patients with CD_4 < 50/mm³, high mycobacterial loads and severely symptomatic disease. Duration of therapy is **lifelong**, consider discontinuation in asymptomatic patients with > 12 months therapy and CD_4 > 100/mm³ for > 6 months in response to ART	Alternative to clarithromycin Azithromycin 500 mg (PO) q24h Alternative 3rd or 4th drug for severe symptoms or disseminated disease Ciprofloxacin 500–750 mg (PO) q12h **or** Levofloxacin 500 mg (PO) q24h **or** Amikacin 10–15 mg/kg (IV) q24h

Clinical Presentation: Typically presents as a febrile wasting illness in advanced HIV disease ($CD_4 < 50/mm^3$). Focal invasive disease is possible, especially in patients with advanced immunosuppression after starting antiretroviral therapy. Focal disease likely reflects restoration of pathogen-specific immune response to subclinical infection ("immune reconstitution inflammatory syndrome" [IRIS]), and typically manifests as lymphadenitis (mesenteric, cervical, thoracic) or rarely disease in the spine mimicking Pott's disease. Immune reconstitution syndrome usually occurs within weeks to months after starting antiretroviral therapy for the first time, but may occur a year or more later.

Diagnostic Considerations: Diagnosis by isolation of organism from a normally sterile body site (blood, lymph node, bone marrow, liver biopsy). Lysis centrifugation (DuPont Isolator) is the preferred blood culture method. Anemia/↑ alkaline phosphatase are occasionally seen.

Pitfalls: Isolator blood cultures may be negative, especially in immune reconstitution inflammatory syndrome initially.

Therapeutic Considerations: Some studies suggest benefit for addition of rifabutin 300 mg (PO) q24h, others do not. Rifabutin may require dosage adjustment with NNRTIs and PIs. For concurrent use with nelfinavir, indinavir, or amprenavir, decrease rifabutin to 150 mg (PO) q24h. For concurrent use with ritonavir, decrease rifabutin to 150 mg (PO) 2–3x/week. For concurrent use with efavirenz, increase rifabutin to 450–600 mg (PO) q24h. The dose of PIs or NNRTIs may need to be increased by 20–25%. Monitor carefully for rifabutin drug toxicity (arthralgias, uveitis, leukopenia). Treat IRIS initially with NSAIDs; if symptoms persist, systemic corticosteroids (prednisone 20–40 mg daily) for 4–8 weeks can be used. Some patients will require a more prolonged course of corticosteroids with a slow taper over months. Azithromycin is often better tolerated than clarithromycin and has fewer drug-drug interactions. Optimal long-term management is unknown, though most studies suggest that treatment can be discontinued in asymptomatic patients with > 12 months of therapy and $CD_4 > 100/mm^3$ for > 6 months.

Prognosis: Depends on immune reconstitution in response to antiretroviral therapy. Adverse prognostic factors include high-grade bacteremia or severe wasting.

Varicella Zoster Virus (VZV)

Infection	Preferred Therapy
Primary VZV infection (chickenpox)	Acyclovir 10 mg/kg (IV) q8h × 7–10 days. Can start with or change to oral therapy with Valacyclovir 1 gm (PO) q8h or Famciclovir 500 mg (PO) q8h after defervescence if no evidence of visceral involvement exists
Local dermatomal herpes zoster	Famciclovir 500 mg (PO) q8h × 7–10 days **or** Valacyclovir 1 gm (PO) q8h × 7–10 days

Varicella Zoster Virus (VZV) *(cont'd)*

Infection	Preferred Therapy
Extensive cutaneous or visceral involvement	Acyclovir 10 mg/kg (IV) q8h until cutaneous and visceral disease has clearly resolved and the patient is clinically improved
Acute retinal necrosis	Acyclovir 10 mg/kg (IV) q8h until progression stops, then Valacyclovir 1 gm (PO) q8h × 6 weeks. Treat in conjunction with close ophthalmologic consultation

Clinical Presentation: Primary varicella (chickenpox) presents as clear vesicles on an erythematous base that heal with crusting and sometimes scarring. Zoster usually presents as painful tense vesicles on an erythematous base in a dermatomal distribution. In patients with HIV, primary varicella is more severe/prolonged, and zoster is more likely to involve multiple dermatomes/disseminate. VZV can rarely cause acute retinal necrosis, which requires close consultation with ophthalmology.

Diagnostic Considerations: Diagnosis is usually clinical. In atypical cases, immunofluorescence can be used to distinguish herpes zoster from herpes simplex.

Pitfalls: Extend treatment beyond 7–10 days if new vesicles are still forming after initial treatment period. Corticosteroids for dermatomal zoster are not recommended in HIV-positive patients.

Therapeutic Considerations: IV therapy is generally indicated for severe disease/cranial nerve zoster.

Prognosis: Usually responds slowly to treatment.

HIV COINFECTIONS (HBV/HCV)

Hepatitis B Virus (HBV)/HIV Coinfection

Preferred Therapy	Alternate Therapy	Additional Considerations
Indication for therapy Initiation: All HIV-positive patients with HBV coinfection should start antiretroviral therapy (ART) irrespective of CD4 cell count Prior to initation of ART, HBV DNA quantitative assay should be obtained Preferred therapy: Patients with HIV/HBV coinfection should receive an NRTI-backbone containing tenofovir alafenamide (TAF) or tenofovir disoproxil fumarate (TDF) in combination with lamivudine (3TC) or emtricitabine (FTC) 3TC-resistant HBV emerges in up to 90% of patients after 4 years; thus, 3TC and FTC should always be used in combination with other anti-HBV drugs Dosing recommendations for normal renal function: Lamivudine (3TC) 300 mg PO daily or emtricitabine (FTC) 200 mg PO daily plus tenofovir (TAF 25 mg PO daily or TDF 300 mg PO daily) plus additional agent[s] active against HIV	If TAF or TDF cannot be utilized: Entecavir 1 mg PO daily can be considered in patients with complete HIV suppression (while on ART): Entecavir has weak HIV activity and may select for the M184V mutation that confers HIV resistance to 3TC and FTC Peginterferon alfa monotherapy for up to 48 weeks can be considered in certain scenarios but should not used in patients with decompensated cirrhosis Telbivudine and adefovir are *not recommended* for patients with HIV/HBV coinfection due to higher rates of treatment failure and toxicities	Duration of therapy: Because of the high rates of relapse, certain specialists recommended continuing therapy indefinitely Abrupt discontinuation or ART modification: Abrupt discontinuation of anti-HBV therapy in persons with HIV/HBV coinfection can lead to serious hepato-cellular damage and decompensation following HBV reactivation If ART requires modification due to HIV viroiogic failure and the patient has HBV suppression, the ARV drugs active against HBV should be continued for HBV treatment in combination with other ARV agents to achieve HIV suppression Additional considerations: Emtricitabine, entecavir, lamivudine, or tenofovir should not be used for the treatment of HBV infection in patients with HIV who are not receiving combination ART Cross-resistance to emtricitabine should be assumed in patients with suspected or proven lamivudine resistance

3TC = lamivudine = **Epivir**; FTC = emtricitabine = **Emtriva**; tenofovir alafenamide = TAF = **Vemlidy**; tenofovir disoproxil fumarate = TDF = **Viread**
Combination dual-NRTI products; tenofovir alafenamide/emtricitabine = TAF/FTC = **Descovy**; tenofovir disoproxil fumarate/emtricitabine = TDF/FTC = **Truvada**; tenofovir disoproxil fumarate/lamivudine= TDF/3TC = **Cimduo**
https://www.assid.org
https://aidsinfo.nih.gov/guidelines

Epidemiology: Hepatitis B virus (HBV) infection is relatively common in patients with HIV, with approximately 60% showing some evidence of prior exposure. Chronic hepatitis B infection interacts with HIV infection in several important ways:

- HBV increases the risk of liver-related death and hepatotoxicity from antiretroviral therapy.
- 3TC, FTC, and tenofovir each have anti-HBV activity. Thus selection of antiretroviral therapy for patients with HBV can have clinical and resistance implications for HBV as well as HIV. This is most notable with 3TC and FTC, as a high proportion of coinfected patients will develop HBV-associated resistance to these drugs after several years of therapy. This resistance reduces response to subsequent non-3TC or FTC anti-HBV therapy.
- Cessation of anti-HBV therapy may lead to exacerbations of underlying liver disease; in some cases, these flares have been fatal.
- Immune reconstitution may lead to worsening of liver status, presumably because HBV disease is immune mediated. This is sometimes associated with loss of HBeAg.
- Entecavir can no longer be recommended for HIV/HBV coinfected patients, as it has anti-HIV activity and may select for HIV resistance mutation M184V. If needed, it should be used only with a fully suppressive HIV regimen.

Diagnostic Consideration: Obtain HBsAb, HBsAg, and HBCAb at baseline in all patients. If negative, hepatitis B vaccination is indicated. If chronic HBV infection (positive HBsAg) is identified, obtain HBEAg, HBEAb, and HBV DNA levels. As with HCV infection, vaccination with hepatitis A vaccine and counseling to avoid alcohol are important components of preventive care. <u>Isolated Hepatitis B Core Antibody</u>: Many patients with HIV have antibody to hepatitis B core (anti-HBc) but are negative for both HBsAg and HBsAb. This phenomenon appears to be more common in those with HCV coinfection (Clin Infec Dis. 2003:36:1602–6). In this scenario, diagnostic considerations include: (1) recently acquired HBV, before development of HBsAb; (2) chronic HBV, with HBsAg below the levels of detection; (3) immunity to HBV, with HBsAb below the levels of detection; (4) false-positive anti-HBV core. As the incidence of HBV is relatively low in most populations and anti-HBc alone is usually a stable phenomenon over years, recent acquisition of HBV is rarely the explanation. We recommend checking HBV DNA in this situation: If positive, this indicates chronic HBV; if negative, then low-level immunity or false-positive anti-HBV core remain as possible explanations; since distinguishing between these possibilities cannot be done, we recommend immunization with the hepatitis B vaccine series. It is useful to measure HBV serologic markers periodically in this population, as improvement in immune status due to ART may lead to increasing titers of HBsAb and subsequently confirm immunity.

Therapeutic Considerations: The optimal treatment for HBV infection is in evolution. Current guidelines suggest treatment of HBV in all patients with active HBV replication, defined as a detectable HBEAg or HBV DNA. Pending long-term studies defining optimal management, the recommendations set forth in the grid above are reasonable. Patients being treated with regimens for HBV should be monitored for ALT every 3–4 months. HBV DNA levels provide a good marker for efficacy of therapy and should be added to regular laboratory monitoring. The goal of therapy is to reduce HBV DNA to as low a level as possible, preferably below the limits of detection. The duration of HBV therapy is not well established; with development of HBEAb, while some individuals without HIV can stop therapy after reversion of HBEAg to negative, there are no clear stopping rules for HIV-coinfected patients.

Hepatitis C Virus (HCV) Treatment

Geno-type(s)	Recommended Regimens for Treatment-Naïve Patients with or without Compensated Cirrhosis	Duration
1a, 1b, 4	Glecaprevir (300 mg)/pibrentasvir (120 mg) **(Mavyret)**[a]	8 weeks[b]
	Ledipasvir (90 mg)/sofosbuvir (400 mg) **(Harvoni)**[c]	12 weeks[d]
	Elbasvir (50 mg)/grazoprevir (100 mg) **(Zepatier)**[e,f]	12 weeks
	Sofosbuvir (400 mg)/velpatasvir (100 mg) **(Epclusa)**[g]	12 weeks
2	Glecaprevir (300 mg)/pibrentasvir (120 mg) **(Mavyret)**[a]	8 weeks[b]
	Sofosbuvir (400 mg)/velpatasvir (100 mg) **(Epclusa)**[g]	12 weeks
3	Glecaprevir (300 mg)/pibrentasvir (120 mg) **(Mavyret)**[a]	8 weeks[b]
	Sofosbuvir (400 mg)/velpatasvir (100 mg) **(Epclusa)**[g,h]	12 weeks
5,6	Glecaprevir (300 mg)/pibrentasvir (120 mg) **(Mavyret)**[a]	8 weeks[b]
	Ledipasvir (90 mg)/sofosbuvir (400 mg) **(Harvoni)**[c]	12 weeks
	Sofosbuvir (400 mg)/velpatasvir (100 mg) **(Epclusa)**[g]	12 weeks

[a] GLE/PIB; 3-tablet coformulated regimen; pangenotypic regimen; administer with food; regimens containing protease inhibitors should be avoided in patients with active or history of decompensated cirrhosis (Child-Turcotte-Pugh B or C); can be utilized in chronic kidney disease and end-stage-renal-disease.

[b] For patients with HCV/HIV coinfection and cirrhosis, duration of GLE/PIB should be extended to 12 weeks.

[c] LED/SOF; single-tablet coformulated regimen; avoid if CrCl <30 mL/min; add ribavirin or extend to 24 weeks in presence of decompensated cirrhosis; requires acid for absorption (avoid acid-reducing medications).

[d] Consider 8 weeks of treatment in patients with Genotype 1 or 4 (non-4r) who are non-cirrhotic, HIV-uninfected, and whose HCV RNA level is <6 million IU/mL.

[e] ELB/GRZ; single-tablet coformulated regimen; regimens containing protease inhibitors should be avoided in patients with active or history of decompensated cirrhosis (Child-Turcotte-Pugh B or C); can be utilized in chronic kidney disease and end-stage-renal-disease.

[f] For Genotype 1a, baseline NS5A resistance testing required prior to use of ELB/GRZ; if resistance present (resistance-associated substitutions at amino acid positions 28, 30, 31, or 93), use alternative regimen.

[g] SOF/VEL; single-tablet coformulated regimen; pangenotypic regimen; avoid if CrCl <30 mL/min; add ribavirin or extend to 24 weeks in presence of decompensated cirrhosis; requires acid for absorption (avoid acid-reducing medications).

[h] For Genotype 3, NS5A resistance testing for Y93H is recommended for cirrhotic patients prior to use of SOF/VEL. If present, ribavirin should be included in the regimen or sofosbuvir/velpatasvir/voxilaprevir (SOF/VEL/VOX) (Vosevi) should be considered.

https://www.hcvguidelines.org/

Recommendations related to HCV medication interactions with HIV antiretroviral medications.

Daclatasvir:

- Daclatasvir requires dose adjustment with ritonavir boosted atazanavir (decrease to 30 mg daily) and etravirine (increase to 90 mg daily).

Fixed-dose combination of Ledipasvir (90 mg)/Sofosbuvir (400 mg):

- Because ledipasvir increase tenofovir levels, when given as tenofovir disoproxil fumarate, concomitant use should be avoided in those with CrCl <60 mL/min. Because potentiation of this effect occurs when tenofovir is used with ritonavir-boosted HIV protease inhibitors, ledipasvir should be avoided with this combination unless antiretroviral regimen cannot be changed and the urgency of treatment is high.

- For combinations expected to increase tenofovir levels, baseline and ongoing assessment for tenofovir nephrotoxicity is recommended.

Daily fixed-dose combination of paritaprevir (150 mg)/ritonavir (100 mg)/ombitasvir (25 mg) plus twice daily dosed dasabuvir (250 mg) (paritaprevir/ritonavir/ombitasvir plus dasabuvir or PrOD).

- Paritaprevir/ritonavir/ombitasvir plus dasabuvir should be used with antiretroviral drugs with which they do not have substantial interactions (atazanavir, dolutegravir, emtricitabine, enfuviride, lamivudine, raltegravir, or tenofovir).

- The dose of ritonavir used for boosting of HIV protease inhibitors may need to be adjusted (or held) when administered with paritaprevir/ritonavir/ombitasvir plus dasabuvir and then restored when HCV treatment is completed. The HIV protease inbhibitor should be administered at the same time as the fixed-dose HCV combination.

Simeprevir:

- Simeprevir should be used with antiretroviral drugs with which it does not have clinically significant interactions (abacavir, emtricitabine, enfuviritide, lamivudine, maraviroc, raltegravir, dolutegravir, rilipivirine, and tenofovir).

Following are NOT recommended or should not be used.

- Antiretroviral treatment interruption to allow HCV therapy is NOT recommended.
- Ledipasvir/sofosbuvir should NOT be used with cobicistat when given with tenofovir disoproxil fumarate.
- Sofosbivir or ledipasvir/sofosbuvir should NOT be used with tipranavir.
- Paritaprevir/ritonavir/ombitasvir plus dasabuvir should NOT be used with daranavir, efavirenz, ritonavir-boosted lopinavir, or rilpivirine.
- Paritaprevir/ritonavir/ombitasvir with/without dasabuvir should NOT be used in HIV/HCV-coinfected individuals who are not taking antiretroviral therapy.
- RBV should NOT be used with didanosine, stavudine, or zidovudine.
- Simeprevir should NOT be used with cobicistat, efavirenz, etravirine, nevirapine, or any HIV protease inhibitor.

Recommended regimens for HIV/HVC coinfected individuals.

- HIV/HCV coinfected persons should be treated and retreated the same as persons without HIV infection, after recognizing and managing interactions with anteritroviral medications.
- Daily daclatasvir (see dose above) and sofosbuvir (400 mg), with/without RBV (refer to Initial Treatment of HCV Infection and Retreatment of Persons Who Failed Therapy sections for duration) is recommended when antiretroviral regimen changes cannot be made to accommodate alternate HCV direct-acting antivirals.

> **The following regimens are NOT recommended for treatment-naïve or experienced HIV/HCV coinfected patients.**

- Treatment courses shorter than 12 weeks, such as the use of 8 weeks of ledipasvir/sofosbuvir.
- Monotherapy with PEG-IFN, RBV, or a direct-acting antiviral.
- PEG-IFN and RBV with/without simeprevir, telaprevir, or boceprevir for 24 weeks to 48 weeks.

Adapted from: http://www.hcvguidelines.org/full-report/unique-patient-populations-hivhcv-coinfection-box-summary-recommendations-hivhcv.

Epidemiology: Hepatitis C virus (HCV) infection is transmitted primarily through blood exposure; sexual and perinatal transmission are also possible but less efficient. A notable exception is sexually transmitted HCV among gay men. Since modes of transmission of HIV and HCV are similar, there are high rates of HCV coinfection in HIV—an estimated 16% of HIV patients overall, including 80% or more of IDUs and 5–10% of gay men. Genotype 1 accounts for 75% of HCV in the United States. HIV accelerates the progression of chronic HCV infection to cirrhosis, liver failure, and hepatocellular carcinoma. Data are conflicting regarding the independent effect of HCV on HIV disease progression, but several studies have shown a markedly higher rate of antiretroviral therapy-induced hepatotoxicity in those with chronic HCV. In some series, liver failure from HCV is one of the leading causes of death in HIV/HCV coinfected individuals.

Clinical Presentation: Persistently elevated liver transaminases; usually asymptomatic.

Diagnostic Considerations: All HIV-positive patients should be tested for HCV antibody. If the antibody test is negative but the likelihood of HCV infection is high (IDU, unexplained increase in LFTs), obtain an HCV RNA since false-negative antibody tests may occur, especially in advanced HIV disease. Since LFT elevation does not correlate well with underlying HCV activity, a liver biopsy is the best way to assess the degree of fibrosis and inflammation.

Therapeutic Considerations: Advise patients to abstain from alcohol and administer vaccinations for hepatitis A and B (if nonimmune). Also obtain HCV RNA levels with genotype assessment. HCV RNA levels do not have prognostic significance for underlying degree of liver disease, but higher levels make treatment for cure less likely. Genotype results also correlate with cure rates (reported cure rates: 60–75% for genotypes 2 and 3; 15–25% for genotype 1). Some clinicians elect to treat HCV without a liver biopsy due to the risks, costs, and discomfort of the test; the potential to underestimate the degree of HCV activity due to sampling error; and the high rate of treatment success for genotypes 2 and 3.

Table 5.8 HIV Pre-Exposure Prophylaxis (PrEP)

Exposure	Preferred Regimen	Comments
HIV	Tenofovir/Emtricitabine (TDF/FTC) **(Truvada)** 1 tablet (PO) q24h × 90 days (recheck HIV status)	Avoid if CrCl <60 mL/min. Avoid if breastfeeding.

HIV Post-Exposure Prophylaxis (PEP)

Exposure	Preferred Regimen	Alternative Regimen
HIV	Tenofovir/Emtricitabine (TDF/FTC) **(Truvada)** 1 tablet (PO) q24h × 4 weeks **plus either** Raltegravir (RAL) **(Isentress)** q12h × 4 weeks **or** Dolutegravir[a] (DTG) **(Tivicay)** (PO) q24h × 4 weeks	Tenofovir/Emtricitbine (TDF/FTC) **(Truvada)** 1 tablet (PO) q24h × 4 weeks **plus** Darunavir/Ritonavir (DRV/r) **(Prezista, Norvir)** (800 mg/100 mg) (PO) q24h × 4 weeks

[a] DTG-based regimens should not be initiated in those who are pregnant and within 12 weeks post-conception, those who are trying to conceive, or those of child bearing potential not using effective contraception, due to risk of neural tube defects.

REFERENCES

Bennett JE, Dolin R, Blaser MJ (eds). Mandell, Douglas, and Bennett's Principles and Practice of Infectious Diseases (9th Ed), Philadelphia, Elsevier, 2019.

Cohen J, Powderly WG, Opal S (eds). Infectious Diseases (4th Ed), Philadelphia, Elsevier, 2016.

Cunha CB, Schlossberg D (eds). Clinical Infectious Disease (3rd Ed), Cambridge University Press, Cambridge, 2020.

Dolin R, Masur H, Saag MS (eds). AIDS Therapy (3rd Ed), Churchill Livingstone, New York, 2008.

Gorbach SL, Bartlett JG, Blacklow NR (eds). Infectious Diseases (3rd Ed), Philadelphia, Lippincott, Williams & Wilkins, 2004.

Sax PE, Cohen CJ, (eds). HIV Essentials (8th Ed), Jones & Bartlett, Sudbury, MA, 2017.

Wormser GP (ed). AIDS (4th Ed), Philadelphia, Elsevier, 2004.

Chapter 6

Prophylaxis and Immunizations

**Pierce Gardner, MD, John L. Brusch, MD,
Jean E. Hage, MD, Ronald L. Nichols, MD,
Staci A. Fischer, MD, Arthur Gran, MD,
Muhammed Raza, MBBS, Gina L. Wu, MD,
Maria D. Mileno, MD, Burke A. Cunha, MD**

SURGICAL PROPHYLAXIS

- Antibiotic prophylaxis is designed to prevent infection for a defined period of time.
- **Prophylaxis is most likely to be effective when given for a short duration against a single pathogen with a known sensitivity pattern,** and least likely to be effective when given for a long duration against multiple organisms with varying/unpredictable sensitivity patterns.
- It is a common misconception that antibiotics used for prophylaxis should not be used for therapy and vice versa.
- **The only difference between prophylaxis and therapy is the inoculum size and the duration of antibiotic administration:** In prophylaxis, there is no infection, so the inoculum is minimal/none and antibiotics are administered only for the duration of exposure/surgical procedure.
- With therapy, the inoculum is large (infection already exists), and antibiotics are continued until the infection is eradicated.

Table 6.1 Factors Affecting the Efficacy of Surgical Antibiotic Prophylaxis

Number of Organisms	Susceptibility Pattern	Duration of Protection	Efficacy of Prophylaxis
Single organism	Predictable	Short	Excellent
Multiple organisms	Predictable	Short	Excellent
Single organism	Unpredictable	Short	Good
Single organism	Predictable	Long	Good
Multiple organisms	Unpredictable	Long	Poor/none

- **Antibiotic prophylaxis is designed to achieve effective antibiotic serum/tissue concentrations at the time of initial surgical incision, and is maintained throughout the "vulnerable period" of the procedure (i.e. time between skin incision and skin closure).**
- If prophylaxis is given too early, antibiotic levels will be suboptimal/nonexistent when protection is needed.
- Properly timed pre-operative antibiotic prophylaxis is desirable for optimal effectiveness since **antibiotics given after skin closure are unlikely to be effective.**
- When no infection exists prior to surgery (clean/clean contaminated surgery), single-dose prophylaxis is preferred.
- When infection is present/likely prior to surgery ("dirty" surgery, e.g., perforated colon, TURP in the presence of positive urine cultures, repair of open fracture), antibiotics are given for > 1 day and represent early therapy, not true prophylaxis.

- Parenteral cephalosporins are commonly used for surgical prophylaxis, and ordinarily given as a bolus injection/rapid IV infusion < 5 minutes prior to the procedure.
- Prophylaxis with vancomycin or gentamicin is given by slow IV infusion over 1 hour, starting 1–2 hours preprocedure.

Table 6.2 Surgical Prophylaxis

Procedure	Usual Organisms	Preferred Prophylaxis	Alternate Prophylaxis	Comments
CNS shunt (VP/VA) placement, craniotomy, open CNS trauma	S. epidermidis (CoNS) S. aureus (MSSA)	MRSA/MRSE unlikely Ceftriaxone 1 gm (IV) × 1 dose MRSA/MRSE likely Linezolid 600 mg (IV) × 1 dose	MRSA/MRSE unlikely Cefotaxime 2 gm (IV) × 1 dose **or** Ceftizoxime 2 gm (IV) × 1 dose MRSA/MRSE likely Linezolid 600 mg (PO) × 1 dose **or** Vancomycin 1 gm (IV) × 1 dose **or** Minocycline 200 mg (IV) × 1 dose	Administer immediately prior to procedure. Vancomycin protects against wound infections, but may not prevent CNS infections. Give vancomycin slowly IV over 1 hour prior to procedure.
Thoracic (non-cardiac) surgery	S. aureus (MSSA)	Cefazolin 1 gm (IV) × 1 dose **or** Ceftriaxone 1 gm (IV) × 1 dose	Cefotaxime 2 gm (IV) × 1 dose **or** Ceftizoxime 2 gm (IV) × 1 dose	Administer immediately prior to procedure.
Cardiac valve replacement surgery	S. epidermidis (CoNS) S. aureus (MSSA/MRSA) Enterobacter	Vancomycin 1 gm (IV) × 1 dose **plus** Gentamicin 120 mg (IV) × 1 dose	Linezolid 600 mg (IV) × 1 dose **plus** Gentamicin 120 mg (IV) × 1 dose	Administer vancomycin and gentamicin slowly IV over 1 hour prior to procedure.
Coronary artery bypass graft (CABG) surgery	S. aureus (MSSA)	Cefazolin 2 gm (IV) × 1 dose **or** Ceftriaxone 1 gm (IV) × 1 dose	Cefotaxime 2 gm (IV) × 1 dose **or** Ceftizoxime 2 gm (IV) × 1 dose	Administer immediately prior to procedure. Except for ceftriaxone, repeat dose intraoperatively for procedures lasting > 6 hours.

Table 6.2 Surgical Prophylaxis *(cont'd)*

Procedure	Usual Organisms	Preferred Prophylaxis	Alternate Prophylaxis	Comments
Biliary tract surgery	E. coli Klebsiella E. faecalis (VSE)	Meropenem 1 gm (IV) × 1 dose **or** Piperacillin/ Tazobactam 3.375 gm (IV) × 1 dose	Ampicillin/ sulbactam 3 gm (IV) × 1 dose	Administer immediately prior to procedure
Hepatic surgery	E. coli Klebsiella E. faecalis (VSE) B. fragilis	Ampicillin/ Sulbactam 3 gm (IV) × 1 dose **or** Piperacillin/ Tazobactam 3.375 gm (IV) × 1 dose	Meropenem 1 gm (IV) × 1 dose **or** Moxifloxacin 400 mg (IV) × 1 dose	Administer immediately prior to procedure.
Stomach, upper small bowel, bariatric surgery	S. aureus (MSSA) Group A streptococci	Ceftriaxone 1 gm (IV) × 1 dose **or** Cefazolin 1 gm (IV) × 1 dose	Cefotaxime 2 gm (IV) × 1 dose **or** Ceftizoxime 2 gm (IV) × 1 dose	Administer immediately prior to procedure.
Distal small bowel, colon surgery	E. coli Klebsiella B. fragilis	Oral Neomycin* **plus either** Erythromycin base* **or** Metronidazole* Parenteral Ertapenem 1 gm (IV) × 1 dose **or** Piperacillin/ Tazobactam 3.375 gm (IV) × 1 dose **or** Cefoxitin 2 gm (IV) × 1 dose	**Combination therapy** Metronidazole 1 gm (IV) × 1 dose **plus either** Ceftriaxone 1 gm (IV) × 1 dose **or** Levofloxacin 500 mg (IV) × 1 dose **or** Gentamicin 120 mg (IV) × 1 dose	Administer immediately prior to procedure. Give gentamicin slowly IV over 1 hour.
Pelvic (OB/GYN) surgery	GNB Anaerobic streptococci B. fragilis	Ceftriaxone 1 gm (IV) × 1 dose **plus** Metronidazole 1 gm (IV) × 1 dose	Cefoxitin 2 gm (IV) × 1 dose **or** Cefotetan 2 gm (IV) × 1 dose	Administer immediately prior to procedure

* Give either neomycin 1 gm (PO) plus erythromycin base 1 gm (PO) at 1 pm, 2 pm, and 11 pm, or give neomycin 2 gm (PO) plus metronidazole 2 gm (PO) at 7 pm and 11 pm the day before an 8 am operation.

Table 6.2 Surgical Prophylaxis *(cont'd)*

Procedure	Usual Organisms	Preferred Prophylaxis	Alternate Prophylaxis	Comments
Orthopedic prosthetic implant surgery (total hip/knee replacement)	S. epidermidis (CoNS) S. aureus (MSSA)	<u>MRSA/MRSE unlikely</u> Cefazolin* <u>MRSA/MRSE likely</u> Vancomycin 1 gm (IV) × 1 dose	<u>MRSA/MRSE unlikely</u> Ceftriaxone 1 gm (IV) × 1 dose <u>MRSA/MRSE likely</u> Linezolid 600 mg (IV) × 1 dose	Administer immediately prior to procedure.
Arthroscopy	S. aureus (MSSA)	Cefazolin 1 gm (IV) × 1 dose	Ceftriaxone 1 gm (IV) × 1 dose	Pre-procedure prophylaxis to cover skin pathogens.
Orthopedic surgery (open fracture)	S. aureus (MSSA) GNB	Ceftriaxone 1 gm (IV) × 1 week	Clindamycin 600 mg (IV) q8h × 1 week **plus** Gentamicin 240 mg (IV) q24h × 1 week	Represents early therapy, not prophylaxis. Duration of post-op antibiotics depends on severity of infection.
Urological implant surgery	S. aureus (MSSA) GNB	Ceftriaxone 1 gm (IV) × 1 dose	Cefotaxime 2 gm (IV) × 1 dose **or** Ceftizoxime 2 gm (IV) × 1 dose	Administer immediately prior to procedure.
TURP, cystoscopy	P. aeruginosa P. cepacia P. maltophilia E. faecalis (VSE) GNB	Levofloxacin 500 mg (IV) × 1 dose **or** Piperacillin/ Tazobactam 3.375 gm (IV) × 1 dose	Ciprofloxacin 400 mg (IV) × 1 dose	Prophylaxis given to TURP patients with positive pre-op urine cultures. Represents early therapy, not true prophylaxis. No prophylaxis needed for TURP if pre-op urine culture is negative.
	E. faecium (VRE)	Linezolid 600 mg (IV) × 1 dose	Quinupristin/ Dalfopristin 7.5 mg/kg (IV) × 1 dose	

MSSA/MRSA = methicillin-sensitive/resistant S. aureus; MSSE/MRSE = methicillin-sensitive/resistant S. epidermidis.
*THR = cefazolin 1 gm (IV) × 1 dose, TKR = cefazolin 2 gm (IV) × 1 dose

POST-EXPOSURE PROPHYLAXIS

Some infectious diseases can be prevented by post-exposure prophylaxis (PEP). To be maximally effective, PEP should be administered within 24 hours of the exposure, since the effectiveness of prophylaxis > 24 hours after exposure decreases over time. PEP is usually reserved for persons with close/intimate contact with an infected individual. Casual contact does not warrant PEP.

Table 6.3 Post-Exposure Prophylaxis

Exposure	Usual Organisms	Preferred Prophylaxis	Alternate Prophylaxis	Comments
Meningitis	N. meningitidis	Any quinolone (PO) × 1 dose	Minocycline 100 mg (PO) q12h × 2 days **or** Rifampin 600 mg (PO) q12h × 2 days	Should be administered within 24 hours of close face-to-face exposure for optimal effectiveness. Otherwise, observe and treat if infection develops.
	H. influenzae	Rifampin 600 mg (PO) q24h × 3 days	Any quinolone (PO) × 3 days	Must be administered within 24 hours of close face-to-face exposure for optimal effectiveness. H. influenzae requires 3 days of prophylaxis.
Influenza	Influenza A or B	Oseltamivir 75 mg (PO) q24h for least 7 days after of contact to an infected person§ **or** Baloxavir 40 mg (40–80 kg) or 80 mg (>80 kg) tablets (PO) × 1 dose **or** Laninamivir 40 mg (via inhaler) × 1 dose	Rimantadine 100 mg (PO) q12h* for duration of outbreak (or at least 7–10 days after close contact to infected person) **or** Amantidine 200 mg (PO) q24h† for 7–10 days or outbreak	Give to non-immunized contacts and high-risk contacts even if immunized. Begin at onset of outbreak or within 3 days of close contact to an infected person. Oseltamivir is active against both influenza A and B; rimantadine and amantadine are only active against influenza A.

§   Dose for CrCl > 30–60 mL/min = 30 mg (PO) q24h; for CrCl >10–30 mL/min = 30 mg (PO) q48h.

Table 6.3 Post-Exposure Prophylaxis *(cont'd)*

Exposure	Usual Organisms	Preferred Prophylaxis	Alternate Prophylaxis	Comments
Avian influenza	Influenza A (H_5N_1)	Oseltamivir (as for influenza, above)	Rimantadine **or** Amantadine[†] (as for influenza, above)	Oseltamivir may be ineffective due to resistance.
Swine influenza	Influenza A (H_1N_1)	Oseltamavir above (as for influenza, above)	None	Amantadine/rimantadine ineffective. Continue PEP for swine influenza (H_1N_1) × 10 days post-close exposure.[‡]
Pertussis	B. pertussis	Erythromycin 500 mg (PO) q6h × 2 weeks	TMP–SMX 1 SS tablet (PO) q12h × 2 weeks **or** Levofloxacin 500 mg (PO) q24h × 2 weeks	Administer as soon as possible after exposure. Effectiveness is greatly reduced after 24 hours.
Diphtheria	C. diphtheriae	Erythromycin 500 mg (PO) q6h × 1 week **or** Benzathine penicillin 1.2 mu (IM) × 1 dose	Azithromycin 500 mg (PO) q24h × 3 days	Administer as soon as possible after exposure. Effectiveness is greatly reduced after 24 hours.
TB	M. tuberculosis	Rifampin 600 mg (PO) q24h × 4 months[§] **or** INH 300 mg (PO) q24h × 9 months	Rifapentine 900 mg (PO) q week **plus** INH 900 mg (PO) q week × 3 months (D.O.T.)	For INH, monitor AST/ALT weekly × 4, then monthly. Mild elevations are common and resolve spontaneously. D/C INH if AST/ALT levels ≥ 5 × normal.

* For elderly, severe liver dysfunction, or CrCl < 10 cc/min, give 100 mg (PO) q24h.

† For age ≥ 65 years, give 100 mg (PO) q24h. For renal dysfunction, give 200 mg (PO) load followed by 100 mg q24h (CrCl 30–50 mL/min), 100 mg q48h (CrCl 15–29 mL/min), or 200 mg weekly (CrCl < 15 mL/min).

‡ *Pediatric prophylaxis*: < 15 kg: 30 mg PO qd for 10 days, > 15–24 kg: 45 mg PO qd for 10 days, 24–40 kg: 60 mg PO qd for 10 days, > 40 kg: same as adults.

§ INH preferred if patient uses contact lens, has HIV, or is taking medications that may interact with rifampin.

Table 6.3 Post-Exposure Prophylaxis *(cont'd)*

Exposure	Usual Organisms	Preferred Prophylaxis	Alternate Prophylaxis	Comments
Gonorrhea (GC)	N. gonor-rhoeae	Ceftriaxone 125 mg (IM) × 1 dose	Spectinomycin 2 gm (IM) × 1 dose **or** Any oral quinolone × 1 dose	Administer as soon as possible after sexual exposure (≤ 72 hours). Ceftriaxone also treats incubating syphilis.
Syphilis	T. pallidum	Benzathine penicillin 2.4 mu (IM) × 1 dose	Doxycycline 100 mg (PO) q12h × 1 week	Administer as soon as possible after sexual exposure. Obtain HIV serology.
Chancroid	H. ducreyi	Ceftriaxone 250 mg (IM) × 1 dose	Azithromycin 1 gm (PO) × 1 dose **or** Any oral quinolone × 3 days	Administer as soon as possible after sexual exposure. Obtain HIV and syphilis serologies.
Non-gonococcal urethritis (NGU)	C. trachomatis U.urealyticum M. genitalium	Azithromycin 1 gm (PO) × 1 dose **or** Doxycycline 100 mg (PO) q12h × 1 week	Any oral quinolone × 1 week	Administer as soon as possible after sexual exposure. Also test for gonorrhea/Ureaplasma.
Varicella (chicken-pox)	VZV	<u>Preferred:</u> For exposure < 72 hours, give varicella-zoster immune globulin (VZIG) 625 mcg (IM) × 1 dose to immuno-compromised hosts and pregnant women (esp. with respiratory conditions). For others or exposure > 72 hours, consider Acyclovir 800 mg (PO) 5x/day × 5–10 days <u>Alternate:</u> Varicella vaccine 0.5 mL (SC) × 1 dose. Repeat in 4 weeks		Administer as soon as possible after exposure (≤ 72 hours). Varicella vaccine is a live attenuated vaccine and should not be given to immunocompromised or pregnant patients. If varicella develops, start Acyclovir treatment immediately.

Table 6.3 Post-Exposure Prophylaxis *(cont'd)*

Exposure	Usual Organisms	Preferred Prophylaxis	Alternate Prophylaxis	Comments
Hepatitis A (HAV)	Hepatitis A virus	HAV vaccine 1 mL (IM) × 1 dose	Immune serum globulin (IG) 0.02 mL/kg (IM) × 1 dose	Give HAV vaccine alone if within 14 days after exposure.
Hepatitis B (HBV)	Hepatitis B virus	<u>Unvaccinated</u> Hepatitis B immune globulin (HBIG) 0.06 mL/kg (IM) × 1 dose **plus** HBV vaccine (40 mcg HBsAg/mL) deep deltoid (IM) at 0, 1, 6 months (can use 10-mcg dose in healthy adults < 40 years)	<u>Previously vaccinated</u> *Known responder* (anti-HBsAg antibody levels ≥ 10 IU/mL): No treatment. *Known non-responder/incompletely vaccinated* (anti-HBsAg antibody levels < 10 IU/mL): Heplisav-B (Hep B – CpG) vaccine 0.5 mL (IM) × 2 doses/month apart. *Antibody status unknown*: Obtain HBsAg antibody levels to determine immunity status. If testing is not possible or results are not available within 24 hours of exposure, give HBIG plus 1 dose of HBV vaccine (booster). Risk of transmission from needle stick HBV = 30% HCV = 3% HIV = 0.3%	
Leptospirosis	L. interrogans	Doxycycline 200 mg (PO) q week **or** Azithromycin 250 mg (PO) q week		
Rocky Mountain spotted fever (RMSF)	R. rickettsia	Doxycycline 100 mg (PO) q12h × 1 week	Any oral quinolone × 1 week	Administer prophylaxis after removal of Dermacentor tick.
Lyme disease	B. burgdor-feri	Doxycycline 200 mg (PO) × 1 dose	Amoxicillin* 1 gm (PO) q8h × 3 days **or** Any oral 1ˢᵗ gen. cephalosporin* × 3 days	If tick is in place ≥ 72 hours or is grossly engorged, prophylaxis may be given after tick is removed. Otherwise, prophylaxis is usually not recommended.

HDCV = human diploid cell vaccine, HRIG = human rabies immune globulin, PCEC = purified chick embryo cells, RVA = rabies vaccine absorbed.

*   All or as much of the full dose of HRIG should be injected into the wound, and the remaining vaccine should be injected IM into the deltoid. Do not give HRIG at the same site or through the same syringe with PCEC, RVA, or HDCV.

Table 6.3 Post-Exposure Prophylaxis *(cont'd)*

Exposure	Usual Organisms	Preferred Prophylaxis	Alternate Prophylaxis	Comments
		* Although experience is limited, single-dose prophylaxis with these agents is probably also effective.		
Plague Anthrax	Y. pestis B. anthracis	Doxycycline 100 mg (PO) q12h for duration of exposure	Any oral quinolone for duration of exposure	Continued for the duration of a naturally-acquired exposure/ outbreak for bioterrorist plague/anthrax recommendations.
Rabies	Rabies virus	<u>No Previous Immunization</u> HRIG 20 IU/kg* **plus either** PCEC 1 mL (IM) in deltoid **or** RVA 1 mL (IM) in deltoid **or** HDCV 1 mL (IM) in deltoid PCEC, RVA, HDCV given on days 0, 3, 7, 14, and 28 post-exposure	<u>Previous Immunization</u> PCEC 1 mL (IM) in deltoid on days 0 and 3 **or** RVA 1 mL (IM) in deltoid on days 0 and 3 **or** HDCV 1 mL (IM) in deltoid on days 0 and 3	Following unprovoked or suspicious dog or cat bite, immediately begin prophylaxis if animal develops rabies during a 10-day observation period. If dog or cat is suspected of being rabid, begin vaccination sequence immediately. Raccoon, skunk, bat, fox, and most wild carnivore bites should be regarded as rabid, and bite victims should be vaccinated against rabies immediately (contact local health department regarding rabies potential of animals in your area). All potential rabies wounds should immediately be thoroughly cleaned with soap and water. Do not inject rabies vaccine IV (may cause hypotension/ shock). Serum sickness may occur with HDCV.

HDCV = human diploid cell vaccine, HRIG = human rabies immune globulin, PCEC = purified chick embryo cells, RVA = rabies vaccine absorbed.

*   All or as much of the full dose of HRIG should be injected into the wound, and the remaining vaccine should be injected IM into the deltoid. Do not give HRIG at the same site or through the same syringe with PCEC, RVA, or HDCV.

Table 6.3 Post-Exposure Prophylaxis *(cont'd)*

Exposure	Usual Organisms	Preferred Prophylaxis	Alternate Prophylaxis	Comments
BIOTERRORIST AGENTS				
Anthrax *Inhalation/ cutaneous*	B. anthracis	Doxycycline 100 mg (PO) q12h × 60 days **or** Levofloxacin 500 mg (PO) q24h × 60 days **or** Ciprofloxacin 500 mg (PO) q12h × 60 days	Amoxicillin 1 gm (PO) q8h × 60 days	Duration of anthrax PEP based on longest incubation period of inhaled spores in nares.
Tularemia pneumonia	F. tularensis	Doxycycline 100 mg (PO) q12h × 2 weeks	Levofloxacin 500 mg (PO) q24h × 2 weeks **or** Ciprofloxacin 500 mg (PO) q12h × 2 weeks	Duration of PEP for tularemia is 2 weeks, not 1 week as for plague.
Pneumonic plague	Y. pestis	Doxycycline 100 mg (PO) q12h × 7 days **or** Levofloxacin 500 mg (PO) q24h × 7 days **or** Ciprofloxacin 500 mg (PO) q12h × 7 days	Chloramphenicol 500 mg (PO) q6h × 7 days	Pneumonic plague should be considered as potential bioterrorism since most natural cases of plague are bubonic plague.
Smallpox	Variola virus	Smallpox vaccine ≤ 4 days after exposure	None	Smallpox vaccine is protective when diluted 1:5.
Viral hemorrhagic fever	Lassa fever	Ribavarin loading dose: 35mg/kg (PO) (not to exceed 2.5 g), then 15 mg/kg (PO) (not to exceed 1g) q8h × 10 days	None	Decrease maintenance dose to 7.5 mg/kg (PO) q8h if CrCl < 50/mL/min.

CHRONIC MEDICAL PROPHYLAXIS

Table 6.4 Chronic Medical Prophylaxis

Disorder	Usual Organisms	Preferred Prophylaxis	Alternate Prophylaxis	Comments
Immuno-suppressive therapy/ steroids[†]	LTB (+ PPD/ Quantiferon), no evidence of active TB	Rifampin 600 mg (PO) q24h × 4 months	INH 300 mg (PO) q24h + pyridoxine 25 mg (PO) q24h × 9 months	Discontinue 1–3 months after stopping immunosuppressive regimen.[ℯ]
	PCP	TMP–SMX 1 DS tablet three times weekly	Atovaquone 1500 mg (PO) q24h **or** Dapsone 100 mg (PO) q24h	Discontinue 1–3 months after stopping immunosuppressive/ steroid therapy.[ℯ]
Asplenia/ impaired splenic function	S. pneumoniae H. influenzae N. meningitidis	Amoxicillin 1 gm (PO) q24h indefinitely	Respiratory quinolone* (PO) q24h indefinitely	Long-term prophylaxis effective. Vaccines may be given but are not always protective. Use amoxicillin in children.
UTIs (recurrent)	GNB VSE	Nitrofurantoin 100 mg (PO) q24h × 6 months	Amoxicillin 500 mg (PO) q24h × 6 mos **or** TMP–SMX 1 SS tablet (PO) q24h × 6 months	Prophylaxis for reinfection UTIs (≥ 3 per year). Relapse UTIs should be investigated for stones, abscesses, or structural abnormalities.
Asympto-matic bacteriuria in pregnancy	GNB VSE	Nitrofurantoin 100 mg (PO) q24h × 1 week	Amoxicillin 1 gm (PO) q24h × 1 week	Prophylaxis prevents symptomatic infections.
Prophylaxis of fungal infections in neutropenic patients[†]	Candida albicans Non-albicans Candida Aspergillus	Posaconazole 200 mg (PO) q8h*	Itraconazole 200 mg (PO) q12h*	Prophylaxis given until neutropenia resolves (absolute neutrophil count ≥ 500 cells/mm³).
Recurrent genital herpes (< 6 episodes/ year)	H. simplex (HSV-2)	Valacyclovir 500 mg (PO) q24h × 5 days	Acyclovir 200 mg (PO) 5x/day × 5 days	Begin therapy as soon as lesions appear. Famciclovir 1 gm (PO) q12h × 1 day ↓ lesion progression by 2 days.

* Until no longer neutropenic
† > 20 mg prednisone/equivalent daily for > 2 weeks
ℯ Depending in the intensity and duration of immunosuppression

Table 6.4 Chronic Medical Prophylaxis (cont'd)

Disorder	Usual Organisms	Preferred Prophylaxis	Alternate Prophylaxis	Comments
Recurrent genital herpes (> 6 episodes/year)	H. simplex (HSV-2)	Valacyclovir 1 gm (PO) q24h × 1 year **or** Famciclovir 250 mg (PO) q12h × 1 year	Acyclovir 400 mg (PO) q12h × 1 year	Suppressive therapy is indicated for frequent recurrences.
Acute exacerbation of chronic bronchitis (AECB)	S. pneumoniae H. influenzae M. catarrhalis	Doxycycline 100 mg (PO) q12h × 5 days **or** Azithromycin 500 mg (PO) × 3 days **or** Moxifloxacin 400 mg **or** Levofloxacin 500 mg **or** Amoxicillin/Clavulanic acid 875 mg (PO) q12h × 5 days **or** Clarithromycin XL 1 gm (PO) q24h × 5 days		Treat each episode individually.
Acute rheumatic fever (ARF)	Group A streptococci (GAS)	Benzathine penicillin 1.2 mu (IM) monthly until age 30	Amoxicillin 500 mg (PO) q24h **or** Azithromycin 500 mg (PO) q72h until age 30	Group A streptococcal pharyngitis and acute rheumatic fever are uncommon after age 30.
Neonatal Group B streptococcal infection (primary prevention)	Group B streptococci (GBS)	Ampicillin 2 gm (IV) q4h at onset of labor until delivery	Clindamycin 600 mg (IV) q8h at onset of labor until delivery **or** Vancomycin 1 gm (IV) q12h at onset of labor until delivery	Indications: previous infant with GBS infection, maternal GBS colonization/infection during pregnancy, vaginal/rectal culture of GBS after week 35 of gestation, delivery ≤ week 37 of gestation without labor/ruptured membranes, ruptured membranes ≥ 12 hrs, or intrapartum temp ≥ 100.4°F.

* Levofloxacin 500 mg (PO) or moxifloxacin 400 mg (PO).
† During induction chemotherapy for acute myelogenous leukemia (AML) or myelodysplastic syndrome (MDS).

Table 6.5 HIV Pre-Exposure Prophylaxis (PrEP)

Exposure	Preferred Regimen	Comments
HIV	Tenofovir/Emtricitabine (TDF/FTC) **(Truvada)** 1 tablet (PO) q24h (recheck HIV status/viral load every 3 months)	Avoid if CrCl < 60 mL/min. Avoid if breastfeeding.

Table 6.6 HIV Post-Exposure Prophylaxis (PEP)

Exposure	Preferred Regimen	Alternate Regimens
HIV	Tenofovir/Emtricitabine (TDF/FTC) **(Truvada)** 1 tablet (PO) q24h × 4 weeks **plus either** Raltegravir (RAL) **(Isentress)** q12h × 4 weeks **or** Dolutegravir (DTG) **(Tivicay)** (PO) q24h × 4 weeks	Tenofovir/Emtricitbine (TDF/FTC) **(Truvada)** 1 tablet (PO) q24h × 4 weeks **plus** Darunavir/Ritonavir (DRV/r) **(Prezista, Norvir)** (800 mg/100 mg) (PO) q24h q24h × 4 weeks

Table 6.7 HIV: Prophylaxis of Opportunistic Infections

Usual Organisms	Indication	Prophylaxis	Alternate Regimens
Pneumocystis (carinii) jiroveci pneumonia (PCP)	**Start:** CD_4 < 200 cells/mm^3 **or** History of AIDS-defining illness **Stop:** CD_4 > 200 cell/mm^3 after > 3 months on ART	TMP-SMX 1 DS (PO) q24h	TMP-SMX 1 DS (PO) three times weekly **or** Dapsone 100 mg (PO) q24h **or** Atovaquone 1500 mg (PO) q24h
Toxoplasma gondii encephalitis	**Start:** Toxoplasma IgG positive with CD_4 < 100 cells/mm^3 **Stop:** CD_4 > 200 cell/mm^3 after >3 months on ART	TMP-SMX 1 DS (PO) q24h	TMP-SMX DS (PO) three times weekly **or** Dapsone 50 mg (PO) q24h + pyrimethamine 50 mg + leucovorin 25 mg) PO weekly **or** Dapsone 200 mg (PO) q24h + pyrimethamine 75 mg + leucovorin 25 mg) PO weekly **or** Atovaquone 1500 mg (PO) q24h

Table 6.7 HIV: Prophylaxis of Opportunistic Infections *(cont'd)*

Usual Organisms	Indication	Prophylaxis	Alternate Regimens
Mycobacterium tuberculosis (TB)	**Start:** Positive screening test for LTB with no evidence of active TB and no prior treatment for active TB or LTB **Stop:** After completion of TB treatment	Rifampin 600 mg (PO) q24h × 4 months **or** Isoniazid (INH) 300 mg (PO) q24h + pyridoxine 25 mg (PO) q24h × 9 months	Isoniazid (INH) 900 mg (PO) twice weekly (by DOT) + pyridoxine 25 mg (PO) q24h × 9 months **or** Rifabutin (dose adjusted based on concomitant ART) × 4 months
Disseminated Myobacterium avium-complex (MAC)	**Start:** CD_4 cells < 50 cells/mm³ after ruling out active disseminated MAC disease **Stop:** CD_4 cells > 100 cell/mm³ after > 3 months on ART	Azithromycin 1200 mg (PO) once weekly **or** Clarithromycin 500 mg (PO) q12h **or** Azithromycin 600 mg (PO) twice weekly	Rifabutin (dose adjusted based on concomitant ART); rule out active TB before starting rifabutin

Table 6.8 Transplant Prophylaxis (BMT/SOT)

Exposure	Usual Organism	Preferred Prophylaxis	Alternate Prophylaxis	Comments
Herpes simplex (HSV)	Herpes simplex	<u>HSV → < 6 recurrences/ year</u> Valacyclovir 500 mg (PO) q24h × 30 days **or** Famciclovir 1 gm (PO) q12 × 30 days	Acyclovir 400 mg (PO) q8h × 30 days post-BMT	<u>Acute prophylaxis</u> Nearly all post-tranplant HSV infections occur < 1 month. Transplants receiving CMV prophylaxis with Ganciclovir, or Valganciclovir are protected against HSV (see CMV prophylaxis).
		<u>HSV → > 6 recurrences/ year</u> Valacyclovir 1 gm (PO) q24h × 90 days	Acyclovir 400 mg (PO) q8h × 90 days post-BMT	<u>Chronic prophylaxis</u> Valacyclovir 500 mg (PO) q12h **or** Famciclovir 500 mg (PO) q12h **or** Acyclovir 400 mg (PO) q8h
Varicella zoster virus (VZV)	Varicella zoster virus	<u>VZV seropositive recipient</u> Valacyclovir 500 mg (PO) q12h post-transplant x 4–24 months	Acyclovir 400 mg (PO) q8h post-transplant x 4–24 months	Post-transplant VZV infections occur later than HSV. > 95% of adults are VZV seropositive. In transplants, most VZV infections are due to reactivation rather than primary infection. Patients may develop shingles after prophylaxis is discontinued.
		<u>VZV seronegative recipient (VZV seropositive graft)</u> Valacyclovir 1 gm (PO) q8h post-transplant x 4–24 months	Acyclovir 800 mg (PO) 5x/day post-transplant x 4–24 months	Transplant recipients on CMV prophylaxis with Gangciclovir or Valganciclovir do not require VZV prophylaxis.

Table 6.8 Transplant Prophylaxis (BMT/SOT) *(cont'd)*

Exposure	Usual Organism	Preferred Prophylaxis	Alternate Prophylaxis	Comments
Cytomegalo-virus (CMV)	SOT (D+/R-, D+/R+, D-/R+)	Valganciclovir 900 mg (PO) q24h × 3–6 months	Ganciclovir 5 mg/kg (IV) q24h × 3–6 months	Alternately, preemptive therapy may be used. When quantitative CMV PCR/pp 65 antigenemia levels become +/↑.

D-/R- patients should receive CMV negative blood and leukocyte depleted RBCs but do not require antiviral prophylaxis. |
PCP	SOT/BMT (with GVHD)	TMP-SMX 1 DS tablet (PO) q week × 12 months	TMP-SMX 1 SS tablet (PO) q24h × 12 months **or** Atova-quone 1500 mg (PO) q24h × 12 months (with a meal)	See Drug Summaries for drug-drug interactions.
Toxoplasmosis	Heart trans-plants	TMP-SMX 1 DS tablet (PO) q24h	Atova-quone 1500 mg (PO) q24h (take with a meal)	See Drug Summaries for drug-drug interactions.
Candida	Liver/pancreas trans-plants	Fluconazole 400 mg (IV/PO) q24h × 4 weeks	Posacon-azole 200 mg (PO) q8h × 4 weeks	See Drug Summaries for drug-drug interactions.
Aspergillus	Allogeneic BMT/lung trans-plants	Voriconazole 200 mg (PO) q12h	Posacon-azole 200 mg (PO) q8h	Until engrafted (BMT); duration in lung transplants unclear. See Drug Summaries in Chapter 11 for drug-drug interactions.

GVHD = graft vs. host disease.

ENDOCARDITIS PROPHYLAXIS

Endocarditis prophylaxis is now recommended only for previous endocarditis, prosthetic cardiac valve or prosthetic cardiac valve material, congenital heart disease (CHD), unrepaired cyanotic CHD, including palliative shunts and conduits, completely repaired congenital heart defects with prosthetic material/devices (placed by surgery or by catheter intervention during the first 6 months post-procedure), repaired CHD with residual defects adjacent to the site of prosthetic patch/device, and cardiac transplantation with cardiac valvupathy.

Table 6.9 Indications for Infective Endocarditis (IE) Prophylaxis*

Subset	Prophylaxis Recommended (Column A)	Prophylaxis Not Recommended (Column B)
Cardiac conditions	• Ostium primum ASD • Prosthetic heart valves, including bioprosthetic and homo graft valves • Previous infective endocarditis • Most congenital cardiac mal formations • Rheumatic valve disease • Hypertrophic cardiomyopathy • MVP with significant valvular regurgitation • Calcific aortic stenosis	• Isolated ostium secundum ASD • Surgical repair without residue beyond 6 months of ostium secundum ASD or PDA • Previous coronary artery bypass surgery • MVP without valvular regurgitation • Physiologic, functional, or innocent murmurs • Previous Kawasaki's cardiac disease or rheumatic fever without valve disease
Procedures	• Dental procedures known to induce gingival/mucosal bleeding, including dental cleaning • Tonsillectomy or adenoidectomy • Surgical operations involving intestinal or respiratory mucosa • Cystoscopy or urethral dilation • Urethral catheterization or urinary tract surgery if UTI is present • Prostate surgery • I & D of infected tissue	• Dental procedures not likely to induce gingival bleeding • Tympanostomy tube insertion • Flexible bronchoscopy ± biopsy • Endotracheal intubation • Endoscopy ± gastrointestinal biopsy • Cesarean section • D & C, IUD insertion/removal, or therapeutic abortion in the absence of infection • Cardiac pacemaker/defibrillator insertion

* Wilson W, et al. Prevention of Infective Endocarditis. Circulation 116:1736–1754, 2007. (PMID: 17446442)

Table 6.9 Indications for Infective Endocarditis (IE) Prophylaxis* *(cont'd)*

Subset	Prophylaxis Recommended (Column A)	Prophylaxis Not Recommended (Column B)
	• Biopsies of infected respiratory mucosa or infected skin/soft tissues • Any surgical procedure involving an infected field	• Coronary stent implantation • Percutaneous transluminal coronary angioplasty (PTCA) • Cardiac catheterization

ASD = atrial septal defect, D & C = dilatation and curettage, I & D = incision and drain, IUD = intrauterine device, MVP = mitral valve prolapse, PDA = patent ductus arteriosus, UTI = urinary tract infection.

* Prophylaxis is indicated for patients with cardiac conditions in Column A undergoing procedures in Column A. Prophylaxis is not recommended for patients or procedures in Column B. See Tables 6.9 and 6.10 for prophylaxis regimens for above-the-waist and below-the-waist procedures, respectively.

Table 6.10 Endocarditis Prophylaxis for Above-the-Waist (Dental, Oral, Esophageal, Respiratory Tract) Procedures*

Prophylaxis	Reaction to Penicillin	Antibiotic Regimen
Oral prophylaxis	None	Amoxicillin 2 gm (PO) 1 hour pre-procedure†
	Non-anaphylactoid	Cephalexin 1 gm (PO) 1 hour pre-procedure
	Anaphylactoid	Clindamycin 300 mg (PO) 1 hour pre-procedure††
IV prophylaxis	None	Ampicillin 2 gm (IV) 30 minutes pre-procedure
	Non-anaphylactoid	Cefazolin 1 gm (IV) 15 minutes pre-procedure
	Anaphylactoid	Clindamycin 600 mg (IV) 30 minutes pre-procedure

* Endocarditis prophylaxis is directed against viridans streptococci, the usual SBE pathogen above the waist. Macrolide regimens are less effective than other regimens; clarithromycin/azithromycin regimens (500 mg PO 1 hour pre-procedure) are of unproven efficacy.
† Some recommend a 3 gm dose of amoxicillin, which is excessive given the sensitivity of viridans streptococci to amoxicillin.
†† Some recommend a 600 mg dose of clindamycin, but a 300 mg dose gives adequate blood levels and is better tolerated (less diarrhea).

Table 6.11 Endocarditis Prophylaxis for Below-the-Waist (Genitourinary, Gastrointestinal) Procedures Involving an Infected Field*†

Prophylaxis	Reaction to Penicillin	Antibiotic Regimen
Oral prophylaxis	None	Amoxicillin 2 gm (PO) 1 hour pre-procedure
	Anaphylactoid	Linezolid 600 mg (PO) 1 hour pre-procedure

Table 6.11 Endocarditis Prophylaxis for Below-the-Waist (Genitourinary, Gastrointestinal) Procedures Involving an Infected Field*† *(cont'd)*

Prophylaxis	Reaction to Penicillin	Antibiotic Regimen
IV prophylaxis	None	Ampicillin 2 gm (IV) 30 minutes pre-procedure **plus** Gentamicin 80 mg (IM) or (IV) over 1 hour 60 minutes pre-procedure
	Anaphylactoid	Vancomycin 1 gm (IV) over 1 hour 60 minutes pre-procedure **plus** Gentamicin 80 mg (IM) or (IV) over 1 hour 60 minutes pre-procedure

*   Endocarditis prophylaxis is directed against E. faecalis, the usual SBE pathogen below the waist.
†   Seto TB. The case for infectious endocarditis prophylaxis. Arch Intern Med 167:327–330, 2007. (PMID:17325292)
     Harrison JL, Hoen B, Prendergast BD. Antibiotic Prophylaxis for Infective Endocarditis. Lancet 371:1317–1319, 2008. (PMID:18424310)

Table 6.12 Q Fever Endocarditis Prophylaxis

Prophylaxis	Antibiotic Regimen
PO prophylaxis (for significant valvulopathy)* in acute Q fever	Doxycycline 100 mg (PO) of q12 h × 12 months **Plus** Hydroxychloroquine 200 mg (PO) q8h × 12 months

* Significant valvulopathy: history of rheumatic fever, aortic bicuspid valve, ≥ 2 valve stenosis/regurgitation, MVP, remodeled/thickened valve.

TRAVEL PROPHYLAXIS

Travelers may acquire infectious diseases from ingestion of fecally-contaminated water/food, exchange of infected body secretions, inhalation of aerosolized droplets, direct inoculation via insect bites, or from close contact with infected birds/animals.

Recommendations to prevent infection in travelers consist of general travel precautions, and specific travel prophylaxis regimens.

Table 6.13 General Infectious Disease Travel Precautions

Exposure	Risk	Precautions
Unsafe water (fecally contaminated)	Diarrhea/ dysentery, viral hepatitis (HAV)	• Avoid ingestion of unbottled/unpotable water. Be sure bottled water has an unbroken seal and has not been opened/refilled with tap water. • Avoid ice cubes made from water of uncertain of origin/handling, and drinking from unclean glasses. • Drink only pasteurized bottled drinks. Be sure bottles/cans are opened by you or in your presence.

Table 6.13 General Infectious Disease Travel Precautions (cont'd)

Exposure	Risk	Precautions
		• Avoid drinking unpasteurized/warm milk; beer, wine, and pure alcoholic beverages are safe 2. • Eat only canned fruit or fresh fruit peeled by you or in your presence with clean utensils. • Avoid eating soft cheeses. • Avoid eating raw tomatoes/uncooked vegetables that may have been exposed to contaminated water • Avoid using hotel water for tooth brushing/rinsing unless certain of purity. Many hotels use common lines for bath/sink water that is unsuitable for drinking. • Avoid wading/swimming/bathing in lakes or rivers.
Food-borne (fecally-contaminated)	Diarrhea/dysentery	• Eat only seafood/poultry/meats that are freshly cooked and served hot. Avoid eating at roadside stands or small local restaurants with questionable sanitary practices. • "Boil it, peel it, or forget it."
Body fluid secretions	Viral hepatitis (HBV, HCV), STDs, HIV	• Do not share utensils/glasses/straws or engage in "risky behaviors" involving body secretion exchange. • Avoid blood transfusion (use blood expanders instead). • Treat dental problems before travel.
Animal bite	Animal bite-associated infections	• Do not pet/play with stray dogs/cats. Rabies and other infections are common in wild (and some urban) animals.
Flying insects	Malaria, arthropod-borne infections	• Avoid flying/biting insects by wearing dark protective clothing (long sleeves/pants) and using insect repellent on clothes/exposed skin, especially during evening hours. • Minimize dawn-to-dusk outdoor exposure. • Use screens/mosquito nets when possible. • Do not use perfume, after shave, or scented deodorants/toiletries that will attract flying insects.

Table 6.14 Travel Prophylaxis Regimens

Exposure	Usual Pathogens	Prophylaxis Regimens	Comments

Water (contaminated)	E. coli
	  ETEC
	  EIEC
	Campylobacter
	Salmonella
	Shigella
	Non-cholera
	  vibrios
	V. cholerae
	Aeromonas
	Rotavirus
	Norovirus
	Enteroviruses
	Giardia lamblia
	Yersinia
	Cryptosporidium
	Cyclospora
	Amebiasis
		Doxycycline 100 mg (PO) q24h for duration of exposure
		or
		Any quinolone (PO) for duration of exposure
		or
		TMP–SMX 1 SS tablet (PO) q24h for duration of exposure
			Observe without prophylaxis and treat mild diarrhea symptomatically with loperamide (2 mg). Persons with medical conditions adversely affected by dehydration caused by diarrhea may begin prophylaxis after arrival in country and continue for 1 day after returning home. Should severe diarrhea/dysentery occur, continue/switch to a quinolone, maximize oral hydration, and see a physician if possible.
			Anti-spasmodics may be used for symptomatic relief of mild, watery diarrhea but are contraindicated in severe diarrhea/dysentery. Bismuth subsalicylate is less effective than antibiotic prophylaxis. Most cases are due to enterotoxigenic E. coli. TMP–SMX is active against some bacterial pathogens and Cyclospora, but not against E. histolytica. Doxycycline is active against most bacterial pathogens and E. histolytica, but misses Campylobacter, Cryptosporidium, Cyclospora, Giardia.

Meningococcal meningitis	N. meningitidis	<u>Pre-travel prophylaxis</u> Meningococcal conjugate vaccine 0.5 mL (IM) ≥ 1 month prior to travel to endemic/epidemic areas	Acquired via close face-to-face contact (airborne aerosol/droplet exposure). Vaccine is highly protective against N. meningitidis serotypes A, C, Y, and W-135, but misses serotype B. For areas with serogroup B may use meningococcal group B vaccine. Alternately, consider chemoprophylaxis.
Hepatitis A (HAV)	Hepatitis A virus	HAV vaccine 1 mL (IM) prior to travel, then follow with a one-time booster 3, 6 months later	HAV vaccine is better than immune globulin for prophylaxis. Take care to avoid direct/indirect ingestion of fecally contaminated water. HAV vaccine is recommended for travel to all developing countries. Protective antibody titers develop after 2 weeks.

Table 6.14 Travel Prophylaxis Regimens (cont'd)

Exposure	Usual Pathogens	Prophylaxis Regimens	Comments
Typhoid fever	S. typhi	ViCPS vaccine 0.5 mL (IM). Booster every 2 years for repeat travelers **or** Oral Ty21a vaccine 1 capsule (PO) q48h × 4 doses. Booster every 5 years for repeat travelers	For the oral vaccine, do not co-administer with antibiotics. Contraindicated in compromised hosts and children < 6 years old. Take oral capsules with cold water. Degree of protective immunity is limited with vaccine. Some prefer chemoprophylaxis the same as for Traveler's diarrhea
Cholera	V. cholera (serotype 01)	Oral vaccine 3 fluid oz (PO) > 10 days before travel	Approved for adults 18–64 years. Side effects: N/V/D, fatigue, anorexia.
Yellow fever (YF)	Yellow fever virus	Yellow fever vaccine 0.5 mL (SC). Booster no longer generally recommended as protection is life long	Vaccine is often required for travel to West Africa. Administer 1 month apart from other live vaccines. Contraindicated in children < 4 months old; caution in children < 1 year old. Reactions may occur in persons with egg allergies. Immunity is probably life long, but a booster suggested for prolonged period in endemic area or travel to areas of an ongoing outbreak or laboratory personnel who routinely handle wild type YF virus.
Japanese encephalitis (JE)	Japanese encephalitis virus	JE vaccine 1 mL (SC) on days 0, 7, and 14 or 30. Booster schedule not established	Recommended for travelers planning prolonged (> 3 weeks) visits during the rainy season to rural, endemic areas of Asia (e.g., Eastern Russia, Indian subcontinent, China, Southeast Asia, Thailand, Korea, Laos, Cambodia, Vietnam, Malaysia, Philippines). Administer 3, 2 weeks before exposure. Children < 3 years may be given 0.5 mL (SC) on same schedule as adults.

Table 6.14 Travel Prophylaxis Regimens *(cont'd)*

Exposure	Usual Pathogens	Prophylaxis Regimens	Comments
Rabies	Rabies virus	HDCV, PCEC, or RVA prolonged period in an YF endemic area, 1 mL (IM) on days 0, 7, and 21 or 28 prior to travel **or** HDCV 0.1 mL (ID) on days 0, 7, and 21 or 28 prior to travel	Avoid contact with wild dogs/animals during travel. Dose of rabies vaccine for adults and children are the same. A booster dose prior to travel is recommended if antibody levels are measured and are low.
Tetanus Diphtheria Pertussis	C. tetani C. diphtheriae B. pertussis	Tdap 0.5 mL (IM)	Tdap also boosts pertussis immunity.

Table 6.15 Malaria Prophylaxis

Drug	Area of Exposure	Adult Dose	Comments
Atovaquone/ proguanil (Malarone)	Prophylaxis in all areas	1 Tablet (250 mg atovaquone/100 mg proguanil) daily	Begin 1 day before travel to malarious areas. Take daily while in malarious areas and daily for 1 week after returning. Contraindicated in persons with severe renal impairment (creatinine clearance < 30 mL/min). Atovaquone/proguanil should be taken with food or a milk drink. Not recommended prophylaxis for pregnant women, and women breastfeeding.
Chloroquine (Aralen)	Prophylaxis in areas with chloroquine-sensitive malaria	300 mg once daily	Begin 1 week before travel to malarious areas. Take daily while in malarious area and daily for 4 weeks after returning.

Table 6.15 Malaria Prophylaxis (cont'd)

Drug	Area of Exposure	Adult Dose	Comments
Doxycycline	Prophylaxis in all areas	100 mg orally, (with food) daily	Begin 1 day before travel to malarious areas. Take daily while in malarious areas and daily for 4 weeks after leaving area. Contraindicated in children < 8 years and in pregnancy.
Tafenoquine	Prophylaxis in all areas	200 mg orally daily × 3 days	Begin 1 day before travel. Repeat weekly while in malarious areas and 1 dose 1 week after returning.
Mefloquine (Lariam)	Prophylaxis in areas with mefloquine-sensitive malaria (mefloquine resistance in SE Asia)	250 mg once weekly	Begin 2½ weeks before travel to malarious areas. Take weekly while in malarious areas and for 4 weeks after returning. Contraindicated in persons allergic to mefloquine or related compounds (e.g., quinine, quinidine) and with depression psychiatric disorders, or seizures or cardiac conduction abnormalities.
Primaquine[†]	Prophylaxis for short-duration travel to areas with principally P. vivax	30 mg orally, daily	Begin 1–2 days before travel to malarious areas. Take daily at the same time each day while in malarious areas and for 7 days after leaving such areas. Contraindicated in persons with G6PD deficiency, pregnancy and breastfeeding unless the infant being breastfed has a documented normal G6PD level.

Table 6.15 Malaria Prophylaxis *(cont'd)*

Drug	Area of Exposure	Adult Dose	Comments
Hydroxy-chloroquine (Plaquenil)	An alternative to chloroquine for prophylaxis only in areas with chloro-quine-sensitive malaria	400 mg orally, once weekly	Begin 1–2 weeks before travel to malarious areas. Take weekly while in the malarious area and for 4 weeks after returning.

HDCV = human diploid cell vaccine, PCEC = purified chick embryo cell vaccine, RVA = rabies vaccine absorbed, RIG = rabies immune globulin.

†   Glucose-6-phosphate dehydrogenase. Those who take primaquine should have a normal G6PD level before starting the medication.

TETANUS PROPHYLAXIS

Current information suggests that immunity lasts for decades/life-time after teta-nus immunization. A tetanus booster should not be routinely given for minor wounds, but is recommended for wounds with high tetanus potential (e.g. massive crush wounds, soil-contaminated wounds, or deep puncture wounds).

Table 6.16 Tetanus Prophylaxis in Routine Wound Management

History of Adsorbed Tetanus Toxoid	Wound Type	Recommendations
Unknown or < 3 doses	Clean, minor wounds	Td‡ or Tdap‡
	Tetanus-prone wounds†	(Td‡ or Tdap‡) plus TIG
≥ 3 doses	Clean, minor wounds	No prophylaxis needed
	Tetanus-prone wounds†	Td‡ if > 10 years since last dose*

DT = diphtheria and tetanus toxoids adsorbed (pediatrics), DTP = diphtheria and tetanus toxoids and pertussis vaccine adsorbed, Td = tetanus and diphtheria toxoids adsorbed (adult), TIG = tetanus immune globulin, Tdap = tetanus and diphtheria toxoids and pertussis vaccine absorbed.

†   For example, massive crush wounds; wounds contaminated with dirt, soil, feces, or saliva; deep puncture wounds; or significant burn wounds or frostbite.

‡   For children < 7 years, DTP (DT if pertussis is contraindicated) is preferred to tetanus toxoid alone. For children ≥ 7 years old and adults, Tdap is preferred to Td or tetanus toxoid alone.

*   More frequent booster doses are unnecessary and can increase side effects. Protection lasts > 20yrs
    Adapted from: Centers for Disease Control and Prevention. MMWR Rep 40 (RR-10):1–28. 1991.

ADULT IMMUNIZATIONS

Immunizations are designed to reduce infections in large populations, and may prevent/decrease the severity of infection in non-immunized individuals. Compromised hosts with altered immune systems may not develop protective antibody titers to antigenic components of various vaccines. **Immunizations are not fully protective, but are recommended** (depending on the vaccine) for most normal hosts, since some protection is better than none.

Table 6.17 Adult Immunizations

Vaccine	Indications	Dosage	Comments
Bacille Calmette Guérin (BCG)	Possibly beneficial for adults at high-risk of multiple-drug resistant tuberculosis.	Primary: 1 dose (intradermal). Booster not recommended.	Live attenuated vaccine induces a positive PPD which may remain positive for years/life. Contraindicated in immuno-compromised hosts. Injection site infection or disseminated infection are rare.
Hemophilus influenzae (type B)	For those at increased risk for invasive disease, e.g., functional or anatomic asplenia, HIV, immunoglobulin deficiency, complement deficiency (C_{1-3}), stem cell transplants, chemotherapy or radiation therapy.	Primary: 0.5 mL dose (IM). Booster not recommended.	Capsular polysaccharide conjugated to diphtheria toxoid. Benefit uncertain. Safety in pregnancy unknown. Mild local reactions in 10%.
Hepatitis A (HAV)	All children beginning age 12 to 23 months and adults at increased risk of HAV.	Primary: 1 mL dose (IM). One-time booster ≥ 6 months later. Booster not routinely recommended.	Inactivated whole virus. Pregnancy risk not fully evaluated. Mild soreness at injection site. Occasional headache/malaise.

Table 6.17 Adult Immunizations *(cont'd)*

Vaccine	Indications	Dosage	Comments
Hepatitis B (HBV)	Those desiring HBV protection or household/ sexual contact with carrier, IV drug use, multiple sex partners (heterosexual), homosexual male activity, blood product recipients, hemodialysis, occupational exposure to blood, residents/ staff of institutions for developmentally disabled, prison inmates, residence ≥ 6 months in areas of high endemicity, others at high risk. Heplisav–B (Hep B–CpG) vaccine.	Primary (3- dose series): Recombivax 10 mcg (1 mL) or Engerix-B 20 mcg (1 mL) IM in deltoid at 0, 1, and 6 months. Alternate schedule for Engerix-B: 4- dose series at 0, 1, 2, and 12 months. Booster not routinely recommended. Primary: 2 doses of 0.5 mL (IM) ≥ 4 weeks apart, Booster not recommended.	Recombinant vaccine comprised of hepatitis B surface antigen. For compromised hosts (including dialysis patients), use specially packaged Recombivax 40-mcg doses (1 mL vial containing 40 mcg/mL). HBsAb titers should be obtained 6 months after 3-dose primary series. Those with non-protective titers (≤ 10 mIU/mL) should receive 1 dose monthly up to a maximum of 3 doses and retest for HbsAb titers. Pregnancy not a contraindication in high-risk females. Twinrix 1 mL (IM) (combination of Hepatitis A inactivated vaccine and Hepatitis B recombinant vaccine) is available for adults on a 0, 1, and 6-month schedule or 0, 7 days, 21–30 days, and 12- month schedules.
Herpes zoster (HZV)	Adults ≥ 60 years to reduce the frequency of shingles/prevent post-herpetic neuralgia (PHN). Use in those with previous H. zoster is not yet defined. Protection best in 60–69 years group; efficacy decreases with increasing age.	Primary: 0.65 mL (SC). Need for revaccination not yet defined. Primary: Two 0.5 mL (IM) doses as 0 and 2–6 months. Shingrix recombinant zoster vaccine (RZV).	Duration of protection is at least 4 years. Injection site reactions common. Contraindicated in immunocompromised hosts (with immunosuppressive disorder or receiving immunosuppressive drug) or untreated TB. Not indicated for therapy of H. zoster or post-herpetic neuralgia. Efficacy ~ 50%. RZV with AS01$_B$ adjuvant highly efficacious >90% for prevention of shingles/PHN in adults > 50 years.

Table 6.17 Adult Immunizations *(cont'd)*

Vaccine	Indications	Dosage	Comments
Influenza	All adults.	Annual standard dose vaccine (SD). Single 0.5 mL dose (IM) before flu season is optimal, but can be given anytime during flu season. (2 A strains + 1 B strain).	High dose (HD) vaccine has $4\times$ the antigen content as the standard dose (SD) vaccine. Quadrivalent (2 A strains + 2 B strain) and trivalent inactivated whole and split virus vaccines available. Contraindications include anaphylaxis to eggs or sensitivity to thimerosal. Mild local reaction common. Malaise/myalgias in some. For pregnancy, administer in 2nd or 3rd trimester during flu season. High titer (HD) inactivated vaccine indicated for adults $\geq$ 65 years. Enhanced protective efficacy (vs. SD), but expensive. Statins may $\downarrow$ efficacy.
Measles	Adults born after 1956 without live-virus immunization or measles diagnosed by a physician or immunologic test. Also indicated for revaccination of persons given killed measles vaccine between 1963 and 1967.	Primary: 0.5 mL dose (SC). A second dose ($\geq$ 1 month later) is recommended for certain adults at increased risk of exposure (e.g., healthcare workers, travelers to developing countries). No routine booster.	Live virus vaccine (usually given in MMR). Contraindicated in compromised hosts, pregnancy, history of anaphylaxis to eggs or neomycin. Ineffective if given 3–11 months after blood products. Side effects include low-grade fever 5–21 days after vaccination, rash, and local reactions in if previously immunized with killed vaccine (1963–67).
Meningococcus (invasive disease)	Patients with splenic dysfunction or with complement defects (C_{7-9}) laboratory workers. May be given to 1st year college students living in dormitories.	Meningococcal conjugate vaccine 0.5 mL (IM). Primary: 0.5 mL (IM) then again at months 2 and 6 (3-dose series) MC (fHBP) vaccine 0.5 mL (IM). Primary 0.5 mL (IM) then again at 2 and 6 months (3-dose series)	Also used in epidemic control of N. meningitidis outbreaks serogroups A, C, Y, and W-135. Use meningococcal group B vaccine in adolescents and young adults at $\uparrow$ risk and group B outbreaks.

Table 6.17 Adult Immunizations *(cont'd)*

Vaccine	Indications	Dosage	Comments
Mumps	Non-immune adults.	Primary: 0.5 mL dose (SC). No routine booster.	Live attenuated vaccine (usually given in MMR). Contraindicated in immunocompromised hosts, pregnancy, history of anaphylaxis to eggs or neomycin.
Papilloma (human) Virus (HPV)	Females up to 26 years of age. Contraindicated in pregnancy. Suggested for males up to 26 years of age.	Primary: 0.5 mL (IM). Second dose: 2 months after 1st dose. Third dose: 6 months after 1st dose.	Quadrivalent HPV vaccine to prevent cervical, vulvar, vaginal and cancers caused by HPV types 6, 11, 16, 18. 9 valent HPV vaccine includes HPV types 52, 58, 31, 33, 45, 6, 11, 16, 18.
Pertussis	Use Tdap instead of Td in booster dose.	A single Tdap booster dose 0.5 mL (IM).	Recommended since adults may get pertussis or transmit it to susceptible infants.
Pneumococcus (S. pneumoniae)	Immunocompetent hosts ≥ 65 years old, or > 19 years old with diabetes, CSF leaks, or chronic cardiac, pulmonary or liver disease. Also for immunocompromised hosts > 19 years old with functional/anatomic asplenia,* leukemia, lymphoma, multiple myeloma, widespread malignancy, chronic renal failure, bone marrow/organ transplant, or on immunosuppressive/steroid therapy.	PCV-13 (conjugate) PPSV-23 (polysaccharide) Primary: 0.5 mL dose (IM). No booster. Primary: 0.5 mL dose (SC or IM). A one-time booster at 5 years is recommended for immuno-compromised hosts > 2 years old and for those who received the vaccine before age 65 for high-risk conditions.	*Pneumococcal vaccine naïve persons aged ≥ 65.* Give PCV-13, then give PPSV-23 6–12 months later (minimal interval 8 weeks). *Persons who previously received PPSV-23 at age ≥ 65.* Give PCV-13 >1 year later after PPSV-23 given. *Persons who previously received PPSV-23 before age 65 years who are now age ≥ 65.* Give PCV-13 when ≥ 65 years give > 1 year later (minimum interval between sequential administration of PCV-13 and PPSV-23 is 8 weeks). If this window is missed, PPSV-23 can be given 6-12 months after PCV-13.

PCV-13 = **13 valent** pneumococcal **conjugate** vaccine (contains strains: 1, 3, 5, 6A, 6B, 7F, 9V, 14, 18C, 19A, 19F, 23F)

PPSV-23 = **23 valent** pneumococcal **polysaccharide** vaccine (contains strains: 1, 2, 3, 4, 5, 6B, 7F, 8, 9N, 9V, 10A, 11A, 12F, 14, 15B, 17F, 18C, 19F, 19A, 20, 22F, 23F, 33F).

*Pneumococcal **polysaccharide vaccine** should be given before splenectomy, but *is ineffective post-splenectomy.* The conjugate vaccine is more effective post-splenectomy.

COLOR ATLAS

CSF, Sputum, and Urine Gram Stains

Paul E. Schoch, PhD
Edward J. Bottone, PhD
Daniel Caplivski, MD

CSF GRAM STAINS

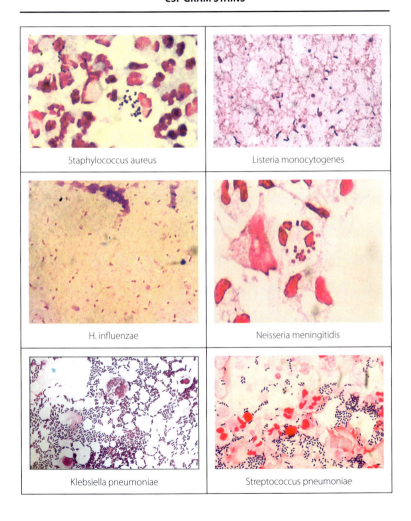

Staphylococcus aureus

Listeria monocytogenes

H. influenzae

Neisseria meningitidis

Klebsiella pneumoniae

Streptococcus pneumoniae

SPUTUM GRAM STAINS

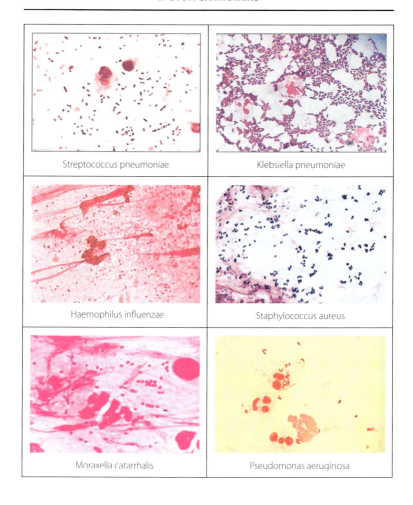

Streptococcus pneumoniae

Klebsiella pneumoniae

Haemophilus influenzae

Staphylococcus aureus

Moraxella catarrhalis

Pseudomonas aeruginosa

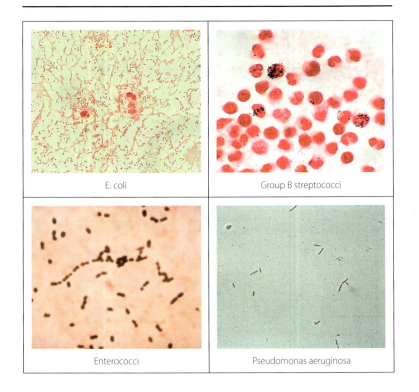

E. coli

Group B streptococci

Enterococci

Pseudomonas aeruginosa

COLOR ATLAS

Fungal Stains

Daniel Caplivski, MD
Edward J. Bottone, PhD

FUNGAL STAINS

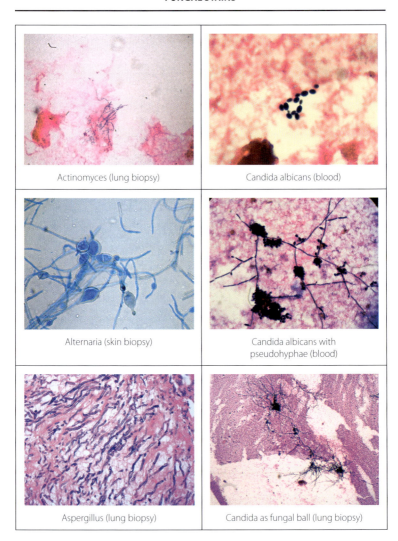

Actinomyces (lung biopsy)

Candida albicans (blood)

Alternaria (skin biopsy)

Candida albicans with pseudohyphae (blood)

Aspergillus (lung biopsy)

Candida as fungal ball (lung biopsy)

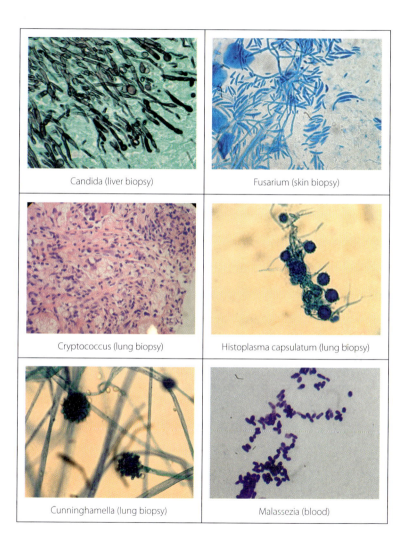

Candida (liver biopsy)

Fusarium (skin biopsy)

Cryptococcus (lung biopsy)

Histoplasma capsulatum (lung biopsy)

Cunninghamella (lung biopsy)

Malassezia (blood)

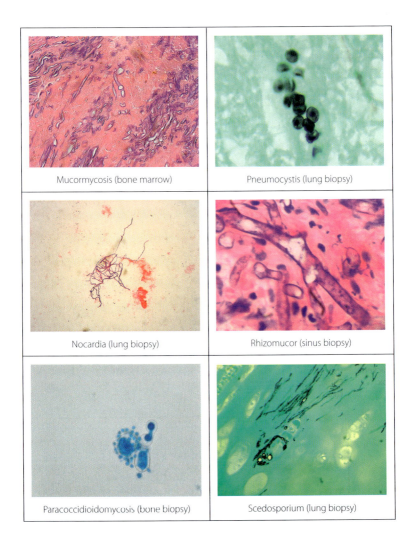

Mucormycosis (bone marrow)

Pneumocystis (lung biopsy)

Nocardia (lung biopsy)

Rhizomucor (sinus biopsy)

Paracoccidioidomycosis (bone biopsy)

Scedosporium (lung biopsy)

Table 6.17 Adult Immunizations *(cont'd)*

Vaccine	Indications	Dosage	Comments
Rubella	Non-immune adults, particularly women of child bearing age.	Primary: 0.5 mL dose (SC). No routine booster.	Live virus (RA 27/3 strain) vaccine (usually given in MMR). Contraindicated in immuno-compromised hosts, pregnancy, history of anaphylactic reaction to neomycin. Joint pains and transient arthralgias in up to 40%, beginning 3–25 days after vaccination and lasting 1–11 days; arthritis in < 2%.
Tetanus-diph-theria (Td)	Adults	Primary: Td two 0.5 mL doses (IM), 1–2 months apart; third dose 6–12 months after second dose. Booster: a single Tdap 0.5 mL (IM) is recommended. Tdap should be substituted for one of the three Td doses.	Adsorbed toxoid vaccine. Contraindicated if hypersensitivity/neurological reaction or severe local reaction to previous doses. Side effects include local reactions, occasional fever, systemic symptoms, Arthus-like reaction in persons with multiple previous boosters, and systemic allergy (rare).
Varicella (VZV) chicken-pox	Non-immune adolescents and adults, especially healthcare workers and others likely to be exposed.	Primary: Two 0.5 mL doses (SC), 4–8 weeks apart. Vaccine must be stored frozen and used within 30 minutes after thawing and reconstitution. No routine booster.	Live attenuated vaccine. Contraindications include pregnancy, active untreated TB, immunocompromised host, malignancy of bone marrow or lymphatic system, anaphylactic reaction to gelatin/neomycin, or blood product recipient within previous 6 months (may prevent development of protective antibody). Mild febrile illness. Injection site symptoms are common. Mild diffuse rash in 5%.

*Kim DK, Hunter P. Advisory Committee on Immunization Practices. Recommended adult immunization schedule. Ann Intern Med. 170:182-92, 2019.

REFERENCES

Bennett JE, Dolin R, Blaser MJ (eds). Mandell, Douglas, and Bennett's Principles and Practice of Infectious Diseases (9th Ed), Philadelphia, Elsevier, 2019.

Brunette GW, Kozarsky P, Magill A, et al (eds). The Yellow Book CDC Health Information for International Travel. Oxford University Press, 2016.

Brusch JL, Endocarditis Essentials. Jones & Bartlett, Sudbury, MA, 2011.

Cohen J, Powderly WG, Opal S (eds). Infectious Diseases (4th Ed). Philadelphia: Elsevier, 2016.

Cunha CB, Schlossberg D (eds). Clinical Infectious Disease (3rd Ed), Cambridge University Press, Cambridge, 2020.

Gorbach SL, Bartlett JG. Blacklow NR Infectious (eds). Diseases (3rd Ed), Lippincott, Williams & Wilkins, Philadelphia, 2004.

Hawker J, Begg N, Blair et al. Communicable Disease Control Handbook (3rd Ed), Malden, Massachusetts, Blackwell Publishing, 2012.

Heymann DL. Control of Communicable Disease Manual (20th Ed), American Public Health Association, 2014.

Keystone JS, Kozarski PE, Freedman DO, et al. Travel Medicine. (3rd Ed), Mosby, Edinburgh, 2013.

Koff R. Hepatitis Essentials. Jones & Bartlett, Sudbury, MA, 2011.

Plotkin SA, Orenstein WA (eds) Vaccines (7th Ed), Philadelphia, W.B. Saunders, 2017.

Sax PE, Cohen CJ. HIV Essentials (7th Ed), Jones & Bartlett, Sudbury, MA, 2017.

Yu VL, Merigan Jr, TC, Barriere SL. Antimicrobial Therapy and Vaccines (2nd Ed), Williams & Wilkins, Baltimore, 2005.

Chapter 7

Pediatric Infectious Diseases and Pediatric Drug Summaries

Leonard R. Krilov, MD,
Asif Noor, MD,
George H. McCracken, Jr, MD

- This chapter pertains to infectious diseases and antimicrobial agents in the pediatric population. It is organized by clinical syndrome, patient subset, and in some cases, specific organism.
- Clinical summaries immediately follow each treatment grid. Therapeutic recommendations are based on antimicrobial effectiveness, reliability, cost, safety, and resistance potential.
- Antimicrobial agents and duration of therapy are listed in the treatment grids; corresponding drug dosages are provided on pages 438–446 and represent the usual dosages for normal renal and hepatic function.
- Drug dosages in infants/children are based on weight, up to adult dosage as maximum.
- Please refer to pediatric drug references and manufacturer's package inserts for dosage adjustments, side effects, and drug interactions.

- "PO Therapy or IV-to-PO Switch" indicates the clinical syndrome can be treated by IV therapy alone, PO therapy alone, or IV followed by PO therapy.
- Most patients on IV therapy able to take oral medications should be switched to PO equivalent therapy after clinical improvement.

Empiric Therapy of CNS Infections

Acute Bacterial Meningitis

Subset (age)	Usual Pathogens	Preferred IV Therapy†	Alternate IV Therapy†
Neonate (≤ 28 days)	Group B streptococci E. coli Listeria monocytogenes Other GNB (e.g., Citrobacter, Serratia) Enterococci	Ampicillin **plus** Gentamicin*	Ampicillin **plus** Cefotaxime* Vancomycin **plus** Cefotaxime
1–3 months	Overlap neonate and > 3 months	Vancomycin **plus either** Cefotaxime **or** Ceftriaxone*	Ampicillin **plus either** Cefotaxime **or** Ceftriaxone*
> 3 months	S. pneumoniae N. meningitidis H. influenzae B (very rare) Non-typable H. influenzae (rare)	<u>Before culture results</u>: Vancomycin **plus either** Ceftriaxone **or** Cefotaxime* <u>After culture results</u> Discontinue vancomycin if penicillin-susceptible S. pneumoniae, N. meningitidis, or H. influenzae isolated	Meropenem* <u>Severe penicillin allergy</u> Vancomycin **plus either** Aztreonam **or** Levofloxacin

Acute Bacterial Meningitis (cont'd)

Subset (age)	Usual Pathogens	Preferred IV Therapy†	Alternate IV Therapy†
CNS shunt infection (Treat initially for S. epidermidis; if later identified as MSSA, treat accordingly)	S. epidermidis S. aureus (MRSA)	Vancomycin ± Rifampin 10 mg/kg (IV or PO) q12h × 7–10 days after shunt removal	Linezolid × 7–10 days after shunt removal If MSSA isolated Nafcillin ± Rifampin 10 mg/kg (PO) q12h × 7–10 days after shunt removal
	S. aureus (MSSA)	Nafcillin × 7–10 days after shunt removal	Vancomycin × 7–10 days after shunt removal
	Enterobacteriaceae	Cefotaxime **or** Ceftriaxone × 7–10 days after shunt removal	Meropenem × 7–10 days after shunt removal

MRSA/MSSA = methicillin-resistant/sensitive S. aureus. Duration of therapy represents total time IV or IV + PO. Most patients on IV therapy able to take PO meds should be switched to PO therapy after clinical improvement.

* Duration of therapy: Group B strep ≥ 14 days (with ventriculitis 4 weeks); E. coli, Citrobacter, Serratia ≥ 21 days; Listeria 10–14 days; Enterococcus ≥ 14 days; S. pneumoniae 10–14 days; H. influenzae ≥ 10 days; N. meningitidis 4–7 days.

† **See p. 436–444 for drug dosages.**

Acute Bacterial Meningitis (Normal Hosts)

Clinical Presentation: Fever, headache, stiff neck (or bulging anterior fontanelle in infants), irritability, vomiting, lethargy, evolving over hours to 1–2 days. The younger the child, the more nonspecific the presentation (e.g., irritability, lethargy, fever, poor feeding).

Diagnostic Considerations: Diagnosis by CSF chemistries, gram stain, culture. CSF findings are similar to those in adults: pleocytosis (100–5000 WBCs/mm³; predominately PMNs), ↑ protein, ↓↓ glucose. Normal CSF values differ by age:

	WBC/mm³ (range); %PMNs	Protein, mg/dL (range)	Glucose, mg/dL (range)
Preterm	9 (0–25); 57% PMNs	115 (65–150)	50 (24–63)
Term newborn	8 (0–22); 61% PMNs	79 (56–102)	52 (34–119)
Child	0 (0–7); 0% PMNs	(5–40)	(40–80)

Modified from *The Harriet Lane Handbook.*

Pitfalls: The younger the child, the more nonspecific the presentation. With prior antibiotic use (e.g., oral therapy for otitis media), partially-treated meningitis (CSF lactic acid levels 4-6 nm/L) is a concern. Especially in the summer season, rapid viral diagnosis (especially enteroviral PCR) can exclude ABM and prevent unnecessary hospitalization and antibiotic use. HSV PCR can also be helpful in excluding ABM.

Therapeutic Considerations: Meningitic doses of antibiotics are required for the *entire* course of treatment. Repeat lumbar puncture (LP) is indicated at 24–48 hours if not responding clinically or in situations where a resistant organism is a concern (e.g., penicillin-resistant S. pneumonia, or neonate with gram-negative bacillary meningitis). Dexamethasone (0.3 mg/kg IV q12h × 2 days) may reduce neurologic sequelae (e.g., hearing loss) in children ≥ 6 weeks of age when given before/with the first dose of antibiotics.

Prognosis: Varies with causative agent and age at presentation. Overall mortality < 5% in US (higher in developing countries). Morbidity 30–35% with hearing loss the most common neurologic sequella. Incidence of neurologic sequelae: S. pneumoniae > H. influenzae > N. meningitidis. Use of H. influenzae (type B) and pneumococcal conjugate vaccines in routine childhood immunizations have greatly reduced the incidence of meningitis caused by these pathogens. Neonates are at increased risk of mortality and major neurologic sequelae, and there is a significant incidence of brain abscesses in neonates with gram-negative meningitis (especially Citrobacter and Serratia infections).

Acute Bacterial Meningitis (CNS Shunt Infections)

Clinical Presentation: Indolent (lethargy, irritability, vomiting) or acute (high fever, depressed mental status).

Diagnostic Considerations: Diagnosis by CSF gram stain/culture, often obtained by shunt tap.

Pitfalls: Blood cultures are usually negative for shunt pathogens and CSF WBCs may be low.

Therapeutic Considerations: High risk of nafcillin resistance with coagulase-negative staphylococcal infection. The addition of rifampin to vancomycin may improve clearance of bacteria. Removal of prosthetic material is usually necessary to achieve a cure.

Prognosis: Good with removal of prosthetic material.

Brain Abscess

Clinical Presentation: May remain asymptomatic for a long period of time until the mass is large enough to cause increase in ICP. Fevers can be absent, however fever, headache and vomiting present in more than half.

Diagnostic Consideration: Contrast enhanced imaging (CT and/or MRI)

Pitfalls: Diagnosis is often delayed as the non-specific presentation with fever headache and vomiting are usually attributed to an earlier viral illness.

Therapeutic consideration: Empiric choice should be based on possible source. A brain abscess can occur from an associated meningitis, contagious spread (dental infection, sinusitis, mastoiditis, foreign body) or from bacteremia/endocarditis (causing multiple abscesses in distribution of middle cerebral artery).

Prognosis: With better imaging and neurosurgical advances, there is a reduction in overall mortality but a high proportion of children develop neurologic deficits.

Other CNS infections treated in a similar fashion are subdural empyema, venous sinus thrombosis/septic thrombophlebitis/infarction.

Brain Abscess

Subset	Usual Pathogens	Preferred IV Therapy	Alternate IV Therapy
Brain abscess (2° to dental work)	Viridans streptococci, oral anaerobes	Ceftriaxone **plus** Metronidazole	Meropenem
Brain abscess (2° to endocarditis)	Streptococcal sp.	Ampicillin **plus** Gentamicin	Vancomycin **plus** Gentamicin particularly for PVE
Brain abscess (2° to chronic otitis, mastoiditis, or sinusitis)	Consider pseudomonas	Cefepime **plus** Metronidazole	Meropenem

Encephalitis

Subset	Usual Pathogens	IV Therapy†	IV-to-PO Switch†
Herpes	HSV-1	Acyclovir × 14–21 days	Treat IV only
Arbovirus	WNV, SLE, Powassan encephalitis, EEE, WEE, VEE, JE, CE, La crosse	No specific therapy	
Mycoplasma	M. pneumoniae	Doxycycline or Minocycline × 2–4 weeks	Doxycycline or minocycline × 2–4 weeks
Respiratory viruses	Influenza, Enteroviruses, Measles	No specific therapy	

WNV = West Nile Virus, SLE = St. Louis encephalitis, EEE = Eastern equine encephalitis, WEE = Western equine encephalitis, VEE = Venezuelan equine encephalitis, JE = Japanese encephalitis, CE = California encephalitis.

† **See p. 436–444 for drug dosages.**

Herpes Encephalitis (HSV-1)

Clinical Presentation: Acute onset of fever and mental status/behavioral changes. High fever with intractable seizures and profoundly depressed sensorium may dominate the clinical picture.

Diagnostic Considerations: Diagnosis by CSF PCR for HSV-1. CSF findings include ↑ RBC/WBC, ↓ glucose, and ↑↑ protein. Classic EEG changes with temporal lobe spikes may be present early. Brain biopsy is rarely, if ever, indicated.

Pitfalls: MRI/CT scan can be normal initially. Delays in diagnosis and therapy adversely affect outcome.

Therapeutic Considerations: HSV is the only treatable viral encephalitis in normal hosts.

Prognosis: Antiviral therapy improves survival based on level of consciousness at presentation. Mortality is 10–20%, and major neurologic sequellae are frequent in survivors.

Arboviral Encephalitis

Clinical Presentation: Acute onset of fever, headache, altered mental status. Usually seasonal (more common in summer/fall), based on vector/travel history. Can be very severe with high mortality. Symptomatic West Nile encephalitis is rare in children.

Diagnostic Considerations: Serological studies are the primary means of diagnosis. PCR "encephalitis panels" are being developed for clinical use.

Therapeutic Considerations: No specific antiviral therapy. Supportive therapy is crucial.

Pitfalls: Be sure to elicit potential exposures/travel history in children with fever/altered mental status.

Prognosis: Varies with agent. Severe residual deficits and high mortality rates can occur, especially with Eastern Equine encephalitis.

Mycoplasma Encephalitis

Clinical Presentation: Acute onset of fever and mental status changes. Prodromal cough, sore throat, respiratory symptoms may occur.

Diagnostic Considerations: CSF shows mild pleocytosis with a predominance of mononuclear cells, normal or mildly ↓ glucose, and mildly ↑ protein. Mycoplasma IgG/IgM titers are elevated.

Pitfalls: CSF findings can be confused with viral encephalitis.

Therapeutic Considerations: Often self-limited illness even without antibiotic therapy. Doxycycline or minocycline penetrate CNS and can be used in children > 8 years of age. Macrolides may treat pulmonary infection but do not penetrate CNS.

Prognosis: Good. Neurologic sequelae are rare.

Empiric Therapy of HEENT Infections

Periorbital (Preseptal) Cellulitis/Orbital Cellulitis

Subset	Usual Pathogens	Preferred IV Therapy†	Alternate IV Therapy†	IV-to-PO Switch†
Periorbital cellulitis	S. pneumoniae H. influenzae M. catarrhalis S. aureus (MSSA)	**Combination Therapy** Nafcillin* **plus either** Ceftriaxone **or** Cefotaxime × 10–14 days	Ampicillin/ Sulbactam × 10–14 days	Amoxicillin/ Clavulanate **or** Cefuroxime **or** Cefpodoxime **or** Cefdinir × 10–14 days
Orbital cellulitis	S. pneumoniae H. influenzae M. catarrhalis S. aureus (MSSA) Oral anaerobes Group A streptococci	**Combination Therapy** Vancomycin **plus** Ceftriaxone × 10–14 days	Piperacillin/ Tazobactam **or** Ampicillin/ Sulbactam **or** Ticarcillin/ Clavulanate × 10–14 days	Amoxicillin/ Clavulanate **or** Cefuroxime **or** Cefpodoxime **or** Cefdinir × 10–14 days

Duration of therapy represents total time IV or IV + PO. Most patients on IV therapy able to take PO meds should be switched to PO therapy after clinical improvement.

*   Clindamycin or Vancomycin if CA-MRSA likely.

†   **See p. 436–444 for drug dosages.**

Clinical Presentation: Periorbital and orbital cellulitis are bacterial infections. Fever, lid swelling, and erythema around the eye often in conjunction with acute sinusitis. In periorbital cellulitis the infection is anterior to the orbital septum. Orbital cellulitis involves the orbit proper, extraocular muscles/nerves, and possibly the orbital nerve. Proptosis and limitation of ocular mobility define orbital cellulitis.

Diagnostic Considerations: CT scan is used to differentiate preseptal from periorbital cellulitis and identify the extent of orbital involvement when present.

Pitfalls: Failure to recognize orbital involvement leading to optic nerve damage or CNS extension/cavernous sinus thrombosis. CT scan cannot differentiate phlegmon from abscess.

Therapeutic Considerations: Orbital cellulitis is more emergent than periorbital cellulitis and should be treated with IV antibiotics initially. Surgical drainage may be indicated if a well defined abscess is present or in more severe disease.

Prognosis: Good with prompt antimicrobial therapy and ophthalmologic surgery if needed.

Sinusitis

Subset	Usual Pathogens	IV Therapy† (Hospitalized)	PO Therapy or IV-to-PO Switch† (Ambulatory)
Acute	S. pneumoniae H. influenzae M. catarrhalis	Ceftriaxone **or** Cefuroxime × 1–2 weeks	Amoxicillin **or** Amoxicillin/Clavulanic acid **or** 2nd or 3rd generation cephalosporin **or** Levofloxacin **or** Azithromycin*
Chronic	Same as acute + oral anaerobes	Requires prolonged antimicrobial therapy (2–4 weeks)	

Duration of therapy represents total time IV, PO, or IV + PO. Most patients on IV therapy able to take PO meds should be switched to PO therapy soon after clinical improvement (usually < 72 hrs).
† **See p. 436–444 for drug dosages.**

Clinical Presentation: Nasal discharge and cough frequently with headache, facial pain, and low-grade fever lasting > 10 days. Can also present acutely with high fever (≥ 104°F) and purulent nasal discharge ± intense headache for ≥ 3 days.

Diagnostic Considerations: Acute sinusitis is a clinical diagnosis. Imaging studies are not routinely indicated. Overlap with acute viral infection and allergic symptoms may make diagnosis difficult.

Pitfalls: Transillumination, sinus tenderness to percussion, and color of nasal mucus are not reliable indicators of sinusitis.

Therapeutic Considerations: Microbiology/antibiotics are similar to acute otitis media, but duration of therapy is 10–14 days. Failure to respond to initial antibiotic therapy suggests a resistant pathogen or an alternative diagnosis. There are insufficient data to support long-course antibiotic treatment. (Rarely, quinolones may be considered as 3rd line alternative.)

Prognosis: Good. For frequent recurrences, consider radiologic studies and ENT/allergy consultation.

Otitis Externa

Subset	Usual Pathogens	Topical Therapy
"Swimmer's ear"	Pseudomonas sp. Enterobacteria-ceae S. aureus	Polymyxin B plus neomycin **plus** hydrocortisone (eardrops) q6h × 7–10 days **or** Ciprofloxacin (otic solution) q12h × 7–10 days **plus** Dexamethasone or hydrocortisone ear drops **or** Ofloxacin (otic solution) q12h × 7–10 days

Clinical Presentation: Ear pain, itching, and sensation of fullness. Pain is exacerbated by tugging on the pinna or tragus of the outer ear. Purulent discharge may be visible in the external ear canal. Fever is generally absent.

Diagnostic Considerations: Otitis externa is a clinical diagnosis. A recent history of swimming or cleaning with cotton swabs is often elicited. Malignant otitis externa, as seen in elderly adults with diabetes mellitus, is extremely rare in children but may be seen in immunocompromised hosts.

Pitfalls: Failure to recognize a ruptured tympanic membrane may lead to a misdiagnosis of otitis externa based on purulence in the canal.

Therapeutic Considerations: Local cleansing (e.g., 2% acetic acid) and topical therapy with corticosporin-polymixin B-neomycin suspension is usually sufficient. Oral antibiotics should be considered for fever/cervical adenitis.

Prognosis: Excellent. Cleansing with 2% acetic acid drops after swimming prevents recurrences.

Acute Otitis Media

Subset	Usual Pathogens	IV/IM Therapy[†]	PO Therapy[†]
Initial uncomplicated bacterial infection	H. influenzae S. pneumoniae M. catarrhalis	Ceftriaxone × 1 dose	Amoxicillin[§] × 10 days **or** Azithromycin[§§] (1, 3, or 5 day regimen) **or** Erythromycin sulfisoxazole × 10 days** **or** TMP–SMX × 10 days**
Treatment failure or resistant organism*	MRSP Beta-lactamase positive H. influenzae	Ceftriaxone q24h × 3 doses	Amoxicillin/Clavulanic acid or oral cephalosporin × 10 days[‡]*

DRSP = drug-resistant S. pneumoniae. Pediatric doses are provided; acute otitis media is uncommon in adults. For chronic otitis media, prolonged antimicrobial therapy is required.

†   **See p. 436–444 for drug dosages.**

*   Treatment failure = persistent symptoms and otoscopy abnormalities 48–72 hours after starting initial antimicrobial therapy. For risk factors for DRSP, see Therapeutic Considerations, below. If still fails after recommended therapy, consider clindamycin for resistant S. pneumoniae or tympanocentesis for gram stain and culture.

**   In children > 6 years of age with mild-moderate acute otitis media, a 5–7-day course of antimicrobial theory may be adequate.

†† ES-600 = 600 mg amoxicillin/5 mL.

‡   10-day course with either cefuroxime axetil 15 mg/kg (PO) q12h or cefdinir 7 mg/kg (PO) q12h or 14 mg/kg (PO) q24h or cefpodoxime 5 mg/kg (PO) q12h may be used.

§   For S-pneumoniae with MIC < 2 mg/mL, use high dose amoxicillin (80–90 mg/kg/day in divided doses q12h.

§§ Macrolides and TMP-SMX may be less effective and should be reserved for penicillin or cephalosporin allergic patients.

Clinical Presentation: Fever, otalgia, hearing loss. Nonspecific presentation is more common in younger children (irritability, fever). Key to diagnosis is examination of the tympanic membrane. Acute otitis media requires evidence of inflammation and effusion. Uncommon in adults.

Diagnostic Considerations: Diagnosis is made by finding an opaque, hyperemic, bulging tympanic membrane with loss of landmarks and decreased mobility on pneumatic otoscopy.

Pitfalls: Otitis media with effusion (i.e., tympanic membrane retracted or in normal position with decreased mobility or mobility with negative pressure; fluid present behind the drum but normal in color) usually resolves spontaneously and should not be treated with antibiotics.

Therapeutic Considerations: American Academy of Pediatrics guidelines suggest initial observation without antibiotics for non-severe otitis media or in children > 6 month of age. Risk factors for infection with drug-resistant S. pneumoniae (DRSP) include antibiotic therapy in past 30 days, failure to respond within 48–72 hours of therapy, day care attendance, and antimicrobial prophylaxis. Quinolones not approved for therapy.

Prognosis: Excellent, but tends to recur. Chronic otitis, cholesteatomas, mastoiditis are rare complications. Tympanostomy tubes/adenoidectomy for frequent recurrences of otitis media are the leading surgical procedures in children.

Mastoiditis

Subset	Usual Pathogens	Preferred IV Therapy[†]	Alternate IV Therapy[†]	PO Therapy or IV-to-PO Switch[†]
Acute	S. pneumoniae S. aureus Group A streptococci H. influenzae	Nafcillin **or** Clindamycin **or** Vancomycin (if CA-MRSA suspected) **plus either** Ceftriaxone **or** Cefotaxime × 10–14 days	Ampicillin Sulbactam × 10–14 days	Amoxicillin/ Clavulanate **or** Cefpodoxime **or** Cefdinir **or** Cefuroxime axetil × 10–14 days
Chronic	Polymicrobial (P. aeruginosa, S. aureus, anaerobes, Enterobacteriaceae)	Piperacillin/ Tazobactam **or** Ticarcillin/Clavulanate × 10–14 days	Meropenem **or** Imipenem × 10–14 days	None

Duration of therapy represents total time IV, IV + PO, or PO. Most patients on IV therapy able to take PO meds should be switched to PO therapy after clinical improvement.

†   **See p. 436–444 for drug dosages.**

Clinical Presentation: Fever and otalgia with postauricular swelling/erythema pushing the ear superiorly and laterally. The presentation may be more subtle (e.g., less toxic, less swelling, Bell's palsy alone) in older children partially treated with antibiotics. Concomitant otitis media is rare.

Diagnostic Considerations: Acute mastoiditis is diagnosed clinically, but CT scan is definitive. Tympanocentesis through intact ear drum for aspirate and insertion of tympanostomy tube are helpful for microbiology and drainage, respectively. Chronic mastoiditis is often polymicrobial, including anaerobes and P. aeruginosa. Tuberculosis rarely presents as chronic mastoiditis.

Pitfalls: Do not overlook mastoiditis in older child with unresponsive otitis. Orbital involvement may lead to optic nerve damage or CNS extension/cavernous sinus thrombosis.

Therapeutic Considerations: Treatment is based on microbiology and requires at least 3 weeks of antibiotics.

Prognosis: Good with early treatment.

Pharyngitis

Subset	Usual Pathogens	IV or IM Therapy†	PO Therapy or IV-to-PO Switch†
Exudative (culture)	Group A streptococci	Benzathine penicillin IM × 1 dose	*Preferred*: Penicillin V **or** Amoxicillin × 10 days. *Alternate*: Azithromycin 12 mg/kg/day × 5 days **or** Cefadroxil **or** Clarithromycin **or** Clindamycin × 10 days
Asymptomatic carrier	Group A streptococci	No treatment indicated	No treatment indicated
Persistent/ recurrent disease	Group A streptococci	Clindamycin	Amoxicillin/Clavulanate × 10 days **or** **Combination Therapy** Penicillin V **or** Amoxicillin × 10 days **plus** Rifampin added on days 7–10
Exudative, sexually active	N. gonorrhoeae*	Ceftriaxone (IM) × 1 dose **plus** Azithromycin 1 gm (PO)	Cefixime 400 mg (PO) **plus** Azithromycin 1 gm (PO)
Lemierre's Syndrome (jugular vein septic thrombophlebitis)‡	Fusobacterium necrophorum	Clindamycin (IV) **or** Penicillin G (IV) × 4–6 weeks	Clindamycin **or** Penicillin VK × 4–6 weeks

* Obtain test of cure after therapy.

Pharyngitis *(cont'd)*

Subset	Usual Pathogens	IV or IM Therapy†	PO Therapy or IV-to-PO Switch†
Vesicular, ulcerative	Enteroviruses HSV 1 or 2	*Primary HSV*: Acyclovir × 5–7 days	*Primary HSV*: Acyclovir × 5–7 days **or** Valacyclovir × 5–7 days

Duration of therapy represents total time IV, IM, IV + PO, or PO. Most patients on IV therapy able to take PO meds should be switched to PO therapy after clinical improvement.
†   **See p. 436–444 for drug dosages.**
‡   Treat only IV or IV-to-PO switch.

Clinical Presentation: Acute sore throat and fever with tender cervical lymphadenitis. Primary clinical consideration is differentiating Group A streptococci (GAS) from viral/other causes (e.g., adenovirus, enterovirus, respiratory viruses, other strep groups [C, G], Arcanobacterium hemolyticum, M. pneumoniae, C. pneumoniae, EBV). GAS is less likely with concomitant coryza, conjunctivitis, hoarseness, cough, acute stomatitis, discrete oral ulcerations, or diarrhea—children with these manifestations should not be cultured routinely.

Diagnostic Considerations: Laboratory testing for GAS is recommended, since clinical differentiation of viral pharyngitis from GAS is not possible. Rapid tests for GAS antigens are reliable with excellent specificities, but due to variable sensitivities of the assays, a negative rapid test should be confirmed by a throat culture. The accuracy of antigen and culture tests is dependent on obtaining a good throat swab containing pharyngeal/tonsillar secretions.

Pitfalls: Be sure to obtain a good throat swab. Post-treatment testing is generally not recommended unless the patient is at high risk for rheumatic fever (e.g., family history, ongoing outbreak) or is still symptomatic after 10 days of therapy. Asymptomatic GAS carriers do not require antibiotic therapy, but identifying a "true carrier" may be difficult. Eradication of GAS carriage should be considered in the following situations: an outbreak of acute rheumatic fever or post-streptococcal glomerulonephritis; an outbreak of GAS in a closed community; a family history of rheumatic fever; multiple episodes of GAS infection within the family for many weeks despite therapy; family anxiety about the presence of GAS; or tonsillectomy is being considered based on persistent carriage. Eradication is achieved using the same antimicrobial regimen as for "persistent/recurrent disease" (see treatment grid p. 417).

Therapeutic Considerations: Penicillin V (or amoxicillin) is the drug of choice for GAS pharyngitis. Erythromycin is still considered the drug of choice for penicillin-allergic individuals, although macrolide-resistant GAS strains are being reported. First-generation cephalosporins are also useful alternatives. Broader spectrum agents, although likely effective, should not be used routinely. Macrolides or sulfonamides may not eradicate GAS pharyngitis. When eradication of carriage is indicated amoxicillin, amoxicillin/clavulanate or clindamycin alone or penicillin plus rifampin may be useful.

Prognosis: Excellent. Rheumatic fever is rare in the US.

Empiric Therapy of Lower Respiratory Tract Infections

Community Acquired Pneumonia

Subset (age)	Usual Pathogens	IV Therapy†	PO Therapy or IV-to-PO Switch†
Community-acquired pneumonia *Birth to 20 days*	Group B streptococci (GBS) GNB	Ampicillin **plus either** Gentamicin **or** Cefotaxime × 10–21 days	Not applicable
3 weeks to 3 months	RSV Parainfluenza (HPIV) Human metapneumo-virus (hMPV)	None (supportive care)	None
	C. trachomatis S. pneumoniae B. pertussis S. aureus	Cefotaxime **or** Ceftriaxone × 10–14 days* **or** Ampicillin **or** Clindamycin*	<u>Afebrile:</u> Erythromycin × 14 days **or** Azithromycin × 5–7 days. <u>Lobar, febrile:</u> Amoxicillin **or** Amoxicillin/Clavulanic acid **or** Cefdinir **or** Cefuroxime **or** Cefpodoxime × 10–14 days
> 3 months to < 5 years	Viruses (RSV, parainfluenza, (HPIV) influenza, adenovirus, rhinoviruses)	<u>RSV:</u> consider Ribavirin.§ For infants at highest risk for severe RSV infection, consider palivizumab 15 mg/kg/month × 1–2 seasons for prevention. <u>Influenza:</u> Oseltamivir (influenza A, B).¶ Routine immunization for all children > 6 months	
	S. pneumoniae H. influenzae M. pneumoniae	Ampicillin** **or** Ceftriaxone **or** Cefotaxime × 10–14 days*	Amoxicillin **or** Amoxicillin/Clavulanate **or** Clarithromycin **or** Azithromycin × 10–14 days
5–15 years	M. pneumoniae C. pneumoniae S. pneumoniae	Ceftriaxone **plus** a macrolide × 10–14 days*	Amoxicillin **plus either** a macrolide **or** Doxycycline (age > 8 years) × 10–14 days

Community Acquired Pneumonia (cont'd)

Subset (age)	Usual Pathogens	IV Therapy[†]	PO Therapy or IV-to-PO Switch[†]
Pertussis	Bordetella sp.[‡] Adenoviruses M. pneumoniae C. trachomatis C. pneumoniae	Azithromycin × 5 days **or** Erythromycin × 14 days	Erythromycin estolate × 14 days **or** Clarithromycin × 7 days **or** Azithromycin × 5 days. If macrolide-intolerant: TMP–SMX × 14 days
Tuberculosis	M. tuberculosis	See pp. 423–425	See pp. 423–425

Duration of therapy represents total time IV or IV, PO, or IV + PO. Most patients on IV therapy able to take PO meds should be switched to PO therapy after clinical improvement.

† **See p. 436–444 for drug dosages.**

* If chronic cough of more insidious onset, consider adding IV or PO macrolide (azithromycin, clarithromycin, erythromycin) to cover Pertussis/C. trachomatis (3 weeks–3 months of age), Mycoplasma (> 5 years of age), or Mycoplasma/C. pneumoniae (5–15 years of age).

** If fully immunized against H. influenzae and S. pneumoniae.

‡ B. pertussis, B. parapertussis, B. bronchiseptica.

§ Use should be limited to the most severely ill with RSV, i.e., transplant patients.

¶ Influenza A strains now circulating are amantadine resistant.

Community Acquired Pneumonia

Clinical Presentation: Fever ± dyspnea, cough, tachypnea with infiltrates on chest x-ray.

Diagnostic Considerations: Usual pathogens differ by age. In neonates, pneumonia is typically diffuse and part of early-onset sepsis. In young infants, there is significant overlap between signs and symptoms of bronchiolitis (primarily due to RSVU) and pneumonia. Severe pneumonia is usually due to bacterial infection, although the organism is frequently not isolated (e.g., blood cultures are positive in only 10–20% of children < 2 years of age with bacterial pneumonia). In young infants, Chlamydia trachomatis can be detected by or culture of nasopharyngeal (NP) secretions. Mycoplasma pneumonia, suggested by high titer cold agglutinins > 1:64. Diagnosis by nucleic acid amplification testing or ↑ IgM titers. Although cases in children < 5 years have been reported. Respiratory viruses (RSV, influenza, adenoviruses, parainfluenza viruses, hMPV) can also be detected by PCR of throat/nasal secretions. If child lives in area with high prevalence of tuberculosis, consider tuberculosis in the differential diagnosis of primary pneumonia.

Pitfalls: Reliance on upper airway specimen for gram stain/culture leads to misdiagnosis and mistreatment, as true deep sputum specimen is rarely obtainable in children.

Therapeutic Considerations: Therapy is primarily empiric based on child's age, clinical/epidemiologic features and chest x-ray findings. Mycoplasma or C. pneumoniae may require 2 weeks of treatment. Routine use of pneumococcal vaccines has decreased the incidence of pneumococcal pneumonia, especially severe disease, empyema.

Prognosis: Varies with pathogen, clinical condition at presentation, and underlying health status. Prognosis is worse in children with chronic lung disease, congenital heart disease, immunodeficiency, neuromuscular disease, hemoglobinopathy.

Lower Respiratory Tract Infections due to Respiratory Viruses

Clinical Presentation: Viruses cause the majority of lower respiratory tract infections (LRTIs) in children. Respiratory syncytial virus (RSV) is the leading cause of LRTI in young infants, manifesting as bronchiolitis/viral pneumonia and causing annual mid-winter epidemics. The risk of secondary bacterial infection (other than possibly otitis media) is very low. Fever is typically low grade and usually improves over 3–5 days, even if hospitalized. Influenza viruses are another major cause of winter epidemic LRTIs in children of all ages. Hospitalization rates in infants under one year of age rival those in the > 65-year- old population. Characteristic findings include high fever and diffuse inflammation of the airways. Young infants may have prominent GI symptoms as well. Secondary bacterial infection (otitis media, pneumonia, sepsis) are frequent complications of influenza. Primary influenza pneumonia, encephalopathy, and myocarditis are rare, severe complications. Other respiratory viruses associated with LRTIs in children include human parainfluenza (HPIV) type 3 (pneumonia), parainfluenza types 1 and 2 (croup), adenoviruses, and human metapneumovirus (hMPV). Influenza in children resembles that in adults, but in children, lymphocytosis is usual. Atypical lymphocytes are common in children, but not in adults. Thrombocytopenia is common in both children and adults.

Diagnostic Considerations: Viral syndromes are often diagnosed based on clinical assessment alone. For confirmation or in more severe cases, rapid diagnosis by PCR.

Pitfalls: Routine use of corticosteroids or bronchodilators in RSV bronchiolitis are not supported by clinical evidence. Overuse of the diagnosis of "flu" (e.g., stomach flu, summer flu) has led to diluted appreciation for true influenza and its severity. Influenza vaccine (RIDT) has been traditionally underutilized in children. As in adults, a negative rapid influenza diagnostic test does not rule out influenza. ILI with negative RIDTs should be retested by PCR for respiratory viruses.

Therapeutic Considerations: For most viral LRTIs treatment is primarily supportive (e.g., adequate hydration, fever control, supplemental oxygen for severe illness). Ribavirin is approved for RSV infection but is very rarely used due to uncertain clinical benefit, high cost, and cumbersome method of administration (prolonged aerosol). For infants at greatest risk of severe RSV disease (e.g., premature infants, infants with underlying chronic lung disease or congenital heart disease), monthly prophylaxis with palivizumab (synagis) 15 mg/kg/month (IM) decreases RSV hospitalization rates. Per American Academy of Pediatrics guidelines, palivizumab is indicated for infants with chronic lung disease and ≤ 32 weeks gestational age (GA) or congenital heart disease who are 12 months of age at start of RSV season. For premature infants, palivizumab is considered for premature infants < 29 weeks GA for a maximum of 5 doses through the winter season are recommended.

Annual influenza vaccination is indicated for all individuals > 6 months of age. All circulating influenza A strains are resistant to amantadine. The neuraminidase inhibitors oseltamivir and zanamivir have pediatric indications for treatment and prophylaxis of influenza (Table 7.1).

Table 7.1 Influenza Antiviral Dosing Recommendations

Antiviral		Treatment	Chemoprophylaxis
Oseltamivir*			
Children (age, 12 months or older), weight:	15 kg or less	60 mg per day divided into 2 doses	30 mg once per day
	15–23 kg	90 mg per day divided into 2 doses	45 mg once per day
	24–40 kg	120 mg per day divided into 2 doses	60 mg once per day
	> 40 kg	150 mg per day divided into 2 doses	75 mg once per day
Zanamivir			
Children		Two 5-mg inhalations (10 mg total) twice per day (age, 7 years or older)	Two 5-mg inhalations (10 mg total) once per day (age, 5 years or older)
Peramivir			
Children		Full-term neonate: IV: 6 mg/kg/dose; 29 to 30 days of life: 6 mg/kg/dose; 31 to 90 days of life: 8 mg/kg/dose and 91 to 180 days of life: 10 mg/kg/dose once daily for 5 to 10 days	
		Children ≥2 years: IV: 12 mg/kg as a single dose (uncomplicated) or 5–10 days for high risk/hospitalized.	
		Adolescents: IV: 600 mg as a single dose (uncomplicated) or 5–10 days for high risk/hospitalized.	

* CDC recommends oseltamivir 3 mg/kg (PO) q12h × 5 days for full term infants <12 months of age. Lower doses recommended for pre-term infants.

Prognosis: Most children with viral LRTIs do well and recover without sequelae. Infants hospitalized with RSV infection have higher rates of wheezing episodes over the next 10 years. The highest rates of hospitalization from influenza occur in children < 2 years of age and in the elderly.

Pertussis

Clinical Presentation: Upper respiratory tract symptoms (congestion, rhinorrhea) over 1–2 weeks (catarrhal stage) progressing to paroxysms of cough (paroxysmal stage) lasting 2–4 weeks, often with a characteristic inspiratory whoop, followed by a convalescent stage lasting 1–2 weeks during which cough paroxysms decrease in frequency and severity. Fever is low grade or absent. In children < 6 months, whoop is frequently absent and apnea may occur. Duration of classic pertussis is 6–10 weeks. Older children and adults may present with persistent cough (without whoop) lasting 2–6 weeks. Complications include seizures, secondary bacterial pneumonia, encephalopathy, death; risk of complications is greatest in children < 1 year.

Diagnostic Considerations: Diagnosis is usually based on nature of cough and duration of symptoms. Laboratory diagnosis may be difficult. A positive culture for Bordetella pertussis from a nasopharyngeal swab inoculated on fresh selective media is diagnostic, but the organism is difficult to recover after 3–4 weeks of illness. PCR of nasal secretions is the best rapid diagnostic test for pertussis.

Pitfalls: Be sure to consider pertussis in older children and adults with prolonged coughing illness. Family contacts of index case should receive post-exposure antimicrobial prophylaxis. Virtually all children should be vaccinated against pertussis. A single booster dose of acellular pertussis is recommended at 11–12 years of age (additional guidelines for catch-up for older adolescents and adults up to 64 years of age). Pregnant women should be vaccinated during the 2nd – 3rd trimester of each pregnancy to protect themselves and provide passive immunity to their infants. Relative precautions to further pertussis immunization include: seizure within 3 days of a dose; persistent, severe, inconsolable crying for ≥ 3 hours within 48 hours of a dose; collapse or shock-like state within 48 hours of a dose; or temperature of ≥ 40.5°C without other cause within 48 hours of a dose.

Therapeutic Considerations: Infants < 6 months frequently require hospitalization. By the paroxysmal stage, antibiotics have minimal effect on the course of the illness but are still indicated to decrease transmission. An association has been made between oral erythromycin and infantile hypertrophic pyloric stenosis in infants < 6 weeks of age; consider an alternative macrolide (azithromycin or clarithromycin) in these cases.

Prognosis: Good. Despite the prolonged course, long-term pulmonary sequelae have not been described after pertussis. Children < 1 year are at greatest risk of morbidity and mortality, although mortality rates remain very low.

Tuberculosis

Subset	Pathogen	PO or IM Therapy (see footnote for drug dosages)
Latent infection (positive PPD, clinically well, negative chest x-ray)	M. tuberculosis	INH × 9 months **or** Rifampin × 6 months (if INH-resistant **or** INH unavailable and child at risk) **or** INH **plus** Rifapentine weekly × 12 weeks
Pulmonary and extrapulmonary TB (except meningitis)	M. tuberculosis	INH **plus** Rifampin **plus** PZA **plus** EMB × 2 months followed by INH **plus** Rifampin × 4 months†

Duration of therapy represents total time IV or IV, PO, or IV + PO. Most patients on IV therapy able to take PO meds should be switched to PO therapy after clinical improvement.

† If drug resistance is a concern, EMB or streptomycin (IM) is added (4-drug regimen in areas where MDR TB is prevalent) to the initial regimen until drug susceptibilities are determined.

Tuberculosis *(cont'd)*

Subset	Pathogen	PO or IM Therapy (see footnote for drug dosages)
Meningitis	M. tuberculosis	INH **plus** Rifampin **plus** PZA **plus either** Streptomycin (IM) **or** Ethionamide × 2 months, followed by INH **plus** Rifampin × 7–10 months (9–12 months total therapy)‡
Congenital	M. tuberculosis	INH **plus** Rifampin **plus** PZA **plus** Streptomycin (IM)

Duration of therapy represents total time IV or IV, PO, or IV + PO. Most patients on IV therapy able to take PO meds should be switched to PO therapy after clinical improvement.

‡ Plus steroids.

TB Drug	Daily Dosage (mg/kg)	Twice Weekly Dosage (mg/kg)
Isoniazid (INH)	10–15	20–30
Rifampin (RIF)	10–20	10–20
Ethambutol (EMB)	15–25	50
Pyrazinamide (PZA)	20–40	50
Streptomycin	20–40 (IM)	–
Ethionamide	15–20 (in 2–3 divided doses/day)	–

Alternative drugs (capreomycin, ciprofloxacin, levofloxacin, cycloserine, kanamycin, para-aminosalicylic acid) are used less commonly and should be administered in consultation with an expert in the treatment of tuberculosis.

Tuberculosis

Clinical Presentation: Most children diagnosed with tuberculosis have asymptomatic infection detected by tuberculin skin testing. Symptomatic disease typically presents 1–6 months after infection with fever, growth delay, weight loss, night sweats, and cough. Extrapulmonary involvement may present with meningitis, lymphadenopathy, bone, joint, or skin involvement.

Diagnostic Considerations: A positive tuberculin skin test indicates likely infection with M. tuberculosis. Tuberculin reactivity develops 2–12 weeks after infection. Children < 8 years old cannot produce sputum for AFB smear and culture. Interferon gamma release assays (IGRAs) may be used to diagnose TB in children > 5 years. Testing recommended only for children or increased risk, e.g., HIV, immigrants from TB endemic areas clinical and those with clinical findings suggestive of TB.

Pitfalls: Tuberculosis may be missed if not considering the diagnosis in children at increased epidemiological risk for exposure. Tuberculous meningitis often presents insidiously with nonspecific irritability and lethargy weeks prior to the development of frank neurological defects.

Therapeutic Considerations: Choice of initial therapy depends on stage of disease and likelihood of resistant organisms (based on index case, geographical region of acquisition). For HIV-infected patients, duration of therapy is prolonged to ≥ 12 months. For tuberculosis meningitis and miliary disease, the addition of corticosteroids to anti-TB therapy is beneficial.

Prognosis: Varies with extent of disease, drug resistance and underlying immune status, but is generally good for pulmonary disease in children. Bone infection may result in orthopedic sequelae (e.g., Pott's disease of the spine with vertebral collapse). The prognosis for meningitis is guarded once focal neurological deficits and persistent depression of mental status occur.

Empiric Therapy of Vascular Infections

Central Venous Catheter (CVC) Infections (Broviac, Hickman, Mediport)

Subset	Usual Pathogens	Preferred IV Therapy[†]	Alternate IV Therapy[†]
Empiric; immuno-compromised host	S. aureus[¶] Enterobacteriaceae Pseudomonas Viridans streptococci Enterococci	Meropenem **or** Piperacillin/ Tazobactam **or** Cefepime × 7–14 days	Piperacillin/Tazobactam **plus** an aminoglycoside × 7–14 days
Isolate-based	S. aureus MSSA	Nafcillin **or** Oxacillin for ≥ 2 weeks	Cefazolin (Vancomycin preferred if severe beta-lactam allergy) for ≥ 2 weeks
	MRSA	Vancomycin ± Gentamicin for ≥ 2 weeks	Linezolid **or** Quinupristin/ Dalfopristin for ≥ 2 weeks (addition of Rifampin may be of benefit for MRSA)
	Enterobacteriaceae Pseudomonas	Piperacillin/Tazo-bactam **or** Ticarcillin/ Clavulanate ± an aminoglycoside* for ≥ 2 weeks	Meropenem **or** Imipenem ± an aminoglycoside[x] for ≥ 2 weeks

Central Venous Catheter Infections (Broviac, Hickman, Mediport) *(cont'd)*

Subset	Usual Pathogens	Preferred IV Therapy†	Alternate IV Therapy†
	ESBL + GNB	Meropenem **or** Ertapenem ± an aminoglycoside* for ≥ 2 weeks	—
	Candida	Amphotericin B × 2–6 weeks‡	Fluconazole **or** Caspofungin **or** liposomal amphotericin (L-amb) × 2–6 weeks‡

MSSA/MRSA = methicillin-sensitive/resistant S. aureus. Duration of therapy represents total time IV.

†   **See p. 436–444 for drug dosages.**
*   Gentamicin, tobramycin, or amikacin.
‡   Based on promptness of line removal, clearance of blood cultures, evidence of metastatic foci.
¶   If severely ill or suspicion of MRSA based on local epidemiology, include vancomycin in initial regimen pending culture results.

Clinical Presentation: Fever ± site tenderness, erythema.

Diagnostic Considerations: Quantitative blood cultures from the peripheral blood/vascular catheter are best used to make the diagnosis. However in clinical practice these are not often obtained, and the diagnosis is based on culture results in conjunction with one or more of the following features: local phlebitis or inflammation at the catheter insertion site; embolic disease distal to the catheter; sepsis refractory to appropriate therapy; resolution of fever after device removal; or clustered infections caused by infusion-associated organisms.

Pitfalls: It may be difficult to differentiate infection from contamination in blood cultures, especially with coagulase-negative staphylococci. Multiple positive cultures with the same organism and/or clinical features noted above suggest infection, not colonization. Semiquantitative culture of the catheter tip yielding ≥ 15 colonies may also be useful in confirming the diagnosis but requires removal of the device.

Therapeutic Considerations: Indications for catheter removal include septic shock, tunnel infection, failure to respond to treatment within 48–72 hours, or infection with Candida, atypical mycobacteria, or possibly S. aureus. Otherwise attempt to retain the catheter while treating with antibiotics (plus systemic and lock therapy). Localized exit site infections (erythema, induration, tenderness, purulence) within 2 cm of the exit site should be treated topically (e.g., Neosporin, Bacitracin, Bactroban) in conjunction with systemic therapy.

Prognosis: Major complications (septic emboli, endocarditis, vasculitis) are rare with aggressive therapy. Recrudescent infection can occur after therapy apparent clearance and can often be successfully treated with additional courses of antibiotics; persistence ultimately requires line removal.

Empiric Therapy of Gastrointestinal Infections

Acute Diarrheal Syndromes (Gastroenteritis)

Subset	Usual Pathogens	Preferred Therapy†	Alternate Therapy†
Community acquired	Viruses (Rotavirus, Norwalk agent, enteric adenovirus, enteroviruses)	No specific therapy indicated	No specific therapy indicated
	Salmonella non-typhi	Ceftriaxone (IV) **or** Cefotaxime (IV) × 10–14 days*	TMP–SMX (IV or PO) **or** Amoxicillin (PO) **or** Cefixime (PO) × 10–14 days
	Shigella	Ceftriaxone (IV) **or** Azithromycin (PO) × 5 days	TMP–SMX (PO) **or** Cefixime (PO) **or** Ampicillin (PO) × 5 days
	Campylobacter	Erythromycin (PO) × 7 days **or** Azithromycin (PO) × 5 days	Doxycycline (PO) (> 8-year-old) × 7 days
	Yersinia enterocolitica	TMP–SMX (PO) × 5–7 days	Cefotaxime (IV) **or** Doxycycline (PO) × 5–7 days
Traveler's diarrhea	E. coli	TMP–SMX (PO) × 3 days	Azithromycin (PO) × 3 days
Typhoid (enteric) fever	Salmonella typhi	Ceftriaxone (IV) **or** Cefotaxime (IV) × 10–14 days	TMP–SMX (IV or PO) **or** Amoxicillin (PO) **or** Cefixime (PO) × 10–14 days
Antibiotic-associated colitis	Clostridium difficile	Metronidazole (PO) × 7–10 days **or** Nitazoxanide (PO) × 3 days	Vancomycin (PO) × 7–10 days

Acute Diarrheal Syndromes (Gastroenteritis) *(cont'd)*

Subset	Usual Pathogens	Preferred Therapy[†]	Alternate Therapy[†]
Chronic watery diarrhea	Giardia lamblia[‡]	Metronidazole (PO) × 5–7 days **or** Nitazoxanide (PO) × 3 days	Tinidazole (PO) × 1 dose **or** Furazolidone (PO) × 7–10 days **or** Albendazole × 5–7 days
	Cryptosporidia[‡]	Nitazoxanide (PO) × 3 days	Human immunoglobulin (PO) **or** bovine colostrum (PO) for immunocompromised hosts
Acute dysentery	E. histolytica	Metronidazole (PO) × 10 days **followed by either** Iodoquinol (PO) × 20 days **or** Paromomycin (PO) × 7 days	Tinidazole (PO) × 3-5 days **followed by either** Iodoquinol (PO) × 20 days **or** Paromomycin (PO) × 7 days
	Shigella**	Ceftriaxone (IV) **or** Azithromycin (PO) × 5 days	TMP–SMX (PO) **or** Cefixime (PO) **or** Ampicillin (PO) × 5 days

†   **See p. 436–444 for drug dosages.**
*   Therapy only indicated in child < 3 to 6 months of age, immunocompromised host, or toxic appearing child.
**   Mild cases acquire no antibiotic therapy. However, antibiotic therapy shortens durations of symptoms and by decreasing the duration of diarrhea limits potential spread.
‡   May also present as acute watery diarrhea.

Acute Gastroenteritis (Community-Acquired)

Clinical Presentation: Typically presents with the acute onset of diarrhea with fever. This is not an indication for antibiotic therapy unless illness is severe ($\geq$ 6 unformed stools/day, fever $\geq$ 102°F, bloody stools). Travel history regarding risk for potential E. coli and parasitic exposures is important.

Diagnostic Considerations: In the absence of blood in the stools viruses are the most common cause of acute community-acquired gastroenteritis. Rotaviruses are the most common cause of acute gastroenteritis in 4–24-month-old children. Enteric adenoviruses, Norwalk-like virus, enteroviruses and astroviruses are common causes of gastroenteritis in older children. Commercially available antigen tests using ELISA or latex agglutination techniques are readily available to detect rotavirus. Testing for the other viral agents may not be as readily available. Inflammatory changes (presence of white blood cells and/or blood) in the stool are more consistent with bacterial infection. When requesting stool cultures, it may be necessary to order special conditions/media for the detection of yersinia or E. coli O157.

Pitfalls: Antimotility drugs may worsen the course of illness in children with colitis. Empiric therapy with antibiotics may prolong the carriage of Salmonella or increase the risk for developing hemolytic uremic syndrome (HUS) with E. coli O157 infection. The benefit of antibiotics in treating diarrhea caused by yersinia is also unproven. Thus, antibiotic therapy is not routinely indicated prior to culture results in most instances of mild diarrheal disease, especially as most such infections are self-limited.

Therapeutic Considerations: As above, pending cultures in the absence of severe symptoms or dysentery antibiotics may not be indicated. Overall, the fluoroquinolones have the most complete spectrum for pathogens causing bacterial diarrhea but are not presently approved for use in children < 18 years of age.

Prognosis: Good. Up to 5–10% of children with E. coli O157 are at risk for hemolytic-uremic syndrome.

Giardiasis (Giardia lamblia)

Clinical Presentation: Giardia lamblia is the most common parasite causing diarrheal illness in children. Giardiasis may present as acute watery diarrhea with abdominal pain and bloating or as a chronic, intermittent illness with foul smelling stools, abdominal distension, and anorexia.

Diagnostic Considerations: Trophozoites or cysts of Giardia lamblia can be identified in direct examination of infected stools with 75%–95% sensitivity on a single specimen. Testing 3 or more stools further increases sensitivity of detection. If giardiasis is suspected with negative stool tests, examination of duodenal contents (Entero- or string test) may be helpful.

Pitfalls: Asymptomatic infection is commonly seen in children in day care; therefore, indications to treat must take into account stool testing results *and* clinical findings.

Therapeutic Considerations: Treatment failures occur commonly, and retreatment with the same initial drug is recommended. Furazolidone is the only pediatric liquid available for treating giardiasis < 3 years of age.

Prognosis: Good.

Cryptosporidiosis

Clinical Presentation: Usually presents as fever, vomiting, and non-bloody, watery diarrhea. Infection may also be asymptomatic. More severe and chronic infection is seen in immunocompromised patients (e.g., HIV infection). Cryptosporidia parasite is resistant to chlorine and maybe transmitted in swimming pools. Transmission can also occur from livestock, and a major outbreak through contamination of a public water supply has been reported.

Diagnostic Considerations: Cryptosporidium cysts are detected by microscopic examination of Kinyoun-stained stool specimens using a sucrose floatation method or formalin-ethyl acetate method to concentrate oocysts. This test is not part of routine stool ova and parasite examination and must be specifically requested. Shedding is intermittent; therefore, 3 stool samples should be submitted for optimal detection.

Pitfalls: The oocysts of cryptosporidium are small and may be missed by an inexperienced exam-iner. A commercially available ELISA test is available but may have false-positive and false-negative results.

Therapeutic Considerations: Treatment failures are frequent. In immunocompromised hosts oral human immune globulin and bovine colostrum are beneficial. Improvement in CD_4 counts with antiretroviral therapy in HIV-infected patients shortens the clinical illness.

Prognosis: Good. Recovery may take months.

Amebiasis (Entamoeba histolytica)

Clinical Presentation: E. histolytica can lead to a spectrum of clinical illnesses from asymptomatic infection to acute dysentery to fulminant colitis. Disseminated disease, primarily manifest as hepatic abscesses, can also occur. E. histolytica is most prevalent in developing countries and is transmitted by the fecal-oral route.

Diagnostic Considerations: Trophozoites or cysts of E. histolytica can be identified in stool specimens. In more severe disease (amebic colitis, hepatic abscesses), serum antibodies can be detected.

Pitfalls: Treatment with steroids or antimotility drugs can worsen symptoms and should not be used.

Therapeutic Considerations: Treatment is two-staged to eliminate tissue-invading trophozoites and organisms in the intestinal lumen. Surgical drainage of large hepatic abscesses may be beneficial.

Prognosis: Good.

Clostridium difficile Colitis

Clinical Presentation: Classically occurs in a child receiving antibiotic therapy and presents as diarrhea, cramping, bloody/mucousy stools, abdominal tenderness, fever, and toxicity. It may also present weeks after a course of antibiotics.

Diagnostic Considerations: C. difficile toxin can be detected with commercially available immunoassays. Endoscopic finding of pseudomembranous colitis is the definitive method of diagnosis although rarely indicated.

Pitfalls: C. difficile may be normal flora in infants < 1 year of age and probably does not cause illness in this age group. The finding of C. difficile toxin in an infant should not be equated with cause and additional evaluations should be perused. Antimotility drugs may worsen symptoms and should be avoided.

Therapeutic Considerations: Cessation of antibiotics is recommended if possible in the presence of significant C. difficile colitis. Patients with severe symptoms or persistent diarrhea × 2–3 days after discontinuing antibiotics should then be treated with oral metronidazole or oral vancomycin. Up to ~25% relapse after a single course; re-treatment using the same initial antibiotic is recommended. For persistent infection alternate therapies such as nitazoxanide, rifaximin, tinidazole, oral immune globulin therapy, toxin binders or repopulating intestinal flora may be considered.

Prognosis: Good.

Empiric Therapy of Bone and Joint Infections

Septic Arthritis

Subset	Usual Pathogens	Preferred IV Therapy†*	Alternate IV Therapy†*	IV-to-PO Switch†
Newborns (≤ 3 months)	S. aureus‡ Group B streptococci (GBS) Enterobacteriaceae N. gonorrhoeae	**Combination Therapy** Nafcillin **or** Vancomycin **plus either** Ceftriaxone **or** Cefotaxime*	**Combination Therapy** Vancomycin **or** Clindamycin **plus either** Ceftriaxone **or** Cefotaxime **or** Gentamicin **or** Tobramycin*	Not applicable
Child (> 3 months to 14 years)	S. aureus‡ Group A streptococci (GAS) S. pneumoniae GNB N. meningitidis (H. influenzae type b if unvaccinated) Kingella (3–36 months)	**Combination Therapy** Nafcillin **or** Vancomycin **plus either** Ceftriaxone **or** Cefotaxime*	**Combination Therapy** Vancomycin **or** Clindamycin **plus either** Ceftriaxone **or** Cefotaxime*	Dicloxacillin **or** Cephalexin **or** Clindamycin
Adolescents (sexually active)	As above plus N. gonorrhoeae (typically 2 or 3 joints involved)	**Combination Therapy** Nafcillin **or** Vancomycin **plus either** Ceftriaxone **or** Cefotaxime*	If GC isolated and penicillin allergy: Azithromycin	GC arthritis with prompt response to IV therapy may switch to Cefixime to complete 7 days of total therapy

Duration of therapy represents total time IV or IV + PO. Most patients on IV therapy able to take PO meds should be switched to PO therapy after clinical improvement. Taper to individual drug therapy once organism isolated and sensitivities are available.

† **See p. 436–444 for drug dosages.**

* Total duration of therapy for non-gonococcal septic arthritis ≥ 3 weeks based on clinical response.

‡ If CA-MRSA is suspected based on clinical presentation/local epidemiology, consider empiric coverage for CA-MRSA with clindamycin, TMP–SMX, doxycycline, or vancomycin pending culture results.

Clinical Presentation: Varies with age of the child. Presentation is often nonspecific in infants (i.e., fever, poor feeding, tachycardia). Physical exam findings can be subtle: asymmetrical tissue folds, unilateral swelling of an extremity, subtle changes in limb/joint position. In older children, signs and symptoms are more localized to the involved joint. Commonly affected joints: hips, elbows, knees.

Diagnostic Considerations: Joint aspiration (large-bore needle) shows 50,000–250,000 WBCs/mm^3 with a marked predominance of PMNs. Gram stain/culture of joint fluid confirm the diagnosis. Toxic synovitis, Lyme arthritis, rheumatoid arthritis, traumatic arthritis, and sympathetic effusion from adjacent osteomyelitis can mimic septic arthritis on presentation, but joint fluid has fewer WBCs and cultures are negative. Multiple joint involvement is more typical of rheumatic/Lyme disease. In young infants, persistence of the nutrient artery can lead to osteomyelitis and septic arthritis. Obtain Kingella PCR in children < 3 years (3–36 months).

Pitfalls: Septic arthritis of the hip is an emergency concomitant condition requiring prompt joint aspiration and irrigation to minimize the risk of femoral head necrosis, which may occur within 24 hours. Toxic synovitis of the hip, which is treated with anti-inflammatory agents and observation, typically causes less fever, pain, and leukocytosis than septic arthritis; however, at times the two can not be differentiated and aspiration of the joint is indicated. In sexually active adolescents, consider N. gonorrhoeae and culture aspirate appropriately.

Therapeutic Considerations: Therapy is recommended for at least 3–4 weeks (IV followed by oral therapy), for a total antibiotic course of 4–6 weeks based on clinical response and laboratory parameters (WBC, ESR, CRP). Intra-articular therapy is not helpful. Empiric coverage is broader than for osteomyelitis in children.

Prognosis: Good with prompt joint aspiration and at least 3 weeks of antibiotics.

Acute Osteomyelitis, Osteochondritis, Diskitis

Subset	Usual Pathogens	Preferred IV Therapy[†]	Alternate IV Therapy[†]	IV-to-PO Switch or PO Therapy[†]
Acute osteomyelitis Newborn (0–3 months)	S. aureus[§] GNB Group B streptococci (GBS)	**Combination therapy** Nafcillin **or** Oxacillin **plus either** Cefotaxime **or** Ceftriaxone × 4–6 weeks	Vancomycin **plus either** Cefotaxime **or** Ceftriaxone × 4–6 weeks	Not applicable

Acute Osteomyelitis, Osteochondritis, Diskitis *(cont'd)*

Subset	Usual Pathogens	Preferred IV Therapy†	Alternate IV Therapy†	IV-to-PO Switch or PO Therapy†
> 3 months*	S. aureus§ Group A strepto-cocci (GAS) GNB (rare) Salmonella (sickle cell disease)	Nafcillin **or** Oxacillin **or** Cefazolin × 4–6 weeks	Clindamycin **or** Ampicillin Sulbactam **or** Vancomycin × 4–6 weeks	Cephalexin **or** Clindamycin **or** Dicloxacillin **or** Cefadroxil × 4–6 weeks
Osteochon-dritis	P. aeruginosa S. aureus§	Ticarcillin Clavulanate × 7–10 days after surgery **or** **Combination Therapy with** Nafcillin **plus** Ceftazidime × 7–10 days after surgery	Piperacillin/Tazobactam **or** Ciprofloxacin × 7–10 days after surgery	Cipro-floxacin** × 7–10 days after surgery
Diskitis	S. aureus, K. kingae Entero-bacteriaceae S. pneumoniae S. epidermidis	<u>PO Therapy:</u> Cephalexin Clindamycin × 3–4 weeks or ESR returns to normal††	**or** **or**	

Duration of therapy represents total time IV, PO, or IV + PO. Most patients on IV therapy able to take PO meds should be switched to PO therapy soon after clinical improvement.

† **See p. 436–444 for drug dosages.**
** Not approved for children but might consider in adolescent.
* Treat only IV or IV-to-PO switch.
†† Add gram-negative coverage only if culture proven.
§ If CA-MRSA is suspected based on clinical presentation/local epidemiology, consider empiric coverage for CA-MRSA with clindamycin, TMP–SMX, doxycycline, or vancomycin pending culture results.

Acute Osteomyelitis

Clinical Presentation: Acute onset of fever and pain/decreased movement around the infected area. Can be difficult to localize, especially in younger children. Occurs primarily via hematogenous spread (vs. direct inoculation) to metaphysis of long bones.

Diagnostic Considerations: Acute phase reactants are elevated (ESR, CRP, WBC). X-rays may not reveal osteolytic lesions for > 7 days, but soft tissue swelling and periosteal reaction may be seen as early as 3 days. Bone scan/MRI reveal changes in the first 24 hours, but bone scans are insensitive in neonates. Blood cultures may be positive, especially in younger children. Definitive diagnosis by bone aspirate for gram stain and culture, but empiric therapy is often initiated based on clinical history and the presence of an acute lytic lesion on MRI, bone scan, or x-ray.

Pitfalls: Bony changes on x-ray may not be present initially. It may be difficult to differentiate cellulitis from osteomyelitis, even on bone scan.

Therapeutic Considerations: Initiate empiric therapy by IV route. Treatment is required ≥ 4 weeks, but children with a prompt clinical response can complete therapy with high-dose oral antibiotics. With adequate treatment, CPR and ESR normalize over 2 weeks and 4 weeks, respectively.

Prognosis: Good with 4–6 weeks of total therapy. Long-term growth of affected bone may be impaired.

Osteochondritis of the Foot ("Puncture Wound Osteomyelitis")

Clinical Presentation: Tenderness, erythema, and swelling several days to weeks after a nail puncture wound through a sneaker/tennis shoe (Pseudomonas found in foam layer between sole and lining of shoe). Fever and other systemic complaints are rare. Develops in 1–2% of puncture wounds of foot.

Diagnostic Considerations: P. aeruginosa is the primary pathogen, although infection with S. aureus is also a concern.

Pitfalls: Antibiotics with surgical debridement of necrotic cartilage.

Therapeutic Considerations: With prompt debridement, 7–10 days of antibiotic therapy is usually sufficient.

Prognosis: Good with debridement and antibiotics.

Diskitis

Clinical Presentation: Typically involves the lumbar region and occurs in children < 6 years old. Presents with gradual onset (over weeks) of irritability and refusal to walk. Fever is low-grade or absent. Older children may be able to localize pain to back, hip, or abdomen. Pain is exacerbated by motion of the spine and can be localized by percussion of the vertebral bodies.

Diagnostic Considerations: ESR is elevated, but WBC count is normal. X-rays are usually normal initially, but later reveal disk space narrowing and sclerosis of the vertebrae. Increased disk space uptake can be seen on bone scan. MRI is very sensitive for assessing disk space involvement.

Therapeutic Considerations: Diskitis is probably a low-grade bacterial infection, but the role of antibiotic therapy is unclear. Bed rest and anti-inflammatory medications are the mainstays of treatment. Immobilization may be required for severe cases. Oral antibiotics are given for 3–4 weeks or until the ESR returns to normal.

Pitfalls: Difficult to isolate an organism, even with needle aspiration of disk space. S. aureus is the most common pathogen, but diskitis can also be caused by coagulase-negative staphylococcus, K. kingae, coliforms, S. pneumoniae.

Prognosis: Fusion of involved vertebrae may occur as the infection resolves. Otherwise, outcome is generally good.

Empiric Therapy of Skin and Soft Tissue Infections

Skin and Soft Tissue Infections

Subset	Usual Pathogens	Preferred IV Therapy†	Alternate IV Therapy†	PO Therapy or IV-to-PO Switch†
Cellulitis, impetigo	S. aureus Group A streptococci (GAS)	Cefazolin **or** Nafcillin **or** Oxacillin × 7–10 days	Clindamycin‡ × 7–10 days	Cephalexin **or** Cefadroxil **or** Dicloxacillin **or** Clindamycin **or** Amoxicillin/ Clavulanate **or** Erythromycin **or** Azithromycin × 7–10 days
Severe pyoder-mas, abscesses	CA-MRSA	Vancomycin **plus** Clindamycin × 7–14 days	Vancomycin **or** Linezolid × 7–14 days	TMP–SMX **or** Doxycycline × 7–14 days**
Animal bite wounds (dog/cat)	Group A streptococci (GAS) P. multocida Capnocyto-phaga S. aureus	Ampicillin Sulbactam × 7–10 days	Piperacillin **or** Ticarcillin/ Clavulanate × 7–10 days <u>Penicillin allergy:</u> Clindamycin **plus** TMP–SMX × 7–10 days (dog bites); **or** Doxycycline **or** Cefuroxime × 7–10 days (cat bites)	Amoxicillin/ Clavulanate **or** Doxycycline × 7–10 days + Metronidazole **or** Clindamycin
Human bite wounds	Oral anaerobes E. corrodens Group A streptococci S. aureus	Ampicillin/ Sulbactam × 5–7 days	Piperacillin **or** Ticarcillin/ Clavulanate × 5–7 days <u>Penicillin allergic:</u> Clindamycin **plus** TMP–SMX × 5–7 days	Amoxicillin/ Clavulanate **or** Doxycycline × 5–7 days **plus either** Metronidazole **or** Clindamycin
Cat scratch disease (CSD)*	Bartonella henselae	Gentamicin × 10–14 days		Azithromycin × 5 days **or** TMP–SMX **or** Ciprofloxacin **or** Rifampin × 10–14 days

† **See p. 436–444 for drug dosages.**
** In childrens > 8 years of age.
* No well-controlled trials of antibiotic treatment for CSD to demonstrate benefit.
‡ Preferred therapy for patients in geographic regions with a high prevalence of MRSA or for those with penicillin/cephalosporin allergy.

Skin and Soft Tissue Infections (cont'd)

Subset	Pathogens	IV Therapy[†]	PO Therapy or IV-to-PO Switch[†]
Chicken pox *Immunocompromised host*	VZV	Acyclovir × 7–10 days	Acyclovir **or** Valacyclovir × 7–10 days
Immunocompetent host	VZV	Acyclovir × 5 days	Acyclovir **or** Valacyclovir × 5 days
H. zoster (Shingles)	VZV	Same as for chicken pox	Acyclovir **or** Valacyclovir × 10 days (for individuals ≥ 12 years of age)

Duration of therapy represents total time IV, PO, or IV + PO. Most patients on IV therapy able to take PO meds should be switched to PO therapy soon after clinical improvement.

† **See p. 436–444 for drug dosages.**

Cellulitis

Clinical Presentation: Erythema, warmth, and tenderness of skin. Impetigo is characterized by a vesiculopapular rash with honey-colored discharge.

Diagnostic Considerations: Primarily a clinical diagnosis. Group A streptococci is the primary pathogens in healthy children. Cellulitis, alone without a pustular component, is caused by streptococci (not staphylococci).

Pitfalls: Differential diagnosis of cellulitis may include hypersensitivity to insect bites. Herpetic whitlow (HSV) may be mistaken for a bacterial skin or paronychial infection.

Therapeutic Considerations: First generation cephalosporin or semi-synthetic penicillin with anti-staphylococcal activity (i.e., dicloxacillin, nafcillin, oxacillin) are drugs of choice. Increasing incidence of community-acquired MRSA may affect treatment decisions.

Prognosis: Excellent. Impetigo may only require topical treatment (Mupirocin).

Bite Wounds

Clinical Presentation: 80% of animal bite wounds in children are from dogs, and 15%–50% of dog bites become infected. More than 50% of cat bites become infected, and due to their long teeth, there is an increased risk of inoculation into bone/joints with development of osteomyelitis/septic arthritis. Human bite wounds are most prone to infection, and 75%–90% of all human bites become infected.

Diagnostic Considerations: Clinical diagnosis. Culture of wound exudate may yield organism.

Pitfalls: Failure to assess depth of infection, especially with cat bites, may result in late identification of bone/joint infection. Macrolides are ineffective against P. multocida.

Therapeutic Considerations: It is important to cover oral anaerobes, S. aureus, and Group A streptococci in human bite wounds. P. multocida is an important pathogen in cat and dog bite wounds. Facial/hand lesions require plastic surgery evaluation. Recurrent debridement may be necessary, especially with human bite wound infections of hand. Assess tetanus immunization status for all bite wounds. For human bites consider the risk of HIV and hepatitis B. For dog bites consider the risk of rabies. Antimicrobial therapy initiated within 8 hours of a bite wound and administered for 2–3 days may decrease the rate of infection.

Prognosis: Good with early debridement and antibiotics.

Cat Scratch Disease (CSD)

Clinical Presentation: Classic presentation is a papular lesion at site of cat scratch with lymphadenitis in the draining region (axillary, epitrochlear, inguinal, cervical most commonly). Frequently associated with fever/malaise 1–2 weeks after scratch. Infection can present with conjunctivitis and ipsilateral preauricular lymph node (Parinaud oculoglandular syndrome). Unusual presentations in normal hosts include encephalitis, hepatitis, microabscesses in liver/spleen, fever of unknown origin, osteolytic lesions.

Diagnostic Considerations: Most often secondary to kitten scratch with Bartonella henselae. Diagnosed using specific serology for B. henselae.

Pitfalls: Failure to obtain history of kitten exposure.

Therapeutic Considerations: Most lesions are self-limited and resolve over 2–4 months. Antibiotic therapy may be helpful in severe cases with hepatosplenomegaly.

Prognosis: Very good with spontaneous resolution over 2–4 months.

Chicken Pox/Shingles (VZV)

Clinical Presentation: Primary illness is chicken pox, a generalized pruritic, vesicular rash with fever that erupts in crops of lesions over 3–5 days followed by crusting and recovery. More severe in adolescents and adults, particularly if immunocompromised. Reactivation disease (shingles) may occur in children and remains localized. Post-herpetic neuralgia occurs less often in children. Reactivation disease in Immunocompromised hosts re-disseminate.

Diagnostic Considerations: The characteristic eruption of chicken pox occurs in waves—multiple stages appear at the same time, characteristic of chickenpox.

Prognosis: Overall prognosis is good with complete recovery.

Pediatric Antimicrobial Drug Dosages

Drug	Dosage in Neonates	Dosage in Infants/Children*
Acyclovir	20 mg/kg (IV) q8h × 14–21 days. Dosing interval may need to be increased for infants < 34 weeks post-maturational age (GA + CA) or if significant renal impairment or liver failure followed by <u>Chronic suppression</u>: 75 mg/kg (PO) q12h × 6 months	<u>HSV encephalitis</u>: 10 mg/kg (IV) q8h × 14–21 days <u>Primary HSV infection</u>: 10–20 mg/kg (PO) q6h × 5–10 days **or** 5 mg/kg/dose (IV) q8h × 5 days <u>Varicella in immunocompromised hosts</u>: 10 mg/kg (IV) q8h × 7–10 days <u>Varicella in immunocompetent hosts</u>: 20 mg/kg (PO) q6h × 5 days (maximum 800 mg/dose)
Albendazole	Not applicable	400 mg (PO) q24h
Amikacin**	<u>*During first week of life* dosing is based on gestational age</u> (administer IV dose over 30 min) • ≤ 27 weeks (or asphyxia, PDA, or indomethacin): 18 mg/kg (IV) q48h • 28–30 weeks: 18 mg/kg (IV) q36h • 31–33 weeks: 16 mg/kg (IV) q36h • ≥ 34 weeks: 15 mg/kg (IV) q24h *After first week of life:* Initial dose of 15 mg/kg, then draw serum concentrations 30 min after end of infusion (peak) and 12–24 hours later (trough) to determine dosing interval. Aim for peak of 20–30 mcg/mL and trough of 2–5 mcg/mL	5–7.5 mg/kg (IV or IM) q8h
Amoxicillin	Not indicated	22.5–45 mg/kg (PO) q12h
Amoxicillin-clavulanate	Not indicated	22.5–45 mg/kg (of amoxicillin component) (PO) q12h
Amphotericin B (conventional)	0.5–1 mg/kg (IV over 2–6 hours) q24-48h (Some authorities recommend an initial test dose of 0.1–0.5 mg/kg IV over 2–6 hours)	
Ampicillin	25–50 mg/kg/dose (IV or IM). <u>Severe Group B streptococcal sepsis</u>: 100 mg/kg/dose. Dosing interval is based on gestational age (GA) and chronological age (CA):	25–50 mg/kg (IV or IM) q6h

* Dosages are generally based on weight (mg/kg), maximum up to adult dose.
** Drug can be given IM but absorption may be variable.

Pediatric Antimicrobial Drug Dosages *(cont'd)*

Drug	Dosage in Neonates			Dosage in Infants/Children*
	GA + CA (weeks)	CA (days)	Interval (hours)	
	≤ 29	0–28 > 28	12 8	
	30–36	0–14 > 14	12 8	
	≥ 37	0–7 > 7	12 8	
Ampicillin-Sulbactam	Not indicated			25–50 mg/kg (of ampicillin component) (IV) q6h
Azithromycin	Not indicated			<u>Otitis media/sinusitis:</u> 30 mg/kg (PO) × 1 dose **or** 10 mg/kg (PO) q24h × 3 days **or** 10 mg/kg (PO) on day 1 followed by 5 mg/kg (PO) q24h on days 2–5 <u>Pharyngitis/tonsillitis:</u> 12 mg/kg (PO) q24h × 5 days
				Community-acquired pneumonia (not indicated for moderate or severe disease): 10 mg/kg (PO) × 5 days **or** 10 mg/kg (IV or PO) on day 1 followed by 5 mg/kg (IV or PO) q24h on days 2–5 <u>Skin/soft tissue infections</u> (including Cat Scratch Disease): 10 mg/kg (PO) on day 1 followed by 5 mg/kg (PO) q24h on days 2–5
Aztreonam	30 mg/kg (IV or IM). See *ampicillin* for dosing interval (p. 438)			30 mg/kg (IV or IM) q6-8h
Caspofungin	70 mg/m² loading dose, then 25 mg/m² (IV) q24h			70 mg/m² loading dose, then 50 mg/m² (IV) q24h (> 3 months)
Cefadroxil	Not indicated			15 mg/kg (PO) q12h
Cefazolin	25 mg/kg (IV or IM). See *ampicillin* for dosing interval (p. 438)			25–100 mg/kg/day (IV or IM) divided q6-q8h
Cefdinir	Not indicated			7 mg/kg (PO) q12h or 14 mg/kg (PO) q24h
Cefepime	50 mg/kg (IV) q12h			33.3–50 mg/kg (IV or IM) q8h

*   Dosages are generally based on weight (mg/kg), maximum up to adult dose.

Pediatric Antimicrobial Drug Dosages *(cont'd)*

Drug	Dosage in Neonates	Dosage in Infants/Children*
Cefotaxime	50 mg/kg (IV or IM). (25 mg/kg/dose is adequate for gonococcal infection). See *ampicillin* for dosing interval (p. 438)	25–50 mg/kg (IV or IM) q6–8h
Cefotetan	Not indicated	20–40 mg/kg (IV or IM) q12h
Cefoxitin	25–33 mg/kg/dose (IV or IM). See *ampicillin* for dosing interval (p. 436)	80–160 mg/kg/day (IV or IM) divided q4–8h
Cefpodoxime	Not indicated	5 mg/kg (PO) q12h
Cefprozil	Not indicated	15 mg/kg (PO) q12h
Ceftazidime	30 mg/kg/dose (IV or IM). See *ampicillin* for dosing interval (p. 436)	25–50 mg/kg (IV or IM) q8h
Ceftibuten	Not indicated	9 mg/kg (PO) q24h
Ceftizoxime	Not indicated	50 mg/kg (IV or IM) q6–8h
Ceftriaxone[‡]	<u>Sepsis and disseminated gonococcal infection:</u> 50 mg/kg (IV or IM) q24h <u>Meningitis:</u> 100 mg/kg loading dose followed by 80 mg/kg (IV or IM) q24h <u>Uncomplicated gonococcal ophthalmia:</u> 50 mg/kg (maximum 125 mg) as a single dose (IV or IM)	50 mg/kg (IV or IM) q24h. <u>Meningitis:</u> 50 mg/kg (IV or IM) q12h or 100 mg/kg (IV or IM) q24h <u>Acute otitis media:</u> 50 mg/kg (IM) × 1 dose (or 3 doses IM q24h in high-risk patients)
Cefuroxime	Not indicated	10–15 mg/kg (PO) q12h 25–50 mg/kg (IV or IM) q8h
Cephalexin	Not indicated	6.25–25 mg/kg (PO) q6h
Cephalothin	Not indicated	25 mg/kg (IV or IM) q4-6h
Clarithromycin	Not indicated	7.5 mg/kg (PO) q12h
Clindamycin	5.0–7.5 mg (IV or PO). Dosing interval is based on gestational age (GA) and chronological age (CA)	5–10 mg/kg (IV or IM) q6-8h or 10–30 mg/kg/day (PO) divided q6-8h

*   Dosages are generally based on weight (mg/kg), maximum up to adult dose.
**   Do not use in presence of hyperbilirubinemia.

Pediatric Antimicrobial Drug Dosages (cont'd)

Drug	Dosage in Neonates			Dosage in Infants/Children*
	GA + CA (weeks)	CA (days)	Interval (hours)	
	< 29	0–28 > 28	12 8	
	30–36	0–14 > 14	12 8	
	37–44	0–7 > 7	8 6	
Dicloxacillin	Not indicated			6.25–12.5 mg/kg (PO) q6h
Doxycycline	Contraindicated			> 45 kg: 100 mg (PO) q12h ≤ 45 kg: 1.1–2.5 mg/kg (PO) q12h Use only in children > 8 years (unless RMSF) 1–2 mg/kg (IV) q12–24h
Erythromycin	<u>Chlamydia pneumonitis/ conjunctivitis or pertussis</u>: 12.5 mg/kg (PO) q6h (E. estolate preferred) <u>Other infections</u>: Erythromycin estolate 10 mg/kg (PO) q8h **or** Erythromycin ethylsuccinate 10 mg/kg (PO) q6h <u>Severe infections and PO not possible</u>: 5–10 mg/kg (IV over ≥ 60 min) q6h			10–12.5 mg/kg (PO) q6–8h 5–12.5 mg/kg (IV) q6h
Ertapenem	Not indicated			15 mg/kg (IV) q12h (not to exceed 1 gm/day)
Ethambutol	See p. 421			See p. 421
Ethionamide	See p. 421			See p. 421

*   Dosages are generally based on weight (mg/kg), up to adult dose as maximum.

Pediatric Antimicrobial Drug Dosages *(cont'd)*

Drug	Dosage in Neonates			Dosage in Infants/Children*
Fluconazole	<u>Systemic infection or meningitis:</u> 12 mg/kg (IV over 30 min or PO) × 1 dose, then 6 mg/kg/dose (IV or PO) with dosing interval based on gestational age (GA) and chronological age (CA) (below) <u>Prophylaxis</u> (e.g., extremely low birth weight infants in NICU with high rates of fungal disease): 3 mg/kg/dose (IV or PO) according to dosing interval grid (below) <u>Thrush:</u> 6 mg/kg (PO) × 1 dose, then 3 mg/kg (PO) q24h			10 mg/kg (IV or PO) loading dose followed by 12 mg/kg (IV or PO) q24h
	GA + CA (weeks)	**CA (days)**	**Interval (weeks)**	
	≤ 29	0–14 >14	72 48	
	30–36	0–14 >14	48 24	
	37–44	0–7 >7	48 24	
Gentamicin**	*During first week of life* dosing is based on gestational age (administer IV dose over 30 min): • ≤ 29 weeks (or asphyxia, PDA, or indomethacin): 5 mg/kg (IV) q48h • 30–33 weeks: 4.5 mg/kg (IV) q48h • 34–37 weeks: 4 mg/kg (IV) q36h • ≥ 38 weeks: 4 mg/kg (IV) q24h *After first week of life:* Initial dose of 4 mg/kg, then draw serum concentrations 30 min after end of infusion (peak) and 12–24 hours later (trough) to determine dosing interval. Aim for peak of 5–12 mcg/mL and trough of 0.5–1 mcg/mL			2–2.5 mg/kg (IV or IM) q8h **or** 4.5–7.5 mg/kg (IV) q24h

*   Dosages are generally based on weight (mg/kg), maximum up to adult dose.
** Drug can be given IM but absorption may be variable.

Pediatric Antimicrobial Drug Dosages *(cont'd)*

Drug	Dosage in Neonates			Dosage in Infants/Children*
Imipenem	20–25 mg/kg (IV) q12h			15–25 mg/kg (IV or IM) q6h
Iodoquinol	No information			10–13.3 mg/kg (PO) q8h
Isoniazid	See p. 424			See p. 424
Linezolid	10 mg/kg (IV) q12h			10 mg/kg (IV) q8h
Liposomal/ Amphotericin preparations	1–5 mg/kg (IV over 2 hours) q24h			3–6 mg/kg (IV) q24h
Meropenem	20 mg/kg (IV) q12h			10 mg/kg (IV) q8h (skin); 20 mg/kg (IV) q8h (intraabdominal); 40 mg/kg (IV) q8h (meningitis). May be used in neonates.
Methenamine mandelate	Not indicated			15–25 mg (PO) q6–8h
Metronida-zole	15 mg/kg (IV or PO) × 1 dose, then 7.5 mg/kg/dose (IV or PO) with dosing interval based on gestational age (GA) and chronological age (CA):			5–12.5 mg/kg (PO) q8h 15 mg/kg (IV) × 1 dose followed by 7.5 mg/kg (IV) q6h
	GA + CA (weeks)	**CA (days)**	**Interval (hours)**	
	≤ 29	0–28 > 28	24 48	
	30–36	0–14 > 14	24 12	
	37–44	0–7 > 7	24 12	
Micafungin	10 mg/kg (IV) of q24h			4–12 mg/kg (IV) q24 (higher dose for patients < 8-year of age
Mupirocin	Not indicated			Nasal cream: ½ of single use tube into nostril q12h × 5 days; Cream: apply q8h × 5–10 days
Nafcillin	25–50 mg/kg/dose (IV). See *ampicillin* for dosing interval (p. 438)			12.5–50 mg/kg (IV or IM) q6h

*   Dosages are generally based on weight (mg/kg), maximum up to adult dose.

Pediatric Antimicrobial Drug Dosages *(cont'd)*

Drug	Dosage in Neonates	Dosage in Infants/Children*
Nitazoxanide	Not applicable	Children 1–3 years old: 100 mg (PO) q12h; children 4–11 years old: 200 mg (PO) q12h
Nitrofuran-toin	Not indicated	<u>UTI:</u> 1.25–1.75 mg/kg (PO) q6h <u>UTI prophylaxis:</u> 1–2 mg/kg (PO) q24h
Nystatin	<u>Oral:</u> 1 mL (preterm) to 2 mL (term) of 100,000 U/mL suspension applied with swab to each side of mouth q6h until 3 days after resolution of lesions <u>Topical:</u> Apply ointment or cream to affected area q6h until 3 days after resolution of lesions.	<u>Suspension:</u> 4–6 mL swish and swallow 4×/day <u>Troche:</u> 1–2 troches 4–5×/ day
Oxacillin	25–50 mg/kg/dose (IV). See *ampicillin* for dosing interval (p. 436)	25–50 mg/kg (IV or IM) q6h
Paromomycin	Not applicable	10 mg/kg (PO) q8h
Penicillin G	25,000–50,000 IU/kg/dose (IV). See *ampicillin* for dosing interval (p. 438) <u>Meningitis:</u> 75,000–100,000 IU/kg (IV) in meningitis (IV). Q8–12h based on GA + CA, See *ampicillin* for dosing interval (p. 415). Crystalline penicillin G: IM: procaine penicillin G q24 hours. <u>Congenital syphilis:</u> Aqueous penicillin G 50,000 IU/kg (slow IV push) q12h × 7 days, then q8h to complete 10–14 days or procaine penicillin G 50,000 IU/kg (IM) q24h × 10–14 days	12,500–75,000 U/kg (IV or IM) q4–6h
Penicillin V	Not indicated	6.25–12.5 mg/kg (PO) q6-8h
Piperacillin	50–100 mg/kg/dose (IV or IM). See *ampicillin* for dosing interval (p. 436)	25–75 mg/kg (IV or IM) q6h; may increase to q4h in severe infection, especially Pseudomonas

* Dosages are based on weight (mg/kg), maximum up to adult dose.

Pediatric Antimicrobial Drug Dosages *(cont'd)*

Drug	Dosage in Neonates	Dosage in Infants/Children*
Piperacillin/ Tazobactam	Not indicated	100–300 mg/kg/day (IV) (of piper-acillin component) divided q6-8h
Pyrazinamide	See p. 421	See p. 421
Quinupristin/ Dalfopristin	No information	7.5 mg/kg (IV) q12h
Rifampin	10–20 mg/kg (PO) q24h **or** 5–10 mg/kg (IV) q24h	20 mg/kg (PO) q24h **or** 10 mg/kg (PO) q12h
		10–20 mg/kg/day (IV) divided q12–24h
Streptomycin	See p. 421	See p. 421
Sulfisoxazole	Contraindicated	30–35 mg/kg (PO) q6h <u>Otitis media prophylaxis:</u> 37.5 mg/kg (PO) q12h
Tetracycline	Contraindicated	5–12.5 mg/kg (PO) q6h. Use only in children > 8 years
Ticarcillin	75–100 mg/kg/dose (IV). See *ampicillin* for dosing interval (p. 438)	25–75 mg/kg (IV or IM) q6h
Ticarcillin/ Clavulanate	75–100 mg/kg/dose (of ticarcillin component) (IV). See *ampicillin* for dosing interval (p. 438)	25–75 mg/kg (of ticarcillin component) (IV or IM) q6h
Tinidazole	Not applicable	50–60 mg/kg (PO) q24h
Tobramycin	Same as gentamicin	2–2.5 mg/kg (IV or IM) q8h or 4.5–7.5 mg/kg (IV) of q24h
Trimetho-prim sulfa methoxazole (TMP–SMX)	Contraindicated	<u>UTI:</u> 4–5 mg/kg (of trimethoprim component) (PO) q12h <u>Pneumocystis carinii pneumonia (PCP)</u> 5 mg/kg (PO) q6h (typically after initial IV therapy) <u>UTI prophylaxis:</u> 2–4 mg/kg (PO) q24h *IV dosing* <u>PCP or severe infection:</u> 5 mg/kg (of trimethoprim component) (IV) q6h <u>Minor infections:</u> 4–6 mg/kg (of trimethoprim component) (IV) q12h

* Dosages are generally based on weight (mg/kg), maximum up to adult dose.

Pediatric Antimicrobial Drug Dosages *(cont'd)*

Drug	Dosage in Neonates			Dosage in Infants/Children*
Vancomycin	<u>Bacteremia</u>: 10 mg/kg/dose (IV) <u>Meningitis</u>: 15 mg/kg/dose (IV). Administer IV dose over 60 min. Dosing interval is based on gestational age (GA) and chronological age (CA):			10–20 mg/kg (IV) q6h
	GA + CA (weeks)	**CA (days)**	**Interval (weeks)**	
	≤ 29	0–14 > 14	18 12	
	30–36	0–14 > 14	12 8	
	37–44	0–7 > 7	12 8	
Voriconazole	Not applicable			7 mg/kg (IV) q12h 8 mg/kg (PO) q12h × 1 day, then 7 mg/kg (PO) q12h

*   Dosages are generally based on weight (mg/kg), up to adult dose as maximum.

REFERENCES

Bergelson J, Zaoutis T, Shah SS (eds). Pediatric Infectious Diseases: Requisites (1st Ed), McGraw-Hill, 2009.

Bradley JS, Nelson JD, Kimberlin DW, et al (eds). Nelson's Pediatric Antimicrobial Therapy (25th Ed), American Academy of Pediatrics, Elk Grove Village IL, 2019.

Cherry J, Demmler GJ, Kaplan SL, et al. Feigin and Cherry's Textbook of Pediatric Infectious Diseases (8th Ed), Saunders, Philadelphia, 2013.

Kimberlin DW, Long SS, Brady MT, Jackson MA, et al. Red Book 2015: Report of the Committee on Infectious Diseases (31st Ed), American Academy of Pediatrics, Elk Grove Village, IL, 2018.

Long SS, Pickering LK, Prober CG (eds). Principles and Practice of Pediatric Infectious Diseases (5th Ed), Saunders, Philadelphia, 2012.

Pickering LK (ed). Red Book: 2012 Report of the Committee on Infectious Diseases (30th Ed), American Academy of Pediatrics, Elk Grove Village, IL, 2015.

Shah S. Pediatric Infectious Disease Practice. New York: McGraw-Hill, 2009.

Steele WR (ed.). Clinical Handbook of Pediatric Infectious Disease (3rd Ed), Informa Healthcare, New York, 2007.

Wilson CB, Nizet V, Maldonado Y, et al. (eds) Infectious Diseases of the Fetus and Newborn Infant (8th Ed), Saunders, Philadelphia, PA, 2010.

Chapter 8
CHEST X-RAY ATLAS

Burke A. Cunha, MD,
Douglas S. Katz, MD,
Robert Moore, MD,
Daniel S. Siegal, MD

Chest X-Ray Patterns

- This atlas has been developed to assist in the DDx of patients who present with respiratory symptoms and chest x-ray abnormalities.
- Eight common chest x-ray patterns are provided.
- Infectious and noninfectious etiologies are followed by clinical features useful in the DDx and help guide empiric therapy.

Unilateral Focal Segmental/Lobar Infiltrate without Effusion

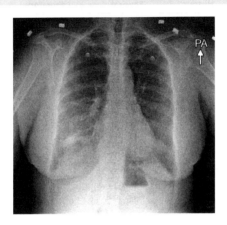

Infectious Causes

	Features (may have some, none, or all)			
Causes	**History**	**Physical**	**Laboratory**	**Chest X-Ray**
S. pneumoniae	Elderly, smokers, COPD, ↓ humoral immunity (multiple myeloma, SLE, CLL, hyposplenism).	Fever/chills, no relative bradycardia. Chest signs related to extent of consolidation.	↑ WBCs, ↓ platelets (overwhelming infection/hyposplenism), normal LFTs. Sputum with abundant PMNs and Gram positive diplococci. Blood cultures usually positive.	Consolidation usually limited to one lobe (RLL most common) ± air bronchogram. Pleural effusion very uncommon, but empyema not uncommon. No cavitation.
H. influenzae	Recent contact with H. influenzae URI.	Fever/chills.	↑ WBCs. Sputum/pleural effusion with Gram negative pleomorphic bacilli. Blood cultures often positive.	Usually RLL with small/moderate effusion. No empyema. No cavitation.

Infectious Causes *(cont'd)*

	Features (may have some, none, or all)			
Causes	**History**	**Physical**	**Laboratory**	**Chest X-Ray**
M. catarrhalis	Chronic/heavy smoker, COPD.	Nonspecific.	Sputum with Gram negative/ variable diplococci. Blood cultures negative.	Usually lower lobe ± consolidation. No pleural effusion or cavitation.
K. pneumoniae	Nosocomial pneumonia or history of alcoholism in patient with community-acquired pneumonia.	Fever/chills, signs of alcoholic cirrhosis, signs of consolidation over involved lobe.	↑WBCs, ↓ platelets, ↑ AST/ALT (2° to alcoholism). "Red currant jelly" sputum with PMNs and plump Gram negative encapsulated bacilli.	"Bulging fissure" sign secondary to expanded lobar volume. Empyema rather than pleural effusion. Cavitation (thick-walled) in 5–7 days.
Legionella	Recent aerosolized water exposure. Most frequent in late summer/ fall. Recent contact with Legionella containing water. Usually elderly. May have watery diarrhea, abdominal pain, mental confusion.	Fever/chills, relative bradycardia. ↓ breath sounds if consolidation or pleural effusion.	↑WBCs, ↑ AST/ ALT, ↓ PO₄⁼, ↓ Na⁺, ↑ CPK, ↑ ESR, ↑ CRP, ↑ ferritin levels, microscopic hematuria. Mucoid/purulent sputum with few PMNs. Sputum culture for Legionella or sputum DFA (before therapy) is diagnostic. ↑ Legionella titers, L. pneumophila antigenuria (serotype 01 only) may not be positive early.	Rapidly progressive multifocal infiltrates clue to Legionella. Consolidation and pleural effusion not uncommon. Cavitation rare.

Infectious Causes *(cont'd)*

Features (may have some, none, or all)				
Causes	**History**	**Physical**	**Laboratory**	**Chest X-Ray**
Psittacosis	Recent bird contact with psittacine birds. Severe headache.	Fever/chills, ± relative bradycardia, Horder's spots on face, ± epistaxis, ± spleno-megaly. Signs of consolidation common.	↓/normal WBCs, ↑ AST/ALT. Sputum with few PMNs. ↑ C. psittaci titers.	Dense infiltrate. Consolidation common. Pleural effusion/cavitation rare.
Q fever	Recent contact with sheep or parturient cats.	Fever/chills, ± relative bradycardia, ± spleno-megaly, ± hepato-megaly.	↑/normal WBC, ↑ AST/ALT. Sputum with no bacteria/few PMNs. Acute Q fever: ↑ in phase II titers (caution: biohazard).	Dense consolidation. Cavitation/pleural effusion rare.

Noninfectious Causes

Features (may have some, none, or all)				
Causes	**History**	**Physical**	**Laboratory**	**Chest X-Ray**
Atelectasis	Ineffectual recurrent cough characteristic of post-operative atelectasis.	Fevers ≤ 102°F. If large, signs of volume loss (↓ respiratory excursion, ↑ diaphragm, mediastinum shift toward affected side). If small, ↓ breath sounds over affected segment/lobe.	↑ WBCs, (left shift), normal platelets. Other lab results related to underlying cause of atelectasis.	Segmental infiltrate. RUL/RML atelectasis obscures right heart border. In LUL atelectasis, may be triangular infiltrate extending to upper anterior mediastinum mimicking malignancy. LLL atelectasis causes ↑ density of heart shadow. No cavitation or pleural effusion.

Noninfectious Causes *(cont'd)*

	Features (may have some, none, or all)			
Causes	History	Physical	Laboratory	Chest X-Ray
Pulmonary embolus/ infarct	Acute onset dyspnea/ pleuritic chest pain. History of lower extremity trauma, stasis or hyperco- agulable disorder.	↑ pulse/ respiratory rate.	↑ fibrin split products (FSP) and D-dimers ± ↑ total bilirubin. Bloody pleural effusion. ECG with RV strain/ p-pulmonale (large embolus). Positive V/Q scan and CT pulmonary angiogram.	Normal or show non-specific pleural based infiltrates resem- bling atelectasis. Focal segmental/ lobar hyperlucency (Westermark's sign) in some. "Hampton's hump" with infarct. Resolving infarcts ↓ in size but maintain shape/density ("melting ice cube").
Lymphoma	Fever, ↓ appetite with weight loss, night sweats, fatigue.	Adenopathy ± splenomegaly.	Normal WBCs, ↑ basophils, eosinophilia, ↓ lymphocytes, ↑ platelets, ↑ ESR, ↑ ACE, ↑ alkaline phosphatase, ↑$\alpha_{1, 2}$ globulins on SPEP.	Unilateral or asym- metrical bilateral hilar adenopathy. Lung infiltrate may appear conti- guous with hilar adenopathy. No "clear channel" between media- stinum and hilar nodes. Small pleural effusions rare.
Alveolar cell carcinoma	Fever, ↓ appetite with weight loss, night sweats.	± dullness over lobe with large lower lobe lesions.	Positive cytology by BAL/lung biopsy.	Well-defined or ill-defined circumscribed peripheral infiltrates ± air bronchograms. May be multifocal/ multilobar. Hilar adenopathy present. Stranding to the hilum ("pleural tail" sign). ± pleural effusion if lower lobe infiltrate. No cavitation.

Noninfectious Causes *(cont'd)*

Features (may have some, none, or all)				
Causes	**History**	**Physical**	**Laboratory**	**Chest X-Ray**
Aspiration pneumonia	Swallowing disorder 2° to CNS/GI disorder; impaired consciousness. Recent aspiration 2° to dental, upper GI, or pulmonary procedure.	Unremarkable.	↑WBCs	Infiltrate usually involves superior segments of lower lobes (or posterior segments of upper lobes if aspiration occurred supine). Focal infiltrate initially, which may be followed in 7 days by cavitation/lung abscess.

Unilateral Focal Segmental/Lobar Infiltrate with Effusion

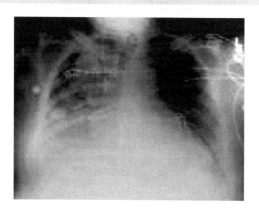

Infectious Causes

	Features (may have some, none, or all)			
Causes	History	Physical	Laboratory	Chest X-Ray
K. pneumoniae	Nosocomial pneumonia or history of alcoholism in patient with community-acquired pneumonia.	Fever/chills, signs of alcoholic cirrhosis, signs of consolidation over involved lobe.	↑ WBCs, ↓ platelets, ↑ AST/ALT (if 2° to alcoholism). "Red currant jelly" sputum with PMNs and plump Gram negative encapsulated bacilli.	"Bulging fissure" sign secondary to expanded lobar volume. Empyema rather than pleural effusion. Usually cavitation in 5–7 days (thick-walled).
H. influenzae	Recent contact with H. influenzae URI.	Fever/chills.	↑ WBCs. Sputum/pleural effusion with Gram negative pleomorphic bacilli. Blood cultures often positive.	Usually RLL with small/moderate effusion. No empyema. No cavitation.

Infectious Causes *(cont'd)*

Features (may have some, none, or all)				
Causes	**History**	**Physical**	**Laboratory**	**Chest X-Ray**
TB (primary)	Recent TB contact.	Unilateral lower lobe dullness related to size of pleural effusion.	PPD – (anergic). Exudative pleural effusion (pleural fluid with ↑ lymphocytes, ↓ glucose, ± RBCs).	Lower lobe infiltrate with small/moderate pleural effusion. No cavitation or apical infiltrates. Hilar adenopathy asymmetrical if present.
Coccidio-mycosis (chronic)	Previous exposure in endemic coccidiomy-cosis areas. Asympto-matic.	± E. nodosum.	Normal WBCs, no eosinophilia in chronic phase. Complement fixation IgG titer ≥ 1:32 indicates active disease.	Thick/thin-walled cavities < 3 cm ± calcifications. Air fluid level rare unless secondarily infected. Cavities usually in anterior segments of upper lobes (vs. posterior segments with TB). No surrounding tissue reaction. Pleural effusion common.
Tularemia	History of recent deer fly, rabbit, or tick exposure. Tularemia pneumonia may complicate any of the clinical presentations of tularemia.	Fever/chills, no relative bradycardia. Chest findings related to extent of infiltrate/ consolidation and pleural effusion.	Normal/↑ WBC, normal LFTs. Sputum/pleural effusion with Gram negative coccobacilli. Bloody pleural effusion. Tularemia serology: ↑ micro-agglutination titer ≥ 1:160 acutely and ≥ 4-fold rise between acute and convalescent titers (caution: biohazard).	Pleural effusion ± hilar adenopathy.

Infectious Causes *(cont'd)*

	Features (may have some, none, or all)			
Causes	**History**	**Physical**	**Laboratory**	**Chest X-Ray**
Adenovirus	Recent URI.	Fever/chills, myalgias. Sore throat and conjunctivitis not always present with adenoviral pneumonia. Chest exam ± signs of consolidation.	↓ WBCs, ↓ platelets, ↑ LFTs, ↑ CPK (in some), mild ↑ cold agglutinins (in some) ↑ adenoviral titers ± positive adenoviral throat cultures or PCR of respiratory secretions.	Usually begins unilaterally, but may progress to bilateral patchy/interstitial infiltrates. Usually ill-defined infiltrate without cavitation and usually no pleural effusion. Only viral cause of focal lobar pneumonia.
Legionella	Recent aerosolized water exposure. Recent contact with Legionella containing water. Usually elderly. May have watery diarrhea, abdominal pain, mental confusion.	Fever/chills, relative bradycardia. ↓ breath sounds if consolidation or pleural effusion.	↑ WBCs, ↑ AST/ALT, ↓ PO₄⁼, ↓ Na⁺, ↑ CPK, ↑ ESR, ↑ CRP, ↑ ferritin, microscopic hematuria. Mucoid/purulent sputum with few PMNs. Sputum culture for Legionella or sputum DFA (before therapy) is diagnostic. ↑ Legionella titers, L. pneumophila antigenuria (serotype 01 only) may not be positive early.	Rapidly progressive asymmetrical multifocal infiltrates clue to Legionella. Consolidation and pleural effusion not uncommon. Cavitation rare.
Group A streptococci (GAS)	Recent exposure or recent blunt chest trauma ± chest pain.	Fever/chills. Physical signs related to size of pleural effusion.	↑ WBCs, Pleural fluid is serosanguineous. Sputum/pleural fluid with Gram positive cocci in pairs/chains. Positive pleural fluid/blood cultures.	Unilateral infiltrate may be obscured by large pleural effusion. No empyema. No cavitation.

Infectious Causes *(cont'd)*

Features (may have some, none, or all)				
Causes	**History**	**Physical**	**Laboratory**	**Chest X-Ray**
Rhodococcus equi	Insidious onset of fever, dyspnea, chest pain, ± hemoptysis. Immuno-suppressed patients with ↓ cell-mediated immunity. Exposure to cattle, horses, pigs.	Unremarkable.	Normal/↑ WBCs, Sputum/pleural fluid with Gram positive pleomorphic weakly acid fast bacilli. Sputum, pleural fluid, blood cultures positive for R. equi.	Segmental infiltrate with upper lobe predominance ± cavitation. Air-fluid levels and pleural effusion common.

Noninfectious Causes

Features (may have some, none, or all)				
Causes	**History**	**Physical**	**Laboratory**	**Chest X-Ray**
Pulmonary embolus/ infarct	Acute onset dyspnea/ pleuritic chest pain. History of lower extremity trauma, stasis or hyperco-agulable disorder.	Fever < 102°F, ↑ pulse/ respiratory rate.	↑ fibrin split products (FSP) and D-dimers ± ↑ total bilirubin. Bloody pleural effusion. ECG with RV strain/p-pulmonale (large embolus). Positive V/Q scan and CT pulmonary angiogram.	Normal or show non-specific pleural-based infiltrates resembling atelectasis. Focal segmental/lobar hyperlucency (Westermark's sign) in some. "Hampton's hump" with infarct. Resolving infarcts ↓ in size but maintain shape/density ("melting ice cube").

Noninfectious Causes *(cont'd)*

	Features (may have some, none, or all)			
Causes	**History**	**Physical**	**Laboratory**	**Chest X-Ray**
Lymphoma	Fever, ↓ appetite with weight loss, night sweats, fatigue.	Adenopathy ± spleno-megaly.	Normal WBCs, ↑ basophils, eosinophilia, ↓ lymphocytes, ↑ platelets, ↑ ESR, ↑ alkaline phosphatase, ↑ ACE, ↑$\alpha_{1,2}$ globulins on SPEP.	Unilateral or asymmetrical bilateral hilar adenopathy. Lung infiltrate contiguous with hilar adenopathy. No "clear channel" between media-stinum and hilar nodes. Small pleural effusions rare.
Alveolar cell carcinoma	Fever, ↓ appetite with weight loss, night sweats.	± dullness over lobe with large lower lobe lesions.	Positive cytology by BAL/lung biopsy.	Well/ill-defined circumscribed peripheral infiltrates ± air bronchograms. May be multifocal/ multilobar. Hilar adenopathy present. Stranding to the hilum ("pleural tail" sign). ± pleural effusion if lower lobe infiltrate. No cavitation.
Radiation pneumonitis	History of mantle radiation for lymphoma, lung cancer, or breast cancer.	Nonspecific.	Nonspecific.	Symmetrical infiltrates in the distribution of radiation therapy after 1 month. Infiltrates have "straight edges". Fibrosis common over radiation field after 9–12 months. Usually no pleural effusions (small, if present).

Unilateral Ill-Defined Infiltrates
without Effusion

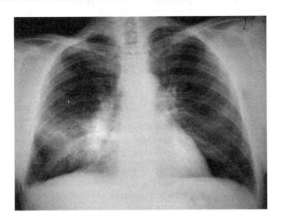

Infectious Causes

| | Features (may have some, none, or all) | | | |
Causes	**History**	**Physical**	**Laboratory**	**Chest X-Ray**
Mycoplasma pneumoniae	Prolonged dry/nonproductive cough. No laryngitis. Mild sore throat/ear. Watery diarrhea.	Usually fevers ≤102°F without relative bradycardia. Myalgias, bullous myringitis or otitis, non-exudative pharyngitis, E. multiforme. Chest exam: rales with no signs of consolidation or effusion.	Normal/↑ WBCs, normal/↑ platelets, normal AST/ALT, ↑ cold agglutinins (early) >1:64. ↑ IgM (not IgG) Mycoplasma pneumoniae titers. Respiratory secretion culture or PCR positive for Mycoplasma pneumoniae.	Ill-defined usually lower lobe indistinct infiltrates. No consolidation or air bronchograms. Small/no pleural effusion.

Infectious Causes *(cont'd)*

Features (may have some, none, or all)				
Causes	**History**	**Physical**	**Laboratory**	**Chest X-Ray**
Chlamydophilia (Chlamydia) pneumoniae	Prolonged "mycoplasma-like" illness with laryngitis.	Low grade fevers, myalgias, non-exudative pharyngitis, laryngitis. No relative bradycardia, ear findings, or rash. Chest exam: without signs of consolidation or pleural effusion.	↑ WBC, normal platelets, normal LFTs. No cold agglutinins. ↑ IgM (not IgG) C. pneumoniae titers. Respiratory secretions culture or PCR positive for C. pneumoniae.	Ill-defined, usually lower lobe indistinct infiltrate(s). May be "funnel shaped." No consolidation, cavitation, or pleural effusion.
Adenovirus	Recent URI.	Fever/chills, myalgias. Sore throat and conjunctivitis not always present with adenoviral pneumonia. Chest exam: ± signs of consolidation.	↓ WBC, ↓ platelets, ↑ AST/ALT, ↑ CPK (in some), mild ↑ cold agglutinins (in some) ↑ adenoviral throat titers ± positive adenoviral cultures or PCR of respiratory secretions.	Usually begins unilaterally, but may progress to bilateral patchy/interstitial infiltrates. Usually ill-defined infiltrate without cavitation ± pleural effusion. Only viral cause of focal lobar pneumonia.

Infectious Causes *(cont'd)*

| | Features (may have some, none, or all) | | | |
Causes	History	Physical	Laboratory	Chest X-Ray
Legionella	Most frequent in late summer/fall. Recent contact with Legionella containing water. Usually elderly. May have watery diarrhea, abdominal pain, mental confusion.	Fever/chills, relative bradycardia. ↓ breath sounds if consolidation or pleural effusion.	↑ WBC, ↑ AST/ALT, ↓ PO$_4^=$, ↓ Na$^+$, ↑ CPK, ↑ ESR, ↑ CRP, ↑ ferritin, microscopic hematuria. Mucoid/purulent sputum with few PMNs. Sputum culture for Legionella or sputum DFA (before therapy) is diagnostic. ↑ Legionella titers, L. pneumophila antigenuria (serotypes 01 only) may not be positive early.	Rapidly progressive asymmetrical infiltrates clue to Legionella. Consolidation and pleural effusion not uncommon. Cavitation rare.
Psittacosis	Recent bird contact with psittacine birds. Severe headache.	Fever/chills, ± relative bradycardia, ± Horder's spots on face, epistaxis, ± splenomegaly. Signs of consolidation common.	↓/normal WBCs, ↑ AST/ALT. Sputum with few PMNs. ↑ C. psittaci titers.	Dense infiltrate. Consolidation common. Pleural effusion/cavitation rare.
Q fever	Recent contact with sheep or parturient cats.	Fever/chills, ± relative bradycardia, ± splenomegaly, ± hepato-megaly.	↑/normal WBCs, ↑ AST/ALT. Sputum with no bacteria/few PMNs. Acute Q fever with ↑ in phase II titers (caution: biohazard).	Dense consolidation. Cavitation/pleural effusion rare.

Infectious Causes (cont'd)

	Features (may have some, none, or all)			
Causes	History	Physical	Laboratory	Chest X-Ray
Nocardia	Fevers, night sweats, fatigue, ↓ cell mediated immunity (e.g., HIV, organ transplants, PAP, immunosuppressive therapy).	Unremarkable. No chest wall sinus tracts	Normal/↑ WBCs, ↑ ESR. Sputum with Gram positive beaded acid fast aerobic bacilli.	Dense large infiltrates. May cavitate and mimic TB, lymphoma, or squamous cell carcinoma. No calcification ± pleural effusion.
Actinomycosis	Recent dental work.	± chest wall sinus tracts.	Normal/↑ WBCs, ↑ ESR. Sputum with Gram positive filamentous anaerobic bacilli.	Dense infiltrates extending to chest wall. No hilar adenopathy. Cavitation rare. ± pleural effusion rare.
Cryptococcus neoformans	Exposure to air conditioner or pigeons.	Unremarkable.	Normal WBCs, Cryptococcal serology with ↑ C. neoformans antigen levels.	Dense lower nodular mass lesions. No calcification or cavitation. ± pleural effusion.
Aspiration pneumonia	Swallowing disorder 2° to CNS/GI disorder; impaired consciousness. Recent aspiration 2° to dental, upper GI, or pulmonary procedure.	Unremarkable.	↑ WBCs	Infiltrate usually involves superior segments of lower lobes (or posterior segments of upper lobes if aspiration occurred supine). Focal infiltrate initially, which may be followed in 7 days by cavitation/lung abscess.

Noninfectious Causes

	Features (may have some, none, or all)			
Causes	**History**	**Physical**	**Laboratory**	**Chest X-Ray**
Bronchogenic carcinoma	Fever, ↓ appetite with weight loss, cough ± hemoptysis. Cough with copious clear/ mucoid sputum in large cell anaplastic carcinoma. Increased risk in smokers, aluminum/ uranium miners, cavitary lung disease (adenocarci-noma), previous radiation therapy from lymphoma/ breast cancer.	Paraneo-plastic syndromes especially with small (oat) cell/ squamous cell carci-noma ± hypertrophic pulmonary osteoarthro-pathy ± clubbing.	Normal/↑ WBCs, ↑ platelets, ↑ ESR, findings related to underlying malignancy.	Small/squamous cell carcinomas present as central lesions/ hilar masses. Adenocarcinoma/ large cell anaplastic carcinomas are usually peripheral initially. "Tumor tendrils" extending into surrounding lung tissue is characteristic. No calcifications (may be present on chest CT). Cavitation with squamous cell carcinoma. ± pleural effusions.
Lymphangitic metastases	History of breast, thyroid, pancreas, cervical, prostate, or lung carcinoma.	Findings related to underlying malignancy.	Normal/↑ WBCs, ↑ ESR.	Interstitial indistinct pulmonary infil-trates (may be reticulonodular) with lower lobe predominance Usually unilateral but may be bilateral. No con-solidation or cavitation ± pleural effusions.
Lung contusion	Recent closed chest trauma, chest pain.	Chest wall contusion over infiltrate.	↑ WBCs, (left shift).	Patchy ill-defined infiltrate(s) ± rib fractures/ pneumothorax in area of infiltrate. Infiltrate clears within 1 week.

Noninfectious Causes (cont'd)

	Features (may have some, none, or all)			
Causes	**History**	**Physical**	**Laboratory**	**Chest X-Ray**
Congestive heart failure	Coronary heart disease, valvular heart disease, cardiomyopathy.	No/low-grade fevers ↑ pulse and respiratory rate, positive jugular venous distension and hepato-jugular reflex, cardio-megaly, S₃, ascites, hepato-megaly, pedal edema.	↑ WBCs, (left shift), normal platelets, mildly ↑ AST/ ALT.	Cardiomegaly, pleural effusion (R > [R + L] > L). Kerley B lines with vascular redistribution to upper lobes. Typically bilateral rather than unilateral.
Alveolar cell carcinoma	Fever, ↓ appetite with weight loss, night sweats.	± dullness over lobe with large lower lobe lesions.	Positive cytology by BAL/lung biopsy.	Well/ill-defined circumscribed peripheral infiltrates ± air bronchograms. May be multifocal/ multilobar. Hilar adenopathy present. Stranding to the hilum ("pleural tail" sign). ± pleural effusion if lower lobe infiltrate. No cavitation.
Lymphoma	Fever, ↓ appetite with weight loss, night sweats, fatigue.	Adenopathy ± spleno-megaly.	Normal WBCs, ↑ basophils, eosinophilia, ↓ lymphocytes, ↑ platelets, ↑ ESR, ↑ ACE, ↑ alkaline phosphatase, ↑α_{1,2} globulins on SPEP.	Unilateral or asym-metrical bilateral hilar adenopathy. Lung infiltrate contiguous with hilar adenopathy. No "clear channel" between media-stinum and hilar nodes. Small pleural effusions rare.

Noninfectious Causes *(cont'd)*

Features (may have some, none, or all)				
Causes	**History**	**Physical**	**Laboratory**	**Chest X-Ray**
Pulmonary hemorrhage	History of closed chest trauma or hemorrhagic disorder.	↑ WBCs, (left shift), ↑ pulse rate, respiratory rate. Signs of closed chest trauma.	Anemia plus findings secondary to underlying hemorrhagic disorder.	Localized or diffuse fluffy alveolar infiltrate(s). No cavitation, consolidation, or effusion.
Systemic lupus erythematosus (SLE)	Fatigue, chest pain. History of SLE.	Fever/ myalgias, alopecia, malar rash, "cytoid bodies" in retina, painless oral ulcers, synovitis, ± spleno-megaly, generalized adenopathy, Raynaud's pheno-menon.	↑ ANA, ↑ DS-DNA, ↓ $C_{3,4}$, polyclonal gammopathy on SPEP, ↑ ferritin. Pleural fluid with ↑ ANA, ↓ C_3.	Migratory ill-defined non-segmental infiltrates ± small pleural effusions. No consolidation or cavitation.
Aspiration pneumonia	Swallowing disorder 2° to CNS/GI disorder; impaired consciousness. Recent aspiration 2° to dental, upper GI, or pulmonary procedure.	Unremark-able.	↑ WBCs	Infiltrate usually involves superior segments of lower lobes (or posterior segments of upper lobes if aspiration occurred supine). Focal infiltrate initially, which may be followed in 7 days by cavitation/ lung abscess.

Unilateral Ill-Defined Infiltrates with Effusion

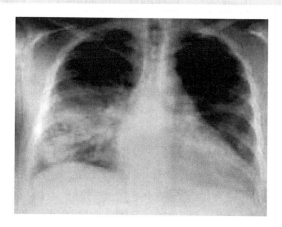

Infectious Causes

Features (may have some, none, or all)				
Causes	History	Physical	Laboratory	Chest X-Ray
TB (primary)	Recent TB contact.	Unilateral lower lobe dullness related to size of pleural effusion.	PPD – (anergic). Exudative pleural effusion (pleural fluid with ↑ lymphocytes, ↑ glucose, ± RBCs).	Lower lobe infiltrate with small/moderate pleural effusion. No cavitation or apical infiltrates. Hilar adenopathy asymmetrical when present.
Nocardia	Fevers, night sweats, fatigue, ↓ cell mediated immunity (e.g., HIV, organ transplant, PAP, immuno-suppressive therapy).	Unremark-able. No chest wall sinus tracts.	Normal/↑ WBCs, ↑ ESR. Sputum: with Gram positive beaded acid fast aerobic bacilli.	Dense large infiltrates. May cavitate and mimic TB, lymphoma, or squamous cell carcinoma. No calcification ± pleural effusion.

Infectious Causes (cont'd)

	Features (may have some, none, or all)			
Causes	**History**	**Physical**	**Laboratory**	**Chest X-Ray**
Legionella	Recent aerosolized water exposure. Most frequent in late summer/fall. Recent contact with Legionella containing water. Usually elderly. May have watery diarrhea, abdominal pain, mental confusion.	Fever/chills, relative brady-cardia. ↓ breath sounds if consoli-dation or pleural effusion.	↑ WBCs, ↑ AST/ALT, ↓ $PO_4^=$, ↓ Na^+, ↑ CPK, ↑ ESR, ↑ CRP, ↑ ferritin, microscopic hematuria. Mucoid/purulent sputum with few PMNs. Sputum culture for Legionella or sputum DFA (before therapy) is diagnostic. ↑ Legionella titers, L. pneumophila antigenuria (serotype 01 only) may not be positive early.	Rapidly progressive asymmetrical infiltrates clue to Legionella. Consolidation and pleural effusion not uncommon. Cavitation rare.

Noninfectious Causes

	Features (may have some, none, or all)			
Causes	**History**	**Physical**	**Laboratory**	**Chest X-Ray**
Lymphangitic metastases	History of breast, thyroid, pancreas, cervical, prostate, or lung carcinoma.	Findings related to underlying malignancy.	Normal/↑ WBCs, ↑ ESR.	Interstitial indi-stinct pulmonary infiltrates (may be reticulonodular) with lower lobe predominance Usually unilateral but may be bilateral. No consolidation or cavitation ± pleural effusions.

Noninfectious Causes (cont'd)

	Features (may have some, none, or all)			
Causes	History	Physical	Laboratory	Chest X-Ray
Pulmonary embolus/ infarct	Acute onset dyspnea/ pleuritic chest pain. History of lower extremity trauma, stasis or hypercoagulable disorder.	Fever <102°F, ↑ pulse/ respiratory rate.	↑ ESR, ↑ fibrin split products (FSP) and D-dimers ± ↑ total bilirubin. Bloody pleural effusion. ECG with RV strain/ p-pulmonale (large embolus). Positive V/Q scan and CT pulmonary angiogram.	Normal or show non-specific pleural-based infiltrates resembling atelectasis. Focal segmental/lobar hyperlucency (Westermark's sign) in some. "Hampton's hump" with infarct. Resolving infarcts ↓ in size but maintain shape/density ("melting ice cube").
Lymphoma	Fever, ↓ appetite with weight loss, night sweats, fatigue.	Adenopathy ± splenomegaly.	Normal WBCs, ↑ basophils, eosinophilia, ↓ lymphocytes, ↑ platelets, ↑ ESR, ↑ ACE, ↑ alkaline phosphatase, ↑$\alpha_{1,2}$ globulins on SPEP.	Unilateral or asymmetrical bilateral hilar adenopathy. Lung infiltrate contiguous with hilar adenopathy. No "clear channel" between mediastinum and hilar nodes. Small pleural effusions rare.

Noninfectious Causes (cont'd)

	Features (may have some, none, or all)			
Causes	**History**	**Physical**	**Laboratory**	**Chest X-Ray**
Bronchogenic carcinoma	Fever, ↓ appetite with weight loss, cough ± hemoptysis. Cough with copious clear/ mucoid sputum in large cell anaplastic carcinoma. Increased risk in smokers, aluminum/ uranium miners, cavitary lung disease (adeno-carcinoma), previous radiation therapy from lymphoma/ breast cancer.	Paraneoplastic syndromes especially with small (oat) cell/ squamous cell carcinoma ± hypertrophic pulmonary osteoarthro-pathy ± clubbing.	Normal/↑ WBCs, ↑ platelets, ↑ ESR, findings related to underlying malignancy.	Small/squamous cell carcinomas present as central lesions/ hilar masses. Adenocarcinoma/ large cell anaplastic carcinomas are usually peripheral initially. "Tumor tendrils" extending into surrounding lung tissue is characteristic. No calcifications (may be present on chest CT). Cavitation with squamous cell carcinoma. ± pleural effusions.
Alveolar cell carcinoma	Fever, ↓ appetite with weight loss, night sweats.	± dullness over lobe with large lower lobe lesions.	Positive cytology by BAL/lung biopsy.	Well/ill-defined circumscribed peripheral infiltrates ± air bronchograms. May be multifocal/ multilobar. Hilar adenopathy present. Stranding to the hilum ("pleural tail" sign). ± pleural effusion if lower lobe infiltrate. No cavitation.

Bilateral Infiltrates without Effusion

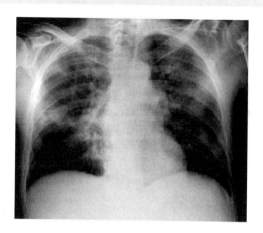

Infectious Causes

	Features (may have some, none, or all)			
Causes	**History**	**Physical**	**Laboratory**	**Chest X-Ray**
Influenza A (human, avian, swine)	Acute onset of fever, myalgias, headache, fatigue, sore throat, rhinorrhea, dry cough, ± pleuritic chest pain.	↑ respiratory rate, cyanosis in severe cases. Chest exam: no rales	↓ WBCs, relative lymphopenia, ↓ platelets, few/no atypical lymphocytes, ↑ AST/ALT, ↑ CPK ↑ A-a gradient. Respiratory secretions culture/PCR + for influenza A.	Early normal/ near normal appearance. (< 48 hours) Later (> 48 hours) diffuse patchy bilateral interstitial infiltrates. No focal/segmental infiltrates unless secondary bacterial pneumonia present. ± small pleural effusions.

Infectious Causes *(cont'd)*

	Features (may have some, none, or all)			
Causes	History	Physical	Laboratory	Chest X-Ray
ILIs HPIV-3 RSV EV 68 hMPV	Recent URI contact, dry cough, ± wheezing (RSV), myalgias	Mild lower respiratory tract infection in normal host. Moderate/severe pneumonia in organ transplants.	Normal WBCs, ↓ pO_2/↑ A-a gradient if severe. ± mildly ↑ cold agglutinins. Respiratory secretion culture/PCR. + for ILI virus	Near normal chest x-ray or bilateral symmetrical patchy infiltrates. Consolidation uncommon. No cavitation or effusion.
SARS	Acute onset of fever/chills, headache myalgias, dry cough ± N/V/D. Biphasic illness	↑ respiratory rate, SOB in severe cases.	N/↓ WBCs, relative lymphopenia, ↓ platelets, ↑ LDH, ↑ AST/ALT, ↓ pO_2, ↑ A-a gradient. SARS – CoV in respiratory secretions by PCR.	Bilateral symmetrical patchy infiltrates. Consolidation uncommon. No cavitation or effusion.
MERS	Acute onset of fever/chills, headache, myalgias, dry cough ± N/V/D Malaise; Hemoptysis	Early fulminant respiratory failure.	Normal WBC count with relative lymphopenia/lymphocytosis, ↑ LDH, ↑ AST/ALT, MERS-CoV in lower respiratory secretions by PCR	Unilateral/bilateral interstitial, nodule dense infiltrate. Consolidation common/± pleural effusions.
COVID-19	Acute onset of fever/chills, headache, myalgias, dry cough, diarrhea	↑ respiratory rate, SOB in severe cases.	Normal WBC count with relative lymphopenia/COVID-19 (SARS-CoV-2) PCR of respiratory specimens. ↑ AST/ALT	Bilateral symmetrical patchy infiltrates.
HSV-1	Fever. Often presents in normal hosts as "failure to wean" from ventilator.	Unremarkable.	↑ WBCs, ↓ pO_2, ↑ A-a gradient. Cytology + for HSV cytopathic effects (CPE).	Minimal bilateral diffuse infiltrates without cavitation or effusion.

Infectious Causes *(cont'd)*

	Features (may have some, none, or all)			
Causes	**History**	**Physical**	**Laboratory**	**Chest X-Ray**
VZV	VZV pneumonia occurs 2–3 days after rash. ↑ risk with pregnancy, smoking.	Healing vesicles, dry cough. Mild pneumonia in normal hosts.	↑ WBCs, ↑ platelets, ↑ basophils; ↓ pO_2/↑ A-a gradient ↑ VZV titers.	Minimal diffuse fluffy interstitial infiltrates. Diffuse small calcifications may develop years later.
CMV	Most common in hosts with ↓ cell mediated immunity (HIV, organ transplants, immunosuppressive therapy). Not uncommon in normal hosts. Increasing dyspnea over 1 week.	Fever ≤ 102°F.	↓ pO_2, ↑ A-a gradient, ↑ AST/ALT CMV "Cowdry Owl eye" inclusion bodies (CPEs) in respiratory secretions or transbronchial/open lung biopsy.	Most HIV patients with PCP also have underlying CMV. Organ transplants with CMV usually do not have underlying PCP.
P. (carinii) jiroveci (PCP)	Not in normal hosts. ↓ cell-mediated immunity (e.g., HIV, immunosuppressive therapy). Increasing dyspnea over 1 week. Chest pain with shortness of breath suggests pneumothorax.	↓ breath sounds bilaterally. Other findings depend on size/location of pneumothorax (if present).	Normal/↑ WBC (left shift), ↑ lymphocytes, ↓ pO_2, ↓ DL_{CO}, ↑ A-a gradient, ↑ LDH, ↑ β 1,3 glucan (GM −), PCP cysts in sputum/respiratory secretions.	Bilateral perihilar symmetrical patchy infiltrates ± pneumothorax. No calcification, cavitation, or pleural effusion.
TB (reactivation)	Fevers, night sweats, normal appetite with weight loss, cough ± hemoptysis.	± bilateral apical dullness.	Normal WBCs, ↑ platelets, ↑ ESR (≤ 70 mm/h). Positive PPD. AFB in sputum smear/culture.	Slowly progressive bilateral infiltrates. No pleural effusion. Usually in apical segment of lower lobes or apical/posterior segments of upper lobes. Calcification common.

Infectious Causes *(cont'd)*

	Features (may have some, none, or all)			
Causes	**History**	**Physical**	**Laboratory**	**Chest X-Ray**
Legionella	Recent aerosolized water exposure. Most frequent in late summer/fall. Recent contact with Legionella containing water. Usually elderly. May have watery diarrhea, abdominal pain, mental confusion.	Fever/chills, relative bradycardia. $\downarrow$ breath sounds if consolidation or pleural effusion.	$\uparrow$ WBC, $\uparrow$ AST/ALT, $\downarrow$ pO$_4^=$, $\downarrow$ Na$^+$, $\uparrow$ CPK, $\uparrow$ ESR, $\uparrow$ CRP, $\uparrow$ ferritin, microscopic hematuria. Mucoid/purulent sputum with few PMNs. Sputum culture for Legionella or sputum DFA (before therapy) is diagnostic. $\uparrow$ Legionella titers, L. pneumophila antigenuria (serotype 01 only) may not be positive early.	Rapidly progressive asymmetrical infiltrates clue to Legionella. Consolidation and pleural effusion not uncommon. Cavitation rare.
Psittacosis	Recent bird contact with psittacine birds. Severe headache.	Fever/chills, $\pm$ relative bradycardia, $\pm$ Horder's spots on face, $\pm$ epistaxis, $\pm$ spleno-megaly. Signs of con-solidation common.	$\downarrow$/normal WBCs, $\uparrow$ AST/ALT. Sputum with few PMNs. $\uparrow$ C. psittaci titers.	Dense infiltrate. Consolidation common. Pleural effusion/cavitation rare.

Infectious Causes (cont'd)

Features (may have some, none, or all)				
Causes	History	Physical	Laboratory	Chest X-Ray
Q fever	Recent contact with sheep or parturient cats.	Fever/chills, ± relative bradycardia, ± spleno-megaly, ± hepato-megaly.	↑/normal WBCs, ↑ AST/ALT. Sputum with no bacteria/few PMNs. Acute Q fever ↑ in phase II titers (caution: biohazard).	Dense consolidation. Cavitation/pleural effusion rare.
Nosocomial pneumonia (hema-togenous)	Fever/pulmonary symptoms ≥ 7 days in hospital. Increased risk with antecedent heart failure in previous 1–2 weeks.	Bilateral rales ± purulent respiratory secretions (tracheo-bronchitis).	↑ WBCs, (left shift). Blood cultures ± positive for bacteremic pulmonary pathogens. Respiratory secretions with WBCs ± cultures positive for P. aeruginosa, Acinetobacter, Enterobacter, Klebsiella, or Serratia (represents upper airway colonization, not lower respiratory tract/lung pathogens). Definitive diagnosis by lung biopsy/culture.	Bilateral symmetrical diffuse infiltrates. May be focal/segmental in aspiration nosocomial pneumonia. ↑ lung volumes (vs. ARDS). P. aeruginosa cavitation in 72 hours. Klebsiella cavitation in 3–5 days; No pleural effusion. CXR – plus purulent respiratory secretions diagnostic of tracheobron-chitis, not NP.

Noninfectious Causes

Features (may have some, none, or all)				
Causes	History	Physical	Laboratory	Chest X-Ray
Adult respiratory distress syndrome (ARDS)	Intubated on ventilator. May be on drugs → acute pancreatitis → ARDS. Sepsis uncommon as ARDS cause.	Fever < 102°F ± rales.	↑ WBCs, (left shift), normal ESR, ↓ pO$_2$, ↓ D$_L$CO, ↑ A-a gradient.	Bilateral fluffy infiltrates appearing ≥ 12 hours after profound hypoxemia. No cardiomegaly or pleural effusion. Reduced lung volumes (vs. nosocomial pneumonia or CHF). Bilateral consolidation ≥ 48 hours after appearance of infiltrates.
Good-pasture's syndrome	Often preceded by a URI. Most common in 20–30-year-old adults. Fever, weight loss, fatigue, cough, hemoptysis, hematuria.	Findings secondary to iron deficiency anemia.	↑ WBCs, anemia, ↑ creatinine, urine with RBCs/RBC casts. Positive pANCA. Linear IgG pattern on alveolar/ glomerular basement membrane.	Bilateral fine reticulonodular infiltrates predominantly in lower lobes. No cavitation.
Wegener's granulomatosis	Most common in middle aged adults. Cough, fever, fatigue.	Findings of chronic sinusitis, bloody nasal discharge.	↑ WBCs, anemia, ↑ platelets, ↑ ESR, ↑ RF, negative ANA, proteinuria, hematuria. Positive cANCA.	Bilateral asymmetrical nodular infiltrates of varying size with irregular margins. Cavitation common. Inner lining of cavities irregular. Air-fluid levels rare. ± pleural effusions. No calcifications.
Pulmonary hemorrhage	History of closed chest trauma or hemorrhagic disorder.	↑ pulse rate, ↑ respiratory rate. Signs of closed chest trauma.	↑ WBCs, (left shift). Anemia plus findings secondary to underlying hemorrhagic disorder.	Localized or diffuse fluffy alveolar infiltrates. No cavitation, consolidation, or effusion.

Noninfectious Causes *(cont'd)*

	Features (may have some, none, or all)			
Causes	History	Physical	Laboratory	Chest X-Ray
Chronic renal failure	Chronic renal failure on dialysis.	Findings related to uremia.	Normal/↑ WBCs, (left shift) plus findings related to renal failure.	Bilateral symmetrical fluffy perihilar infiltrates (butterfly pattern) ± pleural effusions. No cardiomegaly (unlike CHF), but large pericardial effusion can mimic cardiomegaly.
Lung contusion	Recent closed chest trauma, chest pain.	Chest wall contusion over infiltrate.	↑ WBCs, (left shift).	Patchy ill-defined infiltrate(s) ± rib fractures/pneumothorax in area of infiltrate. Infiltrate clears within 1 week.
Fat emboli	1–2 days post-long bone fracture/trauma.	↑ respiratory rate.	Urinalysis with "Maltese crosses."	Bilateral predominantly peripheral lower lobe infiltrates. Usually clears within 1 week.
Loeffler's syndrome	Drug or parasitic exposure.	Unremarkable.	Normal WBCs, eosinophilia, ↑ ESR.	Characteristic "reversed bat-wing" pattern (i.e., peripheral infiltrates). Upper lobe predominance.
Sarcoidosis (Stage III)	Dyspena, fatigue, nasal stuffiness.	Waxy/yellowish papules on face/upper trunk. Funduscopic exam with "candle wax drippings."	↑ ESR, normal LFTs, ↑ creatinine (if renal involvement), ↑ ACE, hypercalciuria, hypercalcemia, polyclonal gammopathy on SPEP. Anergic.	Bilateral nodular infiltrates of variable size without hilar adenopathy. Cavitation/ pleural effusion rare.

Noninfectious Causes *(cont'd)*

	Features (may have some, none, or all)			
Causes	**History**	**Physical**	**Laboratory**	**Chest X-Ray**
Alveolar cell carcinoma	Fever, ↓ appetite with weight loss, night sweats.	± dullness over lobe with large lower lobe lesions.	Positive cytology by BAL/lung biopsy.	Well/ill-defined circumscribed peripheral infiltrates ± air bronchograms. May be multifocal/multilobar. Hilar adenopathy present. Stranding to the hilum ("pleural tail" sign). ± pleural effusion if lower lobe infiltrate. No cavitation.
Metastatic carcinoma	History of breast, thyroid, renal cell, colon, pancreatic cancer or osteogenic sarcoma.	Findings related to underlying malignancy and, when present, to bone, hepatic, CNS metastases.	Secondary to effects of primary neoplasm, metastases, paraneoplastic syndrome.	Nodular lesions that vary in size. Metastatic lesions are usually well circumscribed with lower lobe predominance. Usually no bronchial obstruction (obstruction suggests colon, renal, or melanoma metastases). Usually no cavitation (except for squamous cell metastases). Calcification usually suggests osteosarcoma (rarely adeno-carcinoma). Pleural effusion rare (except for breast cancer).

Noninfectious Causes *(cont'd)*

	Features (may have some, none, or all)			
Causes	History	Physical	Laboratory	Chest X-Ray
Lymphoma	Fever, ↓ appetite with weight loss, night sweats, fatigue.	Adenopathy ± spleno-megaly.	Normal WBCs, ↑ basophils, eosinophilia, ↓ lymphocytes, ↑ platelets, ↑ ESR, ↑ ACE, ↑ alkaline phosphatase, ↑$\alpha_{1,2}$ globulins on SPEP.	Unilateral or asymmetrical bilateral hilar adenopathy. Lung infiltrate contiguous with hilar adenopathy. No "clear channel" between mediastinum and hilar nodes. Small pleural effusions rare.
Leukostasis (AML)	Untreated acute myelogenous leukemia (AML).	Fever, sternal tenderness, petechiae, ecchymosis.	↑ WBCs, (≥ 100 K/mm³) with blasts in peripheral smear/bone marrow, ↓ platelets.	Diffuse symmetrical fluffy infiltrates without pleural effusion.
Drug induced	Exposure to chemo-therapeutic agents (e.g., BCNU, busulfan, methotrexate, cyclophos-phamide, bleomycin) or other drugs (e.g., nitro-furantoin, sulfasalazine, amiodarone, opiates, cocaine).	Unremark-able.	Normal/ ↑ WBCs, ± eosinophilia, normal/ ↑ ESR, ↑ AST/ALT, Eosinophils in pleural effusion.	Bilateral coarse symmetrical patchy infiltrates/fibrosis ± pleural effusions. Hilar adenopathy only with drug-induced pseudolymphoma (secondary to dilantin). No cavitation.

Noninfectious Causes *(cont'd)*

Features (may have some, none, or all)				
Causes	**History**	**Physical**	**Laboratory**	**Chest X-Ray**
Idiopathic pulmonary hemosiderosis (IPH)	Hemoptysis ± cough.	Findings of iron deficiency anemia.	Iron deficiency anemia. Hemosiderin in alveolar macrophages and urine.	Diffuse, bilateral ill-defined opacities or multiple "stellate" shaped infiltrates that clear between attacks. Recent hemorrhage may be superimposed on a fine reticular pattern that occurs after repeated bleeds.
Bronchiolitis obliterans with organizing pneumonia (BOOP)	Dyspnea, cough.	Afebrile (if no other causes of fever). Chest exam: unremarkable.	↑ WBCs, (left shift), ↑ LDH, ↓ pO_2, ↑ A-a gradient.	Classically bilateral patchy peripheral infiltrates. Often lower lobe predominance. No cavitation or pleural effusion.
Pulmonary alveolar proteinosis (PAP)	Asymptomatic if not infected with Nocardia.	Chest exam: unremarkable.	Normal/↑ WBCs, ↑ LDH.	Bilateral granular or peripheral infiltrates in butterfly pattern. No hilar adenopathy, cardiomegaly, or pleural effusion.

Bilateral Infiltrates
with Effusion

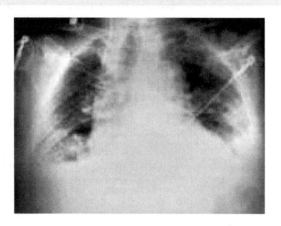

Infectious Causes

	Features (may have some, none, or all)			
Causes	History	Physical	Laboratory	Chest X-Ray
Legionella	Most frequent in late summer/fall. Recent contact with Legionella containing water. Usually elderly. May have watery diarrhea, abdominal pain, mental confusion.	Fever/chills, relative bradycardia. ↓ breath sounds if consolidation or pleural effusion.	↑ WBCs, ↑ AST/ALT, ↓ $PO_4^=$, ↓ Na^+, ↑ CPK, ↑ ESR, ↑ CRP, ↑ ferritin levels, microscopic hematuria. Mucoid/ purulent sputum with few PMNs. Sputum culture for Legionella or sputum DFA (before therapy) is diagnostic. ↑ Legionella titers, L. pneumophila antigenuria (serotype 01 only) may not be positive early.	Rapidly progressive asymmetrical infiltrates clue to Legionella. Consolidation and pleural effusion not uncommon. Cavitation rare.

Infectious Causes *(cont'd)*

	Features (may have some, none, or all)			
Causes	**History**	**Physical**	**Laboratory**	**Chest X-Ray**
Hanta-virus (HPS)	Subacute onset, shortness of breath, sub-sternal chest discomfort. Improvement followed by rapid deterioration.	↑ respiratory rate, cyanosis in severe cases.	↓ WBCs, ↓ platelets ↓ pO_2, ↑ A-a gradient. ↑ hantavirus titers.	Large pleural effusions.
MERS	Recent contact with MERS case or camel contact. Acute onset of fever/chills, headache, myalgias, dry cough ± N/V/D, Malaise, ±/ hemoptysis	Early fulminant respiratory failure.	Normal WBCs, count, relative lymphopenia, ↑ LDH, ↑ LFTs, MERS-CoV in lower respiratory secretions by PCR.	Unilateral (early) or bilateral (late) interstitial, nodular dense infiltrates. Recent contact with MERS case or camel contact. Consolidation common ± pleural effusions.
Measles	Recent airborne exposure.	Measles rash, Koplik's spots (early).	Normal/↑ WBCs, (left shift), normal/↓ platelets, ↑ LFTs, ↑ CPK, normal/↓ pO_2. If ↓ pO_2, then ↑ A-a gradient. ↑ IgM measles titer. Warthin-Finkeldey giant cells (measles CPEs) in nasal secretions.	Bilateral diffuse fine reticulonodular infiltrates ± hilar adenopathy. Lower lobe predominance. Consolidation/ pleural effusion uncommon.
Strongyl-oides	Strongyloides exposure. 1/3 asymptomatic; 2/3 with fever, dyspnea, cough. Hyperinfection syndrome with abdominal pain, diarrhea ± GI bleed.	With hyper-infection syndrome, fever, GNB, abdominal tenderness ± rebound, ± meningitis. ↓ BP	↑ WBCs, (left shift), eosinophilia, ± anemia. Blood/CSF cultures positive for enteric Gram negative bacilli. Rhabditiform larvae in sputum/stool.	Diffuse hilar patchy infiltrates without consolidation or cavitation. Eosinophilic pleural effusion common.

Noninfectious Causes

	Features (may have some, none, or all)			
Causes	**History**	**Physical**	**Laboratory**	**Chest X-Ray**
Congestive heart failure (CHF)	Coronary heart disease, valvular heart disease, cardiomyopathy.	No/low grade fevers, ↑ pulse/ respiratory rate, positive jugular venous distension and hepato-jugular reflex, cardiomegaly, S_3, ascites, hepato-megaly, pedal edema.	↑ WBCs, (left shift), normal platelets, mildly ↑ AST/ ALT.	Cardiomegaly, pleural effusion (R > [R + L] > L). Kerley B lines with vascular redistribution to upper lobes. Typically bilateral rather than unilateral.
Chronic renal failure	Chronic renal failure on dialysis.	Findings related to uremia.	Normal/↑ WBCs, (left shift) plus findings related to renal failure.	Bilateral symmetrical fluffy perihilar infiltrates (butterfly pattern) ± pleural effusions. No cardiomegaly (unlike CHF), but large pericardial effusion can mimic cardiomegaly.
SLE	Fatigue, chest pain. History of SLE.	Fever/myal-gias, alopecia, malar rash, "cytoid bodies" in retina, painless oral ulcers, synovitis, plenomegaly, generalized adenopathy, Raynaud's pheno-menon.	↑ ANA, ↑ DS-DNA, ↓ $C_{3,4}$, polyclonal gammopathy on SPEP, ↑ ferritin. Pleural fluid with ↑ ANA, ↓ C_3.	Migratory ill-defined non-segmental infiltrates. No signs of consolidation or cavitation. ± small pleural effusions.

Noninfectious Causes *(cont'd)*

	Features (may have some, none, or all)			
Causes	**History**	**Physical**	**Laboratory**	**Chest X-Ray**
Good-pasture's Syndrome	Often preceded by a URI. Most common in 20–30 year old adults. Fever, weight loss, fatigue, cough, hemoptysis, hematuria.	Findings secondary to iron deficiency anemia.	↑ WBCs, anemia, ↑ creatinine, urine with RBCs/RBC casts. Positive pANCA. Linear IgG pattern on alveolar/ glomerular basement membrane.	Bilateral fine reticulonodular infiltrates predominantly in lower lobes. No cavitation.
Wegener's granulo-matosis	Most common in middle-aged adults. Cough, fever, fatigue.	Findings of chronic sinusitis, bloody nasal discharge.	↑ WBCs, anemia, ↑ platelets, ↑ ESR, ↑ RF, negative ANA, proteinuria, hematuria. Positive cANCA.	Bilateral asym-metrical nodular infiltrates of varying size with irregular margins. Cavitation common. Inner lining of cavities irregular. Air-fluid levels rare. ± pleural effusions. No calcifications.
Sarcoidosis (Stage III)	Dyspnea, fatigue, nasal stuffiness.	Waxy/ yellowish papules on face/ upper trunk. Funduscopic exam with "candle wax drippings."	↑ ESR, normal LFTs, ↑ creatinine (if renal involvement), ↑ ACE, hyper-calciuria, hyper-calcemia, polyclonal gammopathy on SPEP. Anergic.	Bilateral nodular infiltrates of variable size without hilar adenopathy. Cavitation/pleural effusion rare.

Noninfectious Causes *(cont'd)*

	Features (may have some, none, or all)			
Causes	**History**	**Physical**	**Laboratory**	**Chest X-Ray**
Lymphoma	Fever, ↓ appetite with weight loss, night sweats, fatigue.	Adenopathy ± spleno-megaly.	Normal WBC, ↑ basophils, eosinophilia, ↓ lymphocytes, ↑ platelets, ↑ ESR, ↑ alkaline phosphatase, ↑$\alpha_{1,2}$ globulins on SPEP.	Unilateral or asymmetrical bilateral hilar adenopathy. Lung infiltrate contiguous with hilar adenopathy. No "clear channel" between mediastinum and hilar nodes. Small pleural effusions rare.
Lymphangitic metastases	History of breast, thyroid, pancreas, cervical, prostate, or lung carcinoma.	Findings related to underlying malignancy.	Normal/ ↑ WBCs, ↑ ESR.	Interstitial indistinct pulmonary infiltrates (may be reticulonodular) with lower lobe predominance Usually unilateral but may be bilateral. No consolidation or cavitation ± pleural effusions.
Drug induced	Exposure to chemotherapeutic agents (e.g., BCNU, busulfan, methotrexate, cyclophos-phamide, bleomycin) or other drugs (e.g., nitrofurantoin, sulfasalazine, amiodarone, opiates, cocaine).	Unremark-able.	Normal WBCs, ± eosino-philia, normal/ ↑ ESR, ↑ AST/ALT. Eosinophils in pleural effusion.	Bilateral coarse symmetrical patchy infiltrates/ fibrosis ± pleural effusions. Hilar adenopathy only with drug-induced pseudolymphoma (secondary to dilantin). No cavitation.

Cavitary Infiltrates
(Thick-Walled)

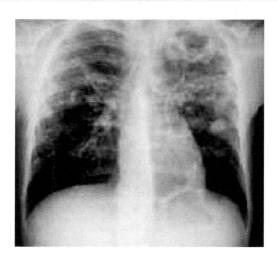

Infectious Causes Based on Speed of Cavitation

Speed of Cavitation	Causes
Very rapid cavitation (3 days)	S. aureus, P. aeruginosa
Rapid cavitation (5–7 days)	K. pneumoniae
Slow cavitation (> 7 days)	Pyogenic lung abscess, septic pulmonary emboli
Chronic cavitation	TB (reactivation), histoplasmosis (reactivation), sporotrichosis, melioidosis, nocardia, actinomycosis, Rhodococcus equi, amebic abscess, alveolar echinococcosis (hydatid cysts)

Infectious Causes

	Features (may have some, none, or all)			
Causes	**History**	**Physical**	**Laboratory**	**Chest X-Ray**
S. aureus	Fever, cough, dyspnea. Recent/ concurrent influenza pneumonia.	↓ breath sounds ± cyanosis.	↑ WBCs, (left shift), ↓ pO_2, ↑ A-a gradient. Purulent sputum positive for S. aureus. ↑ IgM influenza titers or + influenza PCR. Necrotizing vasoinvasive on lung biopsy.	Multiple thick-walled cavitary lesions super-imposed on normal looking lung fields or early minimal infiltrates of influenza A.
P. aeruginosa	Nosocomial pneumonia usually on ventilator. Nearly always rapidly fatal.	Unremark-able.	↑ WBCs, (left shift). Respiratory secretions culture ± for P. aeruginosa. Blood cultures positive for P. aeruginosa (hematogenous nosocomial pneumonia). Necrotizing vasoinvasive on lung biopsy.	Bilateral diffuse infiltrates with rapid cavitation (≤ 72 hours).
Klebsiella pneumoniae	Nosocomial pneumonia or history of alcoholism in patient with community-acquired pneumonia.	Fever/chills, signs of alcoholic cirrhosis, signs of consolidation over involved lobe.	↑ WBCs, ↓ platelets, ↑ AST/ALT (2° to alcoholism). "Red currant jelly" sputum with PMNs and plump Gram negative encapsulated bacilli.	"Bulging fissure" sign secondary to expanded lobar volume. Empyema rather than pleural effusion. Usually cavitation in 5–7 days (thick-walled).
Pyogenic lung abscess	Recent aspiration. weight loss. Swallowing disorder secondary to CNS/GI disorder.	Fevers/chills. Foul (putrid lung abscess) breath.	↑ WBCs, ↑ ESR. Sputum with oropharyngeal anaerobic flora in putrid lung abscess.	Thick walled cavity in portion of lung dependent during aspiration (usually basilar segment of lower lobes if aspiration occurred supine). Cavitation occurs > 7 days.

Infectious Causes *(cont'd)*

	Features (may have some, none, or all)			
Causes	History	Physical	Laboratory	Chest X-Ray
Septic pulmonary emboli	Usually IV drug abuser with fever/chills. Tricuspid regurgitation murmur (2° to TV ABE) or recent OB/GYN surgical procedure.	Fever > 102°F. Tricuspid valve regurgitant murmur with cannon A waves in neck.	Blood cultures positive for acute bacterial endocarditis pathogens.	Multiple peripheral nodules of varying size. Lower lobe predominance. Cavitation > 7 days characteristic of septic pulmonary emboli.
TB (reactivation)	Fevers, night sweats, normal appetite with weight loss, cough ± hemoptysis.	± bilateral apical dullness.	Normal WBCs, ↑ platelets, ↑ ESR (≤ 70 mm/h). Positive PPD. AFB in sputum smear/culture.	Slowly progressive bilateral infiltrates. No pleural effusion. Usually in apical segment of lower lobes or apical/posterior segments of upper lobes. Calcifications common.
Histoplasmosis (reactivation)	Fever, night sweats, cough, weight loss, histoplasmosis exposure (river valleys of Central/ Eastern United States).	± E. nodosum; otherwise Unremarkable.	Normal WBCs, eosinophilia, anemia, ↑ platelets, PPD negative. Immunodiffusion test with positive H precipitin band (diagnostic of active/chronic histoplasmosis). Histoplasma urinary antigen +.	Unilateral/bilateral multiple patchy infiltrates with upper lobe predilection. Bilateral hilar adenopathy uncommon. Calcifications common. No pleural effusion. Chest x-ray resembles reactivation TB.

Infectious Causes *(cont'd)*

	Features (may have some, none, or all)			
Causes	**History**	**Physical**	**Laboratory**	**Chest X-Ray**
Sporotri-chosis	Fever, cough, weight loss. ± hemoptysis. Antecedent lymphocuta-neous or skeletal sporotrichosis, rare.	Only if secondary to residual of lympho-cutaneous sporotri-chosis, ± E. nodosum.	Normal WBCs, No eosinophilia.	Unilateral > bilateral upper lobe nodular densities. Thick or thin-walled cavities. No hilar adenopathy. No pleural effusion.
Melioidosis	Past travel to Asia (usually > 10 years). Fever, cough, hemoptysis. ↑ risk of reactivation/ dissemination with DM, alcoholics, renal failure, leukemias/lym-phomas, steroids, immunosuppres-sives. May occur in normal hosts.	Unremark-able.	↑ WBCs, (left shift), anemia, ↑ ESR, PPD negative. GNBs with bipolar "safety pin" staining in sputum. Sputum/ blood cultures positive for B. (Pseudomonas) pseudomallei.	Resembles reactivation TB, but infiltrates nodular/diffuse (septicemic) or cavitary (chronic) predominantly in middle/lower lung fields. ± air fluid level. No pleural effusion.
Nocardia	Fevers, night sweats, fatigue, ↓ cell mediated immunity (e.g., HIV, organ transplants, PAP, immuno-suppressive therapy).	Unremark-able. No chest wall sinus tracts.	Normal/↑ WBCs, ↑ ESR. Sputum: Gram positive beaded acid fast aerobic bacilli.	Dense large infiltrates. May cavitate and mimic TB, lymphoma, or squamous cell carcinoma. No calcification ± pleural effusion.
Actino-mycosis	Recent dental work.	± chest wall sinus tracts.	Normal/↑ WBCs, ↑ ESR. Sputum with Gram positive filamentous anaerobic bacilli.	Dense infiltrates extending to chest wall. No hilar adenopathy. Cavitation ± pleu-ral effusion rare.

Infectious Causes *(cont'd)*

	Features (may have some, none, or all)			
Causes	History	Physical	Laboratory	Chest X-Ray
Rhodococcus equi	Insidious onset of fever, dyspnea, chest pain, ± hemoptysis. Immuno-suppressed patients with ↓ cell-mediated immunity or exposure to cattle, horses, pigs.	Unremark-able.	Normal/↑ WBCs, Sputum/pleural fluid with Gram positive pleomorphic weakly acid fast bacilli. Sputum, pleural fluid, blood cultures positive for R. equi.	Segmental infiltrate with upper lobe predominance ± cavitation. Air-fluid levels and pleural effusion common.
Amebic cysts	Hepatic amebic abscess. Remote history of usually mild amebic dysentery.	± hepato-megaly.	Normal WBCs, and ESR. ↑ E. histolytica HI titers.	Well-circum-scribed cavitary lesions adjacent to right diaphragm. ± calcifications. Sympathetic pleural effusion above hepatic amebic abscess.
Alveolar echinoco-ccosis (hydatid cysts)	Symptoms related to cyst size/location: 1/3 asymptomatic; 2/3 with fever, malaise, chest pain ± hemoptysis. RUQ abdominal pain may occur.	Hepato-megaly common.	Normal/↑ WBCs, no eosinophilia, ↑ alkaline phosphate/GGT with hepatic cysts. Abdominal ultrasound/CT with calcified hepatic irregularly shaped cysts ("Swiss cheese" calcification characteristic). ↑ E. multilocularis IHA titers.	RLL usual location (hepatic cysts penetrate diaphragm into RLL). Nodules are 70% solitary, 30% multiple. Pleural effusion rare. Endocyst membrane on surface of cyst fluid ("water lilly" sign) is characteristic.

Noninfectious Causes

	Features (may have some, none, or all)			
Causes	History	Physical	Laboratory	Chest X-Ray
Wegener's granulom-atosis	Most common in middle-aged adults. Cough, fever, fatigue.	Findings of chronic sinusitis, bloody nasal discharge.	↑ WBC, anemia, ↑ platelets, ↑ ESR, ↑ RF, negative ANA, proteinuria, hematuria. Positive cANCA.	Bilateral asymmetrical nodular infiltrates of varying size with irregular margins. Cavitation common. Inner lining of cavities irregular. Air-fluid levels rare. ± pleural effusions. No calcifications.
Squamous cell carcinoma	Long-term smoking history.	Clubbing, hypertrophic pulmonary osteoarthro-pathy ± findings 2° to superior vena caval syndrome and CNS/bone metastases.	↑ Ca^{++} (without bone metastases).	Unilateral perihilar mass lesion. Cavitation common. No pleural effusion.
Lymphoma	Fever, ↓ appetite with weight loss, night sweats, fatigue.	Adenopathy ± splenomegaly.	Normal WBC, ↑ basophils, eosinophilia, ↓ lymphocytes, ↑ platelets, ↑ ESR, ↑ ACE, ↑ alkaline phosphatase, ↑$\alpha_{1,2}$ globulins on SPEP.	Unilateral or asymmetrical bilateral hilar adenopathy. Lung infiltrate contiguous with hilar adenopathy. No "clear channel" between mediastinum and hilar nodes. Small pleural effusions rare.

Noninfectious Causes (cont'd)

Features (may have some, none, or all)				
Causes	**History**	**Physical**	**Laboratory**	**Chest X-Ray**
Metastatic carcinoma	History of breast, thyroid, renal cell, colon, pancreatic cancer or osteogenic sarcoma.	Findings related to underlying malignancy and, when present, to bone, hepatic, CNS metastases.	Secondary to effects of primary neoplasm, metastases, paraneoplastic syndrome.	Nodular lesions that vary in size. Metastatic lesions are usually well-circumscribed with lower lobe pre-dominance. Usually no bronchial obstruction (obstruction suggests colon, renal, or melanoma metastases). Usually no cavitation (except for squamous cell metastases). Calcification usually suggests osteosarcoma (rarely adenocarcinoma). Pleural effusion rare (except for breast cancer).
Rheumatoid nodules	Usually in severe rheumatoid arthritis (RA); ± history of silicosis.	Findings secondary to RA. Rheumatoid nodules on extensor surfaces of arms.	Normal WBCs, ↑ ESR, ↑ ANA, ↑ RF (high titer). Pleural fluid with ↓ glucose.	Lung nodules are round and well-circumscribed, predominantly in lower lobes and typically superimposed on interstitial lung disease "rheumatoid lung". Cavitation is common. ± pulmonary fibrosis, pleural effusion. Silicosis + RA nodules = Caplan's syndrome.

Cavitary Infiltrates
(Thin-Walled)

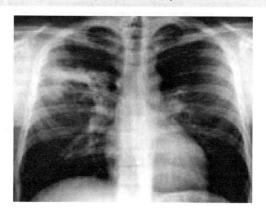

Infectious Causes

	Features (may have some, none, or all)			
Causes	**History**	**Physical**	**Laboratory**	**Chest X-Ray**
Atypical TB (MAI)	Often occurs in setting of previous lung disease.	Unremarkable.	Normal WBCs, ↑ ESR. Weakly positive PPD. Positive sputum AFB/ culture for MAI.	Multiple cavitary lesions ± calci-fications usually involving both lungs. Resembles reactivation TB except that cavities are thln-walled. No pleural effusion.
Coccidio-mycosis (reactivation)	Previous exposure in endemic coccidiomycosis areas (e.g., Southwest USA). Asymptomatic.	± E. nodosum.	Normal WBCs, eosinophilia acutely, but not in chronic phase, and eosinophils in pleural fluid. CF IgG titer ≥ 1:32 indicates active disease.	Thick/thin-walled cavities (< 3 cm) usually in anterior segments of lower lobes ± calci-fications/bilateral hilar adenopathy. Air-fluid levels rare unless secondarily infected. Pleural effusion rare.

Infectious Causes *(cont'd)*

	Features (may have some, none, or all)			
Causes	History	Physical	Laboratory	Chest X-Ray
Paragonimiasis	Ingestion of fresh-water crabs/ crayfish. Acute symptoms (< 6 months): fevers, abdominal pain, diarrhea followed by episodes of pleuritic chest pain. Chronic symptoms (> 6 months): fevers, night sweats, cough ± hemoptysis. Asymptomatic in some.	Wheezing, ± urticaria (acutely).	↑ WBCs, eosinophilia. Eosinophils in pleural fluid. Sputum with Charot-Leyden crystals. Sputum/ feces with operculated P. westermani eggs.	Cavitary patchy or well-defined infiltrates predominantly in mid-lung fields. hydropneumo-thorax common. Calcifications and pleural effusion common.
Sporotrichosis	Fever, cough, weight loss. ± hemoptysis. Antecedent lymphocuta-neous or skeletal sporotrichosis, rare.	Only if secondary to residual of lympho-cutaneous sporotrichosis, ± E. nodosum.	Normal WBCs, No eosino-philia.	Unilateral > bilateral upper lobe nodular densities. Thick or thin-walled cavities. No hilar adenopathy. No pleural effusion.
Pneumato-celes	Common in children but rare in adults with S. aureus pneumonia. Fever, cough, dyspnea. ± antecedent influenza.	Unremarkable unless pneumatocele ruptures, then signs of pneumo-thorax.	↑ WBCs, (left shift).	Multiple thin-walled cavities in areas of S. aureus pneumonia.

Noninfectious Causes

Features (may have some, none, or all)				
Causes	History	Physical	Laboratory	Chest X-Ray
Emphysema (blebs/cyst)	Long history of smoking. Rupture of apical bleb common in males > 30 years. Pneumonia rare in severe emphysema (vs. chronic bronchitis) but may occur early in unaffected areas of lung.	Asthenic "pink puffers." Barrel chest. Diaphragmatic excursions < 2 cm.	Normal WBCs, $\downarrow pO_2$.	$\downarrow$ lung markings ("vanishing lung") $\pm$ blebs. Hyperlucent lungs with upper lobe predominance. Flattened diaphragms, vertically elongated cardiac silhouette, $\uparrow$ retrocardiac and retrosternal airspaces. No infiltrates or pleural effusions. (In upper lobe emphysema, no vascular redistribution to upper lobes with CHF).
Bronchogenic cyst	Congenital anomaly. Usually asymptomatic. Cough if symptomatic.	Unremarkable unless secondarily infected, then signs 2° to mediastinal abscess.	Normal WBCs	Circumscribed cystic lesion originates in lung but appears high in mediastinum. If filled with fluid, appears as solitary tumor. If near the trachea, may rupture into bronchus/trachea and cyst may contain air. If communicates openly with bronchus, appears as thin-walled cavitary nodule. If infected, presents as mediastinal abscess.
Cystic bronchiectasis	Recurrent pulmonary infections with purulent sputum $\pm$ hemoptysis.	Unremarkable unless dextrocardia with sinusitis (Kartagener's syndrome).	$\uparrow$ WBCs	Bilateral large cystic lucencies at lung bases. Upper lobes relatively spared (unless secondary chronic aspiration). Thickened bronchial markings at bases. Bronchiectasis of cystic fibrosis predominantly involves upper lobes.

Noninfectious Causes (cont'd)

	Features (may have some, none, or all)			
Causes	History	Physical	Laboratory	Chest X-Ray
Sequestered lung	Usually asymptomatic. Productive cough ± hemoptysis if communicates with bronchus or if infected.	Unremark-able.	Normal WBCs	Solid nodule unless communicates with bronchus, then thin-walled cavity ± air fluid levels. Usually posterior based segment of lower lobes (LLL > RLL). If > 3 cm, presents as mass lesion,
Histiocytosis X (eosino-philic granuloma, Langerhan's cell histio-cytosis)	Patients usually 20–40 years. Usually asympto-matic. Fever, cough, dys-pnea in some. Diabetes insipidus rare.	Hepato-spleno-megaly, skin lesions, hemoptysis (rare).	Normal WBCs, eosinophilia.	Pneumothorax superimposed on diffuse pulmonary fibrosis. Cystic bone lesions. Usually mid/upper lung fields with nodules/thin-walled cysts or infiltrates. No hilar adenopathy or pleural effusion.

REFERENCES

Burgener FA, Kormano M. Differential Diagnosis in Conventional Radiology (2nd Ed), Stuttgart, Thieme Verlag, 1991.

Chapman S, Nakielny R. Aids to Radiological Differential Diagnosis (2nd Ed), London, Bailliere Tindall, 1990.

Conn RB, Borer WZ, Snyder JW. Current Diagnosis 9. Philadelphia, W. B. Saunders Company, 1997.

Crapo JD, Glassroth J, Karlinsky JB, King TE. Baum's Textbook of Pulmonary Diseases (7th Ed), Philadelphia, Lippincott Williams & Wilkins, 2004.

Cunha BA. Pneumonia Essentials (3rd Ed), Jones & Bartlett, Sudbury MA, 2010.

Eisenberg RL. Clinical Imaging. An Atlas of Differential Diagnosis (2nd Ed), Gaithersburg, Aspen Publishers, Inc., 1992.

Gorbach SL, Bartlett JG, Blacklow NR. Infectious Diseases (3rd Ed), Philadelphia, Lippincott Williams & Wilkins, 2004.

Karetzky M, Cunha BA, Brandstetter RD. The Pneumonias. New York, Springer-Verlag, 1993.

Levison ME. The Pneumonias: Clinical Approaches to Infectious Diseases of the Lower Respiratory Tract. Boston, John Wright, PSG Inc., 1984.

Lillington GA, Jamplis RW. A Diagnostic Approach to Chest Diseases (2nd Ed), Baltimore, Williams & Wilkins Company, 1977.

Mandell GL, Bennet JE, Blaser MJ (eds). Mandell, Douglas, and Bennett's Principles and Practice of Infectious Diseases (8th Ed), Philadelphia, Elsevier, 2015.

Murray JF, Nadel JA. Textbook of Respiratory Medicine (3rd Ed), Philadelphia, W.B. Saunders Company, 2000.

Raoof S, Feigin D, Sung A, et al. Interpretation of Plain Chest Roentgenogram. Chest 141:545–558, 2012.

Reed JC. Chest Radiology. Plain Film Patterns and Differential Diagnoses. (6th Ed). Philadelphia, Elsevier, 2011.

Teplick JE, Haskin ME. Roentgenologic Diagnosis (3rd Ed), Philadelphia, W. B. Saunders Company, 1976.

Wright FW. Radiology of the Chest and Related Conditions. London, Taylor & Francis, 2002.

Chapter 9

Infectious Disease Differential Diagnosis

Cheston B. Cunha, MD,

Burke A. Cunha, MD

Table 9.1 Fever Curves

Finding	Causes
Morning (am) temperature spikes	Infectious: miliary TB, miliary BCG, typhoid fever, Whipple's disease
	Noninfectious: PAN
Relative tachycardia	Infectious: gas gangrene, myocarditis (Coxsackie, RMSF, typhus, diptheria, trichinosis, VLM, influenza)
	Noninfectious: hyperthyroidism, hypoxia, cardiac arrhythmias, anxiety, pulmonary emboli
Relative bradycardia	Infectious: typhoid fever, typhus, leptospirosis, legionnaire's disease, Q fever, psittacosis, RMSF, malaria (after 1 week), babesiosis, ehrlichiosis/anaplasmosis, yellow fever, dengue fever, arboviral hemorrhagic fevers, COVID-19
	Noninfectious: drug fever, CNS lesions, β-blockers, verapamil, diltiazem, lymphoma, factitious fever
Single fever spikes	Infectious: transient bacteremia
	Noninfectious: blood/blood product transfusions
Double quotidian fevers	Infectious: kala-azar, right sided GC ABE, miliary TB, mixed malarial infections
	Noninfectious: adult Still's disease, antipyretics
Camelback fever pattern	Infectious: Colorado tick fever, dengue fever, leptospirosis, brucellosis, LCM, yellow fever, poliomyelitis, smallpox, rat bite fever (Spirillum minus), chikungunya fever, rift valley fever, african hemorrhagic fevers (Marburg, Ebola, Lassa, etc), echovirus (ECHO 9), Coxsackie B_5, ehrlichiosis/anaplasmosis
	Noninfectious: antipyretics

Fever with chills/rigors
Classically, chills/rigors are associated with some infections, diseases, e.g., influenza, bacteremia, malaria, but rare/mild with typhoid fever. Prominent/sustained rigors argues against the diagnosis of typhoid fever.

Fever with night sweats
Night sweats may be present with some chronic infectious diseases, e.g., abscesses, TB, SBE and various malignancies, e.g., lymphomas, leukemias. Other causes include certain medications, e.g., monoclonal antibody therapy (rituximab), HIV drugs. Night sweats are not a feature of rheumatic/inflammatory disorders.

Table 9.2 General Appearance Abnormalities

Finding	Causes
Hypotension/ shock	<u>Infectious</u>: anthrax, plague, typhus, **GI sources**: colon (perforation, colitis, abscess), Vibrio vulnificus; **GU sources**: cystitis (only with SLE, DM, alcoholism, multiple myeloma), CLL, steroids, obstruction: relative (BPH), unilateral (partial) or bilateral/ureteral (partial/total obstruction); kidney (acute pyelonephritis, renal abscess, perinephric abscess, renal calculi); prostate (acute prostatitis, prostatic calculi, prostatic abscess), ureteral stents. **Other sources**: CVC infection, TSS (S. aureus, group A streptococci, C. sordellii), dengue fever, SARS, MERS, HPS, influenza, CAP (with decreased/absent splenic function) or severe cardiopulmonary disease, influenza with CA-MRSA (PVL+), necrotizing fasciitis <u>Noninfectious</u>: myocardial infarction, pulmonary embolism, acute pancreatitis, relative adrenal insufficiency, GI bleed, overzealous diuresis, inadequate volume replacement or hypotonic fluid replacement, aortic dissection, abdominal aneurysm rupture, rectus sheath hematoma
Soft tissue crepitance	<u>Infectious</u>: mixed aerobic/anaerobic infection* <u>Noninfectious</u>: subcutaneous emphysema, recent surgery in area of crepitance
Bullae (vesicles)	<u>Infectious</u>: gas gangrene (hemorrhagic), S. aureus > group A streptococci, V. vulnificus (hemorrhagic), necrotizing fasciitis, bullous impetigo, HSV, VZV, smallpox, disseminated smallpox (hemorrhagic), Coxsackie A (A_6, A_{16}) <u>Noninfectious</u>: pemphigus, pemphigoid, dermatitis herpetiformis, TEN, porphyria, contact dermatitis, E. multiforme, DM, barbiturates
Generalized edema/ nephrotic syndrome	<u>Infectious</u>: malaria (P. malariae), trichinosis, VZV, yellow fever, influenza A, HBV, HIV, EBV, CMV, 2° syphilis, leprosy <u>Noninfectious</u>: drugs, lymphomas, thiamine deficiency (wet beri-beri), kwashiorkor, post-streptococcal glomerulonephritis, DM, PAN, Henoch-Schönlein purpura, SLE, constrictive pericarditis, tricuspid regurgitation, IVC obstruction, myxedema, sickle cell disease, amyloidosis, α-1 antitrypsin deficiency, nail-patella syndrome, Wegener's granulomatosis, sarcoidosis, renal vein thrombosis
Erythroderma	<u>Infectious</u>: human T-cell leukemia virus 1 (HTLV-1), TSS, scarlet fever, dengue fever, chikungunya fever <u>Noninfectious</u>: psoriasis, lymphoma, atopic dermatitis, contact dermatitis, exfoliative dermatitis, drugs, ichthyosis, erythroleukemia, pityriasis, dermatomyositis, Kawasaki's disease, Hodgkin's lymphoma
Hyper-pigmentation	<u>Infectious</u>: kala-azar, Whipple's disease, histoplasmosis <u>Noninfectious</u>: hemochromatosis, PBC, Addison's disease, drugs – brown (bleomycin), blue/gray (busulfan, fluorouracil, chlorpromazine), purple/gray (amiodarone), blue/gray (minocycline)

* Versus gas gangrene (minimal/no gas on auscultation).

Table 9.2 General Appearance Abnormalities *(cont'd)*

Finding	Causes
Jaundice	<u>Infectious</u>: yellow fever, EBV, leptospirosis, ascariasis (in bile/pancreatic duct), arboviral hemorrhagic fevers, viral hepatitis
	<u>Noninfectious</u>: hepatobiliary malignancy, benign biliary obstruction, PBC, cirrhosis, hemolytic anemias, alcoholic hepatitis, drugs, Gilbert's syndrome, pancreatic carcinoma
Vitiligo	<u>Infectious</u>: leprosy, yaws, pinta, HIV
	<u>Noninfectious</u>: DM, hyperthyroidism, hypothyroidism, Hashimoto's thyroiditis
Lizard/elephant skin	<u>Infectious</u>: onchocerciasis
	<u>Noninfectious</u>: ichthyosis
Urticaria	<u>Infectious</u>: strongyloides, dracunculiasis, HBV, F. hepatica, schistosomal dermatitis
	<u>Noninfectious</u>: insect bites/stings, drugs, malignancies, cholinergic urticaria, serum sickness, urticarial vasculitis, cryoglobulinemia, systemic mastocytosis, Schnitzler's syndrome
Rash (only below waist)	<u>Infectious</u>: Parvovirus B19 (stocking/glove)
	<u>Noninfectious</u>: Henoch-Schönlein purpura (HSP)

Table 9.3 Head Abnormalities

Finding	Causes
Prematurely gray hair	<u>Infectious</u>: HIV
	<u>Noninfectious</u>: smoking, pernicious anemia
Temporal muscle wasting	<u>Infectious</u>: HIV
	<u>Noninfectious</u>: myotonic dystrophy
Facial swelling (edema)	<u>Infectious</u>: dengue fever, Zika virus (ZIKV), yellow fever, Lassa virus, trichinosis, leprosy, EEE, onchocerciasis
	<u>Noninfectious</u>: angioneurotic edema, nephrotic syndrome, acute glomerulonephritis, leukemic infiltrates, amyloidosis
Severe seborrheic dermatitis	<u>Infectious</u>: HIV
	<u>Noninfectious</u>: CGD
Facial red spots	<u>Infectious</u>: psittacosis (Horder's spots)
	<u>Noninfectious</u>: Campbell de Morgan spots

Table 9.3 Head Abnormalities *(cont'd)*

Finding	Causes
Localized alopecia	<u>Infectious:</u> leprosy, Tinea capitis, smallpox, blastomycosis, VZV, TB (cutaneous)
	<u>Noninfectious:</u> SLE, DM, scleroderma, common variable immune deficiency (CVID)
Generalized alopecia	<u>Infectious:</u> post-malaria, post-typhoid fever, post-kala-azar, post-yellow fever, 2° syphilis, HIV
	<u>Noninfectious:</u> nutritional deficiencies, drugs, hyperthyroidism
Total/partial eyebrow loss	<u>Infectious:</u> leprosy, syphilis
	<u>Noninfectious:</u> iatrogenic, hereditary, hypothyroidism, hypopituitarism
Long eyelashes	<u>Infectious:</u> kala-azar, trypanosomiasis
	<u>Noninfectious:</u> hereditary, drugs, HIV drugs
Lacrimal gland enlargement *unilateral*	<u>Infectious:</u> Chagas' disease
	<u>Noninfectious:</u> malignancies
bilateral	<u>Infectious:</u> TB
	<u>Noninfectious:</u> Sjögren's syndrome, RA, SLE, sarcoidosis
Facial erythema	<u>Infectious:</u> facial cellulitis, erysipelas, TB (lupus vulgaris), arboviral hemorrhagic fevers (dengue, chikungunya, Zika viruses)
	<u>Noninfectious:</u> dermatomyositis, drugs, rosacea, carcinoid syndrome, SLE
Parotid enlargement	<u>Infectious:</u> mumps, Chagas' disease, rat bite fever (Streptobacillus moniliformis), melioidosis, CMV, EBV, LCM, adenovirus, ECHO 9, Coxsackie A, influenza A, HPIV-1, HPIV-3, HIV
	<u>Noninfectious:</u> Sjögren's syndrome, sarcoidosis, cirrhosis
Scalp nodules	<u>Infectious:</u> myiasis, onchocerciasis
	<u>Noninfectious:</u> bony exostoses, malignancies, benign cysts, pyogenic granuloma, Kimura's disease

Table 9.4 Eye Abnormalities

Finding	Causes
Bilateral upper lid edema	<u>Infectious:</u> EBV (Hoagland's sign)
	<u>Noninfectious:</u> bilateral eye irritation
Bilateral lower lid edema	<u>Infectious:</u> measles
	<u>Noninfectious:</u> bilateral eye irritation
Bilateral lid edema	<u>Infectious:</u> trichinosis, meningococcemia, adenovirus
	<u>Noninfectious:</u> Wegener's granulomatosis

Table 9.4 Eye Abnormalities *(cont'd)*

Finding	Causes
Heliotrope eyelid discoloration	<u>Infectious</u>: cholera (early), influenza A (severe)
	<u>Noninfectious</u>: dermatomyositis
Periorbital edema *unilateral*	<u>Infectious</u>: Chagas' disease, loiasis, gnathostomiasis, sparganosis
	<u>Noninfectious</u>: insect bites, unilateral eye irritation
bilateral	<u>Infectious</u>: RMSF, trichinosis, tularemia, dengue fever, Hantaan (HFRS) virus
	<u>Noninfectious</u>: allergies, Insect bites, TNF-receptor-1-associated periodic syndrome (TRAPS), dermatomyositis
Argyll-Robertson pupils	<u>Infectious</u>: syphilis
	<u>Noninfectious</u>: sarcoidosis
Iritis	<u>Infectious</u>: onchocerciasis, 2° syphilis, relapsing fever, leprosy
	<u>Noninfectious</u>: SLE, dermatomyositis, Behçet's syndrome, Reiter's syndrome, RA
Conjunctivitis *unilateral*	<u>Infectious</u>: TB, HSV, tularemia, adult inclusion conjunctivitis, Chagas' disease, LGV, CSD, loiasis, ocular myiasis, diphtheria, adenovirus (types 8, 19)
	<u>Noninfectious</u>: SLE, eye irritation
bilateral	<u>Infectious</u>: TSS, measles, rubella, meningococcemia, gonorrhea, adenovirus (type 3), plague, RMSF, sparganosis, LGV, listeria, relapsing fever, pertussis, influenza, microsporidia, HHV-6, arboviral hemorrhagic fevers, dengue hemorrhagic fever, Zika virus (ZIKV)
	<u>Noninfectious</u>: Kawasaki's disease, Reiter's syndrome, Steven-Johnson syndrome, adult Still's disease, eye irritation
Hemorrhagic conjunctivitis *unilateral*	<u>Infectious</u>: adenovirus (types 8, 19)
	<u>Noninfectious</u>: trauma
bilateral	<u>Infectious</u>: trichinosis, pertussis, leptospirosis, Coxsackie A (type 24), adenovirus (type 11), enterovirus (type 70), arboviral hemorrhagic fevers
	<u>Noninfectious</u>: trauma, Steven-Johnson syndrome
Subconjunctival hemorrhage	<u>Infectious</u>: SBE, trichinosis, meningococcemia, pertussis, leptospirosis, RMSF
	<u>Noninfectious</u>: severe anemia, Kawasaki's disease
Conjunctival suffusion	<u>Infectious</u>: RMSF, leptospirosis, relapsing fever, ehrlichiosis/anaplasmosis, HPS, influenza, arboviral hemorrhagic fevers, St.LE, measles, ADV
	<u>Noninfectious</u>: bilateral eye irritation

Table 9.4 Eye Abnormalities *(cont'd)*

Finding	Causes
Episcleritis	<u>Infectious</u>: TB, leprosy, 2° syphilis, Lyme disease
	<u>Noninfectious</u>: sarcoidosis, RA, adult Still's disease, SLE, PAN, TA, RE
Scleral nodules	<u>Infectious</u>: loiasis, sparganosis, leprosy, tularemia, TB
	<u>Noninfectious</u>: RA, vitamin A deficiency (Bitot's spots), sarcoidosis
Dry eyes	<u>Infectious</u>: measles
	<u>Noninfectious</u>: vitamin A deficiency, SLE, Sjögren's syndrome, RA, sarcoidosis
Watery eyes	<u>Infectious</u>: bacterial conjunctivitis, adenovirus, measles
	<u>Noninfectious</u>: PAN, allergenic conjunctivitis
Uveitis	<u>Infectious</u>: TB, histoplasmosis, leprosy, syphilis, malaria, HSV, VZV, EBV, TSS, typhus, LGV, CMV, African trypanosomiasis, brucellosis, leptospirosis, RMSF, CSD
	<u>Noninfectious</u>: adult Still's disease, SLE, PAN, sarcoidosis, Behçet's syndrome, Reiter's syndrome, RA, relapsing polychondritis, ankylosing spondylitis, Kawasaki's disease, Wegener's granulomatosis
Corneal haziness	<u>Infectious</u>: adenovirus, leprosy, trachoma, onchocerciasis
	<u>Noninfectious</u>: vitamin A deficiency, cataracts
Keratitis	<u>Infectious</u>: HSV, congenital syphilis, acanthamoeba, TB, toxoplasmosis, histoplasmosis, CMV, trachoma, microsporidia, nocardia, leprosy, onchocerciasis, meliodosis, measles
	<u>Noninfectious</u>: Behçet's syndrome, Reiter's syndrome, Steven-Johnson syndrome, vitamin A deficiency
Corneal ulcers	<u>Infectious</u>: HSV, listeria, acanthamoeba, tularemia, shigella, RMSF
	<u>Noninfectious</u>: trauma, Wegener's granulomatosis
Endophthalmitis	<u>Infectious</u>: miliary TB, candida, aspergillus, toxocara, serratia, S. pneumoniae
	<u>Noninfectious</u>: retinoblastoma
Chorioretinitis	<u>Infectious</u>: toxoplasmosis, CMV, onchocerciasis, congenital syphilis, histoplasmosis, TB, WNE, coccidiomycosis, leptospirosis, chikungunya fever
	<u>Noninfectious</u>: sarcoidosis, SLE, PAN
Cytoid bodies (cotton wool spots)	<u>Infectious</u>: CSD, HIV, CMV, SBE
	<u>Noninfectious</u>: SLE, adult Still's disease, PAN, atrial myxoma, Wegener's granulomatosis, TA

Table 9.4 Eye Abnormalities *(cont'd)*

Finding	Causes
Roth spots	<u>Infectious</u>: SBE, psittacosis, RMSF, malaria
	<u>Noninfectious</u>: PAN, SLE, DM, severe anemia, leukemia, cholesterol emboli syndrome, atrial myxoma, TA, Takayasu's arteritis
Periphlebitis (candle wax drippings)	<u>Infectious</u>: CMV, leptospirosis (Weil's syndrome)
	<u>Noninfectious</u>: sarcoidosis

Table 9.5 Ear Abnormalities

Finding	Causes
Acute deafness	<u>Infectious</u>: ABM, mumps (aseptic meningitis), RMSF, typhus, scrub typhus, murine typhus, Mediterranean spotted fever, brucellosis, Lassa fever, Toscana virus (TOSV), Zika, VZV (Ramsey–Hunt syndrome)
	<u>Noninfectious</u>: sound/barotrauma
External ear lesions	<u>Infectious</u>: cutaneous leishmaniasis (Chiclero ulcer), leprosy, Kaposi's sarcoma, chikungunya fever (local pinna edema), leprosy (pendulous ear lobes)
	<u>Noninfectious</u>: relapsing polychondritis, eczema, carcinoma, contact dermatitis, sarcoidosis, SLE, gout (tophi), keloids, actinic keratosis

Table 9.6 Nasal Abnormalities

Finding	Causes
Purple nose tip/ hyperpigmented	<u>Infectious</u>: Kaposi's sarcoma, TB (Bazin's erythema induratum), chikungunya fever ("Chik sign")
	<u>Noninfectious</u>: vasculitis, lymphoma, drugs, sarcoidosis
Nose tip gangrene	<u>Infectious</u>: Staphylococcus aureus ABE (emboli)
	<u>Noninfectious</u>: SLE, vasculitis
Epistaxis	<u>Infectious</u>: psittacosis, typhoid fever, nasal diphtheria, yellow fever, Colorado tick fever, TBRF, influenza, dengue hemorrhagic fever, arboviral hemorrhagic fevers, acute renal failure, leprosy, leptospirosis, VZV, TB, rhinosporidium, mucocutaneous leishmaniasis
	<u>Noninfectious</u>: Local trauma, sinus malignancies, von Willebrand's disease, polycythemia vera, Waldenstrom's macroglobulinemia, relapsing polychondritis
Nasal septal perforation	<u>Infectious</u>: leprosy, 2° syphilis, mucocutaneous leishmaniasis, blastomycosis, pinta, yaws
	<u>Noninfectious</u>: cocaine, lethal midline granuloma, Wegener's granulomatosis, miasis

Table 9.7 Mouth Abnormalities

Finding	Causes
Trismus	Infectious: tetanus
	Noninfectious: temporomandibular joint dislocation/arthritis, trigeminal neuralgia
Herpes labialis	Infectious: HSV, pneumococcal pneumonia, meningococcal meningitis, malaria
	Noninfectious: contact dermatitis (may mimic H. labialis)
Angular chelitis	Infectious: 2° syphilis, HIV
	Noninfectious: riboflavin deficiency, trauma, contact dermatitis, anemia
Gingivitis	Infectious: trench mouth
	Noninfectious: Wegener's granulomatosis
Tongue tenderness	Infectious: relapsing fever, typhoid fever
	Noninfectious: vitamin deficiencies, pernicious anemia, GCA
Tongue ulcers	Infectious: histoplasmosis, HSV, syphilis
	Noninfectious: aphthous ulcers, chemotherapy, radiation therapy
Leukoplakia	Infectious: HIV (hairy), syphilis
	Noninfectious: lichen planus
Oral ulcers *solitary*	Infectious: syphilis, CMV, histoplasmosis, TB, Leishmania braziliensis, African tick bite fever
	Noninfectious: squamous cell carcinoma, Behçet's syndrome, Wegener's granulomatosis
multiple	Infectious: HSV, HFM disease, herpangina, brucellosis, Lassa fever, African tick bite fever, chickungunya fever, measles
	Noninfectious: SLE*, celiac disease, aphthous ulcers, squamous cell carcinoma, Behçet's syndrome, FAPA syndrome*, hyper IgF (Job's) syndrome, E. multiforme, RE, cyclic neutropenia, hyper IgD syndrome, Sweet's syndrome
Frenal ulcer	Infectious: pertussis
	Noninfectious: trauma
Palatal petechiae	Infectious: Group A streptococci, EBV, CMV, HSV, VZV, toxoplasmosis, rubella, HIV, chikungunya fever, dengue fever, Hantaan (HFRS) virus, Zika virus (ZIKV), tularemia
	Noninfectious: thrombocytopenia (2° to any cause), platelet dysfunction disorders, DIC, Ehlers-Danlos syndrome, Marfan's syndrome

* Painless ulcers.

Table 9.7 Mouth Abnormalities *(cont'd)*

Finding	Causes
Palatal perforation	<u>Infectious</u>: congenital syphilis, histoplasmosis, coccidiomycosis, para-coccidiomycosis, leprosy, TB, kala azar
	<u>Noninfectious</u>: Post-surgical, midline granuloma, SLE, NK cell lymphoma, Wegener's granulomatosis, cocaine
Palatal vesicles	<u>Infectious</u>: ***Anterior***: HSV, VZV, hand-foot-mouth disease (Coxsackie A). ***Posterior***: herpangina (Coxsackie A)
	<u>Noninfectious</u>: bullous pemphigus, Steven-Johnson syndrome (drug-induced)
Uvular edema	<u>Infectious</u>: Group A streptococci
	<u>Noninfectious</u>: Franklin's disease, drugs, angioneurotic edema
Crimson crescents	<u>Infectious</u>: chronic fatigue syndrome (CFS), HIV
	<u>Noninfectious</u>: None
Tonsillar membranes	<u>Infectious</u>: diphtheria, Arcanobacterium hemolyticum
	<u>Noninfectious</u>: None
Tonsillar ulcers	<u>Infectious</u>: tularemia (oropharyngeal), 1° syphilis, Vincent's angina, TB
	<u>Noninfectious</u>: carcinoma, T-cell lymphoma, AML
Hoarseness	<u>Infectious</u>: laryngeal TB, C. pneumoniae, respiratory viruses, pertussis
	<u>Noninfectious</u>: recurrent laryngeal nerve paralysis, laryngeal cancer

Table 9.8 Neck Abnormalities

Finding	Causes
Enlarged greater auricular nerve	<u>Infectious</u>: leprosy
	<u>Noninfectious</u>: none
Bull neck	<u>Infectious</u>: diphtheria, mumps, Ludwig's angina, pertussis, group A streptococcal suppurative lymphangitis
	<u>Noninfectious</u>: angioneurotic edema, subcutaneous emphysema
Jugular vein tenderness	<u>Infectious</u>: suppurative jugular thrombophlebitis (Lemierre's syndrome)
	<u>Noninfectious</u>: thrombophlebitis
Neck sinus tract	<u>Infectious</u>: actinomycosis, TB, atypical TB
	<u>Noninfectious</u>: branchial cleft cyst, CGD
Superior vena cava syndrome	<u>Infectious</u>: actinomycosis
	<u>Noninfectious</u>: lymphoma, squamous cell carcinoma

Table 9.9 Chest Abnormalities

Finding	Causes
Shoulder tenderness	<u>Infectious</u>: subdiaphragmatic abscess, septic arthritis (shoulder)
	<u>Noninfectious</u>: squamous cell carcinoma (Pancoast's tumor), bursitis
Sternal tenderness	<u>Infectious</u>: sternal osteomyelitis (post-open heart surgery)
	<u>Noninfectious</u>: metastatic carcinoma, pre-leukemia, acute leukemia, myeloproliferative disorder, trauma
Costochondral tenderness	<u>Infectious</u>: costochondritis (Coxsackie B)
	<u>Noninfectious</u>: trauma, plasmacytoma
Trapezius tenderness	<u>Infectious</u>: subdiaphragmatic abscess
	<u>Noninfectious</u>: fibromyalgia
Chest wall sinuses	<u>Infectious</u>: TB, actinomycosis, blastomycosis, abscess, M. fortuitum-chelo-nei (post-breast implant surgery), sternal osteomyelitis (post-sternotomy)
	<u>Noninfectious</u>: bronchogenic carcinoma
Spontaneous pneumothorax	<u>Infectious</u>: TB, PCP, Legionnaire's disease, lung abscess, pertussis
	<u>Noninfectious</u>: histiocytosis X (eosinophilic granuloma, Langerhan's cell histiocytosis), osteogenic sarcoma, emphysema, ARDS
Diffuse wheezing	<u>Infectious</u>: RSV, influenza, adenovirus, hMPV, HPIV-3, EV-D68, C. pneumoniae, M. pneumoniae, acute shistosomiasis (S. mansoni > S. haematobium)
	<u>Noninfectious</u>: pulmonary emboli, LVF, asthma, Churg-Strauss granulomatosis, carcinoid syndrome, asthmatic bronchitis, angioedema
Chest dullness *consolidation*	<u>Infectious</u>: bacterial pneumonia, psittacosis, nocardia, Q fever
	<u>Noninfectious</u>: large cell carcinoma
pleural effusion	<u>Infectious</u>: group A streptococci, tularemia, H. influenzae, 1° TB
	<u>Noninfectious</u>: Meig's syndrome, pancreatitis, CHF, malignancies, pulmonary embolism

Table 9.10 Back Abnormalities

Finding	Causes
Spinal tenderness	<u>Infectious</u>: vertebral osteomyelitis, typhoid fever, TB, brucellosis, SBE
	<u>Noninfectious</u>: malignancies, multiple myeloma
D'espine's sign	<u>Infectious</u>: bilateral pneumonia (consolidation), TB
	<u>Noninfectious</u>: sarcoidosis, large cell carcinoma, lymphoma
Unilateral CVA tenderness	<u>Infectious</u>: pyelonephritis, renal/perinephric abscess
	<u>Noninfectious</u>: trauma

Table 9.11 Heart Abnormalities

Finding	Causes
Tachycardia	<u>Infectious</u>: myocarditis (Coxsackie B$_{1-5}$, COVID-19, RMSF, typhus, diphtheria, trichinosis, Toxocara canis/cati (VLM), influenza, dengue), gas gangrene
	<u>Noninfectious</u>: hypovolemia, hypoxia, anxiety, hyperthyroidism, MI, pulmonary embolism, CHF, Kawasaki's disease, substance withdrawal, myocarditis (idiopathic giant cell)
Heart block *Acute*	<u>Infectious</u>: Lyme disease, ABE with paravalvular/septal abscess, diptheria, myocarditis (Coxsackie, influenza, RMSF, COVID-19)
	<u>Noninfectious</u>: acute (inferior) MI, drugs, myocarditis (idiopathic giant cell)
Chronic	<u>Infectious</u>: Chagas' disease
	<u>Noninfectious</u>: AV nodal ablation, sarcoidosis, Lev's/Lenegre's disease
Pericardial effusion	<u>Infectious</u>: viral pericarditis (Coxasackie B$_{1-5}$), TB pericarditis, dengue
	<u>Noninfectious</u>: SLE, uremia, malignancy
Heart murmur	<u>Infectious</u>: SBE, 3° syphilis
	<u>Noninfectious</u>: valvular heart disease, severe anemia, Takayasu's arteritis, SLE (Libman-Sacks), endomyocardial fibroelastosis, atrial myxoma, marantic endocarditis

Table 9.12 Abdominal Abnormalities

Finding	Causes
Abdominal wall tenderness	<u>Infectious</u>: leptospirosis, abdominal wall cellulitis/abscess, trichinosis
	<u>Noninfectious</u>: trauma, rectus sheath hematoma
Abdominal wall sinus tract	<u>Infectious</u>: TB, abscess, ameboma, actinomycosis
	<u>Noninfectious</u>: carcinomas
Rose spots	<u>Infectious</u>: typhoid fever, shigella, trichinosis, rat bite fever, brucellosis, leptospirosis
	<u>Noninfectious</u>: Campbell de Morgan spots
Abdominal tenderness (2° to pancreatitis)	<u>Infectious</u>: Coxsackie virus, echovirus, mumps, ascariasis, EBV, CMV, HBV, HSV, VZV, HIV
	<u>Noninfectious</u>: EtOH, cholelithiasis (+ common pancreatitis duct), tauma, post-ERCP, hyperlipidemia (types I, IV, V), hypertriglyceridemia, TPN, hypercalcemia, SLE, PAN, posterior penetrating duodenal ulcer, drugs (steroids, azathioprine, diuretics, furosemide, thiazides, L-asparaginase, valproic acid, pentamidine)

Table 9.12 Abdominal Abnormalities (cont'd)

Finding	Causes
Right upper quadrant tenderness	<u>Infectious</u>: cholangitis, cholecystitis, pylephlebitis, splenic flexure diverticulitis, emphysematous cholecystitis (Clostridia sp.), hepatic abscess (amebic, echinococcal, bacterial), right lower lobe CAP, brucellosis, leptospirosis, typhoid fever, viral hepatitis, dengue, malaria
	<u>Noninfectious</u>: burns, post-partum, ptosed right kidney, acute pancreatitis, Kawasaki's disease, cholesterol emboli syndrome, acalculous cholecystitis PAN, SLE, total parenteral nutrition, ceftriaxone (pseudo-cholelithiasis)
Right upper quadrant tympany	<u>Infectious</u>: peritonitis (2° to organ perforation)
	<u>Noninfectious</u>: post-abdominal surgery
Right upper quadrant mass	<u>Infectious</u>: bacterial abscess, echinococcal cysts, amebic abscess
	<u>Noninfectious</u>: ptosed right kidney, Reidel's lobe, hepatoma, malignancies, distended gallbladder (Couvoisier's sign)
Right lower quadrant tenderness	<u>Infectious</u>: shigella, typhoid fever, typhoidal EBV, typhoidal tularemia, parvovirus B19, TB, ameboma, typhlitis, actinomycetoma. Pseudo-appendicitis (scarlet fever, Legionnaire's disease, yersinia, campylobacter, pre-eruptive measles, dengue, RMSF), PID, syphilis (luetic crisis), brucellosis, leptospirosis
	<u>Noninfectious</u>: appendicitis, RE, ectopic pregnancy, diverticulitis, hyper IgE (Job's) syndrome, DM crisis, porphyria, pancreatitis, SLE
Left upper abdominal quadrant tenderness (splenic tenderness)	<u>Infectious</u>: SBE, brucellosis, typhoid fever, malaria, splenic abscess, EBV, CMV, HHV-6
	<u>Noninfectious</u>: splenic infarct
Abdominal wall nodules	<u>Infectious</u>: leprosy
	<u>Noninfectious</u>: lipomas, panniculitis, metastatic disease, sarcoidosis
Perubilical purpura (thumb-print sign)	<u>Infectious</u>: strongyloides (hyperinfection syndrome)
	<u>Noninfectious</u>: retroperitoneal hemorrhage (Cullen's sign)
Hepatomegaly	<u>Infectious</u>: viral hepatitis, bacterial liver abscess, amebic abscess, ehrlichiosis/anaplasmosis, babesiosis, brucellosis, leptospirosis (Weil's syndrome), arboviral hemorrhagic fevers, typhus, typhoid fever, malaria, Q fever, EBV, CMV, acute HIV, miliary TB, Castleman's disease (MCD), schistosomiasis

Table 9.12 Abdominal Abnormalities *(cont'd)*

Finding	Causes
	<u>Noninfectious</u>: alcoholic cirrhosis, cholangiocarcinoma, carcinoma of pancreas, constrictive pericarditis, pericholangitis, veno-occlusive disease, autoimmune hepatitis, α-1antitrypsin deficiency, cystic fibrosis, fatty liver, hemangiomas, jejunoileal bypass, Reye's syndrome, multiple myeloma, hepatocellular carcinoma, metastatic carcinoma*, parenteral hyperalimentation (TPN)
Splenomegaly	<u>Infectious</u>: ***Mildly enlarged spleen:*** malaria, babesiosis, kala-azar, dengue, SBE, ehrlichiosis/anaplasmosis, typhoid/enteric fevers, typhus, leptospirosis (Weil's syndrome), ECHO 9, Coxsackie B₅, viral hepatitis, EBV, CMV, relapsing fever, syphilis, toxoplasmosis, psittacosis, brucellosis, Q fever, CSD, schistosomiasis, trypanosomiasis, histoplasmosis, miliary TB, splenic abscess, acute HIV, hydatid cysts, colorado tick fever; Castleman's disease (MCD), ***Moderately enlarged spleen:*** malaria, kala-azar; Castleman's disease (MCD), ***Massively enlarged spleen:*** malaria, kala-azar, Castleman's disease (MCD)
	<u>Noninfectious</u>: ***Mildly enlarged spleen:*** SLE, sarcoidosis, Felty's syndrome, hemochromatosis, Wilson's disease, Budd-Chiari syndrome, megaloblastic anemia, iron deficiency anemia, systemic mastocytosis, angioblastic lymphadenopathy, splenic cysts, splenic trauma/hemorrhage, histiocytosis X (Langerhan's eosinophilic granuloma), hyperthyroidism, serum sickness, amyloidosis, berylliosis, Kawasaki's disease, RE, lymphoma ***Moderately enlarged spleen:*** portal hypertension, hemolytic anemias, myeloproliferative disorders, CLL, Gaucher's disease, Niemann-Pick disease; ***Massively enlarged spleen:*** CML, hairy cell leukemia, lymphoma, myelofibrosis
Hepato-splenomegaly	<u>Infectious</u>: malaria, typhoid/enteric fever, psittacosis, brucellosis, kala-azar, 2° syphilis, EBV, CMV, acute HIV, schistosomiasis, toxoplasmosis, relapsing fever, RMSF, typhus, CSD, histoplasmosis, miliary TB, dengue, babesiosis, ehrlichiosis/anaplasmosis, Q fever, Castleman's disease (MCD), leptospirosis (Weil's syndrome)
	<u>Noninfectious</u>: hypernephroma (RCC), CGD, hyper IgD syndrome, sarcoidosis, myelodysplastic syndrome (MDS), lymphoma
Ascites	<u>Infectious</u>: TB peritonitis, shistosomiasis, filariasis, spontaneous bacterial peritonitis, dengue, Whipple's disease
	<u>Noninfectious</u>: malignancies, Budd-Chiari syndrome, tricuspid regurgitation, constrictive pericarditis, inferior vena cava syndrome, FMF, Henoch-Schönlein purpura, SLE, portal hypertension, pancreatic/bile ascites, CHF, Meig's syndrome

* Usually from lung, colon, pancreas, kidney, breast, stomach, or esophagus.

Table 9.13 Lymph Node Abnormalities

Finding	Causes
Preauricular adenopathy	<u>Infectious:</u> ipsilateral conjunctivitis, tularemia, anterior scalp infections, rat bite fever (Spirillum minus)
	<u>Noninfectious:</u> lymphoma
Occipital adenopathy	<u>Infectious:</u> posterior scalp infections, CSD, rubella
	<u>Noninfectious:</u> lymphoma
Anterior cervical adenopathy	<u>Infectious:</u> pharyngitis, mouth/dental infections, TB (scrofula), HHV-6, toxoplasmosis, CSD, brucellosis, Lyme disease
	<u>Noninfectious:</u> head/neck cancer, Kawasaki's disease, lymphoma, SLE, Kikuchi's disease, Rosai-Dorfman disease
Posterior cervical adenopathy *unilateral*	<u>Infectious:</u> toxoplasmosis, African trypanosomiasis (Winterbottom's sign)
	<u>Noninfectious:</u> posterior scalp infection, Kawasaki's disease, lymphoma, Kikuchi's disease, Rosai-Dorfman disease
bilateral	<u>Infectious:</u> EBV, HHV-6, CMV, Chagas' disease, HAV
	<u>Noninfectious:</u> lymphoma, Kawasaki's disease, Rosai-Dorfman disease, hyper IgD syndrome, sarcoidosis
Supraclavicular adenopathy	<u>Infectious:</u> TB, CSD
	<u>Noninfectious:</u> intra-abdominal malignancy (Virchow's sign), Kikuchi's disease
Infraclavicular adenopathy	<u>Infectious:</u> African trypanosomiasis, CSD
	<u>Noninfectious:</u> lymphoma
Epitrochlear adenopathy	<u>Infectious:</u> 2° syphilis, CSD, brucellosis
	<u>Noninfectious:</u> sarcoidosis, IVDA
Axillary adenopathy	<u>Infectious:</u> CFS (usually left), CSD, B. malayi, rat bite fever (Spirillum minus), brucellosis, Zika virus (ZIKV)
	<u>Noninfectious:</u> lymphoma, CLL, sarcoidosis, Schnitzler's syndrome
Ulcer-node syndromes	<u>Infectious:</u> ***Ulcer > node:*** anthrax, rickettsial fevers (except RMSF), sporotrichosis, cutaneous leishmaniasis (new world). ***Node = ulcer:*** 1° syphilis, chancroid, tularemia (ulceroglandular), rat bite fever (Spirillum minus). ***Node > ulcer:*** syphilis, LGV, chancroid, HSV-2
	<u>Noninfectious:</u> lymphoma
Periumbilical nodule	<u>Infectious:</u> intra-abdominal infection
	<u>Noninfectious:</u> malignancy (Sister Joseph's sign)

Table 9.13 Lymph Node Abnormalities (cont'd)

Finding	Causes
Inguinal adenopathy *unilateral*	<u>Infectious</u>: lower extremity infections, bubonic plague, rat bite fever (Spirillum minus), filariasis, leprosy, tularemia, CSD
	<u>Noninfectious</u>: intra-abdominal malignancy, bilateral lower extremity infection, IVDA
bilateral	<u>Infectious</u>: any infection causing generalized adenopathy, B. malayi, HSV-2, syphilis, LGV, Zika virus (ZIKV)
	<u>Noninfectious</u>: any disorder causing generalized adenopathy, Schnitzler's syndrome
Generalized lympha-denopathy	<u>Infectious</u>: TB, EBV, HHV-6, CMV, rubella, measles, toxoplasmosis, CSD, LGV, brucellosis, group A streptococci, 2° syphilis, HIV, kala-azar, trypanosomiasis (African), arboviral hemorrhagic fevers, Whipple's disease, Castleman's disease (MCD), scrub typhus, Lyme disease
	<u>Noninfectious</u>: SLE, RA, adult Still's disease, pseudolymphoma (Dilantin), Kikuchi's disease, Gaucher's disease, sarcoidosis, serum sickness, hyperthyroidism, ALL, CLL, Kimura's disease

Table 9.14 Genitourinary Abnormalities

Finding	Causes
Epididymoorchitis	<u>Infectious</u>: mumps, TB, blastomycosis, melioidosis, brucellosis, leptospirosis, EBV, W. bancrofti, ECHO 9, Coxsackie B$_5$, S. hematobium, LCM, GC, C. trachomatis (young adults), P. aeruginosa (elderly adults), Colorado tick fever, rat bite fever (Spirillum minus), relapsing fever
	<u>Noninfectious</u>: lymphoma, SLE, PAN, sarcoidosis, FMF, TNF-receptor-1-associated periodic syndrome (TRAPS), trauma, torsion, malignancy
Scrotal enlargement	<u>Infectious</u>: mumps, W. bancrofti (not B. malayi), Fournier's gangrene
	<u>Noninfectious</u>: hydrocele, testicular torsion
Groin mass	<u>Infectious</u>: onchocerciasis (hanging groins), TB, W. bancrofti, shisto-somiasis
	<u>Noninfectious</u>: lymphoma
Perirectal fistula	<u>Infectious</u>: peri-rectal abscess, actinomycosis, LGV
	<u>Noninfectious</u>: RE, malignancies
Perirectal ulcer	<u>Infectious</u>: HSV, amebiasis cutis, 1° syphilis
	<u>Noninfectious</u>: malignancy
Genital ulcers	<u>Infectious</u>: Syphilis (1°), HSV, chancroid, LCV, chikungunya fever, TB
	<u>Noninfectious</u>: Beçhet's syndrome, RE, malignancies
Prostate enlargement/ tenderness	<u>Infectious</u>: prostatitis, prostatic abscess*
	<u>Noninfectious</u>: BPH

* Acute: aerobic GNB, VSE/VRE, Ureoplasma urealyticum, C. trachomatis, B. fragilis (post-transrectal biopsy). Chronic: TB, histoplasmosis, blastomycosis, aspergillus, candida, cryptococcus, meliodosis.

Table 9.15 Extremity Abnormalities

Finding	Causes
Digital gangrene	<u>Infectious</u>: SBE, S. aureus bacteremia/ABE (emboli), meningococcemia, RMSF, typhus
	<u>Noninfectious</u>: SLE, vasculitis, peripheral vascular disease
Splinter hemorrhages	<u>Infectious</u>: SBE, ABE, trichinosis
	<u>Noninfectious</u>: trauma, atrial myxoma, acute leukemia, RA, scurvy, mitral stenosis, severe anemia
Clubbing	<u>Infectious</u>: SBE, lung abscess, TB
	<u>Noninfectious</u>: ulcerative colitis (UC), Crohn's disease (RE), cirrhosis, cyanoic congenital heart disease, bronchogenic carcinoma, PBC, celiac disease, hyperthyroidism, hyperparathyroidism, bronchiectasis, hereditary
Dactylitis	<u>Infectious</u>: kala-azar, 2° syphilis, TB
	<u>Noninfectious</u>: sarcoidosis, sickle cell disease, gout, psoriatic arthritis
Tender fingertips	<u>Infectious</u>: SBE, typhoid fever
	<u>Noninfectious</u>: SLE, vasculitis, radial artery occlusion
Lymphangitis	<u>Infectious</u>: group A streptococci, B. malayi, onchocerciasis, melioidosis
	<u>Noninfectious</u>: IVDA
Nodular lymphangitis	<u>Infectious</u>: sporotrichosis, atypical TB, Erysipelothrix rhusiopathiae, kala-azar, coccidiomycosis, histoplasmosis, blastomycosis, nocardia, Pseudoallescheria boydii, cryptococcus, anthrax, group A streptococci, tularemia
	<u>Noninfectious</u>: ganglion cyst (wrist/hand only)
Painless purple palm/sole lesions	<u>Infectious</u>: ABE (Janeway lesions)
	<u>Noninfectious</u>: trauma
Carpal tunnel syndrome	<u>Infectious</u>: TB, leprosy
	<u>Noninfectious</u>: cirrhosis, RA, scleroderma, SLE, DM, hypothyroidism, sarcoidosis, multiple myeloma, amyloidosis
Verrucous hand/arm lesions	<u>Infectious</u>: TB, leprosy, syphilis, sporotrichosis, kala-azar, bartonellosis (verruga peruana)
	<u>Noninfectious</u>: squamous cell carcinoma, sarcoidosis
Edema of the dorsum of hand/foot	<u>Infectious</u>: RMSF, TSS, loiasis, dengue fever, chikungunya fever, rat bite fever (spirillum minus)*
	<u>Noninfectious</u>: trauma, PMR, Kawasaki's disease

* Unilateral swelling.

Table 9.15 Extremity Abnormalities *(cont'd)*

Finding	Causes
Wrist swelling	<u>Infectious</u>: loiasis, septic arthritis, parvovirus B$_{19}$, rubella, chikungunya fever
	<u>Noninfectious</u>: RA
Arthritis (septic/reactive)	<u>Infectious</u>: septic arthritis, rat bite fever (Streptobacillus moniliformis), Lyme disease, LGV, brucellosis, GC, parvovirus B19, shigella, yersinia, salmonella, campylobacter, Clostridium difficle, mumps, rubella, dengue, Zika virus (ZIKV), Mayaro virus (MAYV), chikungunya fever, HIV, HBV, Whipple's disease
	<u>Noninfectious</u>: FMF, RA, pseudogout, SLE, hyper IgD syndrome, lymphoma, Reiter's syndrome, post-streptococcal RF, Poncet's disease, JRA
Papular axillary lesions	<u>Infectious</u>: hydraadenitis suppurativa, 2° syphilis, yaws, blastomycosis
	<u>Noninfectious</u>: chronic contact dermatitis, acanthosis nigricans, Fox-Fordyce disease, seborrheic dermatitis
Tenosynovitis	<u>Infectious</u>: GC (acute), TB (chronic), atypical TB (acute/chronic)
	<u>Noninfectious</u>: rheumatic diseases
Thigh tenderness (bilateral, anterior)	<u>Infectious</u>: bacteremia (Louria's sign), leptospirosis, ehrlichiosis, endocarditis, parvovirus B$_{19}$
	<u>Noninfectious</u>: myositis, vasculitis, sickle cell crisis
Calf tenderness	<u>Infectious</u>: RMSF
	<u>Noninfectious</u>: myositis
Tender muscles	<u>Infectious</u>: trichinosis
	<u>Noninfectious</u>: myositis
Thrombophlebitis	<u>Infectious</u>: psittacosis, campylobacter
	<u>Noninfectious</u>: Behçet's disease, malignancy
Verrucous foot/leg lesions	<u>Infectious</u>: TB, cutaneous leishmaniasis, paracoccidomycosis, sporotrichosis, leprosy, 2° syphilis, mycetoma
	<u>Noninfectious</u>: lichen planus, squamous cell carcinoma
Foot/leg ulcers	<u>Infectious</u>: M. ulcerans (Buruli ulcer may be anywhere), yaws, cutaneous diphtheria, cutaneous leishmaniasis, TB, rat bite fever (Spirillum minus)
	<u>Noninfectious</u>: sickle cell (medial malleolar ulcers), DM (only sole of foot/between toes), peripheral vascular disease
Leg edema *unilateral*	<u>Infectious</u>: onchocerciasis, B. malayi (below knee)
	<u>Noninfectious</u>: malignancy, Milroy's disease

Table 9.15 Extremity Abnormalities *(cont'd)*

Finding	Causes
bilateral	<u>Infectious</u>: elephantiasis (chronic recurrent erysipelas), Chagas' disease, Zika virus (ankle swelling) (ZIKV), (ankle swelling) <u>Noninfectious</u>: lymphatic obstruction (2° to abdominal/pelvic malignancy), congenital yellow nail syndrome
Nodular arm/leg lesions	<u>Infectious</u>: TB (Bazin's erythema induratum), filariasis, sporotrichosis, cutaneos leishmaniasis, atypical TB, leprosy, HIV <u>Noninfectious</u>: erythema nodosum, PAN, thrombophlebitis, panniculitis, nodular vasculitis, Wegener's granulomatosis, Sweet's syndrome, myiasis
Palpable purpura	<u>Infectious</u>: meningococcemia, RMSF <u>Noninfectious</u>: vasculitis, cryoglobulinemia, Gardner-Diamond syndrome, Sweet's syndrome
Eschar *Single*	<u>Infectious</u>: ecthyma gangrenosum, typhus, rickettsial spotted fevers (except RMSF, rickettsial pox), anthrax, cutaneous diphtheria <u>Noninfectious</u>: burns, drugs, recluse spider bite
Multiple	<u>Infectious</u>: African tick bite fever (multiple eschars) <u>Noninfectious</u>: none
Hemorraghic bullae	<u>Infectious</u>: rat bite fever (streptobacillus moniliformis), V. vulnificus, gas gangrene <u>Noninfectious</u>: trauma
Hyperpigmented shins	<u>Infectious</u>: onchocerciasis <u>Noninfectious</u>: DM (dermopathy)
Cutaneous cold abscesses	<u>Infectious</u>: TB, atypical TB <u>Noninfectious</u>: hyper IgF (Job's) syndrome, CGD
Purple nodules	<u>Infectious</u>: disseminated cryptococcus, aspergillus, candida, trypanosomiasis, Kaposi's sarcoma, HIV <u>Noninfectious</u>: leukemia, lymphoma, melanoma
Painful leg nodules	<u>Infectious</u>: Kaposi's sarcoma <u>Noninfectious</u>: erythema nodosum, superficial thrombophlebitis, PAN, panniculitis, osteogenic sarcoma
Migratory rashes	<u>Infectious</u>: hookworms, dracunculiasis, loiasis, gnathostomiasis, strongyloidiasis, sparganosis <u>Noninfectious</u>: myiasis

Table 9.15 Extremity Abnormalities *(cont'd)*

Finding	Causes
Rash of palms/soles	Infectious: syphilis, RMSF, R. parkeri, EBV, scarlet fever, echo 9, smallpox, monkeypox, chickenpox, rat bite fever (Streptobacillus moniliformis, S. minus), HFM, orf, E. multiforme (M. pneumoniae, HSV) Noninfectious: drug rashes, E. multiforme (drugs)
Rash (purpuric) of hands/feet	Infectious: parvovirus B19, VZV, EBV, CMV, HHV-6, HHV-7, HBV, Coxsackie, rubella, rat bite fever (streptobacillus moniliformis) Noninfectious: trauma
Erythema nodosum	Infectious: TB, group A streptococci, EBV, LGV, psittacosis, coccidio-mycosis, blastomycosis, histoplasmosis, CSD, yersinia, campylobacter Noninfectious: UC, RE, drugs, sarcoidosis, lymphoma, SLE
Erythema multiforme	Infectious: HSV, M. pneumoniae, Coxsackie B Noninfectious: drugs
Plantar hyperkeratoses	Infectious: 3° syphilis, yaws, pinta, HIV, tungiasis Noninfectious: Reiter's syndrome, arsenic
Desquamation of hands/feet	Infectious: erysipelas, scarlet fever, TSS, severe infections, yaws, leptospirosis, influenza, measles, arboviral hemorrhagic fevers, chikungunya fever, dengue fever (palms/soles) Noninfectious: Kawasaki's disease, post-edematous states, radiation therapy, vitamin A excess, pellagra, drugs

Table 9.16 Neurological Abnormalities

Finding	Causes
Mental confusion/ encephalopathy (acute)	Infectious: legionnaire's disease, HSV, EBV, HHV-6, influenza, VZV, RMSF, typhoid fever, scrub typhus (R. tsutsugamuschi), Listeria (waxing/ waning), mycoplasma or adenovirus meningoencephalitis, amebic meningoencephalitis (Negleria Acanthamoeba), trichinosis, VLM (T. solium), brain abscess, anthrax, brucellosis, SBE, ABE, HIV, arboviral encephalitis (EEE, St. LE, VEE, JE, Lacrosse), Ebola, MERS, CSD, Whipple's disease, Q fever, TOSV, POWV, WNE, Colorado tick fever, chikungunya fever, dengue, Heartland virus (HRTV), EV 71, Nipah virus, Zika virus, SFTS, trypanosomiasis, melioidosis, COVID-19 Noninfectious: Wernicke's encephalopathy, toxic/metabolic disorders, Behçet's syndrome, SLE, alcoholism, drugs, CHF, chronic renal failure, hepatic encephalopathy, brain tumor, CNS metastases, meningeal carcinomatosis, celiac disease, cefepime, ciprofloxacin > levofloxacin
Nuchal rigidity	Infectious: meningitis (bacterial, fungal, TB, viral) Noninfectious: meningismus, cervical arthritis

Table 9.16 Neurological Abnormalities (cont'd)

Finding	Causes
General muscle rigidity	<u>Infectious</u>: trichinosis, tetanus, rabies, viral encephalitis, brucellosis
	<u>Noninfectious</u>: malignancies, malignant neuroleptic syndrome, strychnine poisoning, Parkinson's disease
Transient deafness	<u>Infectious</u>: RMSF, mediterranean spotted fever, murine typhus, S. pneumoniae ABM, S. suis ABM, H. influenzae ABM, mumps, measles, VZV (Ramsey-Hunt Syndrome), EEE, TOSV, congenital syphilis, brucellosis, Lassa fever
	<u>Noninfectious</u>: trauma, Susac's syndrome
Cranial nerve (CN) abnormalities *unilateral*	<u>Infectious</u>: 6th CN palsy (TB meningitis, N. meningitidis), 7th CN palsy (see Bell's palsy), TBRF, 8th CN palsy (N. meningitidis), Listeria
	<u>Noninfectious</u>: 7th CN palsy (neurosarcoidosis, meningeal carcinomatosis), 2nd, 6th CN palsy (Wegener's granulomatosis)
bilateral	<u>Infectious</u>: 6th CN palsy (TB)
	<u>Noninfectious</u>: meningeal carcinomatosis
Optic nerve atrophy	<u>Infectious</u>: 3° syphilis, TB, toxoplasmosis, mumps, measles, rubella
	<u>Noninfectious</u>: sickle cell disease, severe anemia, polycythemia vera, drugs, sarcoidosis, TA, Behçet's disease, SLE, PAN, MS, glaucoma
Bell's Palsy	<u>Infectious</u>: Lyme disease, HSV-1, VZV (Ramsay-Hunt syndrome), HIV, St.LE, CSD, mumps, EBV infectious mononucleosis, Mycoplasma pneumoniae, syphilis, otitis media, bacterial meningitis, leprosy
	<u>Noninfectious</u>: sarcoidosis, multiple sclerosis, Guillain-Barre syndrome, B-cell lymphoma, Wegener's granulamatosis, pontine lesions (infarct, tumors, demyelinative lesions), tumor compressing the facial nerve, sphenoid ridge mengiomas, acoustic neuromas, neurofibromatosis (type 2), fibrous dysplasia, osteopetrosis, Paget's disease, scleroderma, Melkersson-Rosenthal syndrome, trauma, drugs (vincristine, HBV vaccination), idiopathic
Tremors	<u>Infectious</u>: WNE, TOSV, WEE, St. LE, CNS TB, Listeria
	<u>Noninfectious</u>: Parkinson's disease, Wilson's disease, hemochromatosis, hyperthyroidism, hypoparathyroidism, para-neoplastic disorders
Anisocoria	<u>Infectious</u>: TB, 3° syphilis, VZV, meningitis, encephalitis, botulism, diphtheria
	<u>Noninfectious</u>: DM, toxins, cavernous sinus thrombosis, glaucoma, brain tumor, intracranial aneurysm
Papilledema	<u>Infectious</u>: meningitis (bacterial, fungal, TB, viral, etc.)
	<u>Noninfectious</u>: pseudotumor cerebri, hypercarbia, brain tumor, DM, subarachnoid bleed, SLE, drugs, central retinal artery occlusion, cavernous sinus thrombosis, hypertensive encephalopathy

Table 9.16 Neurological Abnormalities *(cont'd)*

Finding	Causes
Mononeuritis multiplex	<u>Infectious</u>: leprosy, Lyme disease, HIV
	<u>Noninfectious</u>: DM, amyloidosis, sarcoidosis, lymphomatoid granulomatosis, vasculitis
Transverse myelitis	<u>Infectious</u>: HIV, HTLV-1, EBV, CMV, VZV, HSV, polio, rabies, TB, EV 71, epidural abscess, typhus, brucellosis, shistosomiasis, Lyme disease, syphilis, toxoplasmosis, M. pneumoniae
	<u>Noninfectious</u>: MS, malignancies, vaccines, SLE, sarcoidosis
Guillain-Barré syndrome	<u>Infectious</u>: influenza, Campylobacter jejuni, CMV, EBV, VZV, M. pneumoniae, EV 71, Zika virus (ZIKV), brucellosis
	<u>Noninfectious</u>: influenza vaccine
Flaccid paralysis (acute)	<u>Infectious</u>: polio, WNE, CMV, VZV, rabies, botulism, JE, EV 71, EV D68, Powassan virus (POWV), chikungunya fever, brucellosis
	<u>Noninfectious</u>: CVA, tick bite paralysis, hypocalcemic periodic paralysis
Seizures	<u>Infectious</u>: Brain abscess, subdural empyema, Listeria, neurocysticenosis, ABM, JC disease, PML, VLM, CSD, cerebral malaria, HSV-1, COVID-19
	<u>Noninfectious</u>: Seizure disorders, brain tumor, CNS metatases
Hemiplegia/ hemiparesis	<u>Infectious</u>: SBE, subdural empyema, brain abscess, JE, POWV, brucellosis, post-VZV, Post-dengue, COVID-19
	<u>Noninfectious</u>: TIA, CVA, CNS malignancies, CNS vasculitis, migraine, GCA/TA, SLE, neurosarcoidosis, birth control pills, protein C/S, factor V Leiden deficiency, antiphospholipid syndrome (APS)

Table 9.17 WBC Abnormalities

Finding	Causes
Leukocytosis	<u>Infectious</u>: most acute bacterial infections
	<u>Noninfectious</u>: most acute noninfectious disease disorders, any major stress, steroids, drug fever, daptomycin
Leukopenia	<u>Infectious</u>: miliary TB, typhoid/enteric fever, malaria, babesiosis, dengue fever, chickungunya fever, Zika virus, Mayaro virus (MAYV), tularemia, brucellosis, kala-azar, psittacosis, viral hepatitis, yellow fever, EBV, CMV, HHV-6, VZV, influenza, Colorado tick fever, campylobacter, histoplasmosis, relapsing fever, WNE, VEE, B. miyamotoi (BMD), Heartland virus (HRTV), ehrlichiosis/anaplasmosis, SARS, MERS, COVID-19, adenovirus, SFTS, leptospirosis, HPS
	<u>Noninfectious</u>: drugs, pre/acute leukemias, Felty's syndrome, Gaucher's disease, splenomegaly, pernicious anemia, SLE, cyclic neutropenia, severe combined immunodeficiency disease (SCID), Chediak-Higashi syndrome, Kikuchi's disease, sarcoidosis. Some antibiotics: β-lactams, cephalosporins, sulfonamides, vancomycin, aztreonam/avibactam ganciclovir, acyclovir, amphotericin B.

Table 9.17 WBC Abnormalities *(cont'd)*

Finding	Causes
Relative lymphocytosis	<u>Infectious:</u> Whipple's disease, acute infection (convalescence), TB, brucellosis, pertussis, tularemia, 2° syphilis, histoplasmosis, EBV, CMV, HHV-6, mumps, viral hepatitis, rubella, VZV, kala-azar, toxoplasmosis, RMSF, chickungunya fever, typhoid/enteric fever (non-S. typhi > S. typhi), MERS, coxsackie
	<u>Noninfectious:</u> ALL, CLL, lymphomas, carcinomas, multiple myeloma, RA, Hashimoto's thyroiditis, myxedema, adrenal insufficiency, thyrotoxicosis, vasculitis, Dilantin (DPH), p-aminosalicylic acid (PAS), serum sickness
Relative lymphopenia	<u>Infectious:</u> CMV, HHV-6, HHV-8, HIV, miliary TB, Legionella, typhoid/enteric fever (S. typhi > non-S. typhi), Q fever, brucellosis, malaria, babesiosis, influenza, adenovirus, RMSF, histoplasmosis, Toscana virus (TOSV), dengue fever, chickungunya fever, ehrlichiosis/anaplasmosis, parvovirus B19, HPS, WNE, viral hepatitis (early), Whipple's disease, SARS, MERS, COVID-19
	<u>Noninfectious:</u> cytoxic drugs, steroids, sarcoidosis, SLE, lymphoma, RA, radiation, Wiskott-Aldrich syndrome, severe combine immunodeficiency disease (SCID), common variable immune deficiency (CVID), Di George's syndrome, Nezelof's syndrome, intestinal lymphangiectasia, ataxia-telangiectasia, constrictive pericarditis, tricuspid regurgitation, Kawasaki's disease, idiopathic CD_4 cytopenia, acute/chronic renal failure, hemodialysis, myasthenia gravis, celiac disease, cirrhosis, coronary bypass, Wegener's granulomatosis, CHF, acute pancreatitis, carcinomas (terminal)
Relative monocytosis	<u>Infectious:</u> TB, SBE, RMSF, diphtheria, histoplasmosis, brucellosis, pertussis, kala-azar, 2° syphilis, malaria, typhoid/enteric fever, babesiosis, EBV, CMV, influenza, Zika virus, (ZIKV) influenza A, recovery from infection
	<u>Noninfectious:</u> sarcoidosis, myeloproliferative disorders (↑ pre-AMI), lymphomas, Gaucher's disease, RE, UC, celiac disease, RA, SLE, PAN, TA, hyposplenism, post-splenectomy, pre-AML
Atypical lymphocytes[†]	<u>Infectious:</u> EBV* (Downey type I), CMV* (Downey type II), HHV-6 (Downey type III), Castleman's disease (MCD), viral hepatitis, mumps, measles, rubella, VZV, HSV, toxoplasmosis, brucellosis, pertussis, arboviral hemorrhagic fevers, malaria, dengue, babesiosis, ehrlichiosis/anaplasmosis, coxsackie
	<u>Noninfectious:</u> drug fever, Kikuchi's disease
Immunoblasts	<u>Infectious:</u> HPS
	<u>Noninfectious:</u> lymphomas

Table 9.17 WBC Abnormalities *(cont'd)*

Finding	Causes
Eosinophilia	<u>Infectious</u>: trichinosis, echinococcosis, fascioliasis, paragonimiasis, taeniasis, Strongyloides stercoralis, hookworm, filariasis, loiasis, schistosomiasis, Toxocara, histoplasmosis, coccidioidomycosis, oncocerciasis, filariasis, ascariasis, hydatid cyst (rupture), gnathostomiasis, angiostrongyliasis, clonorchis/opisthorchis cysticercosis, Cystoisosporiasis (Isospora) belli, Dientamoeba fragilis, scarlet fever, leprosy
	<u>Noninfectious</u>: drug fever, asthma, dermatitis herpetiformis, pemphigus vulgaris, eczema, hay fever/allergic rhinitis, psoriasis, atopic dermatitis, mycosis fungoides, myeloproliferative disorders (MPDs), polycythemia vera, CML, eosinophilic leukemia, eosinophilic gastritis, acute leukemias, sickle cell anemia, lymphomas, malignancies, Churg-Strauss granulomatosis, urticaria, hyper IgE syndrome (Job's syndrome), Sweet's syndrome, bronchopulmonary aspergillosis (BPA), angioneurotic edema, serum sickness, eosinophilia-myalgia syndrome, dermatomyositis, PAN, allergic vasculitis, Loffler's syndrome, pulmonary infiltrates eosinophilia (PIE) syndrome, Loffler's endocarditis, Addison's disease, sarcoidosis, Wegener's granulomatosis, Goodpasture's syndrome, UC, RE, Wiskott-Aldrich syndrome, IgA deficiency, allergic vasculitis, Kimura's disease, peritoneal dialysis, radiation
Eosinopenia	<u>Infectious</u>: typhoid/enteric fevers, kala-azar, COVID-19
	<u>Noninfectious</u>: steroids, immunosupressive drugs
Basophilia	<u>Infectious</u>: smallpox, chickenpox (VZV)
	<u>Noninfectious</u>: pre-leukemias, acute leukemias, lymphomas, myeloproliferative disorders (MPDs), post-splenectomy
WBC inclusions	<u>Infectious</u>: ehrlichiosis/anaplasmosis (morula: HGA > HME)
	<u>Noninfectious</u>: staining artifacts

*   May have > 20% atypical lymphocytes.
†   Not seen with malignancies. Abnormal lymphocytes (morphologically monotonous) seen with leukemias.

Table 9.18 RBC Abnormalities

Finding	Causes
Schistocytes (microangiopathic hemolytic anemia)	<u>Infectious</u>: meningococcemia (DIC)
	<u>Noninfectious</u>: DIC (due to any cause), TTP, hemolytic uremic syndrome (HUS), "Waring Blender" syndrome (prosthetic valve), malignant hypertension

Table 9.18 RBC Abnormalities (cont'd)

Finding	Causes
Spherocytes	Infectious: gas gangrene, Castleman's disease (MCD)
	Noninfectious: autoimmune hemolytic anemias, hereditary spherocytosis, severe transfusion reactions, severe burns, cirrhosis
Target cells	Infectious: none
	Noninfectious: post-splenectomy, iron deficiency anemia, cirrhosis, hemoglobulin S or C, thalassemia
RBC inclusions	Infectious: malaria (ring forms, RBC pigment), babesiosis (ring forms, no RBC pigment, "Maltese crosses"/tetrads)
	Noninfectious: Cabot's rings (severe hemolytic anemia, pernicious anemia), Heinz bodies (GGPD deficiency, drug induced, hereditary anemias), Pappenheimer bodies (thalassemia, sideroblastic anemias, lead poisoning), artifacts
Howell-Jolly bodies[†]	Infectious: fulimant pneumococcal sepsis
	Noninfectious: asplenia/hyposplenism*, congenital asplenia, splenectomy, splenic infarcts, splenic neoplasms, megaloblastic anemias, thalassemia, steroids
Hemophago-cytosis	Infectious: HIV, HSV, EBV, CMV, adenovirus, parvovirus B19, malaria, babesiosis, toxoplasmosis, kala-azar, histoplasmosis, cryptococcosis, disseminated candidiasis, typhoid/enteric fever, syphilis, listeria, SBE, Q fever, leprosy, TB, brucellosis, Castleman's disease (MCD)
	Noninfectious: histiocytosis X (eosinophilic granuloma, Langerhan's cell histiocytosis), myeloproliferative disorders (MPDs), SLE, sarcoidosis, RA, lymphomas, acute leukemias, multiple myeloma, Chediak-Higashi syndrome, Dilantin (DPH), familial hemophagocytic histiocytosis
Anemia (acute)	Infectious: Oroya fever, gas gangrene, malaria, babesiosis, M. pneumonlae, CMV
	Noninfectious: ITP, "Waring blender" syndrome (prosthetic heart valve), hemorrhagic/necrotic pancreatitis, hemorrage, drug induced (artesunate)

* Chronic alcoholism, amyloidosis, chronic active hepatitis, IgA deficiency, intestinal lymphangectasia, myeloproliferative disorders, Waldenstrom's macroglobulinemia, NHL, celiac disease, RA, UC, thyroiditis, systemic mastocytosis, sickle cell disease, Fanconi's syndrome, Sezary's syndrome.

† Also "pitted/pocked" RBCs.

Table 9.19 Platelet Abnormalities

Finding	Causes
Thrombocyto-penia	<u>Infectious:</u> acute/severe bacterial infections, measles, rubella, dengue, arboviral hemorrhagic fevers, EBV, CMV, VZV, mumps, influenza, adenovirus, Toscana virus (TOSV), typhus, RMSF, WNE, ehrlichiosis/anaplasmosis, B. miyamotoi (BMD), diphtheria, malaria, babesiosis, trypanosomiasis, TSS, histoplasmosis, kala-azar, HIV, miliary TB, relapsing fever, HPS, brucellosis, campylobacter, SARS, MERS, COVID-19, Zika virus (ZIKV), Mayaro virus (MAYV), R. parkeri, R. phillipi, bourbon virus (Thogotovirus), heartland virus (HRTV)
	<u>Noninfectious:</u> drugs, DIC, fat emboli syndrome, TTP, ITP, hemolytic uremic syndrome (HUS), pre/acute/leukemias, lymphomas, carcinomas, myeloproliferative disorders (MPDs), multiple myeloma, Gaucher's disease, cirrhosis, hemodialysis, some antibiotics (vancomycin, linezolid, rifampin, quinolones, cefepime, piperacillin, piperacillin/tazobactam, meropenem/vaborbactam)
Thrombocytosis	<u>Infectious:</u> miliary TB, chronic infections (e.g., osteomyelitis, abscess), SBE, Q fever, M. pneumoniae
	<u>Noninfectious:</u> Malignancies, myeloproliferative disorders, post-splenectomy, lymphomas, Wegener's granulomatosis, JRA, TA, PAN, Kawasaki's disease, anemia (hemolytic, iron deficiency), some antibiotics (fosfomycin, aztreonam, aztreonam/avibactam, ceftriaxone, oral cephalosporins, carbapenems, β-lactam/β-lactamase inhibitor combinations, miconazole), iron therapy

Table 9.20 Pancytopenia

Finding	Causes
Pancytopenia	<u>Infectious:</u> miliary TB, brucellosis, kala-azar, histoplasmosis, ehrlichiosis/anaplasmosis, POWV, parvovirus B19, HBV, CMV, EBV, HIV
	<u>Noninfectious:</u> myeloproliferative disorders (MPDs), drugs, malignancies, Chediak-Higashi syndrome, megaloblastic anemias, Gaucher's disease, hypersplenism, sarcoidosis, SLE, paroxysmal nocturnal hemoglobinuria (PNH), myelophistic anemias, leukemias, lymphoma

Table 9.21 Serum Test Abnormalities

Finding	Causes
Erythrocyte Sedimentation Rate (ESR) *highly elevated (≥100 mm/hr)*	<u>Infectious:</u> SBE, osteomyelitis, abscess, CAP (Legionnaire's disease, Q fever, S. pneumoniae), non-pulmonary TB, babesiosis, COVID-19 <u>Noninfectious:</u> malignancies, rheumatic disorders, vasculitis, drug fever, PMR/GCA, uremia/chronic renal failure, cirrhosis, Kawasaki's disease, Sweet's syndrome, pulmonary emboli/infarction
low/subnormal	<u>Infectious:</u> trichinosis, CFS, ehrlichiosis/anaplasmosis <u>Noninfectious:</u> severe anemia, cachexia, massive hepatic necrosis, DIC, polycythemia vera, sickle cell anemia, CHF

Table 9.21 Serum Test Abnormalities *(cont'd)*

Finding	Causes
SPEP (polyclonal gammopathy)	<u>Infectious</u>: HIV, malaria, kala-azar, LGV, rat bite fever, Toxocara canis/cati (VLM), Q fever (chronic), Castleman's disease (MCD) <u>Noninfectious</u>: SLE, PAN, cirrhosis, CAH, sarcoidosis, atrial myxoma, Takayasu's arteritis, Rosai-Dorfman disease
SPEP (monoclonal gammopathy)	<u>Infectious</u>: CMV, kala-azar, typhoid/enteric fever, Castleman's disease (MCD) <u>Noninfectious</u>: multiple myeloma, Waldenström's macroglobulinemia, Schnitzler's syndrome, MGUS
↑ ferritin levels[†] *acute*	<u>Infectious</u>: legionnaire's disease, WNE, EBV, CMV, toxoplasmosis, MSSA/MRSA ABE, malaria, babesiosis, ehlichiosis/anaplasmosis, Zika virus (ZIKV), arboviral hemorrhagic fevers, COVID-19 <u>Noninfectious</u>: Kawasaki's disease, Rosai-Dorfman disease, hemophagocytic syndrome (due to any cause), shock liver
chronic	<u>Infectious</u>: HIV, TB, filariasis <u>Noninfectious</u>: malignancies (preleukemias, lymphomas, multiple myeloma, hepatomas, liver/CNS metastases), myeloproliferative disorders (MPDs), RA, adult Still's disease, SLE, TA, Kawasaki's disease, chronic renal failure, hemodialysis, liver transplants, hemochromatosis, cirrhosis, α-1 antitrypsin deficiency, CAH, chronic HCV, cholestatic jaundice, macrophage activation syndrome (MAS), sickle cell anemia, multiple blood transfusions, anemia of chronic disease
↑ cold agglutinins	<u>Infectious</u>: Mycoplasma pneumoniae, EBV, CMV, mumps, measles, malaria, Coxsackie, Q fever, HIV, HCV, influenza, adenovirus, trypanosomiasis, syphilis, scarlet fever, ADV <u>Noninfectious</u>: lymphomas, CLL, CML, multiple myeloma, Waldenstrom's macroglobulinemia, cold agglutinin disease, paroxysmal nocturnal hemoglobinuria (PNH), SLE, Rosai-Dorfman disease
Monospot test (false +)	<u>Infectious</u>: CMV, HSV, HHV-6, malaria, dengue, babesiosis, toxoplasmosis, brucellosis, Mediterranean spotted fever (MSF), rubella, mumps, viral hepatitis, Lyme disease, HIV <u>Noninfectious</u>: SLE, sarcoidosis, AML, drugs, idiopathic
↑ CPK	<u>Infectious</u>: influenza, legionnaire's disease, leptospirosis, myocarditis, RMSF, COVID-19, ADV <u>Noninfectious</u>: malignant hyperthermia, rhabdomyolysis (any cause), MI, seizures, skeletal muscle trauma, SLE, drugs: statins

Table 9.21 Serum Test Abnormalities (cont'd)

Finding	Causes
↑ Lactate dehydrogenase (LDH)	<u>Infectious:</u> malaria, babesiosis, ehrlichiosis/anaplasmosis, viridans streptococcal SBE, amebic liver abscess, PCP, histoplasmosis, disseminated TB, toxoplasmosis, HPS, Oroya fever, gas gangrene, viral myocarditis, rubella, measles, viral hepatitis, CAP/NP, dengue, arboviral hemorrhagic fevers, trichinosis, SARS, MERS, adenovirus, CMV, EBV, influenza, Heartland virus (HRTV), COVID-19 <u>Noninfectious:</u> hemolyzed blood, hemolytic anemia, malignancies, pernicious anemia, megaloblastic anemia, pulmonary emboli, MI, renal infarction, muscle injury, liver injury, DIC, SLE pneumonitis, adult Still's disease, "Waring blender" syndrome (prosthetic heart valve), hemorrhagic/necrotic pancreatitis
↑ Procalcitonin levels (PCT)	<u>Infectious:</u> bacterial pneumonias (CAP, NHAP, NP), legionnaire's disease, bacteremias (Gram – > Gram +), TB, ABM, fungal pneumonias (except PCP), viral hepatitis, toxoplasmosis, osteomyelitis, SBE*, malaria (P. falciparum), B. recurrentis (LRF), COVID-19 <u>Noninfectious:</u> renal insufficiency, alcoholic hepatitis, acute hepatitis, lung cancer (small cell), thyroid cancer, surgery, trauma, burns, cardiogenic shock, Goodpasture's syndrome shock, GVHD, peritoneal dialysis (PD), hypotension, hemorrhagic/necrotic pancreatitis, normal variant (elderly) BMT, febrile neutropenia, drug fever, immunosuppression/steroids, OKT$_3$ therapy
↑ Lactate	<u>Infections:</u> sepsis (bacterial), septic shock, malaria, cholera <u>Noninfectious:</u> cardiogenic shock, hypovolemic shock, hypoperfusion, hypoxia, respiratory insufficiency/failure, renal insufficiency, hepatic insufficiency, hemorrhage, Ringer's lactate, metabolic acidosis (↑ anion gap), seizures, pulmonary emboli, diabetes mellitus, malignancies (leukemias, lymphomas, solid tumors), drugs (salicylates, methanol, ethylene glycol, INH, cyanide, metformin, acetaminophen, lactulose, ethanol, theophylline, niacin, cocaine, methemoglobinemia, severe anemia, carbon monoxide, short bowel syndrome (jejunoileal bypass)
↑ Teichoic acid antibody titer (≥1:4)	<u>Infections:</u> MSSA/MRSA ABE, MSSA/MRSA abscesses, MSSA/MRSA osteomyelitis (chronic/acute) <u>Noninfectious:</u> none

Fungal serum tests	Candida	Aspergillus	Histo	Blasto	PCP	Crypto	Fusaria	Zygomycetes	Penicillium
β 1, 3 D–glucan§ (BG)	+	+	+	–	+	–	+	–	–
Aspergillus galactomannan (GM)	–	+	+	–	–	–	+	–	+

* Viridans streptococci.

† Not an acute phase reactant when highly/persistently ↑ > 2 × normal.

§ False + BG with P. aeruginosa bacteremia, fungal derived antibiotics (amoxicillin/clavulanate, piperacillin/tazobactam), platelet transfusions, IVIG, HD (with cellulose membranes), high serum protein levels (albumin).

Table 9.22 Liver Test Abnormalities

Finding	Causes
↑ Alkaline phosphatase (AP) *mildly elevated*	<u>Infectious</u>: legionnaire's disease, viral hepatitis, liver abscess, EBV, CMV, Q fever, syphilis (2° or tertiary), TSS, hepatic candidiasis, clonorchiasis, ehrlichiosis/anaplasmosis, diphtheria, malaria, trypanosomiasis, histoplasmosis, HIV, miliary TB, relapsing fever, HPS
	<u>Noninfectious</u>: drugs, DIC, fat emboli syndrome, TTP, ITP, hemolytic uremic syndrome, pre/acute/leukemias, lymphomas, carcinomas, myeloproliferative disorders (MPDs), multiple myeloma, Gaucher's disease, cirrhosis, post-hepatic obstruction, alcoholic hepatitis, pregnancy, bone growth (children), osteomalacia, rickets, hyperthyroidism, thyroiditis, UC, drug fever, hepatoma, liver metastases, lymphoma, Erdheim-Chester disease (ECD), mastocytosis, Schnitzler's syndrome, TA, hypernephroma (RCC), PAN, normal variant (elderly)
moderately/ highly elevated	<u>Infectious</u>: liver abscess
	<u>Noninfectious</u>: PBC, post-hepatic obstruction, post-necrotic cirrhosis, Paget's disease, osteogenic sarcoma, hepatoma, TA, bone fractures, tigecycline
↑ Serum transaminases (SGOT/AST, SGPT/ALT) *mildly elevated*	<u>Infectious</u>: legionnaire's disease, psittacosis, Q fever, relapsing fever, (Borrelia), brucellosis, TSS, RMSF, babesiosis, ehrlichiosis/anaplasmosis, B. miyamotoi (BMO), liver abscess, syphilis (2° or tertiary), shigellosis, clonorchiasis, EBV, CMV, HSV-1, VZV (disseminated), HHV-6, anicteric viral hepatitis, bourbon virus (Thogotovirus), gonococcemia, malaria, Gram negative bacteremia, adenovirus, dengue, heartland virus (HRTV), ECHO 9, Coxsackie A_9/B_5, COVID-19
	<u>Noninfectious</u>: drug fever, alcoholic cirrhosis, (SGOT/AST : SGPT/ALT = 2:1), CHF, infarction (myocardial, cerebral, pulmonary), pancreatitis, intrahepatic cholestasis, sickle cell disease, amyloidosis, delirium tremens, intravascular hemolysis, UC, eosinophilia-myalgia syndrome, Kawasaki's disease, adult Still's disease, drugs (statins, INH, RIF)
highly elevated	<u>Infectious</u>: viral hepatitis, HSV hepatitis, yellow fever, arboviral hemorrhagic fevers
	<u>Noninfectious</u>: shock liver, rhabdomyolysis (SGOT/AST 2:1 SGPT/ALT), exercise, drugs (statins, INH, RIF)
↑ Total bilirubin	<u>Infectious</u>: legionnaire's disease, gonococcemia, liver abscess, yellow fever, viral hepatitis, EBV, CMV, pneumococcal bacteremia, malaria
	<u>Noninfectious</u>: hemolysis, Gilbert's syndrome, cirrhosis, alcoholic hepatitis, carcinoma (pancreatic, biliary), choledocholithiasis, amyloidosis, sickle cell disease, Rotor's syndrome, α-1 antitrypsin deficiency, hepatic vein thrombosis, autoimmune (lupoid) hepatitis, hemachromatosis
↑ GGT (GGTP)	<u>Infectious</u>: acute viral hepatitis, EBV
	<u>Noninfectious</u>: cirrhosis, alcoholic hepatitis, PBC, fatty liver, CAH, hepatoma, liver metastases, pancreatitis (acute), myocardial infarction (acute), breast cancer, lung cancer, prostate cancer, melanoma, hypernephroma (RCC), obstructive jaundice, cholestasis, CAH

Table 9.23 Rheumatic Test Abnormalities

Finding	Causes
↑ Rheumatoid factors (RF)	<u>Infectious:</u> SBE, TB, syphilis, kala-azar, EBV, typhoid/enteric fever, HBV, HCV, chickungunya fever, malaria
	<u>Noninfectious:</u> cirrhosis, CAH, ITP, silicosis, asbestosis, asthma, Wegener's granulomatosis, pulmonary fibrosis, Behçet's disease, SLE, RA, Sjögren's, dermatomyositis, sarcoidosis, PBC, B-cell malignancies, normal variant
↑ Anti-nuclear antibody titers (ANA)	<u>Infectious:</u> HIV, EBV, CMV, TB, SBE, leprosy, kala-azar, malaria
	<u>Noninfectious:</u> SLE, scleroderma, MCTD, CREST syndrome, RA, autoimmune (lupoid) hepatitis, CAH, dermatomyositis, subacute thyroiditis, ITP, PBC, multiple sclerosis, sarcoidosis, Wegener's granulomatosis, myasthenia gravis, ESRD on HD, normal variant (elderly)
↑ Double stranded DNA (DS-DNA)	<u>Infectious:</u> CMV, EBV
	<u>Noninfectious:</u> SLE, RA, CAH, PBC
↑ Angiotensin-converting enzyme levels (ACE)	<u>Infectious:</u> TB, leprosy, coccidiomycosis, viral hepatitis
	<u>Noninfectious:</u> sarcoidosis, allergic alveolitis, hyperparathyroidism hyperthyroidism, PBC, Gaucher's disease, DM, ESRD, amyloidosis, multiple myeloma, lymphoma, cirrhosis, psoriasis, silicosis, asbestosis, berylliosis
↑ c-ANCA	<u>Infectious:</u> viridans streptococcal SBE, S. bovis SBE, bartonella SBE, chromomycosis, aspergillosis, amebiasis, legionnaire's disease, leptospirosis, HIV
	<u>Noninfectious:</u> crescentic GMN, Sweet's syndrome, microscopic polyangitis (MPA), PAN, UC, RE, SLE, Churg-Strauss granulomatosis, Wegener's granulomatosis, HSP, TA, Kawasaki's disease, sarcoidosis
↑ Anti-smooth muscle antibodies (ASM)	<u>Infectious:</u> Q fever, HCV (chronic), EBV, typhoid/enteric fever
	<u>Noninfectious:</u> autoimmune (lupoid) hepatitis, Wilson's disease, PBC, TA, normal variant (elderly)

Table 9.24 Urinary Abnormalities

Finding	Causes
Pyuria*§	<u>Infectious:</u> TB, leptospirosis, brucellosis, TSS, diphtheria, candida, GC, trichomonas, cystitis, pyelonephritis, prostatitis, acute urethral syndrome, partially treated UTI, medullary abscess, chlamydia/mycoplasma NGU, balanitis, acute appendicitis, St.LE.
	<u>Noninfectious:</u> interstitial nephritis, GU inflammation, strenuous exercise, SLE, calculi, bladder tumors, chronic interstitial cystitis, RE, diverticulitis, Kawasaki's disease, sarcoidosis

*   Gross pus suggests ruptured renal abscess.
§   WBC casts suggest SLE, nephritis, or acute pyelonephritis.

Table 9.24 Urinary Abnormalities *(cont'd)*

Finding	Causes
Hematuria *gross*	<u>Infectious</u>: ABE (renal septic emboli), malaria (P. falciparum), yellow fever, adenoviral cystitis (type 11), BKV (transplants)
	<u>Noninfectious</u>: renal malignancy, bladder malignancy, BPH, papillary necrosis (DM), trauma
microscopic	<u>Infectious</u>: SBE, renal TB, schistosomiasis (S. hematobium), S. saprophyticus, HPS, legionnaire's disease, Q fever, BKV (transplants), EBV
	<u>Noninfectious</u>: trauma, BPH, prostatitis, malignancy, malignant hypertension, PAN, drug reactions, calculi, urethral stricture, renal vein thrombosis, hydronephrosis, polycystic kidney disease, malakoplakia, strenuous exercise, renal infarction, sarcoidosis
Proteinuria	<u>Infectious</u>: TB, HBV, syphilis, malaria (black water fever), brucellosis, SBE, chronic pyelonephritis, leprosy, shistosomiasis, any acute infection
	<u>Noninfectious</u>: post-streptococcal GMN, malignant hypertension, ATN, amyloidosis, sickle cell disease, polycystic kidney disease, scleroderma, sarcoidosis, PAN, Wegener's granulomatosis, Goodpasture's syndrome, multiple myeloma, lymphomas, RCC, renal trauma, strenuous exercise
Urinary pH *alkaline*	<u>Infectious</u>: Corynebacterium urealyticum, klebsiella (rare), proteus, providencia, S. saprophyticus, Ureaplasma urealyticum
	<u>Noninfectious</u>: systemic alkalosis, postprandial "alkaline tide," alkalinization therapy, old urine, vegetarian diet
acidic	<u>Infectious</u>: TB
	<u>Noninfectious</u>: acidification therapy, systemic acidosis, ketosis
↓ Specific gravity (1.023 – 1.030)	<u>Infectious</u>: pyelonephritis[†]
	<u>Noninfectious</u>: diabetes insipidus, tubo-interstitial renal diseases, sickle cell disease
Nitrite positive	<u>Infectious</u>: most uropathogens**
	<u>Noninfectious</u>: none
Leukocyte esterase[‡‡]	<u>Infectious</u>: acute cystitis, acute pyelonephritis
	<u>Noninfectious</u>: inflammation anywhere in the upper/lower GU tract

† Cystitis is associated with a normal specific gravity. The transient decrease in specific gravity of pyelonephritis corrects to normal following effective treatment.

** Negative urinary nitrite occurs with group B streptococci, group D enterococci, (VSE/VRE) S. saprophyticus, S. aureus, Acinetobacter sp., Gardnerella sp., Corynebacterium urealyticum, Burkholderia sp., Pseudomonas sp., Candida sp.

‡ ≥ 5 WBCs/hpf = positive.

Table 9.24 Urinary Abnormalities *(cont'd)*

Finding	Causes
Eosinophiluria‡	<u>Infectious</u>: Shistosoma hematobium
	<u>Noninfectious</u>: cholesterol emboli syndrome, HSP, drug induced interstital nephritis, renal allograft rejection
Myoglobinuria (2° to rhabdomyolysis)	<u>Infectious</u>: legionnaire's disease, gas gangrene, leptospirosis, Vibrio vulnificus, listeria, S. aureus, group A streptococci, group B streptococci, S. pneumoniae, tularemia, typhoid/enteric fever, echovirus, Coxsackie, influenza, adenovirus, EBV, CMV, HSV, VZV, Heartland virus (HRTV), HIV
	<u>Noninfectious</u>: crush injury, excessive exercise, MI, seizures, malignant hyperthermia, dermatomyositis, burns, polymyositis, SLE, diabetic ketoacidosis, McArdle's syndrome, drugs (statins, alcohol, cocaine, heroin, PCP, neuroleptics, amphetamines, ethylene glycol)
Chyluria	<u>Infectious</u>: W. bancrofti
	<u>Noninfectious</u>: abdominal or chest lymphatic obstruction

‡ ≥ 5 WBCs = positive.

Table 9.25 Pleural Fluid Abnormalities

Pleural Fluid	Causes
↓ Glucose	<u>Infectious</u>: TB, bacterial, cryptococcosis, coccidiomycosis, mycoplasma, empyema
	<u>Noninfectious</u>: carcinoma, rheumatoid lung, lymphoma, esophageal rupture, parapneumonic effusion
↑ Protein	<u>Infectious</u>: TB
	<u>Noninfectious</u>: carcinoma, lymphoma, rheumatoid lung
↑ Amylase	<u>Infectious</u>: None
	<u>Noninfectious</u>: pancreatitis/pseudocyst, adenocarcinoma, esophageal rupture
↑ adenosine deaminase (ADA) levels	<u>Infectious</u>: TB, Legionnaire's disease, Q fever, brucellosis
	<u>Noninfectious</u>: SLE, RA, CLL, mesothelioma, lymphoma
PMNs	<u>Infectious</u>: bacteria, cryptococcosis, coccidiomycosis, empyema, TB (early)
	<u>Noninfectious</u>: pancreatitis, subdiaphragmatic abscess (sympathetic effusion), CHF, idiopathic
Lymphocytes	<u>Infectious</u>: TB
	<u>Noninfectious</u>: carcinoma, lymphoma, rheumatoid lung, SLE

Table 9.26 CSF Abnormalities

Finding	Causes
RBCs in CSF	<u>Infectious</u>: listeria, leptospirosis[†], TB, amebic meningoencephalitis, HSV, POWV, anthrax meningitis
	<u>Noninfectious</u>: traumatic tap, CNS bleed/tumor
Cloudy CSF with negative Gram stain	<u>Infectious</u>: Neisseria meningitidis, Streptococcus pneumoniae, EEE
	<u>Noninfectious</u>: None
CSF with negative Gram stain and predominantly PMNs/decreased glucose	<u>Infectious</u>: PTBM, listeria, HSV, TB (early), parameningeal infection, emboli secondary to SBE, amebic meningoencephalitis, CNS syphilis (early)
	<u>Noninfectious</u>: sarcoidosis, adult Still's disease, posterior-fossa syndrome/intracranial hemorrhage
CSF with negative Gram stain and predominantly *lymphocytes/ normal glucose*	<u>Infectious</u>: PTBM, viral meningitis, Lyme disease, HIV, leptospirosis[†], RMSF, parameningeal infection, TB, fungi, parasitic meningitis
	<u>Noninfectious</u>: sarcoidosis, meningeal carcinomatosis
lymphocytes/ decreased glucose	<u>Infectious</u>: PTBM, CNS TB, CNS fungi, LCM, mumps, enteroviral meningitis, listeria, leptospirosis[†], syphilis
	<u>Noninfectious</u>: neurosarcoidosis, meningeal carcinomatosis
↑ CSF lactic acid levels	<u>Infectious</u>: **< 4 nm/L**, Not acute bacterial meningitis (ABM); **< 4–6 nm/L**, TB, RBCs, HSV, partially treated bacterial meningitis (PTBM), parameningeal infections; **> 6 nm/L**, acute bacterial meningitis (ABM), cerebral malaria (severe)
	<u>Noninfectious</u>: **< 6 nm/L**, neurosarcoidosis, CNS SLE, cerebral anoxia, hepatic encephalopathy; meningeal carcinomatosis; CNS lymphomas, CNS tumor, intracranial hemorrhage, post-craniotomy with EVD
Highly ↑ CSF Protein	<u>Infectious</u>: brain abscess, CNS TB (with subarachnoid block), viral meningitis, viral encephalitis
	<u>Noninfectious</u>: brain tumor, MS, demyelinating CNS diseases
↑ CSF adenosine deaminase (ADA) levels	<u>Infectious</u>: CNS TB, listeria, ABM, neurobrucellosis
	<u>Noninfectious</u>: SAH, CNS malignancy
CSF plasma cells	<u>Infectious</u>: CNS TB, WNE, VZV, HIV, neuroborreliosis, neurosyphilis
	<u>Noninfectious</u>: CNS lymphoma, MS, CNS myeloma, ADEM

[†] Leptospirosis is the only infectious disease with the CSF bilirubin > serum bilirubin.

Table 9.26 CSF Abnormalities *(cont'd)*

Finding	Causes
CSF eosinophils	<u>Infectious</u>: coccidiomycosis, neurocysticercosis, gnathostomiasis, angiostrongyliasis, baylisascariasis, shistosomiasis, paragonamiasis, Toxocara (VLM)
	<u>Noninfectious</u>: CNS lymphomas, CNS leukemias, V-A/VP shunts, myelography (contrast material), CNS vasculitis, drugs (NSAIDs, TMP–SMX), intrathecal drugs

Table 9.27 CSF Diagnostic Criteria for EVD associated ABM

<u>Infectious:</u>

EVD Associated ABM

- <u>Highly elevated CSF lactic acid level</u> (> 6 nmol/L)

    plus

- <u>Marked CSF pleocytosis</u> (> 50 WBCs/hpf)

    plus

- <u>Positive CSF Gram stain</u> (with *same morphology* as the cultured neuropathogen)

    plus

- <u>Positive CSF culture with</u> (*same morphology* as the Gram stain of the neuropathogen)

EVD Associated CSF colonization

- < 4 CSF diagnostic criteria for EVD associated ABM

<u>Noninfectious:</u> CNS malignancy, ICH, SAH, post-craniotomy, brain trauma

LA = CSF lactic acid   ABM = acute bacterial meningitis   EVD = external-ventricular drain

REFERENCES

Bennett JE, Dolin R, Blaser MJ (eds). Mandell, Douglas, and Bennett's Principles and Practice of infectious Diseases (9th Ed), Elsevier Churchill Livingstone, 2019.

Bowden RA, Ljungman P, Snydman DR (eds). Transplant Infections (3rd Ed), Lippincott Williams & Wilkins, Philadelphia, PA, 2010.

Brandstetter R, Cunha BA, Karetsky M (eds). The Pneumonias. Mosby, Philadelphia, 1999.

Brusch, JL. Infective Endocarditis: Management in the Era of Intravascular Devices. Informa Healthcare, New York 2007.

Cohen J, Powderly WG, Opal S (Eds). Infectious Diseases (4th Ed). Elsevier, Philadelphia 2016.

Cunha BA (ed). Tick-Borne Infectious Diseases. Marcel Dekker, New York, 2005.

Cunha CB, Cunha BA (eds). Infectious Disease in Critical Care Medicine (4th Ed), CRC Press, New York, 2020.

Cunha CB, Schlossberg D (eds). Clinical Infections Diseases (3rd Ed), Cambridge University Press, London, 2020.

Farrar J (eds). Manson's Tropical Diseases (23rd Ed). Elsevier Saunders, London, 2014.

Gorbach SL, Bartlett JG, Blacklow NR (eds). Infectious Diseases (3rd Ed), Philadelphia, Lippincott, Williams & Wilkins, 2004.

Guerrant RL, Walker DH, Weller PF (eds). Tropical Infectious Disease: Principles, Pathogens & Practice (3rd Ed), Elsevier, Philadelphia, 2011.

Madkour MM (ed). Tuberculosis. Springer-Verlag, Berlin Germany, 2004.

Raoult D, Parola P. Rickettsial Diseases. Informa Healthcare, New York, 2007.

Chapter 10

Antibiotic Pearls & Pitfalls

Cheston B. Cunha, MD,

Burke A. Cunha, MD

PENICILLIN

- *Penicillin is expensive* because it is made by a single manufacturer.
- PRSP has been associated with TMP–SMX and macrolides, *not penicillin*.
- *Penicillin relatively inactive against VSE*, but is synergistic with gentamicin.

AMPICILLIN

- Unless treating serious systemic infections due to E. faecalis (VSE), *avoid using ampicillin. Ampicillin use results in increased E. coli resistance.*
- Remember ampicillin is the preferred drug to treat serious systemic infections caused by VSE but is *ineffective against nearly all E. faecium (VRE).*
- Because susceptibility is in part "concentration dependent," *do not assume that susceptibilities of ampicillin or amoxicillin are the same.* On a same dose basis, amoxicillin achieves twice the concentrations of ampicillin in body fluids (e.g., middle ear fluid, sinus fluid, bronchial fluid, urine).
- Remember that *unlike ampicillin, amoxicillin is infrequently associated with oral thrush or irritative diarrhea.*
- *Amoxicillin 1 gm (PO) q8h* can be used in ampicillin IV-to-PO switch programs since this dose *provides levels comparable to parenteral (IM) ampicillin.*

AMOXICILLIN/CLAVULANIC ACID

- Clavulanic acid is a beta-lactamase inhibitor which, when added to amoxicillin, restores its activity against beta-lactamase—producing strains of H. influenzae.
- *The newer preparations of amoxicillin/clavulanic acid result in less gastrointestinal symptoms and diarrhea* compared to older preparations with more clavulanate.
- *Ineffective against PRSP due to alterations in PBPs which are not β-lactamase mediated.*

ORAL ANTI-STAPHYLOCOCCAL PENICILLINS

- *Do not rely on oral anti-staphylococcal penicillins* such as dicloxacillin for methicillin-sensitive S. aureus (MSSA) infections since they *are erratically/poorly absorbed and not consistently effective.* When treating MSSA infections orally, a first generation cephalosporin (e.g., cephalexin) is preferable.
- *Dicloxacillin is poorly tolerated due to its metallic taste and belching.*

ORAL ANTI-PSEUDOMONAL PENICILLINS

- *Avoid using indanyl carbenicillin for P. aeruginosa UTIs due to the rapid development of resistance with P. aeruginosa.* Use other oral anti-P. aeruginosa agents for P. aeruginosa lower UTIs, e.g., doxycycline, levofloxacin, or fosfomycin.

PARENTERAL FIRST GENERATION CEPHALOSPORINS

- *Cefazolin has limited activity against H. influenzae.*
- Cefazolin remains *preferred therapy for skin infections due to group A streptococci or MSSA.*
- For treatment of biliary tract infections, cefazolin is active against E. coli and Klebsiella pneumoniae, but is *not active against E. faecalis* (VSE).
- *Cefazolin remains useful prophylaxis for cardiothoracic procedures in hospitals with low prevalence of MRSA.*
- For prophylaxis in orthopedic (THR), gynecologic, and bariatric surgery, 1 gm (IV) push is sufficient in obese patients. Since cefazolin is water soluble (V_d = 0.2 L/kg), increasing the dose to ≥ 2 gm or repeat intra-operative dosing doesn't increase adipose tissue levels. Furthermore, adipose tissue is not infected as a complication of these surgical procedures.

ORAL FIRST GENERATION CEPHALOSPORINS

- *Cephalexin is suboptimal for respiratory tract infections,* i.e., H. influenzae a likely pathogen (otitis media, sinusitis, AECB, community-acquired pneumonia) *since 1st GCs have limited H. influenzae activity.*
- For IV-to-PO switch programs and *cephalexin 1 gm (PO) q6h approximates the serum concentrations of parenteral (IM) cefazolin.*
- Oral 3rd GCs do not have the same degree of anti-S. aureus MSSA activity as cephalexin.

PARENTERAL SECOND GENERATION CEPHALOSPORINS

- Cefoxitin and cefotetan are useful for intra-abdominal infections.
- *Cefuroxime* offers no advantage for bacterial URIs over doxycycline, respiratory quinolones, or 3rd GCs and *does not prevent CNS "seeding" by S. pneumoniae or H. influenzae bacteremia secondary to CAP.*

ORAL SECOND GENERATION CEPHALOSPORINS

- *Oral second generation cephalosporins* include cefaclor, cefprozil, and cefuroxime are *used primarily to treat URIs.*
- *Cefaclor has limited ability to penetrate into respiratory secretions* limiting its efficacy in URIs.
- Among the oral second generation cephalosporins, *cefprozil has the greatest degree of penetration into respiratory secretions.*

PARENTERAL THIRD GENERATION CEPHALOSPORINS

- *Except for cefoperazone, 1st, 2nd, 3rd generation cephalosporins have no anti-E. faecalis (VSE) activity.*
- *Except for ceftriaxone,* third generation cephalosporins may cause C. difficile diarrhea. *Ceftriaxone is associated with non-C. difficile diarrhea* related to changes in colonic flora.
- *Ceftriaxone is associated with pseudo-biliary lithiasis.* Patients developing right upper quadrant pain on ceftriaxone should be suspected as having drug induced pseudo-biliary lithiasis.
- *For CNS infections, give third generation cephalosporins in "meningeal doses."*
- *The only third-generation cephalosporin associated with resistance is ceftazidime with P. aeruginosa.*
- *Ceftazidime predisposes to MDR P. aeruginosa, and increases MRSA prevalence.*
- *Ceftazidime is use associated with increased ESBL K. pneumoniae, E. coli, or Enterobacter agglomerans.*
- *Ceftazidime has little anti-MSSA activity.*
- 3rd GCs *without* anti-B. fragilis activity are *ceftazidime and ceftriaxone.*
- 3rd GCs *without* significant anti-P. aeruginosa activity are *cefotaxime, ceftizoxime, and ceftriaxone.*

ORAL THIRD GENERATION CEPHALOSPORINS

- Cefdinir, cefditoren, cefixime, cefpodoxime and ceftibuten are used for their aerobic anti-GNB activity.
- *The only 3rd GC with good anti-MSSA activity is cefpodoxime.*

PARENTERAL FOURTH GENERATION CEPHALOSPORIN
(Cefepime)

- Cefepime (4th GC) is *an anti-Pseudomonal cephalosporin* that is often active against ceftazidime resistant P. aeruginosa strains.
- For *P. aeruginosa* and MDR GNBs use high dose cefepime, i.e., 2 gm (IV) q8h.

PARENTERAL ANTI-MRSA CEPHALOSPORINS
(Ceftaroline)

- Ceftaroline is the *only cephalosporins active in vivo against both MSSA and MRSA.*
- Ceftaroline is useful for MSSA/MRSA bacteremias, ABE, osteomyelitis

MONOBACTAMS
(Aztreonam)

- *Aztreonam has no Gram-positive activity.*
- Although structurally similar to the beta-lactams, *aztreonam is safe in penicillin-allergic patients.*

CARBAPENEMS
(Imipenem, Meropenem, Ertapenem, Doripenem)

- *Avoid imipenem in patients with seizures/CNS disorders* since imipenem may cause seizures. Also, *renal insufficiency increases imipenem's seizure potential.*
- *Meropenem doesn't cause seizures* in those with or without seizure disorders or with normal or decreased renal function.
- Ertapenem may be used in place of meropenem if activity against VSE or P. aeruginosa is not needed.
- *Ertapenem has no anti-enterococcal activity,* important in biliary tract infections/UTIs.

- *Meropenem and ertapenem may be administered as an IV bolus (< 5 min.), useful in sepsis.*
- Meropenem penetrates the inflamed prostate (acute prostatitis), but not the chronically inflamed prostate (chronic prostatitis).

BETA-LACTAMASE INHIBITOR COMBINATIONS

- *Some strains of MDR Acinetobacter baumannii are susceptible only to sulbactam/ ampicillin.*
- *Tazobactam does not enhance the anti-pseudomonal activity of piperacillin.*
- *Ceftolozane/tazobactam is effective against MDR GNB, but not CRE.*
- *Ceftazidime/avibactam and ceftolozone/tazobactam have some B. fragilis activity, but for clAIs, should be used together with metronidazole.*
- *Meropenem/Vaborbactam and Imipenem/Relebactam are effective against CRE.*

TETRACYCLINES
(Doxycycline, Minocycline, Eravacycline, Omadacycline)

- *While MRSA may be susceptible to doxycycline in vitro, in vivo it frequently fails or the clinical response is delayed/incomplete. Minocycline IV/PO for MSSA/MRSA is more effective than doxycycline.*
- Doxycycline, minocycline, and omadacycline have good anti-B. fragilis activity.
- *At urinary concentrations, doxcycline is effective against P. aeruginosa CAB/lower UTIs, i.e., high urine levels > 300 mcg/mL. Eravacycline not useful for UTIs.*
- Doxycycline one of very few oral drugs effective against urinary CRE pathogens.
- Doxycycline is effective for nearly all non-viral zoonotic infections, *except for babesiosis.*
- *Oral minocycline is useful to treat serious systemic infections due to MSSA/MRSA i.e., ABE, osteomyelitis, meningitis, etc.*

CHLORAMPHENICOL

- Chloramphenicol is *one of few drugs that can be given orally to treat acute bacterial meningitis* due to susceptible organisms.
- *Chloramphenicol when given orally results in higher serum concentrations than when given at the same dose intravenously.*

- *Avoid chloramphenicol for the treatment of hepatobiliary infections and UTIs since chloramphenicol is excreted into the bile as an inactivate metabolite, and urinary levels are low.*

- *Aplastic anemia is a rare idiosyncratic side effect associated with oral/ topical therapy but not IV therapy.*

- *Chloramphenicol induced aplastic anemia is an idiosyncratic reaction and serial CBCs are unhelpful in predicting/avoiding aplastic anemia.*

- *Serial CBCs may be obtained to monitor dose-related side effects (anemia) not idiosyncratic side effects (aplastic anemia).*

- *Prolonged chloramphenicol therapy may cause sequential, dose-related suppression of bone marrow elements. Suppressed blood elements return in reverse sequence when chloramphenicol is discontinued.*

- *Vacuolization on bone marrow biopsy specimens in patients receiving chloramphenicol is a manifestation of chloramphenicol effect, not aplastic anemia.*

- *Chloramphenicol is effective for E. faecium (VRE) systemic infections.*

CLINDAMYCIN

- *Clindamycin misses approximately 15% of coagulase-negative S. epidermidis (CoNS), the most common pathogen in foreign body/implant-related infections.*

- *Clindamycin is one of the few antibiotics able to penetrate/dissolve staphylococcal biofilms.* Clindamycin may be useful adjunctively in treating foreign body associated infections when the prosthetic device cannot be removed.

- The *incidence of C. difficile diarrhea is greater with PO > IV clindamycin.*

- *Clindamycin is not active against group D enterococci (VSE/VRE).*

- With CA-MRSA, *inducible clindamycin resistance should be suspected if erythromycin is resistant and clindamycin is susceptible.* A positive "D test" confirms clindamycin resistance.

- Clindamycin anti-toxin properties may be useful in severe GAS infections, e.g., necrotizing fasciitis.

AMINOGLYCOSIDES
(Gentamicin, Tobramycin, Amikacin, Plazomicin)

- Among aminoglycosides, *gentamicin has the most anti-gram positive coccal activity.*

- *Among the aminoglycosides, amikacin has optimal PK/PD concentration dependent kinetics.*

- Gentamicin and tobramycin have 6 loci that may be inactivated by acetylating, acetylating and phosphorylating enzymes. Amikacin has only 1 locus that may be attacked by these enzymes, making P. aeruginosa resistance rare.

- *Avoid aminoglycoside monotherapy in the treatment of nosocomial pneumonia since aminoglycoside activity is diminished in the presence of tissue hypoxia, WBC debris and local acidosis, prominent in nosocomial pneumonia.*

- *Avoid aminoglycosides via nebulizer since aerosolized aminoglycosides may predispose to resistance. If aerosolized aminoglycoside therapy is used, aerosolized amikacin has the lowest resistance potential.*

- *Avoid administering aminoglycosides in split-daily doses.* A single daily dose is optimal since *aminoglycosides obey "concentration-dependent" killing kinetics.*

- When aminoglycosides are used in *renal insufficiency, begin therapy with the usual initial dose, then give the maintenance dose in proportion to the* creatinine clearance.

- *If aminoglycosides are being used for synergy, use half the therapeutic dose* (synergy dose).

- *Aminoglycosides given on a once-daily basis optimize aminoglycoside antibacterial killing while minimizing nephrotoxic potential and eliminate the need for aminoglycoside levels.*

- *Aminoglycoside ototoxicity may occur with extremely high/prolonged peak levels.* Episodic elevated peak levels are not associated with ototoxicity.

- *Aminoglycoside nephrotoxicity should not be assessed by serum creatinines.* Aminoglycoside nephrotoxicity is best *assessed using rinary renal cast counts indicators of renal tubular damage.*

- *Limiting aminoglycoside therapy to 2 weeks once-daily dosing minimizes the risk of aminoglycoside nephrotoxicity. Once daily dosing essentially eliminates nephrotoxicity.*

- *Amikacin, among the aminoglycosides, has the highest degree of anti-P. aeruginosa activity.*

- *Aminoglycosides appear to be active against streptococci by in-vitro* susceptibility testing, but *aminoglycosides have no inherent activity against streptococci,* i.e., groups A, B, C, G, D.

- Aminoglycosides (e.g., gentamicin) are *only active against E. faecalis (VSE) when combined with penicillin or vancomycin.*

- *Avoid, if possible, using aminoglycosides for peritoneal lavage* since the peritoneum provides a very large cross-sectional area for drug absorption, *increasing the risk for neuromuscular blockade/respiratory arrest.*

- For *CNS infections, aminoglycosides must be administered intrathecally* (IT) since they do not cross the blood brain barrier in sufficient concentrations to be therapeutic.

TMP–SMX

- *TMP–SMX has the same spectrum as ceftriaxone* (no P. aeruginosa coverage).

- *Avoid using TMP–SMX to treat serious systemic K. pneumoniae infections.* Isolates sensitive to TMP–SMX *in-vitro* often ineffective *in-vivo*.

- *In patients with hypersensitivity reactions to TMP–SMX, it is always the sulfa component, not the TMP component, which is responsible.* If continued treatment is desired with TMP–SMX, therapy may be completed with the TMP component alone.

- *Although TMP–SMX is an excellent antibiotic against MSSA it is inactive against most streptococci.*

- For the *treatment of hydradenitis suppurativa due to MSSA, TMP–SMX is preferred* because of its ability to penetrate into infected sebaceous glands.

- For aerobic GNB bacteremias (other than P. aeruginosa), use TMP–SMX 10 mg/kg/day (IV/PO) given in 4 equally divided doses q6h.

- *For CNS penetration and the treatment of unusual organisms (e.g., PCP), use TMP–SMX 20 mg/kg/day (IV/PO) given in 4 equally divided doses q6h.*

- *Avoid TMP–SMX for respiratory tract infections since it's use is associated with S. pneumoniae resistance.*

- *Also avoid TMP–SMX for UTIs since it's use is associated with E. coli resistance.*

- *TMP-SMX may falsely increase creatinine levels, but does not decrease renal function.*

QUINOLONES
(Ciprofloxacin, Ofloxacin, Levofloxacin, Moxifloxacin, Delafloxacin)

- *Levofloxacin at a dose of 750 mg IV/PO is preferred to ciprofloxacin for treatment of serious systemic P. aeruginosa infections.*

- *With the exception of ciprofloxacin, quinolones do not lower the seizure threshold/cause seizures.*

- *Moxifloxacin is the only quinolone with a hepatobiliary mode of excretion; dose does not need to be modified and renal insufficiency but concentrations in the urine for lower UTIs may be suboptimal.*

- *For meningococcal prophylaxis, quinolones are equally effective* (quinolones penetrate well into respiratory secretions/have a high degree of anti-meningococcal activity).

- *Delafloxacin is the only quinolone with activity against MRSA.*

- *Only levofloxacin and delafloxacin have activity against Pseudomonas aeruginosa.*
- *Ciprofloxacin has less activity against S. pneumoniae and S. aureus than moxifloxacin, levofloxacin, or delafloxacin.*
- *Among the quinolones, only moxifloxacin and delafloxacin have anti-B fragilis activity.*

NITROFURANTOIN

- *Nitrofurantoin is an ideal oral agent to treat acute uncomplicated cystitis (AUC) or CAB.*
- *If the CrCL < 30 mL/min, nitrofurantoin may not be effective for AUC/CAB.*
- If pre-emptive treatment of on AUC/CAB is desired in immunocompromised hosts, e.g., diabetics, SLE, myeloma, CLL, steroids, neutropenia, *nitrofurantoin is an ideal oral agent is active against the usual GNB uropathogens, group D enterococci (VSE/VRE), and has a low resistance potential.*
- Nitrofurantoin is effective *against ESBL + and MDR GNB uropathogens including CRE strains (NDM-1), but not except P. aeruginosa, Serratia marcesens, or Proteus sp.*

VANCOMYCIN

- If vancomycin is combined with a nephrotoxic drug and nephrotoxicity occurs, it *should be ascribed to the nephrotoxic drug* and not vancomycin.
- Vancomycin is a *"concentration-dependent"* drug (with MSSA/MRSA with MICs > 1 mcg/mL), but a *"time dependent"* drug (with MSSA/MRSA MICs < 1 mcg/mL).
- Other drugs preferable to vancomycin to treat cSSIs and bacteremias/ABE due to MSSA.
- *No need for vancomycin levels for usual vancomycin dosing.* However, vancomycin levels may be useful in patients with unusually high volume of distribution (V_d) (e.g., edema/ascites, trauma, burns).
- Vancomycin "tolerance" is *common among staphylococci and enterococci.*
- Vancomycin is *alone is inadequate therapy for* E. faecalis (VSE) bacteremia/SBE. Add gentamicin for optimal VSE activity.
- Vancomycin *may cause cell wall thickening ("permeability-mediated" resistance) manifested by* ↑ MICs to vancomycin as well as other antibiotics.
- *Vancomycin penetrates well into bone, but not synovial fluid.*
- *Vancomycin IV predisposes to VRE,* but PO vancomycin does *not.*
- *Oral vancomycin is preferred over oral metronidazole for C. difficile diarrhea, but metronidazole is preferred for C. difficile colitis.*

OXAZOLIDINONES
(Linezolid, Tedizolid)

- Linezolid is highly active against the major Gram positive pathogens, including MSSA, MRSA, VSE, and VRE.
- Linezolid is *equally efficacious when administered PO or IV.*
- Unlike vancomycin, *linezolid does not increase E. faecium (VRE) prevalence.*
- Because linezolid is eliminated by hepatic mechanisms, *no dosing adjustment is necessary in renal insufficiency.*
- Tedizolid, like linezolid, may be given IV/PO.
- Once daily dosing IV/PO effective with tedizolid ($t_{1/2}$ = 11 hrs).
- Linezolid is *one of the few PO antibiotics that can be used to treat CNS infections due to Gram positive ABM pathogens (MSSA, MRSA, CoNS, Listeria).*

QUINUPRISTIN/DALFOPRISTIN

- Quinupristin/dalfopristin is active against E. faecium (VRE) but *not E. faecalis (VSE).*
- *Quinupristin/dalfopristin is highly effective against MSSA and MRSA.*

LIPOPEPTIDE
(Daptomycin)

- Daptomycin is more *active against MSSA/MRSA than* VSE/VRE (mean MSSA/MRSA MICs = 0.5 mcg/mL vs. mean VSE/VRE MICs = 1.0 mcg/mL). *If daptomycin is used to treat VSE/VRE, a higher dose is recommend (dose for MSSA/MRSA bacteremia: 6 mg/kg/day dose for VSE/VRE bacteremia: 12 mg/kg/day).*
- Daptomycin is *inactivated by calcium in alveolar surfactant fluid and should not* be used for pneumonias, but is useful for septic pulmonary emboli or lung abscesses.
- Following vancomycin therapeutic failures with MSSA/MRSA bacteremias/ABE, *daptomycin resistance may occur during therapy.*
- *An initial dose of gentamicin may increase intracellular entry/effectiveness of daptomycin when treating MSSA/MRSA infections.*

TIGECYCLINE

- Tigecycline may be given safely to patients with penicillin or sulfa drug allergy but *avoid in patients with tetracycline allergy.*
- Tigecycline (hepatobiliary elimination) does *not need to be adjusted in renal insufficiency.*
- With A. baumannii, E testing shows falsely high MICs with tigecycline.
- Tigecycline is highly active against *MDR K. pneumoniae* and may be the *only antibiotic effective against such strains.*
- *Tigecycline is one of only a few antibiotics effective against CRE (including NDM-1 strains).*

MACROLIDES
(Erythromycin, Azithromycin, Clarithromycin)

- *Macrolides have been largely responsible for PRSP and MDRSP. Use instead doxycycline or a "respiratory quinolone."*
- IV erythromycin lactobionate is the macrolide *most* likely to be associated with QTc prolongation. Macrolides with *lower serum levels* (e.g., azithromycin) are not associated with QTc prolongation.
- Macrolides may cause an "irritative" diarrhea, but not C. difficile diarrhea.
- Erythromycin estolate may cause cholestatic jaundice in adults, but not in children.
- Due to widespread group A streptococci and MSSA resistance to macrolides, avoid macrolides for the treatment of skin/soft tissue infections.

METRONIDAZOLE

- Metronidazole (IV) is *preferred therapy for C. difficile colitis.*
- Metronidazole (PO) *frequently fails and is inferior to PO vancomycin for C. difficile diarrhea.*
- A underecognized/untoward effect of metronidazole (PO) use for *C. difficile diarrhea is increased VRE* prevalence.
- Metronidazole has a long serum half life ($t_{1/2}$) of approximately 7 hr which permits *once daily dosing,* i.e., 1 g (IV) q24h. Except for C. difficile *colitis,* there is little rationale for dosing metronidazole 500 mg (IV) on a q6 or q8h basis.

- Metronidazole is *one of the few hepatically eliminated antibiotics that requires a dosing adjustment in severe renal insufficiency* (CrCl < 10 mL/min).

- *Don't combine metronidazole and moxifloxacin for intraabdominal infections* (no rationale for double B. fragilis coverage).

LIPOGLYCOPEPTIDES
(Telavancin, Oritavancin, Dalbavancin)

- Lipoglycopeptides with long $t_{1/2}$ permits infrequent dosing, e.g., telavancin ($t_{1/2}$ = 8 hrs) q 24 hrs dosing; oritavancin ($t_{1/2}$ = 245 hrs) single dose; dalbavancin ($t_{1/2}$ = 346 hrs) q weekly dosing, and are ideal for OPAT.

- Dalbavancin effective therapy for MSSA/MRSA acute osteomyelitis.

- Telavancin is not removed by HD (protein binding = 90%), and *like some other antibiotics, may have decreased efficacy with CrCl < 50 mL/min.*

- *Falsely elevated INR, PT, PTT may occur with telavancin.*

- Oritavancin may cause local abscesses.

FOSFOMYCIN

- *Fosfomycin is highly active against most MDR uropathogens (as well as VSE/VRE) and may be used orally to treat lower UTIs/CAB due to susceptible organisms.*

- *Fosfomycin is one of the few oral antibiotics effective against most MDR GNB uropathogens including CRE.*

- *Longer fosfomycin treatment courses may be needed to eradicate some MDR GNB uropathogens particularly in compromised hosts.*

- *High urinary concentrations minimizes potential GNB resistance.*

- *Fosfomycin penetrates well into the inflamed and non-inflamed prostate in therapeutic concentrations.*

- *Fosfomycin is one of the few oral antibiotics effective in treating acute (inflamed prostate) prostatitis and chronic (non-inflamed) prostatitis due to MDR GNB.*

- *Duration of fosfomycin therapy in chronic prostatitis (due to MDR GNB) may need to be prolonged (weeks).*

- *As with other antibiotics used for the treatment of chronic prostatitis, fosfomycin therapy (high dose/prolonged therapy) may fail in the setting of prostate cancer, radioactive prostate seeds, or prostatic calcifications.*

- *May be used in combination therapy to treat MDR GNB or CRE strains.*

- If prostatic calcifications are present, they should if possible be removed (TURP). *If prostatic calcifications cannot be resected, fosfomycin (high dose/prolonged) may be effective ± if doxycycline is added to the regimen.*
- *Fosfomycin urinary concentrations are 1000–4,000 mcg/mL after a 3 gm (PO) dose,* and urine levels > 200 mcg/mL maintained for > 48 hours.
- *Fosfomycin is more active against GNB than VSE/VRE (MICs = 48–64 mcg/mL).*
- IV fosfomycin is effective in treating serious systemic infections due to GNB (including MDR and CRE strains).
- Fosfomycin (IV/PO) is one of the few antibiotics useful in IV-to-PO switch programs in the treatment of MDR GNB and CRE.

COLISTIN AND POLYMYXIN B

- *Colistin and Polymyxin B have same spectrum of activity, but differ in activity, e.g., Polymyxin B has greater activity against P. aeruginosa than colistin.*
- Colistin and Polymyxin B and colistin are active against most aerobic GNBs but *have no activity against Proteus, Providencia, Morganella, Serratia, or B. cepacia.*
- *Polymyxin B and colistin are two of the very few antibiotics effective against NDM-1 strains.*
- Polymyxin B is less nephrotoxic than colistin and is more rapidly effective (colistin is a prodrug that requires time to become effective).

NITAZOXANIDE

- *Nitazoxanide is active against anaerobic bacteria, e.g., C. difficile, H. pylori and B. fragilis.*
- *Oral nitazoxanide is more effective against C. difficile than metronidazole for either C. difficile diarrhea or C. difficile colitis.*
- Nitazoxanide is effective against B, fragilis strains with decreased susceptibility/resistance to metronidazole.
- Nitazoxanide has no activity against aerobic GPC and GNB.
- *Nitazoxanide has some activity against viral pathogens, e.g., norovirus, rotavirus, adenovirus,* SARS-CoV-2.

Chapter 11

Antimicrobial Drug Summaries

**Burke A. Cunha, MD, Damary C. Torres, PharmD,
Cheston B. Cunha, MD, Sigridh Muñoz-Gomez, MD,
Jean E. Hage, MD, David W. Kubiak, PharmD,
Nardeen Mickail, MD, Arthur Gran, MD, Muhammed Raza, MBBS,
Jamie Chin, PharmD, Julia Sessa, PharmD,
Diane M. Parente, PharmD, Veronica B. Zafonte, PharmD,
Sharon Blum, PharmD, Shan Wang, PharmD, Mark H. Kaplan, MD,
John H. Rex, MD**

DRUG SUMMARIES:

- **Drugs are listed alphabetically by generic name;** trade names follow in parentheses. To search by trade name, consult the index. Each drug summary contains the following information:
- **All orally administered antibiotics should be taken with food** unless otherwise specified (noted after usual oral dose).
- **Usual dose represents the dose to treat susceptible pathogens in adults with normal hepatic and renal function.**
- **Loading doses** are necessary for optimal therapy with doxycycline, fluconazole, itraconazole, voriconazole, caspofungin, tigecycline, and other antimicrobials (*see Table 11.1*).
- **Antibiotics with high bioavailability** (> 90% absorbed from the GI tract) are ideal for IV to PO switch or oral therapy.
- **Excreted unchanged.** Refers to the *percentage of drug excreted unchanged*, but is not an **estimate of drug concentration in urine.**
- **Serum half-life** (normal/ESRD). The serum half-life ($t_{1/2}$) is the time (in hours) in which serum concentrations fall by 50%. Serum half-life ($t_{1/2}$) is useful in determining the dosing interval. The *half-life of drugs eliminated by the kidneys is prolonged in renal disease, and the total daily dose is reduced in proportion to the degree of renal dysfunction.* If the half-life in renal insufficiency is similar to the normal half-life, then the total daily dose does not change.
- **Plasma protein binding.** Expressed as the percentage of drug reversibly bound to serum albumin. *It is the unbound (free) portion of a drug that imparts antimicrobial*

activity. Plasma protein binding is not typically a factor in antimicrobial effectiveness unless protein binding 95%.

- **Decreases in serum albumin** (nephrotic syndrome, liver disease) or competition for protein binding sites from other drugs or endogenously produced substances (uremia, hyperbilirubinemia) *increases the percentage of free drug available,* and *may require a decrease in dosage.*
- **Increases in serum binding proteins** (trauma, surgery, critical illness) *decreases the percentage of free drug available,* and *may require an increase in dosage.*
- **Volume of distribution (V_d).** Represents the apparent volume into which the drug is distributed, and is calculated as the amount of drug in the body divided by the serum concentration in L/kg. V_d is related to total body water distribution (V_d H_2O = 0.7 L/kg).
  Water soluble (hydrophilic) drugs are restricted to extracellular fluid have a $V_d \leq 0.7$ L/kg.
  Lipid soluble drugs penetrate most fluids/tissues of the body and have a large V_d (V_d >0.7 L/kg).
  **For water soluble drugs, *increases* in V_d may occur with burns, heart failure, dialysis, sepsis, cirrhosis, or mechanical ventilation; *decreases* in V_d may occur with trauma, hemorrhage, pancreatitis (early), or GI fluid losses. Increases in V_d *may require an increase in total daily drug dose decreases in V_d may require a decrease in drug dose.*
  Tissue penetration of adipose tissue is not increased by increasing the dose of (water soluble V_d ~0.7 L/kg) antibiotics. e.g., cephalosporins.
- **Mode of elimination.** Refers to the *primary route of inactivation/excretion* of the antibiotic, which **impacts dosing adjustments in renal/hepatic failure.**
- **Dosage adjustments.** Each Drug Summary grid provides dosing adjustment recommendations based on renal and hepatic function.
  In renal insufficiency (*for renally eliminated antibiotics*), **the *initial dose* is the *same* as with normal renal function**; but the ***maintenance dose is decreased* ~ ↓ CrCl.**
  Antimicrobial dosing for hemodialysis (HD)/peritoneal dialysis (PD) *between HD/PD is the same as for CrCl < 10 mL/min.*
  Antimicrobials removed by HD require a supplemental dose after hemodialysis (post–HD)/peritoneal dialysis (post–PD). *Following the post–HD or post–PD supplemental dose, antimicrobial dosing should resume as for a CrCl < 10 mL/min.*
  Dosing recommendations are based on pharmacokinetic data, drug studies, and clinical experience.
  CVVH dosing recommendations are general guidelines, since *antibiotic removal is dependent on area/type of filter, ultrafiltration rates, and sieving coefficients.*
  Slow extended daily dialysis (SLEDD) is less likely to remove molecules > 1000 Daltons as compared to CVVH. However increasing flow rate to 300 mL/min increases the clearance during dialysis to 170 mL/min. Therefore, *doses during SLEDD may be the same as for normal renal function.*

Clearances for SLEDD are comparable to CVVH except over a shorter period, when no information is available, dosage adjustments are as for CVVH.

Creatinine clearance (CrCl) is used to gauge the degree of renal insufficiency, and can be estimated by the following calculation: CrCl (mL/min) = [(140 – age) × weight (kg)] / [72 × serum creatinine (mg/dL)]. The calculated value is multiplied by 0.85 for females.

It is important to recognize that due to age dependent decline in renal function. i.e., **elderly patients with "normal" serum creatinines may have low CrCls** requiring dosage adjustments.

- **Drug Interactions.** Refers to common/important drug-drug interactions.
- **Adverse Side Effects.** Side effects are common, uncommon, rare listed as such. Potentially serious side effects are underlined.
- **Allergic Potential.** Described as low or high, **refers to the likelihood of a hypersensitivity reaction.**
- **Safety in pregnancy.** Designated by the U.S. Food and Drug Administration's (USFDA) by use in **pregnancy letter code** (Table 11.3).
- **Cerebrospinal fluid penetration.** Expressed as a % of simultaneous peak serum concentration. **Meningeal doses are listed under CSF penetration.** *No meningeal dose is given if CSF penetration is inadequate for treatment of meningitis.*
- **Biliary tract penetration.** Expressed as a % of simultaneous serum concentration.
- **Additional Pharmacokinetic Considerations** boxed in each Drug Summary.
- **Additional Clinical Considerations** boxed in each Drug Summary.

Clinical Importance of the Loading Dose in Treating Serious Infections

Particularly important when treating serious infections, certain antibiotics *optimally* should be initially given as a "loading dose" (fluconazole) or a "loading regimen" (doxycycline).

- **It takes 4–5 serum half lives ($t_{1/2}$) to achieve maximum therapeutic effect/ steady state (SS) levels.** *Without a loading dose, it takes days to achieve therapeutic levels.*

  Antibiotics optimally requiring an initial "loading dose" rapidly achieve steady state (SS)/therapeutic concentrations are those with *long serum half lives* ($t_{1/2}$).

- *Doxycycline* ($t_{1/2}$ of 18–22h) *if given without a "loading regimen", i.e., 100 mg (IV/PO) q12h takes 4–5 days to achieve therapeutic effect.*
- *If a rapid therapeutic effect is needed with doxycycline,* e.g., in treating Legionnaire's disease, *then a "loading regimen", i.e., 200 mg (IV/PO) q12h × 3 days achieves maximum therapeutic effect rapidly.*

A "loading dose" *is not the same as the initial dose used in renal insufficiency.* In renal insufficiency, it is *the maintenance dose* that is ↓ in proportion CrCl, i.e., the **first dose is the usual dose and is not a "loading dose".**

Table 11.1 Antibiotics Optimally Given with an Initial Loading Dose*

Antibiotics requiring loading doses	Serum half life ($t_{1/2}$)
• Fluconazole	$t_{1/2}$ = 27 h
• Caspofungin	$t_{1/2}$ = 10 h
• Anidulafungin	$t_{1/2}$ = 40–50 h
• Dalbavancin	$t_{1/2}$ = 346 h
• Azithromycin	$t_{1/2}$ = 68 h
• Doxycycline/Minocycline	$t_{1/2}$ = 18–22 h/15–23 h
• Tigecycline	$t_{1/2}$ = 42 h
• Omadacycline	$t_{1/2}$ = 13.5–16.8 h
• Isuvuconazole	$t_{1/2}$ = 67–104 h
• Itraconazole	$t_{1/2}$ = 21–64 h
• Posaconazole	$t_{1/2}$ = 35 h
• Voriconazole	$t_{1/2}$ = 6 h

*See individual Drug Summaries for Loading Doses (LD) and Maintenance Doses (MD)

Relationship of urinary levels to % of serum levels excreted into urine.

- **Urinary levels are not simply a % of serum levels excreted into urine.**
- Bladder urinary levels are determined by **both** *serum levels (% excreted into the kidneys)* **plus** *antibiotic concentration* in bladder urine.

Doxycycline (example)

Usual dose = 100 mg (IV/PO) → serum level = 4 mcg/mL
40% of serum level (= 1.6 mcg/mL) → presented to the **kidneys**
- **Renal** urinary levels = 1.6 mcg/mL (40% of serum levels)
- **Bladder** urinary levels = 300 mcg/mL **after renal concentration**

Clinical Relevance to Antibiotic Tissue Penetration: Volume of Distribution (Vd)

V_d estimates antibiotic distribution in fluid compartments, *but does not predict individual tissue levels.*
- **Low V_d** (V_d < 0.7 L/kg): antibiotic concentrates in *extracellular* (*water soluble*), compartments e.g., cefazolin: V_d = 0.2 L/kg
- **High V_d** (V_d > 0.7 L/kg): antibiotic concentrates in *intracellular* (*lipid soluble*), compartments e.g., minocycline: V_d = 1.5 L/kg
- Increasing serum levels of *water soluble* antibiotics (low V_d), e.g., β-lactams *does not increase levels in adipose tissue.*

Table 11.2 Antibiotics and Cytochrome P450 Isoenzymes

Antibiotics that are **not** involved in CYP450 system	Antibiotics that **are** involved in CYP450 system either as inducer or inhibitor
Tigecycline, Daptomycin, Clindamycin, Linezolid, Vancomycin, Minocycline, Cephalosporins, Carbapenems, Nitrofurantoin, Colistin, Polymyxin B, Penicillins, Oxacillin, Aztreonam, Moxifloxacin, Aminoglycosides, Tedizolid, Telavancin, Dalbavancin, Ceftolozane/Tazobactam, Ceftazidime/ Avibactam, Meropenem/Vaborbactam, Imipenem/Relebactam, Fosfomycin	Nafcillin, Quinupristin/Dalfopristin, Macrolides, Telithromycin, Fluoroquinolones (except Moxifloxacin), Azoles, Rifampin, INH, TMP–SMX, Tetracycline, Doxycycline, Eravacycline, Omadacycline, Metronidazole, Chloramphenicol, Oritavancin

Table 11.3 USFDA Use in Pregnancy Letter Code

Category	Interpretation
A	**Controlled studies show no risk.** Adequate, well-controlled studies in pregnant women have not shown a risk to the fetus in any trimester of pregnancy.
B	**No evidence of risk in humans.** Adequate, well-controlled studies in pregnant women have not shown increased risk of fetal abnormalities despite adverse findings in animals, or, in the absence of adequate human studies, animal studies show no fetal risk. The chance of fetal harm is remote, but remains a possibility.
C	**Risk cannot be ruled out.** Adequate, well-controlled human studies are lacking, and animal studies have shown a risk to the fetus or are lacking. There is a chance of fetal harm if the drug is administered during pregnancy, but potential benefit from use of the drug may outweigh potential risk.
D	**Positive evidence of risk.** Studies in humans or investigational or post-marketing data have demonstrated fetal risk. Nevertheless, potential benefit from use of the drug may outweigh potential risk. For example, the drug may be acceptable if needed in a life-threatening situation or serious disease for which safer drugs cannot be used or are ineffective.
X	**Contraindicated in pregnancy.** Studies in animals or humans or investigational or post-marketing reports have demonstrated positive evidence of fetal abnormalities or risk which clearly outweigh any possible benefit to the patient.

Abacavir (Ziagen) ABC

Drug Class: HIV NRTI (nucleoside reverse transcriptase inhibitor).
Usual Dose: 300 mg (PO) q12h.
Pharmacokinetic Parameters:
Peak serum level: 3 mcg/mL
Bioavailability: 83%
Excreted unchanged (urine): 1.2%
Serum half-life (normal/ESRD): 1.5/8 hrs
Plasma protein binding: 50%
Volume of distribution (V_d): 0.86 L/kg
Primary Mode of Elimination: Hepatic
Dosage Adjustments*

CrCl < 10 mL/min	No change
Post–HD dose	None
Post–PD dose	None
CVVH/CVVHD/CVVHDF dose	No change
Mild hepatic insufficiency	200 mg (PO) q12h
Moderate—severe hepatic insufficiency	Avoid

Drug Interactions: Methadone (↑ methadone clearance with abacavir 600 mg bid); ethanol (↑ abacavir serum levels/half-life and may ↑ toxicity).
Adverse Effects:
Common
- Abdominal pain diarrhea
- Nausea/vomiting/diarrhea
- Headache
- Leukopenia

Uncommon
- Sleep disorders/bad dreams
- Anorexia
- Weakness
- ↑ ALT/AST
- Drug fever/rash
- Hyperglycemia
- Hypertriglyceridemia

Rare

- Hypersensitivity reactions

- Lactic acidosis with hepatic steatosis (potentially life-threatening toxicity with NRTI's)

Allergic Potential: High (~5%)
Safety in Pregnancy: C

Additional Clinical Considerations:
- Discontinue abacavir and do not restart in patients with signs/symptoms of hypersensitivity reactions.
- Ethanol increases abacavir levels by 41%.
- Use with caution in patients with serious risk of coronary disease.

Cerebrospinal Fluid Penetration:
27–33%

SELECTED REFERENCES:
Bedimo RJ, Westfall AO, Drechsler H, et al. Abacavir use and risk of acute myocardial infarction and cerebrovascular events in the highly active antiretroviral therapy era. Clin Infect Dis 53:83–94, 2011. (PMID:21653308)
Carr A, Workman C, Smith DE, et al. Abacavir substitution for nucleoside analogs in patients with HIV lipoatrophy. A randomized trial. JAMA 288:207–15, 2002. (PMID:12095385)

———— = serious side effect [ ] = black box warning. ND = no data. NR = not recommended. s = spectrum inadequate (at site). a = activity or experience inadequate. p = tissue penetration inadequate. *based on peak serum concentration after usual adult dose. †applicable to adult uncomplicated lower UTIs (CrCl > 30 mL/min).

Keating MR. Antiviral agents. Mayo Clin Proc 67:160–78, 1992. (PMID:1347578)

Sax PE, Tierney C, Collier AC, et al. Abacavir/lamivudine versus tenofovir DF/emtricitabine as part of combination regimens for initial treatment of HIV: final results. J Infect Dis 204:1191–201, 2011. (PMID: 21967892)

Website: www.pdr.net

Abacavir + Lamivudine (Epzicom) ABC/3TC

Drug Class: HIV NRTI combination.
Usual Dose: Epzicom tablet = abacavir 600 mg + lamivudine 300 mg. Usual dose: 1 tablet q24h.
Pharmacokinetic Parameters:
Peak serum level: 4.06/2.04 mcg/L
Bioavailability: 86/86%
Excreted unchanged (urine): 1.2/71%
Serum half-life (normal/ESRD): (1.5/8)/(5-7/20) hrs
Plasma protein binding: 50/36%
Volume of distribution (V_d): 0.86/1.3 L/kg
Primary Mode of Elimination: Hepatic/Renal
Dosage Adjustments*

CrCl < 50 mL/min	Avoid
Post–HD dose	Avoid
Post–PD dose	Avoid
CVVH/CVVHD/CVVHDF dose	Avoid
Mild hepatic insufficiency	Contraindicated
Moderate—severe hepatic insufficiency	Contraindicated

Drug Interactions: Methadone (↑ methadone clearance with abacavir 600 mg bid); ethanol (↑ abacavir serum levels/half-life; may ↑ toxicity); didanosine, zalcitabine (↑ risk of pancreatitis); TMP–SMX (↑ lamivudine levels); zidovudine (↑ zidovudine levels).
Adverse Effects:
Common
- Insomnia
- Nausea/vomiting/diarrhea
- Headache
- Weakness
- Cough
- Myalgias
- Abdominal pain
- Peripheral neuropathy
- Leukopenia
- Pancreatitis
- ↑ AST/ALT

Uncommon
- Depression
- Drug fever/rash
- Sleep disorders/bad dreams
- Anorexia
- Dizziness
- Hyperglycemia
- Hypertriglyceridemia

Rare
- Anemia
- Redistribution of body fat
- Immune reconstitution syndrome (IRIS)

- Hypersensitivity reactions

- Lactic acidosis with hepatic steatosis (potentially life-threatening toxicity with use of NRTI's)

───── = serious side effect ☐ = black box warning. ND = no data. NR = not recommended. s = spectrum inadequate (at site). a = activity or experience inadequate. p = tissue penetration inadequate. *based on peak serum concentration after usual adult dose. †applicable to adult uncomplicated lower UTIs (CrCl > 30 mL/min).

Allergic Potential: High (~5%)/Low
Safety in Pregnancy: C

Additional Clinical Considerations:
- In patients with signs/symptoms of hypersensitivity reactions discontinue and do not restart.
- Severe acute exacerbations of hepatitis B may occur in patients who are co-infected with HBV and HIV and have discontinued Epivir.
- Hepatic function should be monitored closely for at least several months in patients who discontinue Epivir.

Cerebrospinal Fluid Penetration: 30%/15%

SELECTED REFERENCE:
Website: www.pdr.net

Abacavir + Lamivudine + Zidovudine (Trizivir) ABC/3TC/ZDV

Drug Class: HIV NRTI combination.
Usual Dose: Trizivir tablet = abacavir 300 mg + lamivudine 150 mg + zidovudine 300 mg. Usual dose = 1 tablet (PO) q12h.
Pharmacokinetic Parameters:
Peak serum level: 3/1.5/1.2 mcg/mL
Bioavailability: 86/86/64%
Excreted unchanged (urine): 1.2/90/16%
Serum half-life (normal/ESRD): [1.5/6/1.1] / 8/20/2.2] hrs
Plasma protein binding: 50/36/20%
Volume of distribution (V_d): 0.86/1.3/ 1.6 L/kg

Primary Mode of Elimination: Hepatic/Renal
Dosage Adjustments*

CrCl < 50 mL/min	Avoid
Post–HD or Post–PD	Avoid
CVVH/CVVHD/ CVVHDF dose	Avoid
Moderate—severe hepatic insufficiency	Avoid

Drug Interactions: Amprenavir, atovaquone (↑ zidovudine levels); clarithromycin (↓ zidovudine levels); cidofovir (↑ zidovudine levels, flu-like symptoms); doxorubicin (neutropenia); stavudine (antagonistic to zidovudine; avoid combination); TMP–SMX (↑ lamivudine and zidovudine levels); zalcitabine (↓ lamivudine levels). May exacerbate neutropenia in combination with gangcyclovir.

Adverse Effects:
Common
- Headache
- Anorexia
- Malaise/fatigue
- Nausea/vomiting/diarrhea
- Insomnia
- Myalgias
- Fever/chills
- Pancreatitis
- ↑ AST/ALT

Uncommon
- Leukopenia
- Anemia

——— = serious side effect ⬚ = black box warning. ND = no data. NR = not recommended. s = spectrum inadequate (at site). a = activity or experience inadequate. p = tissue penetration inadequate. *based on peak serum concentration after usual adult dose. †applicable to adult uncomplicated lower UTIs (CrCl > 30 mL/min).

- Drug rash
- Hyperglycemia
- Hypertriglyceridemia
- ↑ CPK
- ↑ Aldolase
- Peripheral neuropathy
- Myopathy

Rare

- <u>Immune reconstitution syndrome (IRIS)</u>
- Redistribution of body fat

- Hypersensitivity reactions

- Lactic acidosis with hepatic steatosis (potentially life-threatening toxicity with use of NRTI's)

Allergic Potential: High (~5%)
Safety in Pregnancy: C

Additional Clinical Considerations:

- Avoid in patients with CrCl < 50 mL/min.
- HBV hepatitis may relapse if lamivudine is discontinued.

SELECTED REFERENCE:
Website: www.pdr.net

Acyclovir (Zovirax)

Drug Class: Antiviral (HSV, VZV).
Usual Dose:
HSV-1/2: <u>Herpes labialis</u>: 400 mg (PO) 5x/day × 5 days.
<u>Genital herpes</u>: *Initial therapy*. 200 mg (PO) 5x/day × 10 days. *Recurrent/intermittent therapy* (< 6 episodes/year): 200 mg (PO) 5x/day × 5 days. *Chronic suppressive*

therapy (> 6 episodes/year): 400 mg (PO) q12h × 1 year.
<u>Mucosal/genital herpes</u>: 5 mg/kg (IV) q8h × 7 days or 400 mg (PO) 5x/day × 7 days.
<u>Nosocomial pneumonia</u> 5 mg/kg (IV) q8h × 10 days or 400 mg (PO) 5x/day × 7 days.
<u>Meningitis/encephalitis</u>: 10 mg/kg (IV) q8h × 10 days*. PO not recommended.
*Severe HSV encephalitis may require 14–21 days.
VZV: <u>Chickenpox</u>: 10 mg/kg (IV) q8h × 5 days or 800 mg (PO) q6h × 5 days.
<u>VZV pneumonia</u>: 5–10 mg/kg (IV) q8h × 10 days (normal hosts) 10 mg/kg (IV) q8h × 10 days (compromised hosts).
<u>Herpes zoster (shingles)</u>: *Dermatomal/Disseminated*: 10 mg/kg (IV) q8h × 7–10 days or 800 mg (PO) 5x/day × 7–10 days.
<u>VZV meningitis/encephalitis</u>: 10 mg/kg (IV) q8h × 10 days. PO not recommended.

Pharmacokinetic Parameters:
Peak serum level: 7.7 mcg/mL
Bioavailability: 30%
Excreted unchanged (urine): 70%
Serum half-life (normal/ESRD): 3/5 hrs
Plasma protein binding: 30%
Volume of distribution (V_d): 0.7 L/kg
Primary Mode of Elimination: Renal
Dosage Adjustments* for HSV/VZV

CrCl 10–25 mL/min	No change/ 800 mg (IV/PO) q8h
CrCl < 10 mL/min	400 mg (IV/PO) q12h/ 800 mg (IV/PO) q12h
Post–HD dose	None
Post–PD dose	None

―――― = serious side effect [ ] = black box warning. ND = no data. NR = not recommended. s = spectrum inadequate (at site). a = activity or experience inadequate. p = tissue penetration inadequate. *based on peak serum concentration after usual adult dose. †applicable to adult uncomplicated lower UTIs (CrCl > 30 mL/min).

CVVH/CVVHD/ CVVHDF dose	5 mg/kg(IV) q24h/ 10 mg/kg(IV) q24h 400 mg (PO) q8h/ 800 mg (PO) q8h
Moderate— severe hepatic insufficiency	No change

Drug Interactions: Cimetidine, probenecid, theophylline (↑ acyclovir levels); nephrotoxic drugs (↑ nephrotoxicity); zidovudine (lethargy); theophylline (↑ levels).

Adverse Effects:

Common
- Malaise

Uncommon
- Nausea/vomiting/diarrhea
- Injection site/inflammation/phlebitis
- Crystalluria
- ATN (with IV formulation)

Rare
- HUS
- Seizures/tremors (dose related)
- Encephalopathy

Allergic Potential: Low

Safety in Pregnancy: B

Additional Clinical Considerations:
- CSF levels may be increased with probenecid.

***Highly active** against HSV and VZV.*
***Some activity** against CMV.*
***No activity** against EBV, RSV or adenoviruses.*

Cerebrospinal Fluid Penetration: 20%

Meningeal dose = HSV or VZV encephalitis dose.

SELECTED REFERENCES:

Cunha BA, Baron J. The pharmacokinetic basis of oral valacyclovir treatment of herpes simplex virus (HSV) or varicella zoster virus (VZV) meningitis, meningoencephalitis or encephalitis in adults. J Chemo 4: epub, 2015. (PMID:26239190)

Cunha BA, Baron J. Oral valacyclovir treatment of Herpes simplex virus (HSV) or Varicella zoster virus (VZV) Meningitis, Meningoencephalitis or Encephalitis: A Pharmacokinetic Perspective. Journal of Chemotherapy 29:122–125, 2017. (PMID:29522431)

Vanpouille C, Lisco A, Introini A, et al. Exploiting the anti-HIV-1 activity of acyclovir: suppression of primary and drug-resistant HIV isolates and potentiation of the activity by ribavirin. Antimicrob Agents Chemother 56:2604–2611, 2012. (PMID: 22314523)

Vanpouille C, Lisco A, Margolis L. Acyclovir: a new use for an old drug. Curr Opin Infect Dis 22:583–587, 2009. (PMID: 19726982)

Whitley RJ, Gnann JW Jr. Acyclovir: a decade later. N Engl J Med 327:782–3, 1992. (PMID:1288525)

Website: www.pdr.net

Adefovir dipivoxil (Hepsera)

Drug Class: Antiviral (HBV).

Usual Dose: 10 mg (PO) q24h.

Pharmacokinetic Parameters:
Peak serum level: 18 ng/mL
Bioavailability: 59%
Excreted unchanged (urine): 45%
Serum half-life (normal/ESRD): 7.5/9 hrs
Plasma protein binding: 4%
Volume of distribution (V_d): 0.4 L/kg

Primary Mode of Elimination: Renal

Dosage Adjustments*

———— = serious side effect ☐ = black box warning. ND = no data. NR = not recommended. s = spectrum inadequate (at site). a = activity or experience inadequate. p = tissue penetration inadequate. *based on peak serum concentration after usual adult dose. †applicable to adult uncomplicated lower UTIs (CrCl > 30 mL/min).

CrCl ≥ 50 mL/min	10 mg (PO) q24h
CrCl 20–50 mL/min	10 mg (PO) q48h
CrCl 10–20 mL/min	10 mg (PO) q72h
Hemodialysis	10 mg (PO) q7days
Post–HD or PD dose	10 mg (PO)
CVVH/CVVHD/ CVVHDF dose	10 mg (PO) q72h
Moderate—severe hepatic insufficiency	No change

Drug Interactions: No significant interaction with lamivudine, TMP–SMX, acetaminophen, ibuprofen.

Adverse Effects:

Common
- Headache
- Asthenia
- Diarrhea
- Abdominal pain

Uncommon
- Nausea
- GI upset
- Flatulence

Allergic Potential: Low

Safety in Pregnancy: C

> **Additional Clinical Considerations:**
> - May be taken with or without food.
> - Does not inhibit CP450 isoenzymes
> - Do not discontinue abruptly to avoid exacerbation of HBV hepatitis.
>
> **Cerebrospinal Fluid Penetration:** No data

SELECTED REFERENCES:
Buti M, Esteban R. Adefovir dipivoxil. Drugs of Today 39:127–35, 2003. (PMID:12698207)

Cundy KC, Burditch-Crovo P, Walker RE, et al. Clinical pharmacokinetics of adefovir in human HIV-1 infected patients. Antimicrob Agents Chemother 35:2401–2405, 1995. (PMID:8585716)

Segovia MC, Chacra W, Gordon SC. Adefovir dipivoxil in chronic hepatitis B: history and current uses. Expert Opin Pharmacother 13:245–254, 2012. (PMID:22242973)

Yang HJ, Lee JH, Kim YJ, et al. Antiviral efficacy of combination therapy with entecavir and adefovir for entecavir/lamivudine-resistant hepatitis B virus with or without adefovir resistance. J Med Virol 84:424–430, 2012. (PMID:22246827)

Website: www.pdr.net

Amantadine (Symmetrel)

Drug Class: Antiviral (influenza A and B).

Usual Dose: 200 mg (PO) q24h.

Pharmacokinetic Parameters:
Peak serum level: 0.5 mcg/mL
Bioavailability: 90%
Excreted unchanged (urine): 90%
Serum half-life (normal/ESRD): 16/192 hrs
Plasma protein binding: 67%
Volume of distribution (V_d): 6.6 L/kg

Primary Mode of Elimination: Renal

Dosage Adjustments*

CrCl > 30 mL/min	100 mg (PO) q24h
CrCl 15–30 mL/min	100 mg (PO) q48h
CrCl < 15 mL/min	200 mg (PO) q week
Post–HD	None
Post–PD	None
CVVH/CVVHD/ CVVHDF dose	100 mg (PO) q48h
Moderate— severe hepatic insufficiency	No change

—— = serious side effect ☐ = black box warning. ND = no data. NR = not recommended. s = spectrum inadequate (at site). a = activity or experience inadequate. p = tissue penetration inadequate.
*based on peak serum concentration after usual adult dose. †applicable to adult uncomplicated lower UTIs (CrCl > 30 mL/min).

Drug Interactions: Alcohol ($\uparrow$ CNS effects); benztropine, trihexyphenidyl ($\uparrow$ interacting drug effect: dry mouth, ataxia); CNS stimulants (additive stimulation); digoxin ($\uparrow$ digoxin levels); trimethoprim ($\uparrow$ amantadine and trimethoprim levels); scopolamine ($\uparrow$ scopolamine effect: blurred vision, slurred speech, toxic psychosis).

Adverse Effects:
Uncommon
- Nausea
- Confusion
- Hallucinations
- Insomnia
- Dysarthia
- Ataxia
- Anticholinergic effects (dry month, blurry vision, orthostatic hypotension, urinary retention, constipation)
- Livedo reticularis
- Peripheral edema

Rare
- $\uparrow$ QTc

Allergic Potential: Low
Safety in Pregnancy: C

Additional Clinical Considerations:
- May precipitate heart failure.
- Avoid co-administration with anti-cholinergics, MAO inhibitors, or antihistamines.
- Resistance to amantadine widespread, but may improve peripheral airway function/oxygenation in ventilated patients with severe influenza (human, avian, swine).
Highly active against influenza A.
No activity against other viruses.

SELECTED REFERENCES:
Cunha BA, Amantadine may be lifesaving in severe influenza A. Clin Infect Dis 43:1372–3, 2006. (PMID:17051511)
Gubareva LV, Kaiser L, Hayden FG. Influenza virus neuraminidase inhibitors. Lancet 355:827–5, 2000. (PMID:10711940)
Jackson RJ, Cooper KL, Tappenden P, et al. Oseltamivir, zanamivir and amantadine in the prevention of influenza: A systematic review. J Infect 62:14–25, 2011. (PMID:20950645)
Keyser LA, Karl M, Nafziger AN, et al. Comparison of central nervous system adverse effects of amantadine and rimantadine used as sequential prophylaxis of influenza A in elderly nursing home patients. Arch Intern Med 160:1485–8, 2000. (PMID:10826462)
Website: www.pdr.net

Amikacin (Amikin)

Drug Class: Aminoglycoside.
Usual Dose: 1 gm or 15 mg/kg (IV) q24h (preferred to q12h dosing).

Spectrum Synopsis*
Hits
  Gram + : MSSA, VSE, all non-enterococcal streptococci
  Gram – : All aerobic GNB (including P. aeruginosa)
  Problem pathogens:
    Listeria, Nocardia, Acinetobacter
Misses
  Gram + : MRSA, VRE
  Gram – : B. fragilis
  Problem pathogens:
    S. maltophilia, B. cepacia
Urine Spectrum
- Same as serum spectrum
- Optimal urinary pH = 6–7
- Urinary levels = 1,500 mcg/mL

――― = serious side effect ☐ = black box warning. ND = no data. NR = not recommended. s = spectrum inadequate (at site). a = activity or experience inadequate. p = tissue penetration inadequate. *based on peak serum concentration after usual adult dose. †applicable to adult uncomplicated lower UTIs (CrCl > 30 mL/min).

(Full **Susceptibility Profiles** p. 208).
Resistance Potential: Low
Pharmacokinetic Parameters:

*Peak serum level 65–75 mcg/mL (q24h
dosing): 20–30 mcg/mL (q12h dosing)
Bioavailability: Not applicable
Excreted unchanged (urine): 95%
Serum half-life (normal/ESRD): 2/50 hrs
Plasma protein binding: < 5%
Volume of distribution (V_d): 0.25 L/kg*

Primary Mode of Elimination: Renal
Dosage Adjustments*

CrCl 50–80 mL/min	500 mg (IV) q24h or 7.5 mg/kg (IV) q24h
CrCl 10–50 mL/min	500 mg (IV) q48h or 7.5 mg/kg (IV) q48h
CrCl < 10 mL/min	250 mg (IV) q48h or 3.75 mg/kg (IV) q48h
Post–HD dose	500 mg (IV) or 7.5 mg/kg (IV)
Post–HFHD dose	500 mg (IV) or 7.5 mg/kg (IV)
Post–PD dose	250 mg (IV) or 3.75 mg/kg (IV)
CVVH/CVVHD/CVVHDF dose	500 mg (IV) q48h or 7.5 mg/kg (IV)
Moderate—severe hepatic insufficiency	No change

Drug Interactions: Amphotericin B, cephalothin, cyclosporine, enflurane, methoxyflurane, NSAIDs, polymyxin B, radiographic contrast, vancomycin (↑ nephrotoxicity); cis-platinum (↑ nephrotoxicity, ↑ ototoxicity); loop diuretics (↑ ototoxicity); neuromuscular blocking agents (↑ apnea, prolonged paralysis); non-polarizing muscle relaxants (↑ apnea).

Adverse Effects:
Uncommon
- Reversible non-oliguric renal failure (ATN)
- Vestibular toxicity (2/3 of ototoxicity) develops before ototoxicity (typically manifests as tinnitus)

- *Ototoxicity associated only with prolonged/extremely high peak serum levels* (usually irreversible), Cochlear toxicity (1/3 of ototoxicity) manifestsas decreased high frequency hearing but deafness is unusual

- Neuromuscular blockade with rapid infusion/absorption, e.g., IP

- *Nephrotoxicity only with prolonged/extremely high serum trough levelS*

Allergic Potential: Low
Safety in Pregnancy: D

Additional Clinical Considerations:
- **Synergy dose:** 500 mg (IV) q24h or 7.5 mg/kg (IV) q24h.
- **Single daily dosing virtually eliminates nephrotoxic/ototoxic potential.**
- IV infusion should be given slowly over 30 minutes. May be given IM.
- Intraperitoneal infusion ↑ risk of neuromuscular blockade.

- Avoid intratracheal/aerosolized intrapulmonary instillation, which may predispose to antibiotic resistance.
- V_d increases with edema/ascites, trauma, burns, cystic fibrosis; may require ↑ dose.
- V_d decreases with dehydration, obesity; may require ↓ dose.
- **Renal cast counts are the best indicator of aminoglycoside nephrotoxicity, not serum creatinine**.
- Dialysis removes ~ 50% of amikacin from serum.
- **CAPD dose:** 10–20 mg/L in dialysate (IP) with each exchange.
- **Therapeutic Serum Concentrations** (for therapeutic efficacy, not toxicity): **Peak** (q24h/q12h dosing): 65–75/20–30 mcg/mL **Trough** (q24h/q12h dosing): 0.4–8 mcg/mL

May inhibit antibiotic induced LPS (endotoxin) release from GNB potentially minimizing endotoxin mediated tissue damage.

Additional Pharmacokinetic Considerations*

Non-CSF	% of Serum Levels
Peritoneal fluid	40%
Bile	20%
Synovial fluid	NR(a)
Bone	ND
Prostate	NR(p)
Urine[†]	> 1000%
CSF	
Non-inflamed meninges	15%
Inflamed meninges (ABM)	20%

Meningeal dose = NR(p)
Intrathecal dose =10–40 mg (IT) q24h (must be given with systemic IV therapy: 1 g(IV) q24h or 15 mg/kg (IV) q24h)

(also see **Antibiotic Pearls & Pitfalls** p. 531).

SELECTED REFERENCES:
Cunha BA. New uses for older antibiotics: nitrofurantoin, amikacin, colistin, polymyxin B, doxycycline, and minocycline revisited. Med Clin North Am 90:1089–107, 2006. (PMID:17116438)
Cunha BA. Pseudomonas aeruginosa: Resistance and therapy. Semin Respir Infect 17:231–9, 2002. (PMID:12226802)
Cunha BA. Aminoglycosides: Current role in antimicrobial therapy. Pharmacotherapy 8:334–50, 1988. (PMID:3146747)
De Winter S, Wauters J, Meersseman W, et al. Higher versus standard amikacin single dose in emergency department patients with severe sepsis and septic shock: a randomised controlled trial. Int J Antimicrob Agents 51:562-70,2018. (PMID: 29180278)
Edson RS, Terrel CL. The Aminoglycosides. Mayo Clin Proc 74:519–28, 1999. (PMID:10319086)
Hassan NA, Awdallah FF, Abbassi MM, et al. Nebulized versus IV Amikacin as Adjunctive Antibiotic for Hospital and Ventilator-Acquired Pneumonia Postcardiac Surgeries: A Randomized Controlled Trial. Crit Care Med 46:45-52, 2018. (PMID: 28857848)
Taccone FS. Optimizing amikacin regimens in septic patients. Int J Antimicrob Agents. 39:264–264, 2012. (PMID:2218798)
Website: www.pdr.net

Amoxicillin (Amoxil, A-cillin, Polymox, Trimox, Wymox)

Drug Class: Aminopenicillin.
Usual Dose: 1 gm (PO) q8h or 875 mg (PO) q12h for suppressive therapy

---

——— = serious side effect [   ] = black box warning. ND = no data. NR = not recommended. s = spectrum inadequate (at site). a = activity or experience inadequate. p = tissue penetration inadequate. *based on peak serum concentration after usual adult dose. [†]applicable to adult uncomplicated lower UTIs (CrCl > 30 mL/min).

Spectrum Synopsis*
Hits
  Gram + : Most streptococci, PRSP (in high doses), VSE
  Gram – : Most E. coli, H. influenzae (β-lactamase –)
  Problem pathogens:
    Listeria, Oral anaerobes
Misses
  Gram + : MSSA, MRSA, VRE
  Gram – : Most GNB, P. aeruginosa, B. fragilis
  Problem pathogens:
    Nocardia, Acinetobacter, S. maltophilia, B. cepacia
Urine Spectrum
  • Same as serum spectrum (plus most ampicillin resistant E. coli.)
  • Urinary pH = no effect on activity
  • Urine levels = 1000 mcg/mL

(Full **Susceptibility Profiles** p. 196).
Resistance Potential: Low
Pharmacokinetic Parameters:
  Peak serum level: 14 mcg/mL
  Bioavailability: 90%
  Excreted unchanged (urine): 60%
  Serum half-life (normal/ESRD): 1.3/16 hrs
  Plasma protein binding: 20%
  Volume of distribution (V_d): 0.26 L/kg
Primary Mode of Elimination: Renal
Dosage Adjustments* (based on 1 gm (PO) q8h)

CrCl 50–80 mL/min	500 mg (PO) q8h
CrCl 10–50 mL/min	500 mg (PO) q12h
CrCl < 10 mL/min	500 mg (PO) q24h
Post–HD or post–PD	500 mg

| CVVH/CVVHD/ CVVHDF dose | 500 mg (PO) q24h |
| Moderate—severe hepatic insufficiency | No change |

Drug Interactions: Allopurinol (↑ risk of rash).
Adverse Effects:
Common
  • Nausea/vomiting/diarrhea
Uncommon
  • Drug fever/rash (↑ with EBV in)
  • ↑ AST/ALT
Rare
  • <u>Stevens-Johnson syndrome</u>
  • <u>Toxic epidermal necrolysis (TEN)</u>
Allergic Potential: High
Safety in Pregnancy: B

  Additional Clinical Considerations:
  • No diarrhea with 1 gm (PO) q8h dose due to nearly complete proximal GI absorption.
  • 2 gm amoxicillin effective against most strains of PRSP.

Additional Pharmacokinetic Considerations*

Non-CSF	% of Serum Levels
Peritoneal fluid	100%
Bile	30%
Synovial fluid	NR(p)
Bone	30%
Prostate	NR(p)
Urine†	> 300%
CSF	
Non-inflamed meninges	1%
Inflamed meninges (ABM)	8%

—— = serious side effect ⬜ = black box warning. ND = no data. NR = not recommended. s = spectrum inadequate (at site). a = activity or experience inadequate. p = tissue penetration inadequate. *based on peak serum concentration after usual adult dose. †applicable to adult uncomplicated lower UTIs (CrCl > 30 mL/min).

Bile Penetration: 3000%

Cerebrospinal Fluid Penetration:
  Non-inflamed/meninges 1%
  Inflamed meninges 8%

(**Antibiotic Pearls & Pitfalls** p. 526).

SELECTED REFERENCES:
Addo-Yobo E, Chisaka N, Hassan M, et al. Oral amoxicillin versus injectable penicillin for severe pneumonia in children age 3 to 59 months: a randomized multicentre equivalency study. Lancet 364:1141–48, 2004. (PMID: 15451221)
Camacho MT, Casal J, AGuilar L, et al. Very high resistance to amoxicillin in Streptococcus pneumoniae: an epidemiological fact or a technical issue? Journal of Chemotherapy 18:303–06, 2006. (PMID: 17129842)
Curtin-Wirt C, Casey JR, Murray PC, et al. Efficacy of penicillin vs. amoxicillin in children with group A beta hemolytic streptococcal tonsillopharyngitis. Clin Pediatr 42:219–24, 2003. (PMID: 12739920)
File Jr. TM, Clinical implications and treatment of multiresistant Streptococcus pneumoniae pneumonia. Clin Microbiol Infect 12:31–41, 2006. (PMID: 16669927)
Website: www.pdr.net

Amoxicillin/Clavulanic Acid (Augmentin)

Drug Class: Aminopenicillin/β-lactamase inhibitor.
Usual Dose: 500/125 mg (PO) q8h or 875/125 mg (PO) q12h for severe infections or respiratory tract infections.

Spectrum Synopsis*
Hits
  Gram + : Most streptococci, MSSA, VSE
  Gram – : Some GNB, H. influenzae (β-lactamase +), B. fragilis
  Problem pathogens:
    ESBL + Klebsiella, Enterobacter, E. coli
Misses
  Gram + : MRSA, PRSP, VRE
  Gram – : Most GNB
  Problem pathogens:
    Nocardia, Acinetobacter, S. maltophilia, B. cepacia, CRE
Urine Spectrum
  • Same as serum spectrum
  • Urinary pH = no effect on activity
  • Urinary levels = 500 mcg/mL

(Full **Susceptibility Profiles** p. 196).
Resistance Potential: Low
Pharmacokinetic Parameters:
  Peak serum level: 10.0/2.2 mcg/mL
  Bioavailability: 90/60%
  Excreted unchanged (urine): 80/40%
  Serum half-life (normal/ESRD): [1.3/16]/ [½] hrs
  Plasma protein binding: 18/25%
  Volume of distribution (V_d): 0.26/0.3 L/kg
Primary Mode of Elimination: Renal
Dosage Adjustments* (based on 500 mg q8h)

= serious side effect ⬚ = black box warning. ND = no data. NR = not recommended. s = spectrum inadequate (at site). a = activity or experience inadequate. p = tissue penetration inadequate. *based on peak serum concentration after usual adult dose. †applicable to adult uncomplicated lower UTIs (CrCl > 30 mL/min).

CrCl 10–50 mL/min	500/125 mg (PO) q12h
CrCl < 10 mL/min	250/125 mg (PO) q24h
Post–HD dose	250/125 mg (PO)
Post–PD dose	250/125 mg (PO)
CVVH/CVVHD/ CVVHDF dose	500/125 mg (PO) q24h
Moderate— severe hepatic insufficiency	No change

Drug Interactions: Allopurinol (↑ risk of rash).

Adverse Effects:

Common
- C. difficile diarrhea

Uncommon
- Drug fever/rash (↑ risk with EBV)
- ↑ AST/ALT

Rare
- ↑ AST/ALT
- <u>Steven-Johnson syndrome</u>
- <u>TEN</u>

Resistance Potential: Low
Allergic Potential: High
Safety in Pregnancy: B

Additional Clinical Considerations:
- 875/125 mg formulation should not be used in patients with CrCl < 30 mL/min.

Additional Pharmacokinetic Considerations*

Non-CSF	% of Serum Levels
Peritoneal fluid	100/275%
Bile	3000%
Synovial fluid	NR(s)
Bone	30/15%
Prostate	NR(p)
Urine†	25/40%
CSF	
Non-inflamed meninges	1/1%
Inflamed meninges (ABM)	5/4%

(also see **Antibiotic Pearls & Pitfalls** p. 526).

SELECTED REFERENCES:

Cunha BA. Amoxicillin/clavulanic acid in respiratory infections: microbiologic and pharmacokinetic considerations. Clinical Therapeutics 14:418–25, 1992. (PMID:1638583)

File TM Jr, Lode H, Kurz H, et al. Double-blind, randomized study of the efficacy and safety of oral pharmacokinetically enhanced amoxicillin-clavulanic (2,000/125 milligrams) versus those of amoxicillin-clavulanic (875/125 milligrams), both given twice daily for 7 days, in treatment of bacterial community-acquired pneumonia adults. Antimicrob Agents Chemother 48:3323–31, 2004. (PMID:15328092)

Malingoni MA, Song J, Herrington J, et al. Randomized controlled trial of moxifloxacin compared with piperacillin-tazobactam and amoxicillin-clavulanate for the treatment of complicated intra-abdominal infections. Ann Surg 244:204–11, 2006. (PMID:16858182)

Vons C, Barry C, Maitre S, et al. Amoxicillin plus clavulanic acid versus appendicectomy for treatment of acute uncomplicated appendicitis: an open-label, non-inferiority, randomized controlled trial. Lancet 377:1573–1579, 2011. (PMID:21550483)

Website: www.pdr.net

_____ = serious side effect [ ] = black box warning. ND = no data. NR = not recommended. s = spectrum inadequate (at site). a = activity or experience inadequate. p = tissue penetration inadequate. *based on peak serum concentration after usual adult dose. †applicable to adult uncomplicated lower UTIs (CrCl > 30 mL/min).

Amoxicillin/Clavulanic Acid ES-600 (Augmentin ES-600)

Drug Class: Aminopenicillin/β-lactamase inhibitor.

Usual Dose: 90 mg/kg/day oral suspension in 2 divided doses (see comments).

Spectrum Synopsis*

Hits

  Gram + : Most streptococci, MSSA, VSE

  Gram – : Some GNB, H. influenzae (β-lactamase +), B. fragilis

  Problem pathogens:
    ESBL + Klebsiella, Enterobacter, E. coli

Misses

  Gram + : MRSA, PRSP, VRE

  Gram – : Most GNB

  Problem pathogens:
    Nocardia, Acinetobacter, S. maltophilia, B. cepacia, CRE

Urine Spectrum

• Same as serum spectrum
• Urinary pH = no effect on activity

(Full **Susceptibility Profiles** p. 196).

Resistance Potential: Low

Pharmacokinetic Parameters:

  Peak serum level: 15.7/1.7 mcg/mL
  Bioavailability: 90/60%
  Excreted unchanged (urine): 70/40%
  Serum half-life (normal/ESRD): [1.4/16]/[1.1/2] hrs
  Plasma protein binding: 18%/25%
  Volume of distribution (V_d): 0.26/0.3 L/kg

Primary Mode of Elimination: Renal

Dosage Adjustments*

CrCl < 30 mL/min	Avoid
Moderate—severe hepatic insufficiency	Use with caution

Drug Interactions: Allopurinol (↑ risk of rash).

Adverse Effects

• Drug fever/rash, diarrhea
• ↑ AST/ALT
• Rash potential same as ampicillin.

Allergic Potential: High

Safety in Pregnancy: B

Additional Clinical Consideration:

• Take with meals to minimize GI upset.
• May give false + BG.

Volume of ES-600 to provide 90 mg/kg/day:

Weight	Volume (q12h)	Weight	Volume (q12h)
8 kg	3.0 mL	24 kg	9.0 mL
12 kg	4.5 mL	28 kg	10.5 mL
16 kg	6.0 mL	32 kg	12.0 mL
20 kg	7.5 mL	36 kg	13.5 mL

Bile Penetration: 3000%

Cerebrospinal Fluid Penetration:

  Non-Inflamed meninges 1%
  Inflamed meninges   1%

(also see **Antibiotic Pearls & Pitfalls** p. 526).

―――― = serious side effect ☐ = black box warning. ND = no data. NR = not recommended. s = spectrum inadequate (at site). a = activity or experience inadequate. p = tissue penetration inadequate. *based on peak serum concentration after usual adult dose. †applicable to adult uncomplicated lower UTIs (CrCl > 30 mL/min).

SELECTED REFERENCES:

Chung KP, Huang YT, Lee LN, et al. Alarmingly decreasing rates of amoxicillin-clavulanate susceptibility among clinical isolates of Haemophilus influenzae from 2001 to 2009 in a medical center in Taiwan. J Infect 62:185–187, 2011. (PMID: 21145354)

Website: www.pdr.net

Amoxicillin/Clavulanic Acid XR (Augmentin XR)

Drug Class: Aminopenicillin/β-lactamase inhibitor.

Usual Dose: 2000/125 mg (2 tablets) (PO) q12h (see comments).

Spectrum Synopsis*
Hits
  Gram + : Most streptococci, VSE
  Gram – : Some GNB, H. influenzae
    (β-lactamase +), B. fragilis
  Problem pathogens:
    ESBL + Klebsiella, Enterobacter,
    E. coli
Misses
  Gram + : MRSA, PRSP, VRE
  Gram – : Most GNB
  Problem pathogens:
    Nocardia, Acinetobacter,
    S. maltophilia, B. cepacia, CRE
Urine Spectrum
  · Same as serum spectrum
  · Urinary pH = no effect on activity

(Full *Susceptibility Profiles* p. 196).
Resistance Potential: Low

Pharmacokinetic Parameters:
  Peak serum level: 17/2 mcg/mL
  Bioavailability: 90/60%
  Excreted unchanged (urine): 70/40%
  Serum half-life (normal/ESRD): [1.3/16]/ [½] hrs
  Plasma protein binding: 18/25%
  Volume of distribution (V_d): 0.26/0.3 L/kg

Primary Mode of Elimination: Renal

Dosage Adjustments*

CrCl > 30 mL/min	No change
CrCl < 30 mL/min	Avoid
Post–HD/PD dose	Avoid
CVVH/CVVHD/ CVVHDF dose	Avoid
Moderate— severe hepatic insufficiency	Use with caution

Drug Interactions: Allopurinol (↑ risk of rash); may ↓ effectiveness of oral contraceptives.

Adverse Effects:
Common
  · Nausea
  · Non-C. difficile diarrhea
Uncommon
  · Abdominal pain
  · Drug fever
  · Rash (rash potential same as ampicillin)
Rare
  · ↑ AST/ALT
  · Steven-Johnson syndrome
  · TEN

Allergic Potential: High

——— = serious side effect [ ] = black box warning. ND = no data. NR = not recommended. s = spectrum inadequate (at site). a = activity or experience inadequate. p = tissue penetration inadequate. *based on peak serum concentration after usual adult dose. †applicable to adult uncomplicated lower UTIs (CrCl > 30 mL/min).

Safety in Pregnancy: B

Additional Clinical Considerations:

- Amoxicillin/clavulanic acid XR is a time-released formulation.
- Do not crush tablets.
- Take with food to ↑ absorption.
- XR formulation contains a different ratio of amoxicillin/clavulanic acid; do not use interchangably. With other formulations.
- May cause false + BG.

(also see **Antibiotic Pearls & Pitfalls** p. 526).

SELECTED REFERENCES:

Augmentin XR. Med Lett Drugs Ther. 45:5–6, 2003. (PMID:12571540)

Benninger MS. Amoxicillin/clavulanate potassium extended release tablets: a new antimicrobial for the treatment of acute bacterial sinusitis and community-acquired pneumonia. Expert Opin Pharmacother. 4:1839–46, 2003. (PMID:14521493)

Kaye C, Allen A, Perry S, et al. The clinical pharmacokinetics of a new pharmacokinetically enhanced formulation of amoxicillin/clavulatate. Clin Therapeutics 23:578–584, 2001. (PMID:11354391)

Website: www.pdr.net

Amphotericin B (Fungizone)

Drug Class: Antifungal.
Usual Dose: 0.5–0.8 mg/kg (IV) q24h.
Pharmacokinetic Parameters:
 Peak serum level: 1–2 mcg/mL
 Bioavailability: Not applicable
 Excreted unchanged (urine): 5%
 Serum half-life (normal/ESRD): 15/48 days
 Plasma protein binding: 90%
 Volume of distribution (V_d): 4 L/kg
Primary Mode of Elimination:
 Metabolized
Dosage Adjustments*

CrCl 10–50 mL/min	No change
Post–HD or post–PD	None
Post–HFHD dose	No change
CVVH/CVVHD/ CVVHDF dose	No change
Moderate—severe hepatic insufficiency	No change

Drug Interactions: Adrenocorticoids (hypokalemia); aminoglycosides, cyclosporine, polymyxin B (↑ nephrotoxicity); digoxin (↑ digitalis toxicity due to hypokalemia); flucytosine (↑ flucytosine levels if amphotericin B produces renal dysfunction); neuromuscular blocking agents (↑ neuromuscular blockade due to hypokalemia).

Adverse Effects:
Common
- Fevers/chills
- Hypotension
- RTA
- Anemia

Uncommon
- Flushing
- Thrombophlebitis
- Bradycardia

Rare
- Seizures
- Pancreatitis

= serious side effect ☐ = black box warning. ND = no data. NR = not recommended. s = spectrum inadequate (at site). a = activity or experience inadequate. p = tissue penetration inadequate. *based on peak serum concentration after usual adult dose. †applicable to adult uncomplicated lower UTIs (CrCl > 30 mL/min).

Allergic Potential: Low
Safety in Pregnancy: B

Additional Clinical Considerations:
- Higher doses (1–1.5 mg/kg q24h) may be needed in life-threatening situations but are nephrotoxic and should only be administered under expert supervision.
- Give by slow IV infusion over 2 hours initially.
- Aggressive hydration (1–2 liters/d) may reduce nephrotoxicity.
- **Test dose unnecessary.**
- Amphotericin B with granulocyte colony stimulating factor (GCSF) may result in ARDS.
- **Fevers/chills may be reduced by meperidine, aspirin, NSAIDs, hydrocortisone or acetaminophen, if given 30–60 minutes before infusion.**
- **Bladder irrigation dose:** 50 mg/L until cultures are negative.

**Highly active** against Candida
(↓ susceptibility to C. glabrata, C. krusei**), Cryptococcus, Histoplasmosis, Blastomycosis, Sporotrichosis, Penicillum marneffei, Paracoccidiomycosis, Coccidiomycosis.**
**Some activity** against Fusarium, Naegleria, Leishmania, Malassezia or Mucor.
**No activity** against C. lusitaniae, Pseudallescheria/Scedosporium or Trichosporon.

Cerebrospinal Fluid Penetration: < 10%

Meningeal dose = usual dose plus 0.5 mg 3–5x/week (IT) via Ommaya reservoir.

SELECTED REFERENCES:
Cruz JM, Peacock JE Jr., Loomer L, et al. Rapid intravenous infusion of amphotericin B: A pilot study. Am J Med 93:123–30, 1992. (PMID:1497057)

Deray G. Amphotericin B nephrotoxicity. J Antimicrob Chemother 49 Suppl 1:37–41, 2002. (PMID:11801579)

Gallis HA, Drew RH, Pickard WW. Amphotericin B: 30 years of clinical experience. Rev Infect Dis 12:308–29, 1990. (PMID:2184499)

Gubbins PO, Heldenbrand S. Clinically relevant drug interactions of current antifungal agents. Mycoses 53:95–113, 2010. (PMID:20002883)

Moosa MY, Alangaden GJ, Manavathu E. Resistance to amphotericin B does not emerge during treatment for invasive aspergillosis. J Antimicrob Chemother 49:209–13, 2002. (PMID:11751792)

Perfect JR, Dismukes WE, Dromer F, et al. Clinical Practice guidelines for the management of cryptococcal disease: 2010 update by the Infectious Disease Society of America. Clin Infect Dis 50:291–322, 2010. (PMID:20047480)

Safdar A, Ma J, Saliba F, et al. Drug-induced nephrotoxicity caused by amphotericin B lipid complex and liposomal amphotericin B: a review and meta-analysis. Medicine (Baltimore) 89:236–244, 2010. (PMID:20616663)

Website: www.pdr.net

Amphotericin B Lipid Complex (Abelcet) ABLC

Drug Class: Antifungal.
Usual Dose: 5 mg/kg (IV) q24h.
Pharmacokinetic Parameters:
Peak serum level: 1.7 mcg/mL
Bioavailability: Not applicable
Excreted unchanged (urine): 5%
Serum half-life (normal/ESRD): 173/ 173 hrs

———— = serious side effect ☐ = black box warning. ND = no data. NR = not recommended. s = spectrum inadequate (at site). a = activity or experience inadequate. p = tissue penetration inadequate. *based on peak serum concentration after usual adult dose. †applicable to adult uncomplicated lower UTIs (CrCl > 30 mL/min).

Plasma protein binding: 90%
Volume of distribution (V_d): 131 L/kg
Primary Mode of Elimination:
Metabolized
Dosage Adjustments*

CrCl < 50 mL/min	No change
Post–HD/PD dose	None
Post–HFHD dose	None
CVVH/CVVHD/ CVVHDF dose	No change
Moderate—severe hepatic insufficiency	No change

Drug Interactions: Adrenocorticoids (hypokalemia); aminoglycosides, cyclosporine, polymyxin B ($\uparrow$ nephrotoxicity); digoxin ($\uparrow$ digitalis toxicity due to hypokalemia); flucytosine ($\uparrow$ flucytosine effect); neuromuscular blocking agents ($\uparrow$ neuromuscular blockade due to hypokalemia).

Adverse Effects:
Common
- Fevers/chills
- $\uparrow$ Creatinine

Uncommon
- Flushing
- Thrombophlebitis
- Bradycardia
- Hypotension
- Renal failure
- Anemia

Rare
- RTA
- Seizures

Allergic Potential: Low
Safety in Pregnancy: B

Additional Clinical Considerations:
- Useful in patients unable to tolerate amphotericin B or in patients with amphotericin B nephrotoxicity.

Highly active against Candida
($\downarrow$ susceptibility to *C. glabrata, C. krusei*), ***Cryptococcus, Histoplasmosis, Blastomycosis, Sporotrichosis, Penicillum marneffei, Paracoccidio- mycosis, Coccidiomycosis.***

Some activity against Fusarium, Naegleria, Leishmania, Malassezia or Mucor.

No activity against C. lusitaniae, Pseudallescheria/Scedosporium or Trichosporon.

Cerebrospinal Fluid Penetration: <10%

SELECTED REFERENCES:

Arikan S, Rex JH. Lipid-based antifungal agents: current status. Curr Pharm Des 7:393–415, 2001. (PMID:11254895)

Dupont B. Overview of the lipid formulations of amphotericin B. J Antimicrob Chemother 49 Suppl 1:31–6, 2002. (PMID:11801578)

Hiemenz JW, Walsh TJ. Lipid formulations of amphotericin B: Recent progress and future directions. Clin Infect Dis 2:133–44, 1996. (PMID:8722841)

Mondal S, Bhattacharya P, Ali N. Current diagnosis and treatment of visceral leishmaniasis. Expert Rev Anti Infect Ther 8:919–944, 2010. (PMID:20695748)

Website: www.pdr.net

―――― = serious side effect ☐ = black box warning. ND = no data. NR = not recommended. s = spectrum inadequate (at site). a = activity or experience inadequate. p = tissue penetration inadequate. *based on peak serum concentration after usual adult dose. †applicable to adult uncomplicated lower UTIs (CrCl > 30 mL/min).

Amphotericin B Liposomal (AmBisome) L-amb

Drug Class: Antifungal.
Usual Dose: 3–6 mg/kg (IV) q24h (see comments).
Pharmacokinetic Parameters:
Peak serum level: 17–83 mcg/mL
Bioavailability: Not applicable
Excreted unchanged (urine): 5%
Serum half-life (normal/ESRD): 153 hrs/ no data
Plasma protein binding: 90%
Volume of distribution (V_d): 131 L/kg
Primary Mode of Elimination:
Metabolized
Dosage Adjustments*

CrCl < 50 mL/min	No change
Post-HD/PD dose	None
Post-HFHD dose	None
CVVH/CVVHD/ CVVHDF dose	No change
Moderate—severe hepatic insufficiency	No change

Drug Interactions: Adrenocorticoids (hypokalemia); aminoglycosides, cyclosporine, polymyxin B (↑ nephrotoxicity); digoxin (↑ digitalis toxicity due to hypokalemia); flucytosine (↑ flucytosine effect); neuromuscular blocking agents (↑ neuromuscular blockade due to hypokalemia).

Adverse Effect:
Common
- Fever/chills
- Nausea/vomiting/diarrhea
- Hypertension
- Hypotension
- Rash
- ↑ Creatinine
- ↑ AST/ALT

Uncommon
- Flushing
- Bradycardia
- ARF
- Electrolyte abnormalities (hypernatremia, acidosis, hyperchloremia, hyperkalemia, hypermagnesemia, hyperphosphatemia, hypophosphatemia)

Allergic Potential: Low
Safety in Pregnancy: B

Additional Clinical Considerations:
- Less nephrotoxicity than amphotericin B and other amphotericin lipid preparations.
- **Empiric therapy of fungemia dose:** 3 mg/kg (IV) q24h can be used.
- **Suspected/known Aspergillus dose:** 5 mg/kg (IV) q24h.

Highly active **against Aspergillus, Candida** (↓ *susceptibility to C. glabrata, C. krusei*), **Cryptococcus, Histoplasmosis, Blastomycosis, Sporotrichosis, Penicillum marneffei, Paracoccidiomycosis, Coccidiomycosis.**

Some activity **against Fusarium, Naegleria, Leishmania, Malassezia or Mucor.**

No activity **against C. lusitaniae, Pseudallescheria/Scedosporium or Trichosporon.**

Cerebrospinal Fluid Penetration: <10%
Cryptococcal meningitis dose = 6 mg/kg (IV) q24h.

——— = serious side effect ☐ = black box warning. ND = no data. NR = not recommended. s = spectrum inadequate (at site). a = activity or experience inadequate. p = tissue penetration inadequate. *based on peak serum concentration after usual adult dose. †applicable to adult uncomplicated lower UTIs (CrCl > 30 mL/min).

SELECTED REFERENCES:

Chopra R. AmBisome in the treatment of fungal infections: the UK experience. J Antimicrob Chemother 49 Suppl 1:43–7, 2002. (PMID: 11801580)

Chu P, Sadullah S. The current role of amphotericin B lipid complex in managing systemic fungal infections. Curr Med Res Opin 25:3011–3020, 2009. (PMID:19849324)

Hiemenz JW, Walsh TJ. Lipid formulations of amphotericin B: Recent progress and future directions. Clin Infect Dis 2:133–44, 1996. (PMID:8722841)

Jarvis JN, Leeme TB, Molefi M, et al. Short-course high-dose Liposomal Amphotericin B for human immunodeficiency virus-associated Cryptococcal meningitis: A Phase 2 randomized controlled trial. Clin Infect Dis. 68:393-401, 2019. (PMID: 29945252)

Kuse ER, Chetchotisakd P, da Cunha CA, et al. Micafungin versus liposomal amphotericin B for candidaemia and invasive candidosis: a phase III randomised double-blind trial. Lancet 369:1519–1527, 2007. (PMID:17482982)

Safdar A, Ma J, Saliba F, et al. Drug-induced nephrotoxicity caused by amphotericin B lipid complex and liposomal amphotericin B: a review and meta-analysis. Medicine (Baltimore) 89:236–244, 2010. (PMID:20616663)

Website: www.pdr.net

Amphotericin B Cholesteryl Sulfate Complex (Amphotec), ABCD (amphotericin B colloidal dispersion)

Drug Class: Antifungal.
Usual Dose: 3–4 mg/kg (IV) q24h.
Pharmacokinetic Parameters:
Peak serum level: 2.9 mcg/mL
Bioavailability: Not applicable
Excreted unchanged (urine): 5%
Serum half-life (normal/ESRD): 39/29 hrs
Plasma protein binding: 90%
Volume of distribution (V_d): 4 L/kg

Primary Mode of Elimination:
Metabolized
Dosage Adjustments*

CrCl < 50 mL/min	No change
Post–HD/PD dose	None
Post–HFHD dose	None
CVVH/CVVHD/CVVHDF dose	None
Moderate—severe hepatic insufficiency	No change

Drug Interactions: Adrenocorticoids (hypokalemia); aminoglycosides, cyclosporine, polymyxin B ($\uparrow$ nephrotoxicity); digoxin ($\uparrow$ digitalis toxicity due to hypokalemia); flucytosine ($\uparrow$ flucytosine effect); neuromuscular blocking agents ($\uparrow$ neuromuscular blockade due to hypokalemia).

Adverse Effects:
Common
- Fevers/chills
- Vomiting
- Hypotension
- Tachycardia
- Hypokalemia
- $\uparrow$ Creatinine

Uncommon
- Anemia
- Electrolyte abnormalities (hyperglycemia, hypocalcemia, hypomagnesemia, hypophosphatemia)

Rare
- ARF

Allergic Potential: Low
Safety in Pregnancy: B

─── = serious side effect ▭ = black box warning. ND = no data. NR = not recommended. s = spectrum inadequate (at site). a = activity or experience inadequate. p = tissue penetration inadequate. *based on peak serum concentration after usual adult dose. †applicable to adult uncomplicated lower UTIs (CrCl > 30 mL/min).

Additional Clinical Considerations:

- Do not co-administer with in same IV line with other drugs.

- Give by slow IV infusion over 2 hours (1 mg/kg/hr).

- Test dose unnecessary.

__Highly active__ against Aspergillos Candida ($\downarrow$ susceptibility to C. glabrata C. krusei), *Cryptococcus, Histoplasmosis, Blastomycosis, Sporotrichosis, Penicillum marneffei, Paracoccidiomycosis, Coccidiomycosis.*

__Some activity__ against Fusarium, Naegleria, Leishmania, Malassezia or Mucor.

__No activity__ against C. lusitaniae, Pseudallescheria/Scedosporium or Trichosporon.

Cerebrospinal Fluid Penetration: <10%

SELECTED REFERENCES:

De Marie S. Clinical use of liposomal and lipid-complexed amphotericin B. J Antimicrob Chemother 33:907–16, 1994. (PMID:8089064)

Rapp RP, Gubbins PO, Evans ME. Amphotericin B lipid complex. Ann Pharmacother 31:1174–86, 1997. (PMID:9337444)

Safdar A, Ma J, Saliba F, et al. Drug-induced nephrotoxicity caused by amphotericin B lipid complex and liposomal amphotericin B: a review and meta-analysis. Medicine (Baltimore) 89:236–244, 2010. (PMID:20616663)

Website: www.pdr.net

Ampicillin (various)

Drug Class: Aminopenicillin.
Usual Dose: 2 gm (IV) q4h, 500 mg (PO) q6h.

Spectrum Synopsis*
Hits
  Gram + : Most streptococci, VSE
  Gram – : Some GNB, H. influenzae
    (β-lactamase -)
Misses
  Gram + : MSSA, MRSA, VRE
  Gram – : Most GNB, B. fragilis
Problem pathogens:
  Nocardia, Acinetobacter, S. maltophilia, B. cepacia
Urine Spectrum
- Same as serum spectrum
- Opitimal urinary pH = 5–6
- Urine levels = 600 mcg/mL

(Full **Susceptibility Profiles** p. 196)

Resistance Potential: High (MSSA, aerobic GNBs)
Pharmacokinetic Parameters:
Peak serum level: 48 (IV)/5 (PO) mcg/mL
Bioavailability: 50%
Excreted unchanged (urine): 90%
Serum half-life (normal/ESRD): 0.8/10 hrs
Plasma protein binding: 20%
Volume of distribution (V_d): 0.25 L/kg
Primary Mode of Elimination: Renal
Dosage Adjustments*

CrCl 50–80 mL/min	1 gm (IV) q4h 500 mg (PO) q6h
CrCl 10–50 mL/min	1 gm (IV) q8h 250 mg (PO) q8h
CrCl < 10 mL/min	1 gm (IV) q12h 250 mg (PO) q12h
Post–HD dose	1 gm (IV) 500 mg (PO)
Post–PD dose	1 gm (IV) 250 mg (PO)

——— = serious side effect ☐ = black box warning. ND = no data. NR = not recommended. s = spectrum inadequate (at site). a = activity or experience inadequate. p = tissue penetration inadequate. *based on peak serum concentration after usual adult dose. †applicable to adult uncomplicated lower UTIs (CrCl > 30 mL/min).

CVVH/CVVHD/ CVVHDF dose	1 gm (IV) q8h 250 mg (PO) q12h
Moderate— severe hepatic insufficiency	No change

Drug Interactions: Allopurinol (↑ frequency of rash); warfarin (↑ INR).

Adverse Effects:

Common
- GI upset/diarrhea

Uncommon
- Drug fever/rash
- Leukopenia
- Eosinophilia
- Anemia
- Thrombocytopenia

Rare
- Hairy tongue
- ↑ AST/ALT
- C. difficile diarrhea/colitis
- Agranulocytosis

Allergic Potential: High
Safety in Pregnancy: B

Additional Clinical Considerations:
• Incompatible with amphotericin erythromycin, aminoglycosides, or metronidazole

May increase LPS (endotoxin) release from GNB potentially increasing endo-toxin mediated tissue damage

Pharmacokinetic Considerations*	
Non-CSF	**% of Serum Levels**
Peritoneal fluid	10%
Bile	200%
Synovial fluid	60%
Bone	10%

Prostate	NR
Urine†	150%
CSF	
Non-inflamed meninges	1%
Inflamed meninges (ABM)	10%
Meningeal dose = 2 gm (IV) q 4 h	

(also see **Antibiotic Pearls & Pitfalls** p. 526).

SELECTED REFERENCES:

Sakoulas G, Bayer AS, Pogliano J, et al. Ampicillin enhances daptomycin- and cationic host defense peptide-mediated killing of ampicillin- and vancomycin-resistant Enterococcus faecium. Antimicrob Agents Chemother. 56:838–844, 2012. (PMID: 22123698)
Website: www.pdr.net

Ampicillin/Sulbactam (Unasyn)

Drug Class: Aminopenicillin/β-lactamase inhibitor.
Usual Dose: 1.5–3 gm (IV) q6h (see comments).

Spectrum Synposis*
Hits
Gram + : Most streptococci, MSSA, VSE
Gram – : Some GNB (including Klebsiella), H. influenzae, B. fragilis
Problem pathogens:
Listeria, Acinetobacter, animal bite pathogens
Misses
Gram + : MRSA, VRE
Gram – : Most aerobic GNB

——— = serious side effect ☐ = black box warning. ND = no data. NR = not recommended. s = spectrum inadequate (at site). a = activity or experience inadequate. p = tissue penetration inadequate. *based on peak serum concentration after usual adult dose. †applicable to adult uncomplicated lower UTIs (CrCl > 30 mL/min).

Problem pathogens:
  Nocardia, S. maltophilia, B. cepacia
Urine Spectrum
  • Same as serum spectrum
  • Optimal urinary pH = 5–6

(Full *Susceptibility Profiles* p. 196).

Resistance Potential: Low
  (pseudoresistance with E. coli/
  Klebsiella)
Pharmacokinetic Parameters:
  Peak serum level: 109-150/48-88 mcg/mL
  Bioavailability: Not applicable
  Excreted unchanged (urine): 80/80%
  *Serum half-life (normal/ESRD): [1/9]/
  [1/9] hrs*
  Plasma protein binding: 28/38%
  *Volume of distribution (V_d): 0.25/
  0.38 L/kg*
Primary Mode of Elimination: Renal/
  Hepatic
Dosage Adjustments*
(based on 3 gm (IV) q6h)

CrCl 30–80 mL/min	1.5 gm (IV) q6h
CrCl 15–30 mL/min	1.5 gm (IV) q12h
CrCl < 15 mL/min	1.5 gm (IV) q24h
Post–HD dose	1.5 gm (IV)
Post–PD dose	None
CVVH/CVVHD/ CVVHDF dose	1.5–3 gm (IV) q12h
Moderate—severe hepatic insufficiency	No change

Drug Interactions: Probenecid
(↑ ampicillin/sulbactam levels);
allopurinol (↑ rash).

Adverse Effects:
Common
  • Injection site reactions
Uncommon
  • Drug fever/rash
  • Thrombophlebitis
  • Non-C. difficile diarrhea
Rare
  • AIHA
  • ↑ AST/ALT
  • <u>C. difficile diarrhea/colitis</u>
Allergic Potential: High
Safety in Pregnancy: B

Additional Clinical Considerations:
  • **Mild/moderate Infection Dose:**
    1.5 gm (IV) q6h.

May increase LPS (endotoxin) release
from GNB *potentially increasing endotoxin mediated tissue damage*

**Additional Pharmacokinetic
Considerations***

Non-CSF	**% of Serum Levels**
Peritoneal fluid	90%
Bile	<1/<3%
Synovial fluid	$NR_{(s)}$
Bone	$NR_{(s)}$
Prostate	$NR_{(p)}$
Urine†	80%
CSF	
Non-inflamed meninges	3/11%
Inflamed meninges (ABM)	39/34%

Meningeal dose = 4.5 gm (IV) q6h

(also see **Antibiotic Pearls & Pitfalls**
p. 530).

—— = serious side effect ☐ = black box warning. ND = no data. NR = not recommended. s = spectrum inadequate (at site). a = activity or experience inadequate. p = tissue penetration inadequate. *based on peak serum concentration after usual adult dose. †applicable to adult uncomplicated lower UTIs (CrCl > 30 mL/min).

SELECTED REFERENCES:

Itokazu GS, Danziger LH. Ampicillin-sulbactam and ticarcillin-clavulanic acid: A comparison of their in vitro activity and review of their clinical efficacy. Pharmacotherapy 11:382–414, 1991. (PMID:1745624)

Sensakovic JW, Smith LG. Beta-lactamase inhibitor combinations. Med Clin North Am 79:695–704, 1995. (PMID:7791417)

Wood GC, Hanes SD, Croce MA, et al. Comparison of ampicillin-sulbactam and imipenem-cilastatin for the treatment of Acinetobacter ventilator-associated pneumonia. Clin Infect Dis 34:1425–30, 2002. (PMID: 12015687)

Wright AJ. The penicillins. Mayo Clin Proc 73:290–307, 1999. (PMID:12015687)

Website: www.pdr.net

Anidulafungin (Eraxis, Ecalta)

Drug Class: Echinocandin antifungal.
Usual Dose: **Loading Dose:** 200 mg (IV) × 1 dose, then **Maintenance Dose:** 100 mg (IV) q24h.
Pharmacokinetic Parameters:
  Peak serum level: 4.2 mcg/mL (100/50 mg dose)/7.2 mcg/mL (200/100 mg dose)
  Bioavailability: Not applicable
  Excreted unchanged (urine): < 1%
  Serum half-life (normal/ESRD): 40–50 hours/40–50 hours
  Plasma protein binding: 99%
  Volume of distribution (V_d): 30 L/kg
Primary Mode of Elimination: Fecal (30%)
Dosage Adjustments*

CrCl < 50 mL/min	No change
Post–HD dose	None
Post–PD dose	None
CVVH/CVVHD/ CVVHDF dose	No change
Moderate— severe hepatic insufficiency	No change

Drug Interactions: No significant interactions.
Adverse Effects:
Common
  • Nausea/vomiting/diarrhea
  • Drug fever
  • Hypotension/hypertension
  • Peripheral edema
  • Hypokalemia
  • Hypomagnesemia
  • ↑ Alkaline phosphatase
Uncommon
  • ↑ AST/ALT
Rare
  • Rash
  • Pruritus
  • Uricaria
Allergic Potential: Histamine-related symptoms
Safety in Pregnancy: C

Additional Clinical Considerations:
  • Not an inducer, inhibitor, or substrate of CYP450 system. Rate of infusion should not exceed 1.1 mg/min.
  • Do not infuse with other medications.

—— = serious side effect ☐ = black box warning. ND = no data. NR = not recommended. s = spectrum inadequate (at site). a = activity or experience inadequate. p = tissue penetration inadequate. *based on peak serum concentration after usual adult dose. †applicable to adult uncomplicated lower UTIs (CrCl > 30 mL/min).

***Highly active** against **Candida albicans, non-albicans Candida** ($\downarrow$ susceptibility to C. parasilosis).*
Some activity** against **Aspergillus.
No activity** against **Cryptococcus, Fusarium, Pseudallescheria/ Scedosporium, Trichosporon, Rhodotorula** or **Mucor.

Cerebrospinal Fluid Penetration: No data

SELECTED REFERENCES:

Cohen-Wolkowiez M, Benjamin Jr. DK, Steinbach WJ, Smith PB. Anidulafungin: A new Echinocandin for the Treatment of Fungal Infections. Drugs of Today. 42:533–44, 2006. (PMID:16969430)

de la Torre P, Reboli AC. Anidulafungin: a new echinocandin for candidal infections. Expert Rev Anti Infect Ther 5:45–52, 2007. (PMID:17266452)

Dowell JA, Stogniew M, Krause D, et al. Anidulafungin does not require dosage adjustment in subjects with varying degrees of hepatic or renal impairment. J Clin Pharmacol 47:461–470, 2007. (PMID:17389555)

Kofla G, Ruhnke M. Pharmacology and metabolism of anidulafungin, caspofungin, and micafungin in the treatment of invasive candidosis: review of the literature. Eur J Med Res 16:159–166, 2011. (PMID:21486730)

Pfaller MA, Diekema DJ, Boyken L. Effectiveness of anidulafungin in eradicating candida species in invasive candidiasis. Antimicrob Agents Chemother 49:4795–97, 2005. (PMID:16251335)

Raasch RH. Anidulafungin: review of a new echinocandin antifungal agent. Expert Rev Anti Infect Ther 2:499–508, 2004. (PMID:15482216)

Reboli AC, Rotstein C, Pappas PG, et al. Anidulafungin versus fluconazole for invasive candidiasis. N Engl J Med 356:2472–2482, 2007. (PMID:17568028)

Vazquez JA, Sobel JD. Anidulafungin: a novel echinocandin. Clin Infect Dis 43:215–22, 2006. (PMID:16779750)

Wilke M. Treatment and prophylaxis of invasive candidiasis with anidulafungin, caspofungin,

and micafungin and its impact on use and costs: review of the literature. Eur J Med Res 16:180–186, 2011. (PMID:21486732)
Website: www.pdr.net

Atazanavir (Reyataz) ATV

Drug Class: HIV protease inhibitor.
Usual Dose: 300 mg (PO) q24h with ritonavir 100 mg (PO) q24h or 400 mg (PO) q24h *with food* if unable to tolerate ritonavir.
Treatment Experienced Patients: 300 mg with ritonavir 100 mg once daily *with food.*

Pharmacokinetic Parameters:

Peak serum level: 3152 ng/mL; with ritonavir: 5233 ng/mL
Bioavailability: No data
Excreted unchanged (urine) (urine/feces): 7%/20%
Serum half-life (normal/ESRD): 6.5 hrs; with ritonavir: 8.6 hrs/no data
Plasma protein binding: 86%
Volume of distribution (V_d): No data

Primary Mode of Elimination: Hepatic
Dosage Adjustments*

CrCl < 50 mL/min	No change
Post–HD or PD dose	None
CVVH/CVVHD/ CVVHDF dose	No change
Moderate hepatic insufficiency	300 mg (PO) q24h without ritonavir
Severe hepatic insufficiency	Avoid

── = serious side effect ☐ = black box warning. ND = no data. NR = not recommended. s = spectrum inadequate (at site). a = activity or experience inadequate. p = tissue penetration inadequate. *based on peak serum concentration after usual adult dose. †applicable to adult uncomplicated lower UTIs (CrCl > 30 mL/min).

Antiretroviral Dosage Adjustments

Delavirdine	No data
Didanosine	Give atazanavir 2 hrs before didanosine with food
Efavirenz	Treatment naive: atazanavir 400 mg q24h + ritonavir 100 mg q24h + efavirenz 600 mg q24h Treatment experienced: not recommended
Indinavir	Avoid combination
Nevirapine	No data
Ritonavir	Atazanavir 300 mg/d + ritonavir 100 mg/d as single daily dose with food
Saquinavir	↑ saquinavir (soft-gel) levels; no information
Rifampin	Avoid
Rifabutin	150 mg q48h or 3x/week

Drug Interactions: Antacids or buffered medications (↓ atazanavir levels; give atazanavir 2 hours before or 1 hour after); H$_2$-receptor blockers (↓ atazanavir levels). In treatment-naïve patients taking an H$_2$-receptor antagonist, give either atazanavir 400 mg once daily with food at least 2 hours before and at least 10 hours after the H$_2$-receptor antagonist, or give atazanavir 300 mg once daily with ritonavir 100 mg once daily with food, without the need for separation from the H$_2$-receptor antagonist. In treatment-experienced patients, give atazanavir 300 mg once daily with ritonavir 100 mg once daily with food at least 2 hours before and at least 10 hours after the H$_2$-receptor antagonist); antiarrhythmics (↑ amiodarone, systemic lidocaine, quinidine levels; prolongs PR interval; monitor antiarrhythmic levels); antidepressants (↑ tricyclic antidepressant levels; monitor levels); calcium channel blockers (↑ calcium channel blocker levels, ↑ PR interval; ↓ diltiazem dose by 50%; use with caution; consider ECG monitoring); clarithromycin (↑ clarithromycin and atazanavir levels; consider 50% dose reduction; consider alternate agent for infections not caused by MAI); cyclosporine, sirolimus, tacrolimus (↑ immunosuppressant levels; monitor levels); ethinyl estradiol, norethindrone (↑ oral contraceptive levels; use lowest effective oral contra-ceptive dose); lovastatin, simvastatin (↑ risk of myopathy, rhabdomyolysis; avoid combination); sildenafil (↑ sildenafil levels; do not give more than 25 mg q48h); tadalafil (max. 10 mg/72 hours); vardenafil (max. 2.5 mg/72 hours); St. John's wort (avoid combination); warfarin (↑ warfarin levels; monitor INR); tenofovir (tenofovir reduces systemic exposure to atazanavir).

Contraindications: Avoid use with cisapride, pimozide, rifampin, irinotecan, midazolam, triazolam, lovastatin, simvastatin, bepridil, some ergot

---

——— = serious side effect ⬜ = black box warning. ND = no data. NR = not recommended. s = spectrum inadequate (at site). a = activity or experience inadequate. p = tissue penetration inadequate. *based on peak serum concentration after usual adult dose. †applicable to adult uncomplicated lower UTIs (CrCl > 30 mL/min).

derivatives, indinavir, PPIs, St. John's wort, rifapentine, boceprevir.

Adverse Effects:

Common

- Headache
- Dizziness
- Anorexia
- Nausea/vomiting/diarrhea
- Abdominal pain
- Asthenia

Allergic Potential: Low

Safety in Pregnancy: B

Additional Clinical Considerations:

- Take 400 mg (two 200 mg capsules) once daily with food. Bioavailability is enhanced with food.
- Monitor LFTs in patients with HBV, HCV.
- In moderate liver disease reduce dose to 200 mg once daily.
- Not recommended in patients with severe liver impairment.

SELECTED REFERENCES:

Cossarini F, Salpietro S, Galli L, et al. Monotheraphy with atazanavir as a simplification strategy: results from an observational study. J Acquir Immune Defic Syndr 60:101–3, 2012. (PMID:22728751)

Foca E, Ripamonti D, Motta D, et al. Unboosted atazanavir for treatment of HIV infection: rationale and recommendations for use. Drugs 72:1161–73, 2012. (PMID:22646049)

Gandhi M, Ameli N, Bacchetti P, et al. Atazanavir concentration in hair is the strongest predictor of outcomes on antiretroviral therapy. Clin Infect Dis 52:1267–1275, 2011. (PMID:21507942)

Havlir DV, O'Marro SD. Atazanavir: new option for treatment of HIV infection. Clin Infect Dis 38:1599–604, 2004. (PMID:15156449)

Website: www.pdr.net

Atovaquone (Mepron)

Drug Class: Antiprotozoal, PCP.

Usual Dose: PCP treatment dose: 750 mg (PO) q12h. **PCP prophylaxis dose:** 1500 mg (PO) q24h

Pharmacokinetic Parameters:

Peak serum level: 12–24 mcg/mL
Bioavailability: 30% (47% with food; food ↑ bioavailability by 2-fold)
Excreted unchanged (feces): 94%
Serum half-life (normal/ESRD): 2.9/2.9 days
Plasma protein binding: 99.9%
Volume of distribution (V_d): 0.6 L/kg

Primary Mode of Elimination: Hepatic

Dosage Adjustments*

CrCl < 80 mL/min	No change
Post–HD/PD dose	None
CVVH/CVVHD/CVVHDF dose	No change
Mild-moderate hepatic insufficiency	No change
Severe hepatic insufficiency	No change

Drug Interactions: Rifabutin, rifampin (↓ atovaquone effect); zidovudine (↑ zidovudine levels). Rifampin decreases atovaquone levels by 50%.

= serious side effect ☐ = black box warning. ND = no data. NR = not recommended. s = spectrum inadequate (at site). a = activity or experience inadequate. p = tissue penetration inadequate. *based on peak serum concentration after usual adult dose. †applicable to adult uncomplicated lower UTIs (CrCl > 30 mL/min).

Adverse Effects:
Common
- Headache
- Drug fever/rash
- Nausea/vomiting/diarrhea

Uncommon
- Dizziness
- Anemia
- ↑ AST/ALT
- ↑ Amylase

Allergic Potential: Low
Safety in Pregnancy: C

Additional Clinical Considerations:
Active against T. gondii, PCP, Plasmodia, and Babesia.

Cerebrospinal Fluid Penetration: < 1%

SELECTED REFERENCES:
Artymowicz RJ, James VE. Atovaquone: A new anti-pneumocystis agent. Clin Pharmacol 12:563–70, 1993. (PMID:8222520)
Baggish AL, Hill DR. Antiparasitic agent atovaquone. Antimicrob Agents Chemother 46:1163–73, 2002. (PMID:11959541)
Bonoan JT, Johnson DH, Schoch PE, Cunha BA. Life threatening babesiosis treated by exchange transfusion with azithromycin and atovaquone. Heart & Lung 27:42–8, 1998. (PMID:9835673)
Haile LG, Flaherty JF. Atovaquone: a review. Ann Pharmacother 27:1488–94, 1993. (PMID:8305784)
Wormser GP, Prasad A, Neuhaus E, et al. Emergence of resistance to azithromycin-atovaquone in immunocompromised patients with babesia microti infection. Clin Infect Dis 50:381–386, 2010. (PMID:20047477)
Website: www.pdr.net

Atovaquone + Proguanil (Malarone)

Drug Class: Antimalarial.

Usual Dose: Malaria prophylaxis: 1 tablet (250 mg/100 mg) (PO) q24h for 2 days before entering endemic area, daily during exposure, and daily × 1 week post-exposure. Malaria treatment: 4 tablets (1000 mg/400 mg) (PO) as single dose × 3 days.

Pharmacokinetic Parameters:
Peak serum level: 38 mcg/mL
Bioavailability: 23/90%
Excreted unchanged (feces): 94/50%
Serum half-life (normal/ESRD):
[60/60]/[21/no data] hrs
Plasma protein binding: 99/75%
Volume of distribution (V_d): 3.5/42 L/kg

Primary Mode of Elimination:
Metabolized

Dosage Adjustments*

CrCl > 30 mL/min	No change
CrCl 10–30 mL/min	Avoid (for prophylaxis)
CrCl < 10 mL/min	Avoid (for prophylaxis)
Post–HD/PD dose	Avoid
CVVH/CVVHD/ CVVHDF dose	Avoid
Mild-moderate hepatic insufficiency	No change
Severe hepatic insufficiency	No change

Drug Interactions: Chloroquine (↑ incidence of mouth ulcers); metoclopramide, rifabutin, rifampin, tetracycline (↓ atovaquone + proguanil effect); ritonavir (↑ or ↓ atovaquone +

——— = serious side effect ☐ = black box warning. ND = no data. NR = not recommended. s = spectrum inadequate (at site). a = activity or experience inadequate. p = tissue penetration inadequate. *based on peak serum concentration after usual adult dose. †applicable to adult uncomplicated lower UTIs (CrCl > 30 mL/min).

proguanil effect); typhoid vaccine (↓ typhoid vaccine effect).

Adverse Effects:

Common
- Nausea/vomiting/diarrhea
- Abdominal pain

Uncommon
- Headache
- Dizziness
- ↑ AST/ALT
- ↑ Amylase

Rare
- Anemia

Allergic Potential: Low
Safety in Pregnancy: C

Additional Clinical Considerations:
- Malarone tablet = 250 mg atovaquone + 100 mg proguanil.
- Effective against chloroquine sensitive/resistant strains of P. falciparum,
No activity against **P. ovale, P. vivax, P. malariae.**

Cerebrospinal Fluid Penetration: < 1%

SELECTED REFERENCES:
Marra F, Salzman JR, Ensom MH. Atovaquone-proguanil for prophylaxis and treatment of malaria. Ann Pharmacother 37:1266–75, 2003. (PMID:12921511)

McKeage K, Scott L. Atovaquone/proguanil: a review of its use for the prophylaxis of Plasmodium falciparum malaria. Drugs 63:597–623, 2003. (PMID:12656656)

Thapar MM, Ashton M, Lindegardh N, et al. Time-dependent pharmacokinetics and drug metabolism of atovaquone plus proguanil (Malarone) when taken as chemoprophylaxis. Eur J Clin Pharmacol 15:19–27, 2002. (PMID:11956669)

Website: www.pdr.net

Azithromycin (Zithromax)

Drug Class: Macrolide (azolide).
Usual Dose: Loading dose: 500 mg (IV/PO) × 1 dose, then **Maintenance dose:** 250 mg (IV/PO) q24h.

Spectrum Synopsis*

Hits

Gram + : Some GAS, some MSSA, some S. pneumoniae, VSE

Gram – : Some H. influenzae
   Problem pathogens:
      Bordetella

Misses

Gram + : Most GAS, most S. pneumoniae, most MSSA, MRSA, VRE

Gram – : Most GNB, most H. influenzae
   Problem pathogens:
      Listeria, Nocardia, Acinetobacter, S. maltophilia, B. cepacia

---

(Full **Susceptibility Profiles** p. 196).

Resistance Potential: High
   (S. pneumoniae, c. pneumoniae, GAS, MSSA)

Pharmacokinetic Parameters:
Peak serum level: 1.1 (IV)/0.2 (PO) mcg/mL
Bioavailability: 35%
Excreted unchanged (urine): 6%
Serum half-life (normal/ESRD): 68/68 hrs
Plasma protein binding: 50%
Volume of distribution (V_d): 31 L/kg

Primary Mode of Elimination: Hepatic
Dosage Adjustments*

CrCl 10–50 mL/min	No change
CrCl < 10 mL/min	Use with caution

―――― = serious side effect ☐ = black box warning. ND = no data. NR = not recommended. s = spectrum inadequate (at site). a = activity or experience inadequate. p = tissue penetration inadequate. *based on peak serum concentration after usual adult dose. †applicable to adult uncomplicated lower UTIs (CrCl > 30 mL/min).

Post–HD/PD dose	None
CVVH/CVVHD/ CVVHDF dose	No change
Moderate— severe hepatic insufficiency	No change

Drug Interactions: Amiodarone, carbamazepine, cisapride, clozapine, corticosteroids, midazolam, triazolam, valproic acid (not studied/not reported); cyclosporine (↑ cyclosporine levels with toxicity); digoxin (↑ digoxin levels); pimozide (may ↑ QT interval, torsade de pointes).

Adverse Effects:

Common
- Nausea/GI upset/diarrhea

Uncommon
- ↑ QTc
- Torsades de pointes

Rare
- Rash
- ↑ incidence cardiac/non-cardiac sudden deaths after 5 days of therapy

Allergic Potential: Low

Safety in Pregnancy: B

Additional Clinical Considerations:
- CSF levels low, but brain levels high.
- C. trachomatis urethritis dose: 1 gm (PO) × 1 dose.
- **N. gonorrhoea urethritis dose:** 2 gm (PO) × 1 dose.
- **MAC prophylaxis dose:** 1200 mg (PO) weekly.
- **MAC therapy dose:** 600 mg (PO) q24h.

- **COVID-19:** azithromycin plus hydroxychloroquine highly effective against COVID-19. May also be used with remdesavir.

Additional Pharmacokinetic Considerations*

Non-CSF	% of Serum Levels
Peritoneal fluid	NR(s)
Bile	100%
Synovial fluid	NR(s)
Bone	NR(s)
Prostate	NR(s)
Urine	5%
CSF	
Non-inflamed meninges	0%
Inflamed meninges (ABM)	1%

(also see ***Antibiotic Pearls & Pitfalls*** p. 536)

SELECTED REFERENCES:
Bergman M, Huikko S, Huovinen P, et al. Macrolide and azithromycin use are linked to increased macrolide resistance in Streptococcus pneumoniae. Antimicrob Agents Chemother 50:3646–3650, 2006. (PMID:16940064)

Centers for Disease Control. Neisseria gonorrhoeae with reduced susceptibility to azithromycin. Morb Mortal Wkly Rep 60:579–581, 2011. (PMID:21566558)

Cunha BA, Cunha CB. Pharmacokinetic considerations in antibiotic selection for the optimal therapy of mycoplasma pneumoniae encephalitis. European Journal of Medical Microbiology & Infectious Disease 38: (In press) 2019. (PMID: 30680554)

Daneman N, McGeer A, Green K, et al. Macrolide resistance in bacteremic pneumococcal disease.: Implications for patient management. Clin Infect Dis 43:432–438, 2006. (PMID:16838230)

DuPont HL. Azithromycin for the self-treatment of traveler's diarrhea. Clin Infect Dis 44:347–349, 2007. (PMID:17582576)

─── = serious side effect ☐ = black box warning. ND = no data. NR = not recommended. s = spectrum inadequate (at site). a = activity or experience inadequate. p = tissue penetration inadequate. *based on peak serum concentration after usual adult dose. †applicable to adult uncomplicated lower UTIs (CrCl > 30 mL/min).

Frenck RW, Mansour A, Nakhla I, et al. Short-course azithromycin for the treatment of uncomplicated typhoid fever in children and adolescents. Clin Infect Dis 38:951–7, 2004. (PMID:15034826)

Griffin AT, Peyrani P, Wiemken T, et al. Macrolides versus quinolones in Legionella pneumonia: results from the Community-Acquired Pneumonia Organization international study. Int J Tuberc Lung Dis 14:495–499, 2010. (PMID:20202309)

Horner P, Ingle SM, Garrett F, et al. Which azithromycin regimen should be used for treating Mycoplasma genitalium? A meta-analysis. Sex Transm Infect 94:14-20, 2018. (PMID: 28717050)

Jain R, Danzinger LH. The macrolide antibiotics: a pharmacokinetic and pharmacodynamic overview. Curr Pharm Des 10:3045–53, 2004. (PMID:15544496)

Kim Y-S, Yun H-J, Shim SK, et al. A comparative trial of a single dose of azithromycin versus doxycycline for the treatment of mild scrub typhus. Clin Infect Dis 39:1329–35, 2004. (PMID:15494910)

Phillips P, Chan K, Hogg R, et al. Azithromycin prophylaxis for Mycobacterium avium complex during the era of highly active antiretroviral therapy: evaluation of a provincial program. Clin Infect Dis 34:371–8, 2002. (PMID:11774085)

Pichichero ME, Hoeger WJ, Casey JR. Azithromycin for the treatment of pertussis. Pediatr Infect Dis J 22:847–9, 2003. (PMID:14515842)

Plouffe JF, Breiman RF, Fields BS, et al. Azithromycin in the treatment of Legionella pneumonia requiring hospitalization. Clin Infect Dis 37:1475–80, 2003. (PMID:14614670)

Saiman L, Marshall BC, Mayer-Hamblett N, et al. Azithromycin in patients with cystic fibrosis chronically infected with Pseudomonas aeruginosa: a randomized controlled trial. JAMA. 290:1749–5, 2003. (PMID:14519709)

Savaris RF, Teixeira LM, Torres TG, et al. Comparing ceftriaxone plus azithromycin or doxycycline for pelvis inflammatory disease: a randomized controlled trial Obstet Gynecol 110:53–60, 2007. (PMID:17601896)

Suzuki S, Yamazaki T, Narita M. Clinical evaluation of macrolide-resistant Mycoplasma pneumoniae. Antimicrobial Agents and Chemotherapy. 50:709–12, 2006. (PMID:16436730)

To KK, Chan KH, Fung YF, et al. Azithromycin treatment failure in macrolide-resistant Mycoplasma pneumoniae pneumonia. Eur Respir J 36:969–971, 2010. (PMID:20889469)

Wilson R, Wells AU. Azithromycin in bronchiectasis: when should it be used? Lancet. 380:627–629, 2012. (PMID:22901872)

Wormser GP, Prasad A, Neuhaus E, et al. Emergence of resistance to azithromycin-atovaquone in immunocompromised patients with Babesia microti infection. Clin Infect Dis 50:381–386, 2010. (PMID:20047477)

Website: www.pdr.net

Aztreonam (Azactam)

Drug Class: Monobactam.
Usual Dose: 2 gm (IV) q8h (see comments).

Spectrum Synopsis*
Hits
Gram + : None
Gram – : Most aerobic GNBs
Problem pathogens:
CRE
Misses
Gram + : All
Gram – : B. fragilis
Problem pathogens:
S. maltophilia, B. cepacia
P. aeruginosa, Acinetobacter
Urine Spectrum
• Same as serum spectrum
• Optimal urinary pH = ND
• Urine levels = 2000 mcg/mL

―――― = serious side effect ☐ = black box warning. ND = no data. NR = not recommended. s = spectrum inadequate (at site). a = activity or experience inadequate. p = tissue penetration inadequate. *based on peak serum concentration after usual adult dose. †applicable to adult uncomplicated lower UTIs (CrCl > 30 mL/min).

(Full *Susceptibility Profiles* p. 208).
Resistance Potential: Low
Pharmacokinetic Parameters:
Peak serum level: 204 mcg/mL
Bioavailability: Not applicable
Excreted unchanged (urine): 60–70%
Serum half-life (normal/ESRD): 1.7/7 hrs
Plasma protein binding: 56%
Volume of distribution (V_d): 0.2 L/kg

Primary Mode of Elimination: Renal
Dosage Adjustments* (based on 2 gm IV q8h)

CrCl 10–50 mL/min	1 gm (IV) q8h
CrCl < 10 mL/min	500 mg (IV) q8h
Post–HD dose	500 mg (IV)
Post–PD dose	500 mg (IV)
CVVH/CVVHD/CVVHDF dose	1–2 gm (IV) q12h
Moderate hepatic insufficiency	No change
Severe hepatic insufficiency	No change

Drug Interactions: None.
Adverse Effects:
Common
- Injection site pain
- Neutropenia
- ↑ AST/ALT
Uncommon
- ↑ Creatinine
- Thrombocytosis
Rare
- Drug fever/rash
- Eosinophilia
Allergic Potential: Low
Safety in Pregnancy: B

Additional Clinical Considerations:
- Incompatible in solutions containing vancomycin or metronidazole.
- No cross allergenicity with penicillins, β-lactams; safe to use in penicillin allergic patients.
- **CAPD dose:** 1 gm (IP), then 250 mg/L of dialysate (IP) with each exchange.

May increase LPS (endotoxin) release from GNB potentially increasing endotoxin mediated tissue damage.

Additional Pharmacokinetic Considerations*

Non-CSF	% of Serum Levels
Peritoneal fluid	10%
Bile	300%
Synovial fluid	40%
Bone	10%
Prostate	10%
Urine†	60–70%
CSF	
Non-inflamed meninges	1%
Inflamed meninges (ABM)	40%

Meningeal dose = 2 gm (IV) q6h

(also see *Antibiotic Pearls & Pitfalls* p. 529).

SELECTED REFERENCES:
Assael BM. Aztreonam inhalation solution for suppressive treatment of chronic Pseudomonas aeruginosa lung infection in cystic fibrosis. Expert Rev Anti Infect Ther 9:967–973, 2011. (PMID:22029514)
Brogden RN, Heal RC. Aztreonam: A review of its antibacterial activity, pharmacokinetic properties, and therapeutic use. Drugs 31:96–130, 1986. (PMID:3512234)

⎯⎯⎯ = serious side effect ☐ = black box warning. ND = no data. NR = not recommended. s = spectrum inadequate (at site). a = activity or experience inadequate. p = tissue penetration inadequate. *based on peak serum concentration after usual adult dose. †applicable to adult uncomplicated lower UTIs (CrCl > 30 mL/min).

Cunha BA. Aztreonam: A review. Urology 41:249–58, 1993. (PMID:8442309)

Johnson, Cunha BA. Aztreonam. Med Clin North Am 79:733–43, 1995. (PMID:7791420)

Jordan EF, Nye MB, Luque AE. Successful treatment of Pasteurella multocida meningitis with aztreonam. Scand J Infect Dis 39:72–74, 2007. (PMID:17366017)

Zeitler K, Salvas B, Stevens V, et al. Aztreonam lysine for inhalation: new formulation of an old antibiotic. Am J Health Syst Pharm 69:107–115, 2012. (PMID:22215556)

Website: www.pdr.net

Aztreonam/Avibactam (ATM/AVI)

Drug Class: Monobactam/β-lactamase inhibitor.
Usual Dose: 2 gm (IV) q8h.

Spectrum Synopsis*

Hits

Gram + : None

Gram – : Serratia, Klebsiella, Enterobacter, E. coli

Problem pathogens:

S. maltophilia, P. aeruginosa, CRE

Misses

Gram + : All

Gram – : B. fragilis

Problem pathogens:

B. cepacia, Acinetobacter

Urine Spectrum

- Same as serum spectrum
- Optimal urinary pH = *ND*
- Urine levels = 2000/14 mcg/mL

(Full *Susceptibility Profiles* p. 208).
Resistance Potential: Low ↑
Pharmacokinetic Parameters:

Peak serum level: Aztreonam:/ Avibactam: 204/36 mcg/mL
Bioavailability: Not applicable
Excreted unchanged (urine): Aztreonam: 60–70%/Avibactam: 85%
Serum half-life (normal/ESRD): Aztreonam: 1.7/7 hrs/Avibactam: 2/22.8 hrs
Plasma protein binding: Aztreonam: 56%/Avibactam: 8%
Volume of distribution (V_d): Aztreonam: 0.2 L/kg/Avibactam: 0.32 L/kg

Primary Mode of Elimination: Renal
Dosage Adjustments*

CrCl 10–50 mL/min	1 gm (IV) q8h/*ND*
CrCl < 10 mL/min	500 mg (IV) q8h/*ND*
Post–HD dose	500 mg (IV)/*ND*
Post–PD dose	500 mg (IV)/*ND*
CVVH/CVVHD/CVVHDF dose	1–2 gm (IV) q12h/*ND*
Mild of moderate hepatic insufficiency	No change
Severe hepatic insufficiency	No change

Drug Interactions: None.
Adverse Effects:

Common

- Injection site pain
- Neutropenia
- ↑ AST/ALT

Uncommon

- ↑ Creatinine
- Thrombocytosis

—— = serious side effect ☐ = black box warning. ND = no data. NR = not recommended. s = spectrum inadequate (at site). a = activity or experience inadequate. p = tissue penetration inadequate.
*based on peak serum concentration after usual adult dose. †applicable to adult uncomplicated lower UTIs (CrCl > 30 mL/min).

Rare
- Drug fever/rash
- Eosinophilia

Allergic Potential: Low

Additional Clinical Considerations:
- Probably safe in pregnancy.
- Useful in penicillin allergic patients.

Additional Pharmacokinetic Considerations*

Non-CSF	% of Serum Levels
Peritoneal fluid	10%/ND
Bile	300%/ND
Synovial fluid	40%/ND
Bone	10%/ND
Prostate	10%/ND
Urine[†]	60–70%
CSF	
Non-inflamed meninges	1%/ND
Inflamed meninges (ABM)	40%/ND

Meningeal dose = ND

(also see **Antibiotic Pearls & Pitfalls** p. 530).

SELECTED REFERENCES:

Biedenbach DJ, Kazmeirczak KM, Bouchillon SK, et al. In vitro activity of aztreonam-avibactam against a global collection of gram-negative pathogens from 2012-2013. Antimicrob Agents Chemother 59: doi: 10.1128/AAC.00206-15, 2015. (PMID: 25963984)

Karlowsky JA, Kazmierczak KM, de Jonge BLM, et al. In vitro activity of aztreonam-avibactam against Enterobacteriaceae and Pseudomonas aeruginosa isolated by clinical laboratories in 40 countries from 2012-2015. Antimicrob Agents Chemother 61: pii: e00472-17. doi: 10.1128/ACC.00472-17, 2017. (PMID: 28630192)

Mojica MF, Papp-Wallace KM, Taracila MA, et al. Avibactam restores the susceptibility of clinical isolates of Stenotrophomas maltophilia to aztreonam. Antimicrob Agents Chemother 61: pii: e00777-17. doi: 10.1128/AAC.00777-17, 2017. (PMID: 28784669)

Tarral A, Merdjan H. Effect of age and sex on the pharmacokinetics and safety of avibactam in healthy volunteers. Clin Ther 37:877-886, 2015. (PMID: 25769615)

Website: www.pdr.net

Baloxavir (Xofluza)

Drug Class: Antiviral (influenza A and B) polymerase acidic (PA) endonuclease inhibitor

Usual Dose: 40-79 kg: 40 mg (PO) × 1 dose
≥ 80 kg: 80 mg (PO) × 1 dose.
(take without food)

Pharmacokinetic Parameters:
 Peak serum level: .0964-0.107 mcg/mL
 Bioavailability: ND
 Excreted unchanged: 3%
 Serum half-life (normal): 79 hrs
 Plasma protein binding: 93–94%
 Volume of distribution (V_d): 0.27 L/kg

Primary Mode of Elimination: Metabolic

Dosage Adjustments*

CrCl ≥ 50 mL/min	No change
CrCl < 50 mL/min	ND
Post–HD dose	ND
Post–PD dose	ND
CVVH dose	ND
Mild-to-moderate hepatic insufficiency	No change
Severe hepatic insufficiency	ND

"Usual dose" assumes normal renal/hepatic function. * For renal insufficiency, give usual dose × 1 followed by maintenance dose per CrCl. For dialysis patients, dose the same as for CrCl < 10 mL/min and give supplemental (post-HD/PD dose) immediately after dialysis. CrCl = creatinine clearance; CVVH = continuous veno-venous hemofiltration; HD/PD = hemo-dialysis/peritoneal dialysis.

Drug Interactions: Polyvalent cations (calcium, aluminum, magnesium) (↓ baloxavir levels).
Adverse Effects:
Common
- Diarrhea
- Bronchitis
Uncommon
- Headache
- Nausea
- Nasopharyngitis
Allergic Potential: Low

Additional Clinical Considerations:
- Most effective if patient symptomatic < 48 hours.
- Single dose therapy of influenza.
- Effective against oseltamivir resistant strains.
- Clinical improvement in 2 days.
- Decreases viral shedding more rapidly than oseltamivir.

SELECTED REFERENCES:
Antiviral drugs for treatment and prophylaxis of seasonal influenza 2018-2019. Med Lett Drugs Ther. 61:e11-e12. 2019. (PMID: 30681664)
Antiviral drugs for treatment and prophylaxis of seasonal influenza. Med Lett Drugs Ther. 61(1563):1-4. 2019. (PMID: 30681660)
Baloxavir marboxil (Xofluza) for treatment of influenza. Med Lett Drugs Ther. 60(1561):193-196. 2018. (PMID: 30653474)
Ng KE. Xofluza (Baloxavir Marboxil) for the treatment of acute uncomplicated influenza. PT. 9-11. 2019. (PMID: 3067506)
Website. www.pdr.net

Capreomycin (Capastat)

Drug Class: TB drug.
Usual Dose: 1 gm (IM) q24h.

Pharmacokinetic Parameters:
Peak serum level: 30 mcg/mL
Bioavailability: Not applicable
Excreted unchanged (urine): 50%
Serum half-life (normal/ESRD): 5/30 hrs
Plasma protein binding: No data
Volume of distribution (V_d): 0.4 L/kg
Primary Mode of Elimination: Renal
Dosage Adjustments*

CrCl 50–80 mL/min	500 mg (IM) q24h
CrCl 10–50 mL/min	500 mg (IM) q48h
CrCl < 10 mL/min	500 mg (IM) q72h
Post–HD dose	500 mg (IM)
Post–PD dose	None
CVVH/CVVHD/CVVHDF dose	500 mg (IM) q48h
Moderate hepatic insufficiency	No change
Severe hepatic insufficiency	No change

Drug Interactions: None.
Adverse Effects:
Common
- Ototoxicity
- ↑ BUN
Uncommon
- Drug fever/rash
- Eosinophilia
Allergic Potential: Moderate
Safety in Pregnancy: C

Additional Clinical Considerations:
- Pain/phlebitis at IM injection site.
- Additive toxicity with aminoglycosides/viomycin.

Cerebrospinal Fluid Penetration: <10%

"Usual dose" assumes normal renal/hepatic function. * For renal insufficiency, give usual dose × 1 followed by maintenance dose per CrCl. For dialysis patients, dose the same as for CrCl < 10 mL/min and give supplemental (post-HD/PD dose) immediately after dialysis. CrCl = creatinine clearance; CVVH = continuous veno-venous hemofiltration; HD/PD = hemodialysis/peritoneal dialysis.

SELECTED REFERENCES:
Caminero JA, Sotgiu G, Zumla A, et al. Best
   drug treatment for multidrug-resistant and
   extensively drug-resistant tuberculosis. Lancet
   Infect Dis 10:621–629, 2010. (PMID:20797644)
Website: www.pdr.net

Caspofungin (Cancidas)

Drug Class: Echinocandin antifungal.
Usual Dose: *Loading Dose:* 70 mg (IV) ×
1 dose, then *Maintenance Dose:* 50 mg
(IV) q24h (see comments).
Pharmacokinetic Parameters:
   *Peak serum level: 70 mg: 12.1 (single
   dose)/14.83 mcg/mL (multiple dose)
   50 mg: 7.6/8.7 mcg/mL (multiple dose)
   Bioavailability: Not applicable
   Excreted unchanged (urine): 1.4%
   Serum half-life (normal/ESRD): 10/10 hrs
   Plasma protein binding: 97%
   Volume of distribution (V_d): 9.6 L/kg*
Primary Mode of Elimination: Hepatic
Dosage Adjustments*

CrCl < 10 mL/min	No change
Post–HD/PD dose	None
CVVH/CVVHD/ CVVHDF dose	None
Moderate hepatic insufficiency	35 mg (IV) q24h (maintenance dose after 70 mg (IV) loading dose)
Severe hepatic insufficiency	Use with caution

Drug Interactions: Carbamazepine,
rifampin, dexamethasone, efavirenz,
nelfinavir, nevirapine, phenytoin

(↓ caspofungin levels; ↑ caspofungin
maintenance dose to 70 mg/day);
cyclosporine (↑ caspofungin levels,
↑ AST/ALT; co-administration is
discouraged unless careful monitoring
can be ensured and unless the benefit
of caspofungin outweighs the risk of
hepatotoxicity); tacrolimus (↓ tacrolimus
levels, ↑ AST/ALT).
Adverse Effects:
Common
   • Nausea/vomiting/diarrhea
   • Fever/chills
   • Drug fever/rash
   • Headache
   • Hypotension
   • Anemia
   • ↑ AST/ALT
Allergic Potential: Low
Safety in Pregnancy: C

Additional Clinical Considerations:
   • Administer by slow IV infusion
      over 1 hour.
   • Do not mix/co-infuse with
      glucose solutions
   • **Highly-resistant organisms dose:**
      70 mg (IV) q24h.
   • **Esophageal candidiasis dose:**
      begin therapy with 50 mg dose.
Highly active against Candida albicans
   *and non-albicans Candida,
   Hansenula.*
Some activity against C. parapsilosis,
   Aspergillus.
No activity against Cryptococcus,
   *Fusarium, Pseudallescheria/
   Scedosporium, Rhodotorula,
   Trichosporon, or Mucor.*

Cerebrospinal Fluid Penetration: 20%

———— = serious side effect ⬜ = black box warning. ND = no data. NR = not recommended. s = spectrum inadequate (at site). a = activity or experience inadequate. p = tissue penetration inadequate.
*based on peak serum concentration after usual adult dose. †applicable to adult uncomplicated lower UTIs (CrCl > 30 mL/min).

SELECTED REFERENCES:

Armstrong-James D, Stebbing J, John L, et al. A trial of caspofungin salvage treatment in PCP pneumonia. Thorax 66:537–538, 2011. (PMID:20880871)

Bennett JE, Echinocandins for candidemia in adults without neutropenia. N Engl J Med 355:1154–9, 2006. (PMID:16971721)

Colombo AL, Ngai AL, Bourque M, et al. Caspfungin use in patients with invasive candidiasis caused by common non-albicans Candida species: review of the caspofungin database. Antimicrob Agents Chemother 54:1864–1871, 2010. (PMID:20231388)

Deresinski SC, Stevens DA. Caspofungin. Clin Infect Dis 36:1445–57, 2003. (PMID:12766841)

Falagas ME, Ntziora F, Betsi GI, et al. Caspofungin for the treatment of fungal infections: a systematic review of randomized controlled trials. Int J Animicrob Agents 29:136–143, 2007. (PMID:17207609)

Hiemenz JW, Raad II, Maertens JA, et al. Efficacy of caspofungin as salvage therapy for invasive aspergillosis compared to standard therapy in a historical cohort. Eur J Clin Microbiol Infect Dis 29:1387–1394, 2010. (PMID:20703506)

Hope WW, Shoham S, Walsh TJ. The pharmacology and clinical use of caspofungin. Expert Opin Drug Metab Toxicol 3:263–274, 2007. (PMID:17428155)

Kofia G, Ruhnke M. Pharmacology and metabolism of anidulafungin, caspofungin, and micafungin in the treatment of invasive candidosis: review of the literature. Eur J Med Res 16:159–166, 2011. (PMID:21486730)

Lortholary O, Desnos-Ollivier M, Sitbon K, et al. Recent exposure to caspofungin or fluconazole influences the epidemiology of candidemia: a prospective multicenter study involving 2,441 patients. Antimicrob Agents Chemother 55:532–538, 2011. (PMID:21078946)

Maertens J, Raad I, Petrikkos G, et al. Efficacy and safety of caspofungin for treatment of invasive aspergillosis in patients refractory to or intolerant of conventional antifungal therapy. Clin Infect Dis 39:1563–71, 2004. (PMID:15570352)

Nguyen TH, Hoppe-Tichy T, Geiss HK, et al. Factors influencing caspofungin plasma concentrations in patients of a surgical intensive care unit. J Antimicrob Chemother 60:100–106, 2007. (PMID:17525052)

Pappas PG, Rotstein CM, Betts RF, et al. Micafungin versus caspofungin for treatment of candidemia and other forms of invasive candidiasis. Clin Infect Dis 45:883–893, 2007. (PMID:17806055)

Sobel JD, Bradshaw SK, Lipka CJ, et al. Caspofungin in the treatment of symptomatic candiduria. Clin Infect Dis 44:e46–e49, 2007. (PMID:17278048)

Steinmann J, Buer J, Rath PM. Caspofungin: cross-reactivity in the Aspergillus antigen assay. J Clin Microbiol 48:2313, 2010. (PMID:20357214)

Wiederhold NP, Najvar LK, Bocanegra RA, et al. Caspofungin dose escalation for invasive candidiasis due to resistant Candida albicans. Antimicrob Agents Chemother 55:3254–3260, 2011. (PMID:21502632)

Wilke M. Treatment and prophylaxis of invasive candidiasis with anidulafungin, caspofungin, and micafungin and its impact on use and costs: review of the literature. Eur J Med Res 16:180–186, 2011. (PMID:21486732)

Winkler M, Pratschke J, Schulz U, et al. Caspofungin for post solid organ transplant invasive fungal disease: results of a retrospective observational study. Transpl Infect Dis 12:230–237, 2010. (PMID:20070619)

Website: www.pdr.net

Cefaclor (Ceclor)

Drug Class: 2nd generation oral cephalosporin.
Usual Dose: 500 mg (PO) q8h.

Spectrum Synopsis*
Hits
  Gram + : All non-enterococcal streptococci, MSSA
  Gram – : Many GNB (including Klebsiella, H. influenzae)
  Problem pathogens: None
Misses
  Gram + : MRSA, VSE, VRE
  Gram – : Most GNB (including Proteus), P. aeruginosa, B. fragilis
  Problem pathogens: Listeria, Nocardia, Acinetobacter, S. maltophilia, B. cepacia

(Full **Susceptibility Profiles** p. 201).

─── = serious side effect ☐ = black box warning. ND = no data. NR = not recommended. s = spectrum inadequate (at site). a = activity or experience inadequate. p = tissue penetration inadequate. *based on peak serum concentration after usual adult dose. †applicable to adult uncomplicated lower UTIs (CrCl > 30 mL/min).

Resistance Potential: Low

Pharmacokinetic Parameters:

Peak serum level: 13 mcg/mL
Bioavailability: 80%
Excreted unchanged (urine): 60–85%
Serum half-life (normal/ESRD): 0.8/3 hrs
Plasma protein binding: 25%
Volume of distribution (V_d): 0.30 L/kg

Primary Mode of Elimination: Renal

Dosage Adjustments*

CrCl < 10 mL/min	250 mg (PO) q8h
Post–HD dose	250 mg (PO)
Post–PD dose	None
CVVH/CVVHD/CVVHDF dose	No change
Moderate—severe hepatic insufficiency	No change

Drug Interactions: None.

Adverse Effects:

Common
- GI upset
- Drug fever/rash

Uncommon
- C. difficile diarrhea/colitis

Allergic Potential: High

Safety in Pregnancy: B

Additional Clinical Considerations:
- Limited penetration into respiratory secretions.
- Ceclor CD 500 mg (PO) q12h is equivalent to cefaclor 250 mg (PO) q8h, not cefaclor 500 mg (PO) q8h.
- Ceclor CD 500 mg (PO) q12h is equivalent to 250 mg (PO) q8h of cefaclor.

(also see ***Antibiotic Pearls & Pitfalls*** p. 528).

SELECTED REFERENCES:

Cazzola M, Di Perna F, Boveri B. Interrelationship between the pharmacokinetics and pharmacodynamics of cefaclor advanced formulation in patients with acute exacerbation of chronic bronchitis. J Chemother 12:216–22, 2000. (PMID:10877516)

Mazzei T, Novelli A, Esposito S, et al. New insight into the clinical pharmacokinetics of cefaclor: Tissue penetration. J Chemother 12:53–62, 2000. (PMID:10768516)

Meyers BR. Cefaclor revisited. Clin Ther 22:154–66, 2000. (PMID:10743978)

Website: www.pdr.net

Cefadroxil (Duricef, Ultracef)

Drug Class: 1st generation oral cephalosporin.

Usual Dose: 1000 mg (PO) q12h.

Spectrum Synopsis*

Hits
  Gram + : All non-enterococcal streptococci, MSSA
  Gram – : Many GNB (including Klebsiella, H. influenzae)
  Problem pathogens:
    None

Misses
  Gram + : MRSA, VSE, VRE
  Gram – : Most GNB (including Proteus, P. aeruginosa), B. fragilis
  Problem pathogens:
    Listeria, Nocardia, Acinetobacter, S. maltophilia, B. cepacia

(Full ***Susceptibility Profiles*** p. 201).

Resistance Potential: Low

Pharmacokinetic Parameters:

Peak serum level: 16 mcg/mL
Bioavailability: 99%

―――― = serious side effect ☐ = black box warning. ND = no data. NR = not recommended. s = spectrum inadequate (at site). a = activity or experience inadequate. p = tissue penetration inadequate. *based on peak serum concentration after usual adult dose. †applicable to adult uncomplicated lower UTIs (CrCl > 30 mL/min).

Excreted unchanged (urine): 85%
Serum half-life (normal/ESRD): 0.5/22 hrs
Plasma protein binding: 20%
Volume of distribution (V_d): 0.31 L/kg
Primary Mode of Elimination: Renal
Dosage Adjustments*

CrCl 10–25 mL/min	500 mg (PO) q24h
CrCl < 10 mL/min	500 mg (PO) q36h
Post–HD dose	500 mg (PO)
Post–PD dose	250 mg (PO)
CVVH/CVVHD/ CVVHDF dose	500 mg (PO) q24h
Moderate hepatic insufficiency	No change
Severe hepatic insufficiency	No change

Drug Interactions: None.
Adverse Effects:
Common
 • Non-C. difficile diarrhea
Uncommon
 • Drug fever/rash
 • <u>Clostridium difficile diarrhea/colitis</u>
Allergic Potential: High
Safety in Pregnancy: B

Additional Clinical Considerations:
 • Penetrates oral/respiratory secretions well.
Bile Penetration: 20%
Cerebrospinal Fluid Penetration: < 10%

(also see ***Antibiotic Pearls & Pitfalls*** p. 527).

SELECTED REFERENCES:
Gustaferro CA, Steckelberg JM. Cephalosporins: Antimicrobic agents and related compounds. Mayo Clin Proc 66:1064–73, 1991. (PMID:1921490)
Website: www.pdr.net

Cefamandole (Mandol)

Drug Class: 2nd generation cephalosporin.
Usual Dose: 2 gm (IV) q6h.

Spectrum Synopsis*
Hits
Gram + : All non-enterococcal streptococci, MSSA
Gram – : Some GNB (including Klebsiella)
Problem pathogens: None
Misses
Gram + : MRSA, VSE, VRE
Gram – : Enterobacter, Serratia, P. aeruginosa, B. fragilis
Problem pathogens: Listeria, Nocardia, Acinetobacter, S. maltophilia, B. cepacia

(Full ***Susceptibility Profiles*** p. 201)

Resistance Potential: High
 (H. influenzae, Enterobacter sp.)
Pharmacokinetic Parameters:
Peak serum level: 240 mcg/mL
Bioavailability: Not applicable
Excreted unchanged (urine): 85%
Serum half-life (normal/ESRD): 1/11 hrs
Plasma protein binding: 76%
Volume of distribution (V_d): 0.29 L/kg

——— = serious side effect ☐ = black box warning. ND = no data. NR = not recommended. s = spectrum inadequate (at site). a = activity or experience inadequate. p = tissue penetration inadequate. *based on peak serum concentration after usual adult dose. †applicable to adult uncomplicated lower UTIs (CrCl > 30 mL/min).

Primary Mode of Elimination: Renal
Dosage Adjustments*

CrCl 50–80 mL/min	1 gm (IV) q6h
CrCl 10–50 mL/min	1 gm (IV) q6h
CrCl < 10 mL/min	1 gm (IV) q12h
Post–HD dose	1 gm (IV)
Post–PD dose	1 gm (IV)
CVVH/CVVHD/ CVVHDF dose	1 gm (IV) q6h
Moderate—severe hepatic insufficiency	No change

Drug Interactions: Alcohol (disulfiram-like reaction); antiplatelet agents, heparin, thrombolytics, warfarin ($\uparrow$ risk of bleeding).
Adverse Effects:
Common
• Drug fever/rash
Uncommon
• <u>C. difficile diarrhea/colitis</u>
• <u>$\uparrow$ INR</u>
• Disulfiram reactions (with EtOH)
Allergic Potential: High
Safety in Pregnancy: B

Additional Clinical Considerations:
• Contains MTT side chain, *but no increase in clinical bleeding.*

Additional Pharmacokinetic Considerations*

Non-CSF	% of Serum Levels
Peritoneal fluid	NR(s)
Bile	70%
Synovial fluid	NR(s)
Bone	5%
Prostate	NR(p)
Urine	50%

CSF	
Non-inflamed meninges	1%
Inflamed meninges (ABM)	<10%

(also see ***Antibiotic Pearls & Pitfalls*** p. 528).

SELECTED REFERENCE:
Website: www.pdr.net

Cefazolin (Ancef, Kefzol)

Drug Class: 1st generation cephalosporin.
Usual Dose: 1 gm (IV) q8h.

Spectrum Synopsis*
Hits
  Gram + : All non-enterococcal streptococci, MSSA, most CoNS
  Gram – : Some GNB (including Klebsiella)
  Problem pathogens:
    None
Misses
  Gram + : MRSA, some CoNS, VSE, VRE
  Gram – : H. influenzae, Enterobacter, Serratia, P. aeruginosa, B. fragilis
  Problem pathogens:
    Listeria, Nocardia, Acinetobacter, S. maltophilia, B. cepacia

(Full ***Susceptibility Profiles*** p. 201).

Resistance Potential: Low
Pharmacokinetic Parameters:
Peak serum level: 185 mcg/mL
Bioavailability: Not applicable
Excreted unchanged (urine): 96%
Serum half-life (normal/ESRD): 1.8/40 hrs
Plasma protein binding: 85%
Volume of distribution (V_d): 0.2 L/kg

―――― = serious side effect ☐ = black box warning. ND = no data. NR = not recommended. s = spectrum inadequate (at site). a = activity or experience inadequate. p = tissue penetration inadequate. *based on peak serum concentration after usual adult dose. †applicable to adult uncomplicated lower UTIs (CrCl > 30 mL/min).

Primary Mode of Elimination: Renal
Dosage Adjustments*

CrCl 35–55 mL/min	1 gm (IV) q12h
CrCl 10–35 mL/min	500 mg (IV) q12h
CrCl < 10 mL/min	500 mg (IV) q24h
Post–HD dose	1 gm (IV)
Post–HFHD dose	2 gm (IV)
Post–PD dose	500 mg (IV)
CVVH/CVVHD/ CVVHDF dose	500 mg (IV) q12h
HD q 48–72h dose	2 gm (IV) q HD*
Moderate—severe hepatic insufficiency	No change

*Give at end of HD.
Drug Interactions: None.
Adverse Effects:
Common
- Drug fever/rash
Uncommon
- Thrombocytopenia
- AIHA
- C. difficile diarrhea/colitis
Allergic Potential: High
Safety in Pregnancy: B

Additional Clinical Considerations: [†]
- Incompatible in solutions containing erythromycin, aminoglycosides.

Additional Pharmacokinetic Considerations*

Non-CSF	% of Serum Levels
Peritoneal fluid	30%
Bile	300%
Synovial fluid	15%
Bone	25%

Prostate	NR(p)
Urine	100%
CSF	
Non-inflamed meninges	1%
Inflamed meninges (ABM)	<10%

(also see **Antibiotic Pearls & Pitfalls** p. 527).

SELECTED REFERENCES:

Adembri C, Ristori R, Chelazzi C, et al. Cefazolin bolus and continuous administration for elective cardiac surgery: improved pharmacokinetic and pharmacodynamic parameters. J Thorac Cardiovasc Surg 140:471–475, 2010. (PMID:20570290)

Chen X, Brathwaite C, Cunha BA, et al. Optimal Cefazolin Prophylactic Dosing for Bariatric Surgery: No Need for Higher Doses or Intraoperative Redosing. Obesity Surgery 27:626-629, 2017. (PMID: 27520693)

Cunha BA, Gossling HR, Pasternak HS, et al. Penetration of cephalosporins into bone. Infection 12:80–4, 1984. (PMID:6735481)

Gentry LO, Zeluff BJ, Cooley DA. Antibiotic prophylaxis in open-heart surgery: A comparison of cefamandole, cefuroxime, and cefazolin. Ann Thorac Surg 46:167–71, 1988. (PMID:3401076)

Marshall WF, Blair JE. The cephalosporins. Mayo Clin Proc 74:187–95, 1999. (PMID:10069359)

Nightingale CH, Klimek JJ, Quintiliani R. Effect of protein binding on the penetration of nonmetabolized cephalosporins into atrial appendage and pericardial fluids in open-heart surgical patients. Antimicrob Agents Chemother 17:595–8, 1980. (PMID:7396452)

Quintiliani R, Nightingale CH. Cefazolin. Ann Intern Med 89:650–6, 1978. (PMID:362999)

Turnidge JD. Cefazolin and Enterobacteriaceae: rationale for revised susceptibility testing breakpoints. Clin Infect Dis 52:917–924, 2011. (PMID:21427400)

Website: www.pdr.net

——— = serious side effect ☐ = black box warning. ND = no data. NR = not recommended. s = spectrum inadequate (at site). a = activity or experience inadequate. p = tissue penetration inadequate. *based on peak serum concentration after usual adult dose. [†] applicable to adult uncomplicated lower UTIs (CrCl > 30 mL/min).

Cefdinir (Omnicef)

Drug Class: 3rd generation oral cephalosporin.
Usual Dose: 600 mg (PO) q24h.

Spectrum Synopsis*
Hits
  Gram + : All non-enterococcal
     streptococci, MSSA
  Gram – : Some GNB
  Problem pathogens:
     None
Misses
  Gram + : MSSA, MRSA, VSE, VRE
  Gram – : Most GNB, B. fragilis
  Problem pathogens:
     Listeria, Nocardia, Acinetobacter,
     S. maltophilia, B. cepacia

(Full **Susceptibility Profiles** p. 201).

Resistance Potential: Low
Pharmacokinetic Parameters:
  Peak serum level: 2.9 mcg/mL
  Bioavailability: 16% (tab) /
  25%(suspension)
  Excreted unchanged (urine): 11–18%
  Serum half-life (normal/ESRD): 1.7/3 hrs
  Plasma protein binding: 70%
  Volume of distribution (V_d): 0.35 L/kg
Primary Mode of Elimination: Renal
Dosage Adjustments*

CrCl < 30 mL/min	300 mg (PO) q24h
Post–HD dose	300 mg (PO)
Post–PD dose	None
CVVH/CVVHD/ CVVHDF dose	300 mg (PO) q24h
Moderate—severe hepatic insufficiency	No change

Drug Interactions: Probenecid (↑ cefdinir levels).
Adverse Effects:
Common
  • Non-C. difficile diarrhea
Uncommon
  • Drug fever/rash
  • <u>C. difficile diarrhea/colitis</u>
Allergic Potential: High
Safety in Pregnancy: B

Additional Clinical Considerations:
  • Good activity against bacterial respi-
    ratory pathogens.
  • Available as capsules or suspension.
  • **CAP dose:** 300 mg (PO) q12h
  • **Other respiratory infections dose:**
    600 mg (PO) q24h**.**

(also see **Antibiotic Pearls & Pitfalls**
p. 529).

SELECTED REFERENCES:
Cefdinir: A new oral cephalosporin. Med Lett Drugs
   Therap 40:85–7, 1998. (PMID:9731242)
Guay DR. Cefdinir: an advanced-generation, broad-
   spectrum oral cephalosporin. Clin Ther 24:473–
   89, 2002. (PMID:12017394)
Hedrick JA. Community-acquired upper respiratory
   tract infections and the role of third-generation
   oral cephalosporins. Expert Rev Anti Infect Ther
   8:15–21, 2010. (PMID:20014898)
Perry CM, Scott LJ. Cefdinir: a review of its use
   in the management of mild-to-moderate
   bacterial infections. Drugs 64:1433–64, 2004.
   (PMID:15212560)
Website: www.pdr.net

Cefditoren (Spectracef)

Drug Class: 3rd generation oral cephalosporin.
Usual Dose: 400 mg (PO) q12h.

—— = serious side effect ☐ = black box warning. ND = no data. NR = not recommended. s = spec-trum inadequate (at site). a = activity or experience inadequate. p = tissue penetration inadequate. *based on peak serum concentration after usual adult dose. †applicable to adult uncomplicated lower UTIs (CrCl > 30 mL/min).

Spectrum Synopsis*
Hits
  Gram + : All non-enterococcal
     streptococci
  Gram − : Some GNB
     (including Serratia)
  Problem pathogens:
     None
Misses
  Gram + : MSSA, MRSA, VSE, VRE
  Gram − : Most GNB, B. fragilis
  Problem pathogens:
     Listeria, Nocardia, Acinetobacter,
     S. maltophilia, B. cepacia

(Full *Susceptibility Profiles* p. 201).

Resistance Potential: Low
Pharmacokinetic Parameters:
  Peak serum level: 1.8 mcg/mL
  Bioavailability: 16%
  Excreted unchanged (urine): 20%
  Serum half-life (normal/ESRD): 1.5/5 hrs
  Plasma protein binding: 88%
  Volume of distribution (V_d): 0.13 L/kg
Primary Mode of Elimination: Renal
Dosage Adjustments*

CrCl 50–80 mL/min	No change
CrCl 30–50 mL/min	200 mg (PO) q12h
CrCl < 30 mL/min	200 mg (PO) q24h
Post–HD dose	200 mg (PO)
Post–PD dose	None
CVVH/CVVHD/ CVVHDF dose	200 mg (PO) q24h
Moderate— severe hepatic insufficiency	No change

Drug Interactions: H_2 receptor
antagonists, Al^{++}, Mg^{++}) antacids
($\downarrow$ absorption of cefditoren); Probenecid
($\downarrow$ elimination of cefditoren).
Adverse Effects:
Common
  • Non-C. difficile diarrhea
Uncommon
  • Drug rash/fever
  • Hematuria
  • Vaginal candidiasis
  • C. difficile diarrhea/colitis
Allergic Potential: Low
Safety in Pregnancy: B

Additional Clinical Considerations:
  • Serum concentrations increased ~
    50% if taken without food.
  • Contains Na+ caseinate; avoid in
    patients with casein hypersensitivity.

(also see *Antibiotic Pearls & Pitfalls*
p. 529).

SELECTED REFERENCES:
Darkes MJ, Plosker GL. Cefditoren pivoxil. Drugs
  62:319–36, 2002. (PMID:11817976)
Guay DR. Review of cefditoren, an advanced-
  generation, broad-spectrum oral cephalosporin.
  Clin Ther 23:1924–37, 2002. (PMID:11813929)
Tempera G, Furneri PM, Carlone NA, et al. Antibiotic
  susceptibility of respiratory pathogens recently
  isolated in Italy: focus on cefditoren. J Chemother
  22:153–159, 2010. (PMID:20566418)
Wellington K, Curran MP. Cefditoren pivoxil: a
  review of its use in the treatment of bacterial
  infections. Drugs 64:2597–618, 2004.
  (PMID:15516158)
Website: www.pdr.net

─────── = serious side effect 🗌 = black box warning. ND = no data. NR = not recommended. s = spectrum inadequate (at site). a = activity or experience inadequate. p = tissue penetration inadequate.
*based on peak serum concentration after usual adult dose. †applicable to adult uncomplicated lower UTIs (CrCl > 30 mL/min).

Cefepime (Maxipime)

Drug Class: 4th generation cephalosporin.
Usual Dose: 2 gm (IV) q12h (see comments).

Spectrum Synopsis*
Hits
  Gram + : All non-enterococcal streptococci, MSSA, Most CoNS
  Gram – : Most aerobic GNB (including P. aeruginosa)
  Problem pathogens:
    ESBL + Klebsiella, Enterobacter, E. coli, B. cepacia
Misses
  Gram + : MRSA, VSE, VRE
  Gram – : B. fragilis
  Problem pathogens:
    Listeria, Nocardia, S. maltophilia, CRE
Urine Spectrum
  • Same as serum spectrum
  • Optimal urinary pH = 5.5–6

(Full *Susceptibility Profiles* p. 201).

Resistance Potential: Low
Pharmacokinetic Parameters:
  Peak serum level: 163 mcg/mL
  Bioavailability: Not applicable
  Excreted unchanged (urine): 80%
  Serum half-life (normal/ESRD): 2.2/18 hrs
  Plasma protein binding: 20%
  Volume of distribution (V_d): 0.29 L/kg
Primary Mode of Elimination: Renal
Dosage Adjustments*

CrCl 30–60 mL/min	2 gm (IV) q12h
CrCl 10–30 mL/min	2 gm (IV) q24h
CrCl < 10 mL/min	1 gm (IV) q24h
Post–HD dose	2 gm (IV)
Post–HFHD dose	2 gm (IV)
Post–PD dose	1 gm (IV)
CAPD	2 gm (IV) q48h
CVVH/CVVHD/ CVVHDF dose	1 gm (IV) q12h
HD q 48–72h dose	2 gm (IV) q HD*
Moderate— severe hepatic insufficiency	No change

*Give at end of HD.

Drug Interactions: None.
Adverse Effects:
Common
  • AIHA
Uncommon
  • Drug fever/rash
  • C. difficile diarrhea/colitis
Rare
  • Encephalopathy
  • Non-convulsive status epilecticus
  • Myoclonus
Allergic Potential: Moderate
Safety in Pregnancy: B

Additional Clinical Considerations:
  • Breakpoints for P. aeruginosa ≤ 8 mcg/ml (susceptible) and ≥16 mcg/ml (resistant).

―――― = serious side effect ☐ = black box warning. ND = no data. NR = not recommended. s = spectrum inadequate (at site). a = activity or experience inadequate. p = tissue penetration inadequate. *based on peak serum concentration after usual adult dose. †applicable to adult uncomplicated lower UTIs (CrCl > 30 mL/min).

- For ESBL + Enterobacteriaceae susceptible dose dependant (S-DD) break point (MIC 4–8 mcg/mL), for proven serious systemic P. aeruginosa infections, febrile neutropenia, or cystic fibrosis, use 2 gm (IV) q8h.
- For aerobic GNB bacteremias use 2 gm (IV) q12h.

May increase LPS (endotoxin) release from GNB *potentially increasing endotoxin mediated tissue damage.*

Additional Pharmacokinetic Considerations*

Non-CSF	% of Serum Levels
Peritoneal fluid	<10%
Bile	NR(s)
Synovial fluid	ND
Bone	45%
Prostate	50%
Urine[†]	1900%
CSF	
Non-inflamed meninges	1%
Inflamed meninges (ABM)	15%
Meningeal dose = 2 gm (IV) q8h	

(also see ***Antibiotic Pearls & Pitfalls*** p. 529).

SELECTED REFERENCES:

Akhabue E, Synnestvedt M, Weiner MG, et al. Cefepime-resistant Pseudomonas aeruginosa. Emerg Infect Dis 17:1037–1043, 2011. (PMID:21749765)

Al-Hassan MN, Eckel-Passow JE, Baddour LM. Cefepime effectiveness in Gram-negative bloodstream infections. J Antimicrob Chemother 66:1156–1160, 2011. (PMID:21393128)

Altshuler J, et al. Treatment of extended-spectrum beta-lactamase Enterobacteriaceae with cefepime: the dose matters, too. Clin Infect Dis 57:915–916, 2013. (PMID:23784927)

Altshuler J, Guervil DJ, Ericsson CD, et al. Clinical Outcomes in patients with gram-negative infections treated with optimized dosing cefepime over various minimum inhibitory concentrations. J Pharm Pract 31:34-9, 2018. (PMID: 29278990)

Bazan JA, Martin SI, Kaye KM. Newer beta-lactam antibiotics: doripenem, ceftobiprole, ceftaroline fosamil, and cefepime. Med Clin North Am 95:743–760, 2011. (PMID:21679790)

Chapman TM, Perry CM. Cefepime: a review of its use in the management of hospitalized patients with pneumonia. Am J Respir Med 2:75–107, 2003. (PMID:14720024)

Cunha BA, Gill MV. Cefepime. Med Clin North Am 79:721–32, 1995. (PMID:7791419)

Fugate JE, Kalimullah EA, Hocker SE. Cefepime neurotoxicity in the intensive care unit: a cause of severe, underappreciated encephalopathy. Crit Care 17:R264, 2013. (PMID:24200036)

Gangireddy VG, Mitchell LC, Coleman T. Cefepime neurotoxicity despite renal adjusted dosing. Scand J Infect Dis 43:827–829, 2011. (PMID:21604923)

Kassel LE, Van Matre ET, Foster CJ, et al. A Randomized pharmacokinetic and pharmacodynamic evaluation of every 8-hour and 12-hour dosing strategies of vancomycin and cefepime in neurocritically ill patients. Pharmacotherapy 38:921-34, 2018. (PMID: 29906310)

Montalar J, Segura A, Bosch C, et al. Cefepime monotherapy as an empirical initial treatment of patients with febrile neutropenia. Med Oncol 19:161–6, 2002. (PMID:12482126)

Perez KK, Hughes DW, Maxwell PR, et al. Cefepime for Gram-negative bacteremia in long-term hemodialysis: a single-center experience. Am J Kidney Dis 59:740–742, 2012. (PMID:22440135)

Picao RC, Jones RN, Mendes RE, et al. Klebsiella pneumoniae carbapenemase-producing enterobacteriaceae testing susceptible to cefepime by reference methods. Clin Micro 51:2388-2390, 2013. (PMID:23616458)

Tamma PD, Girdwood SCT, Gopaul R, et al. The use of cefepime for treating AmpC β-lactamase-producing Enterobacteriaceae. Clin Infect Dis 57:781–788, 2013. (PMID:23759352)

Ugai T, Morisaki K, Tsuda K. Cefepime induced encephalopathy in patients with haematological malignancies: clinical features and risk factors. Scand J Infect Dis. 46:272-279, 2014. (PMID:24506579)

―――― = serious side effect ▭ = black box warning. ND = no data. NR = not recommended. s = spectrum inadequate (at site). a = activity or experience inadequate. p = tissue penetration inadequate. *based on peak serum concentration after usual adult dose. [†]applicable to adult uncomplicated lower UTIs (CrCl > 30 mL/min).

Yahave D, Paul M, Fraser A, et al. Efficacy and safety of cefepime: a systematic review and meta-analysis. Lancet Infect Dis 7:338–348, 2007. (PMID:17448937)

Wilson FP, Bachhuber MA, Caroff D, et al. Low cefepime concentrations during high blood and dialysate flow continuous venovenous hemodialysis. Antimicrob Agents Chemother 56:2178–2180, 2012. (PMID:22290968)

Website: www.pdr.net

Cefiderocol (Fetroja) CFDC

Drug Class: Siderophore cephalosporin.
Usual Dose: 2 gm (IV) q8h.

Spectrum Synopsis*
Hits
  Gram + : None
  Gram – : Pseudomonas,
    B. cepacia, S. maltophilia
  Problem pathogens:
    Acinetobacter, CRE
Misses
  Gram + : Anaerobic streptococci
  Gram – : B. fragilis
  Problem pathogens:
    MSSA, MRSA, VRE, VSE, Listeria
Urine Spectrum
• ND
• Optimal urinary pH = *ND*
• Urine levels = *ND*

(Full *Susceptibility Profiles* p. 201).

Resistance Potential: Low
Pharmacokinetic Parameters:
  Peak serum level: 81 mcg/mL
  Bioavailability: Not applicable
  Excreted unchanged: 62–68%
  Serum half-life (normal/ESRD): 3/9 hrs
  Plasma protein binding: 58%
Volume of distribution (V_d): 0.19 L/kg

Primary Mode of Elimination: Renal
Dosage Adjustments*

CrCl 30–59 mL/min	1.5 gm (IV) q8h
CrCl 15–29 mL/min	1 gm (IV) q8h
CrCl < 15 mL/min	0.75 gm (IV) q12h
Post–HD dose	0.75 gm (IV) Post-*HD*
Post–PD dose	*ND*
CVVH dose	2 g (IV) q6h
Mild-to-moderate hepatic insufficiency	*ND*
Severe hepatic insufficiency	*ND*

Drug Interactions: None
Adverse Effects:
Uncommon
• Nausea
• Rash
• Urticaria
• Myalgia
• Dizziness
• Constipation
• Phlebitis
Allergic Potential: Low

Additional Clinical Considerations:
• Probably safe in pregnancy

Additional Pharmacokinetic Considerations*

Non-CSF	**% of Serum Levels**
Organ	ND
CSF	
Meningeal dose	ND

——— = serious side effect ☐ = black box warning. ND = no data. NR = not recommended. s = spectrum inadequate (at site). a = activity or experience inadequate. p = tissue penetration inadequate. *based on peak serum concentration after usual adult dose. †applicable to adult uncomplicated lower UTIs (CrCl > 30 mL/min).

SELECTED REFERENCES:

Hackel MA, Tsuji M, Yamano Y, et al. In vitro activity of the siderophore cephalosporin, cefiderocol, against a recent collection of clinically relevant gram-negative bacilli from North America and Europe, including carbapenem-nonsusceptible isolates (SIDERO-WT-2014 Study). Antimicrob Agents Chemother: pii: e00093-17. doi: 10.1128/AAC.00093-17, 2017. (PMID: 28630181)

Katsube T, Echols R, Arjona Ferreira JC, et al. Cefiderocol, a siderophore cephalosporin for gram-negative bacterial infections: pharmacokinetics and safety in subjects with renal impairment. J Clin Pharmacol 57:584-591, 2017. (PMID: 27874971)

Katsube T, Wajima T, Ishibashi T, et al. Pharmacokinetic/pharmacodynamic modeling and simulation of cefiderocol, a parenteral siderephore cephalosporin, for dose adjustment based on renal function. Antimicrob Agents Chemother 61:pii: e01381-16. doi: 10.1128/AAC.01381-16, 2016. (PMID: 277952374)

Saisho Y, Katsube T, White S, et al. Pharmacokinetics, safety, and tolerability of cefiderocol, a novel siderophore cephalosporin for gram-negative bacteria, in healthy subjects. Antimicrob Agents Chemother 23: pii: e02163-17. doi: 10.1128/AAC.02163-17, 2018. (PMID: 29311072)

Zhnel GG, Golden AR, Zelenitsky AR, et al. Cefiderocol: a siderophore cephalosporin with activity against carbapenem-resistant gram-negative bacilli. Drugs. doi: 10.1007/s40265-019-1055-2 [e-pub ahead of print], 2019. (PMID: 30712199)

Website: www.pdr.net

Cefixime (Suprax)

Drug Class: 3rd generation oral cephalosporin.
Usual Dose: 400 mg (PO) q12h.

Spectrum Synopsis*
Hits
  Gram + : All non-enterococcal streptococci
  Gram – : Some GNB
  Problem pathogens: None
Misses
  Gram + : MSSA, MRSA, VSE, VRE
  Gram – : Most GNB, B. fragilis
  Problem pathogens: Listeria, Nocardia, Acinetobacter, S. maltophilia, B. cepacia

(Full **Susceptibility Profiles** p. 201).

Resistance Potential: Low
Pharmacokinetic Parameters:
Peak serum level: 3.7 mcg/mL
Bioavailability: 50%
Excreted unchanged (urine): 50%
Serum half-life (normal/ESRD): 3.1/11 hrs
Plasma protein binding: 65%
Volume of distribution (V_d): 0.1 L/kg
Primary Mode of Elimination: Renal
Dosage Adjustments*

CrCl 20–50 mL/min	400 mg (PO) q24h
CrCl < 20 mL/min	200 mg (PO) q24h
Post–HD dose	400 mg (PO)
Post–PD dose	200 mg (PO)
CVVH/CVVHD/CVVHDF dose	200 mg (PO) q12h
Moderate hepatic insufficiency	No change
Severe hepatic insufficiency	No change

——— = serious side effect ☐ = black box warning. ND = no data. NR = not recommended. s = spectrum inadequate (at site). a = activity or experience inadequate. p = tissue penetration inadequate. *based on peak serum concentration after usual adult dose. †applicable to adult uncomplicated lower UTIs (CrCl > 30 mL/min).

Drug Interactions: Carbamazepine (↑ carbamazepine levels).
Adverse Effects:
Common
- GI upset
- Non-C. difficile diarrhea

Rare
- Drug fever/rash
- <u>C. difficile diarrhea/colitis</u>

Allergic Potential: High
Safety in Pregnancy: B

Additional Clinical Considerations:
- **PRNG dose:** 400 mg (PO) × 1 dose.
- Also useful for quinolone-resistant GC.
- **Little/no activity against S. aureus (MSSA).**

(also see ***Antibiotic Pearls & Pitfalls*** p. 529).

SELECTED REFERENCES:

Chisholm SA, Mouton JW, Lewis DA, et al. Cephalosporin MIC creep among gonococci: time for a pharmacodynamic rethink? J Antimicrob Chemother 65:2141–2148, 2010. (PMID:20693173)

Quintiliani R. Cefixime in the treatment of patients with lower respiratory tract infections: results of US clinical trials. Clinical Therapeutics 18:373–90, 1996. (PMID:8829015)

Website: www.pdr.net

Cefoperazone (Cefobid)

Drug Class: 3rd generation cephalosporin.
Usual Dose: 2 gm (IV) q12h.

Spectrum Synopsis*
Hits
   Gram + : All non-enterococcal streptococci, MSSA, CoNS, VSE
   Gram – : Most GNB (including P. aeruginosa), B fragilis
   Problem pathogens: Nocardia, B. cepacia
Misses
   Gram + : MRSA, VRE
   Gram – : Few GNB
   Problem pathogens: Listeria, Nocardia, Acinetobacter, S. maltophilia
Urine Spectrum
- Same as serum spectrum

(Full ***Susceptibility Profiles*** p. 201).

Resistance Potential: Low
Pharmacokinetic Parameters:
   Peak serum level: 240 mcg/mL
   Bioavailability: Not applicable
   Excreted unchanged (urine): 20%
   Serum half-life (normal/ESRD): 2.4/2.4 hrs
   Plasma protein binding: 90%
   Volume of distribution (V_d): 0.17 L/kg
Primary Mode of Elimination: Hepatic
Dosage Adjustments*

CrCl < 10 mL/min	No change
Post–HD dose	None
Post–PD dose	None
CVVH/CVVHD/CVVHDF dose	No change
Moderate hepatic insufficiency	No change
Severe hepatic insufficiency	1 gm (IV) q12h

"Usual dose" assumes normal renal/hepatic function. * For renal insufficiency, give usual dose × 1 followed by maintenance dose per CrCl. For dialysis patients, dose the same as for CrCl < 10 mL/min and give supplemental (post-HD/PD dose) immediately after dialysis. CrCl = creatinine clearance; CVVH = continuous veno-venous hemofiltration; HD/PD = hemodialysis/peritoneal dialysis.

Drug Interactions: Alcohol (disulfiram-like reaction); antiplatelet agents, heparin, thrombolytics, warfarin (↑ risk of bleeding).

Adverse Effects:

Common
- Non-C. difficile diarrhea

Uncommon
- Drug fever/rash

Rare
- Disulfiram reactions (with EtOH)
- ↑ INR

Allergic Potential: Low
Safety in Pregnancy: B

Additional Clinical Considerations:
- One of the few antibiotics to penetrate into an obstructed biliary tract.
- May be administered IM.
- Concentration dependent serum half life.

May increase LPS (endotoxin) release from GNB potentially increasing endotoxin mediated tissue damage.

Additional Pharmacokinetic Considerations*

Non-CSF	% of Serum Levels
Peritoneal fluid	ND
Bile	1200%
Synovial fluid	ND
Bone	15%
Prostate	NR(p)
Urine	1300%
CSF	
Non-inflamed meninges	1%
Inflamed meninges (ABM)	10%

Meningeal dose = 2 gm (IV) q8h

(also see ***Antibiotic Pearls & Pitfalls*** p. 528).

SELECTED REFERENCES:
Cunha BA. 3rd generation cephalosporins: A review. Clin Ther 14:616–52, 1992. (PMID:1468084)
Klein NC, Cunha BA. Third-generation cephalosporins. Med Clin North Am 79:705–19, 1995. (PMID:7791418)
Marshall WF, Blair JE. The cephalosporins. Mayo Clin Proc 74:187–95, 1999. (PMID:10069359)
Website: www.pdr.net

Cefotaxime (Claforan)

Drug Class: 3rd generation cephalosporin.
Usual Dose: 2 gm (IV) q6h.

Spectrum Synopsis*

Hits

Gram + : All non-enterococcal streptococci, MSSA, most CoNS

Gram – : Most GNB, B fragilis

Problem pathogens: Nocardia, B. cepacia

Misses

Gram + : MRSA, VSE, VRE

Gram – : P. aeruginosa

Problem pathogens: Listeria, Acinetobacter, S. maltophilia

Urine Spectrum
- Same as serum spectrum

(Full ***Susceptibility Profiles*** p. 201).

Resistance Potential: Low
Pharmacokinetic Parameters:
Peak serum level: 214 mcg/mL
Bioavailability: Not applicable
Excreted unchanged (urine): 20–36%; 15–25% excreted as active metabolite
Serum half-life (normal/ESRD): 1/15 hrs

―――― = serious side effect ☐ = black box warning. ND = no data. NR = not recommended. s = spectrum inadequate (at site). a = activity or experience inadequate. p = tissue penetration inadequate. *based on peak serum concentration after usual adult dose. †applicable to adult uncomplicated lower UTIs (CrCl > 30 mL/min).

Plasma protein binding: 37%
Volume of distribution (V_d): 0.25 L/kg
Primary Mode of Elimination: Renal
Dosage Adjustments*

CrCl 10–50 mL/min	1 gm (IV) q12h
CrCl < 10 mL/min	1 gm (IV) q24h
Post–HD dose	1 gm (IV)
Post–PD dose	1 gm (IV)
CVVH/CVVHD/ CVVHDF dose	2 gm (IV) q12h
Moderate hepatic insufficiency	No change
Severe hepatic insufficiency	No change

Drug Interactions: None.
Adverse Effects:
Uncommon
• Injection site reaction
• Drug fever/rash
• C. difficile diarrhea/colitis
Allergic Potential: Moderate
Safety in Pregnancy: B

Additional Clinical Considerations:
• Incompatible in solutions containing, metronidazole, or aminoglycosides.
• **Desacetyl metabolite** (t1/2 = 1.5 hrs) synergistic with cefotaxime against S. aureus/B. fragilis.
• Gallbladder wall levels very low vs. bile levels
• Cefotaxime is converted to less active desacetyl cefotaxime by the choroid plexus.

May increase LPS (endotoxin) release from GNB potentially increasing endotoxin mediated tissue damage.

Additional Pharmacokinetic Considerations*

Non-CSF	% of Serum Levels
Peritoneal fluid	<10%
Bile	75%
Synovial fluid	20%
Bone	<10%
Prostate	NR(p)
Urine†	1500%
CSF	
Non-inflamed meninges	1%
Inflamed meninges (ABM)	10%

Meningeal dose = 3 gm (IV) q6h

(also see **Antibiotic Pearls & Pitfalls** p. 528).

SELECTED REFERENCES:
File Jr. TM, Clinical implications and treatment of multiresistant Streptococcus pneumoniae pneumonia. Clin Microbiol Infect 12:31–41, 2006. (PMID:16669927)
Klein NC, Cunha BA. Third-generation cephalosporins. Med Clin North Am 79:705–19, 1995. (PMID:7791418)
Marshall WF, Blair JE. The cephalosporins. Mayo Clin Proc 74:187–95, 1999. (PMID:10069359)
Patel KB, Nicolau DP, Nightingale CH, et al. Comparative serum bactericidal activities of ceftizoxime and cefotaxime against intermediately penicillin-resistant Streptococcus pneumoniae. Antimicrob Agents Chemother 40:2805–8, 1996. (PMID:9124845)
Website: www.pdr.net

Cefotetan (Cefotan)

Drug Class: 2nd generation cephalosporin (Cephamycin).
Usual Dose: 2 gm (IV) q12h.

—— = serious side effect ☐ = black box warning. ND = no data. NR = not recommended. s = spectrum inadequate (at site). a = activity or experience inadequate. p = tissue penetration inadequate. *based on peak serum concentration after usual adult dose. †applicable to adult uncomplicated lower UTIs (CrCl > 30 mL/min).

Spectrum Synopsis*
Hits
>   **Gram + :** All non-enterococcal
>   streptococci, MSSA
>   **Gram – :** Most GNB, B. fragilis
>   **Problem pathogens:**
>   None

Misses
>   **Gram + :** MRSA, VSE, VRE
>   **Gram – :** P. aeruginosa, B. fragilis
>   (D.O.T. subspecies)
>   **Problem pathogens:**
>   Listeria, Nocardia, Acinetobacter,
>   S. maltophilia, B. cepacia

(Full *Susceptibility Profiles* p. 201).

Resistance Potential: Low
Pharmacokinetic Parameters:
>   *Peak serum level: 237 mcg/mL*
>   *Bioavailability: Not applicable*
>   *Excreted unchanged (urine): 50–80%*
>   *Serum half-life (normal/ESRD): 4/10 hrs*
>   *Plasma protein binding: 88%*
>   *Volume of distribution (V_d): 0.17 L/kg*

Primary Mode of Elimination: Renal
Dosage Adjustments*

CrCl 30–80 mL/min	2 gm (IV) q12h
CrCl 10–30 mL/min	2 gm (IV) q24h
CrCl < 10 mL/min	2 gm (IV) q48h
Post–HD dose	1 gm (IV)
Post–PD dose	1 gm (IV)
CVVH/CVVHD/ CVVHDF dose	750 mg (IV) q12h
Moderate— severe hepatic insufficiency	No change

Drug Interactions: Alcohol
(disulfiram-like reaction); antiplatelet
agents, heparin, thrombolytics, warfarin
($\uparrow$ risk of bleeding).
Adverse Effects:
Uncommon
>   • $\uparrow$ AST/ALT

Rare
>   • Disulfiram reactions (with EtOH)
>   • Drug fever/rash
>   • Hemolytic anemia
>   • $\uparrow$ INR
>   • <u>C. difficile diarrhea/colitis</u>

Allergic Potential: Low
Safety in Pregnancy: B

Additional Clinical Considerations:
>   • Less effective than cefoxitin against
>   B. fragilis D.O.T subspecies.

**Additional Pharmacokinetic
Considerations***

Non-CSF	**% of Serum Levels**
Peritoneal fluid	27%
Bile	20%
Synovial fluid	NR(s)
Bone	NR(s)
Prostate	NR(p)
Urine†	1400%
CSF	
Non-inflamed meninges	<1%
Inflamed meninges (ABM)	10%

(also see *Antibiotic Pearls & Pitfalls*
p. 528).

SELECTED REFERENCES:
Moes GS, MacPherson BR. Cefotetan induced
    hemolytic anemia: A case report and a review of
    the literature. Arch Pathol Lab Med 124:1344–6,
    2000. (PMID:10975934)

———— = serious side effect ☐ = black box warning. ND = no data. NR = not recommended. s = spectrum inadequate (at site). a = activity or experience inadequate. p = tissue penetration inadequate.
*based on peak serum concentration after usual adult dose. †applicable to adult uncomplicated lower UTIs
(CrCl > 30 mL/min).

Ray EK, Warkentin TE, O'Hoski PL. Delayed onset of life-threatening immune hemolysis after perioperative antimicrobial prophylaxis with cefotetan. Can J Surg 43:461–2, 2000. (PMID:11129837)
Website: www.pdr.net

Cefoxitin (Mefoxin)

Drug Class: 2nd generation cephalosporin (cephamycin).
Usual Dose: 2 gm (IV) q6h.

Spectrum Synopsis:*
Hits
Gram + : All non-enterococcal streptococci, MSSA, some CoNS
Gram – : Many GNB, B. fragilis (including D.O.T. subspecies)
Problem pathogens: Enterobacter, Serratia
Misses
Gram + : MRSA, VSE, VRE
Gram – : Proteus, P. aeruginosa
Problem pathogens: Listeria, Nocardia, Acinetobacter, S. maltophilia, B. cepacia

(Full *Susceptibility Profiles* p. 201).

Resistance Potential: Low
Pharmacokinetic Parameters:
Peak serum level: 221 mcg/mL
Bioavailability: Not applicable
Excreted unchanged (urine): 85%
Serum half-life (normal/ESRD): 1/21 hrs
Plasma protein binding: 75%
Volume of distribution (V_d): 0.12 L/kg
Primary Mode of Elimination: Renal
Dosage Adjustments*

CrCl 30–50 mL/min	2 gm (IV) q12h
CrCl 10–30 mL/min	1 gm (IV) q12h
CrCl < 10 mL/min	1 gm (IV) q24h
Post–HD dose	2 gm (IV)
Post–PD dose	1 gm (IV)
CVVH/CVVHD/CVVHDF dose	2 gm (IV) q12h
Moderate hepatic insufficiency	No change
Severe hepatic insufficiency	No change

Drug Interactions: None.
Adverse Effects:
Common
- Non-C. difficile diarrhea
Uncommon
- Drug fever/rash
Rare
- ↑ Creatinine
- ↑ AST/ALT
- C. difficile diarrhea/colitis
Allergic Potential: Low
Safety in Pregnancy: B

Additional Clinical Considerations:
• **Effective against B. fragilis, including D.O.T. strains** (B. distasonis, B. ovatus, B. thetaiotaomicron).
May increase LPS (endotoxin) release from GNB potentially increasing endotoxin mediated tissue damage.

Additional Pharmacokinetic Considerations*	
Non-CSF	**% of Serum Levels**
Peritoneal fluid	86%
Bile	NR(s)

———— = serious side effect ☐ = black box warning. ND = no data. NR = not recommended. s = spectrum inadequate (at site). a = activity or experience inadequate. p = tissue penetration inadequate. *based on peak serum concentration after usual adult dose. †applicable to adult uncomplicated lower UTIs (CrCl > 30 mL/min).

Synovial fluid	ND
Bone	ND
Prostate	NR(p)
Urine[†]	1500%
CSF	
Non-inflamed meninges	<1%
Inflamed meninges (ABM)	<10%

- Cefoxitin penetrates into bile even in the presence of obstruction from the gallbladder wall into the obstructed bile.
- Does not penetrate into encapsulated intra-abdominal abscesses (<2% of serum levels)

(also see **Antibiotic Pearls & Pitfalls** p. 528).

SELECTED REFERENCES:
Donowitz GR, Mandell GL. Beta-lactam antibiotics. N Engl J Med 318:419–26 and 318:490–500, 1993. (PMID:3277054)
Website: www.pdr.net

Cefpodoxime (Vantin)

Drug Class: 3rd generation oral cephalosporin.
Usual Dose: 200 mg (PO) q12h (see comments).

Spectrum Synopsis*
Hits
  Gram + : All non-enterococcal streptococci, MSSA
  Gram – : Many aerobic GNB (including Serratia)
  Problem pathogens:
    S. maltophilia
Misses
  Gram + : MRSA, P. aeruginosa, VSE, VRE
  Gram – : Some GNB (including Enterobacter), B. fragilis

Problem pathogens:
  Listeria, Nocardia, Acinetobacter, B. cepacia

(Full **Susceptibility Profiles** p. 201).

Resistance Potential: Low
Pharmacokinetic Parameters:
  Peak serum level: 2.3 mcg/mL
  Bioavailability: 50%
  Excreted unchanged (urine): 30%
  Serum half-life (normal/ESRD): 2.3/9.8 hrs
  Plasma protein binding: 21–33%
  Volume of distribution (V_d): 0.9 L/kg
Primary Mode of Elimination: Renal
Dosage Adjustments*

CrCl 30–80 mL/min	No change
CrCl < 30 mL/min	200 mg (PO) q24h
Post–HD dose	200 mg (PO)
Post–PD dose	200 mg (PO)
CVVH/CVVHD/ CVVHDF dose	200 mg (PO) q12h
Moderate hepatic insufficiency	No change
Severe hepatic insufficiency	No change

Drug Interactions: None.
Adverse Effects:
Common
  - GI upset
  - Drug fever/rash
Rare
  - Pulmonary infiltrates with eosinophilia
  - ↑ AST/ALT
  - C. difficile diarrhea/colitis
Allergic Potential: High
Safety in Pregnancy: B

―――― = serious side effect ☐ = black box warning. ND = no data. NR = not recommended. s = spectrum inadequate (at site). a = activity or experience inadequate. p = tissue penetration inadequate. *based on peak serum concentration after usual adult dose. †applicable to adult uncomplicated lower UTIs (CrCl > 30 mL/min).

Additional Clinical Considerations:
- Only oral 3rd generation cephalosporin active against S. aureus (MSSA).
- **PPNG dose:** 400 mg (PO) × 1 dose
- **cSSSI dose:** 400 mg (PO) q12h.

Bile Penetration: 100%
Cerebrospinal Fluid Penetration: < 10%

(also see **Antibiotic Pearls & Pitfalls** p. 529).

SELECTED REFERENCES:
Cohen R. Clinical efficacy of cefpodoxime in respiratory tract infection. J Antimicrob Chemother 50 (Suppl):23–7, 2002. (PMID:12077157)
Schatz BS, Karavokiros KT, Taeubel MA, et al. Comparison of cefprozil, cefpodoxime proxetil, loracarbef, cefixime, and ceftibuten. Ann Pharmacother 30:258–68, 1996. (PMID:8833562)
Website: www.pdr.net

Cefprozil (Cefzil)

Drug Class: 2nd generation oral cephalosporin.
Usual Dose: 500 mg (PO) q12h.

Spectrum Synopsis*
Hits
  Gram + : All non-enterococcal streptococci (including S. pneumoniae), MSSA
  Gram – : Some GNB (including Klebsiella, H. influenzae)
  Problem pathogens:
Misses
  Gram + : MRSA, VSE, VRE
  Gram – : Most GNB (including Proteus, P. aeruginosa), B. fragilis)
  Problem pathogens:
    Listeria, Nocardia, Acinetobacter, S. maltophilia, B. cepacia

(Full **Susceptibility Profiles** p. 201).

Resistance Potential: Low
Pharmacokinetic Parameters:
  Peak serum level: 10 mcg/mL
  Bioavailability: 95%
  Excreted unchanged (urine): 60%
  Serum half-life (normal/ESRD): 1.3/5.9 hrs
  Plasma protein binding: 36%
  Volume of distribution (V_d): 0.23 L/kg
Primary Mode of Elimination: Renal
Dosage Adjustments*

CrCl < 30 mL/min	250 mg (PO) q12h
Post–HD dose	500 mg (PO)
Post–PD dose	250 mg (PO)
CVVH/CVVHD/CVVHDF dose	500 mg (PO) q24h

Drug Interactions: None.
Adverse Effects:
Uncommon
  - GI upset
  - Drug fever/rash
Rare
  - ↑ AST/ALT
  - C. difficile diarrhea/colitis
Allergic Potential: Low
Safety in Pregnancy: B

Additional Clinical Considerations:
- Penetrates oral/respiratory secretions well.
- No respiratory pathogen resistance.

(also see **Antibiotic Pearls & Pitfalls** p. 528).

SELECTED REFERENCES:
Schatz BS, Karavokiros KT, Taeubel MA, et al. Comparison of cefprozil, cefpodoxime, proxetil, loracarbef, cefixime, and ceftibuten. Ann Pharmacother 30:258–68, 1996. (PMID:8833562)
Website: www.pdr.net

—— = serious side effect ☐ = black box warning. ND = no data. NR = not recommended. s = spectrum inadequate (at site). a = activity or experience inadequate. p = tissue penetration inadequate. *based on peak serum concentration after usual adult dose. †applicable to adult uncomplicated lower UTIs (CrCl > 30 mL/min).

Ceftaroline fosamil (Teflaro)

Drug class: Anti-MRSA cephalosporin.
Usual dose: 600 mg (IV) q12h.

Spectrum Synopsis*
Hits
Gram + : All non-enterococcal streptococci, MSSA, MRSA, CoNS
Gram – : Some GNB, (including Enterobacter, Serratia)
Problem pathogens: VISA
Misses
Gram + : VSE, VRE
Gram – : B. fragilis
Problem pathogens: Listeria, Nocardia, Acinetobacter, S. maltophilia, B. cepacia

(Full *Susceptibility Profiles* p. 201).

Resistance Potential: Low
Pharmacokinetic Parameters:
Peak serum level: 19 mcg/mL
Bioavailability: not applicable
Excreted unchanged: 64%
Serum half-life (normal/ESRD): 2.7 hours/ 6.16 hours
Plasma protein binding: 20%
Volume of distribution (V_d): 20.3 L/kg
Primary Mode of Elimination: Renal
Drug Interactions: None.
Adverse Effects:

Common
- Direct coombs

Uncommon
- Nausea/vomiting
- Drug fever/rash
- Non-C. difficile diarrhea

- Constipation
- ↑ AST/ALT
- Phlebitis
- C. difficile diarrhea/colitis
- Hypokalemia

Rare
- Agranulocytosis

Dosage Adjustments:

CrCl[a] > 50	No change
CrCl > 30 to ≤ 50	400 mg (IV) (over 1 hour) q12h
CrCl ≥ 15 to ≤ 30	300 mg (IV) (over 1 hour) q12h
ESRD on HD*	200 mg (IV) (over 1 hour) q12h*
Moderate hepatic insufficiency	No change
Severe hepatic insufficiency	No change

* should be administered after HD on hemodialysis days.

Safety in Pregnancy: B

Additional Clinical Considerations:
• The only one of two cephalosporin clinically effective against MRSA.
• Effective in MSSA/MRSA bacteremias.

Cerebrospinal Fluid Penetration: < 10%

(also see *Antibiotic Pearls & Pitfalls* p. 529).

SELECTED REFERENCES:
Casapao AM, Steed ME, Levine DP, et al. Ceftaroline fosamil for community-acquired bacterial pneumonia and acute bacterial skin and skin structure infection. Expert Opin Pharmacother 13:1177–1186, 2012. (PMID:22594846)

──── = serious side effect ☐ = black box warning. ND = no data. NR = not recommended. s = spectrum inadequate (at site). a = activity or experience inadequate. p = tissue penetration inadequate. *based on peak serum concentration after usual adult dose. †applicable to adult uncomplicated lower UTIs (CrCl > 30 mL/min).

Chauzy A, Nadji A, Combes JC, et al. Cerebrospinal fluid pharmacokinetics of ceftaroline in neurosurgical patients with an external ventricular drain. J Antimicrob Chemother [Epub ahead of print]. 2018. (PMID: 30535190)

Cheng K, Pypstra R, Yan JL, et al. Summary of the safety and tolerability of two treatment regimens of ceftaroline fosamil: 600 mg every 8h versus 600 mg every 12h. J Antimicrob Chemother [Epub ahead of print]. 2018. (PMID: 30597021)

File TM Jr, Low DE, Edckburg PB, et al. Efficacy and safety of ceftaroline fosamil versus ceftriaxone in patients with community-acquired pneumonia. Clin Infect Dis 51:1395–1405, 2011. (PMID:21067350)

Kaushik D, Rathi S, Jain A. Ceftaroline: a comprehensive update. Int J Antimicrob Agents 37:389–395, 2011. (PMID:21420284)

Koeth LM, Matuschek E, Kahlmeter G, et al. Development of EUCAST zone diameter breakpoints and quality control range for Staphylococcus aureus with ceftaroline. Eur J Clin Microbiol Infect Dis 33:1511-1517, 2014. (PMID:24744220)

Laudano JB, Ceftaroline fosamil: a new broad-spectrum cephalosporin. J Antimicrob Chemother 66:11–18, 2011. (PMID:21482565)

Lim L, Sutton E, Brown J. Ceftaroline: A new broad-spectrum cephalosporin. Am J Health Syst Pharm 15:491–4198, 2011. (PMID:21378297)

Nannini Ec, Stryjewskin ME, Corey GR. Ceftaroline for complicated skin and skin-structure infections. Expert Opin Pharmacother 11:1197–1206, 2010. (PMID:20402556)

Panagiotidis G, Backstrom T, Asker-Hagelberg C, et al. Effect of ceftaroline on normal human intestinal microflora. Antimicrob Agents Chemother 54:1811–1814, 2010. (PMID:20231399)

Poon H, Chang MH, Fung HB. Ceftaroline fosamil: a cephalosporin with activity against methicillin-resistant Staphylococcus aureus. Clin Ther 34:743–765, 2012. (PMID:22444785)

Saravolatz LD, Pawlak J, Johnson L. In vitro activity of ceftaroline against community-associated methicillin-resistant, vancomycin-intermediate, vancomycin-resistant, and daptomycin-nonsusceptible Staphylococcus aureus isolates. Antimicrob. Agents Chemother 54:3027–3030, 2010. (PMID:20404122)

Saravolatz LD, Stein GE, Johnson LB. Ceftaroline: A novel cephalosporin with activity against methicillin-resistant Staphylococcus aureus. Clin Infect Dis 52:1156–1163, 2011. (PMID:21467022)

Website: www.pdr.net

Ceftazidime (Fortaz, Tazicef, Tazidime)

Drug Class: 3rd generation cephalosporin.
Usual Dose: 2 gm (IV) q8h (see comments).

Spectrum Synopsis*
Hits
Gram + : All non-enterococcal streptococci, some MSSA
Gram – : Most GNB (including P. aeruginosa)
Problem pathogens: Acinetobacter, B. cepacia
Misses
Gram + : MSSA, MRSA, VSE, VRE
Gram – : Some GNB
Problem pathogens: Listeria, Nocardia, S. maltophilia
Urine Spectrum
• Same as serum spectrum

(Full *Susceptibility Profiles* p. 201).

—— = serious side effect ☐ = black box warning. ND = no data. NR = not recommended. s = spectrum inadequate (at site). a = activity or experience inadequate. p = tissue penetration inadequate. *based on peak serum concentration after usual adult dose. †applicable to adult uncomplicated lower UTIs (CrCl > 30 mL/min).

Resistance Potential: High
(P. aeruginosa, Klebsiella pneumoniae;
↑ prevalence of MRSA)

Pharmacokinetic Parameters:
Peak serum level: 170 mcg/mL
Bioavailability: Not applicable
Excreted unchanged (urine): 80–90%
Serum half-life (normal/ESRD): 1.9/21 hrs
Plasma protein binding: 10%
Volume of distribution (V_d): 0.36 L/kg

Primary Mode of Elimination: Renal

Dosage Adjustments*

CrCl 30–80 mL/min	2 gm (IV) q12h
CrCl 10–30 mL/min	2 gm (IV) q24h
CrCl < 10 mL/min	1 gm (IV) q48h
Post–HD dose	1 gm (IV)
Post–PD dose	500 mg (IV)
CVVH/CVVHD/ CVVHDF dose	2 gm (IV) q12h
HD q48–72h dose	2 gm (IV) q HD*
Moderate hepatic insufficiency	No change
Severe hepatic insufficiency	No change

*Give at end of HD.

Drug Interactions: None.

Adverse Effects:

Uncommon
• Drug fever/rash
• Phlebitis
• Eosinophilia
• <u>C. difficile diarrhea/colitis</u>

Allergic Potential: High
Safety in Pregnancy: B

Additional Clinical Considerations:
• ***Use increases MRSA prevalence and P. aeruginosa resistance.***
• ***Potent inducer of Klebsiella/ Enterobacter/E. coli ESBLs.***
• **CAPD dose:** 125 mg/L of dialysate (IP) with each exchange.

May increase LPS (endotoxin) release from GNB *potentially increasing endotoxin mediated tissue damage.*

Additional Pharmacokinetic Considerations*

Non-CSF	% of Serum Levels
Peritoneal fluid	25%
Bile	30%
Synovial fluid	15%
Bone	10%
Prostate	NR(p)
Urine	700%
CSF	
Non-inflamed meninges	1%
Inflamed meninges (ABM)	15%

Meningeal dose = 2 gm (IV) q8h

(also see ***Antibiotic Pearls & Pitfalls*** p. 528).

SELECTED REFERENCES:
Klein NC, Cunha BA. Third-generation cephalosporins. Med Clin North Am 79:705–19, 1995. (PMID:7791418)
Owens JC, Jr, Ambrose PG, Quintiliani R. Ceftazidime to cefepime formulary switch: Pharmacodynamic rationale. Conn Med 61:225–7, 1997. (PMID:9149489)
Rains CP, Bryson HM, Peters DH. Ceftazidime: An update of its antibacterial activity, pharmacokinetic properties, and therapeutic efficacy. Drugs 49:577–617, 1995. (PMID:7789291)
Website: www.pdr.net

—— = serious side effect ☐ = black box warning. ND = no data. NR = not recommended. s = spectrum inadequate (at site). a = activity or experience inadequate. p = tissue penetration inadequate. *based on peak serum concentration after usual adult dose. †applicable to adult uncomplicated lower UTIs (CrCl > 30 mL/min).

Ceftazidime/Avibactam (Avycaz) CAZ/AVI

Drug Class: Anti-pseudomonal cephalosporin/β-lactamase inhibitor.
Usual Dose: 2.5 gm (IV) q8h

Spectrum Synopsis*
Hits
 Gram + : None
 Gram – : Most GNB
 Problem pathogens:
  B. cepacia, MDR
  P. aeruginosa, CRE
Misses
 Gram + :
  VSE, VRE, MSSA, MRSA
 Gram – : B. fragilis
 Problem pathogens:
  Acinetobacter, S. maltophilia,
  Some CRE metallo-β-lactamases
  (MBL)
Urine Spectrum
 • Same as serum spectrum
 • Optimal urinary pH = 5–6
 • Urine levels = 74/14 mcg/mL

(Full *Susceptibility Profiles* p. 201)

Resistance Potential: Low
Pharmacokinetic Parameters:
 Peak Serum level: 170 mcg/mL/15 mcg/mL
 Bioavailability: Not applicable
 Excreted unchanged: 80–90%/85%
 Serum half-life (normal/ESRD): [1.9h/21 h]/[2.0h/22.82 h]
 Plasma protein binding: 10%/8.2%
 Volume of distribution (V_d): 0.36 L/kg/ 0.32 L/kg

Primary Mode of Elimination: Renal
Dosage Adjustments*

CrCl 31–50 mL/min	1.25 gm (IV) q8h
CrCl 16–30 mL/min	0.94 gm (IV) q12h
CrCl 6–15 mL/min	0.94 gm (IV) q24h
CrCl < 5 mL/min	0.94 gm (IV) q48h
Post–HD dose	0.94 gm (IV) q48h
Post-PD dose	ND
CrCl 31–50 mL/min	1.25 gm (IV) q8h
CrCl 16–30 mL/min	0.94 gm (IV) q12h
CrCl 6–15 mL/min	0.94 gm (IV) q24h
CrCl < 5 mL/min	0.94 gm (IV) q48h
Post–HD dose	0.94 gm (IV) q48h
Post-PD dose	ND
CVVH dose	1.25 gm (IV) q12h
Hepatic insufficiency	No change

Drug Interactions: Probenecid (↑ CAZ/AVI levels)
Adverse Effects:
Uncommon
 • Headache
 • Dizziness
 • Insomnia
 • Nausea/vomiting
 • Abdominal pain
 • Non-C. difficile diarrhea
 • Drug fever/rash
 • Phlebitis
 • ↑ AST/ALT
 • C. difficile diarrhea/colitis
 • Eosinophilia

───── = serious side effect ☐ = black box warning. ND = no data. NR = not recommended. s = spectrum inadequate (at site). a = activity or experience inadequate. p = tissue penetration inadequate. *based on peak serum concentration after usual adult dose. †applicable to adult uncomplicated lower UTIs (CrCl > 30 mL/min).

Allergic Potential:
Safety in Pregnancy: B

Additional Clinical Considerations:
- Avibactam is a novel, β-lactamase inhibitor, which acts a reversible inhibitor (compared to irreversible action of other β-lactamase inhibitors) and has an expanded spectrum of β-lactamase inhibition including: class A (includes Klebsiella pneumoniae carbapenemase-KPC), class C, some class D.
- Avibactam's spectrum does not include class B β-lactamases (metallo-β-lactamases) (MBL).
- Use of avibactam with ceftazidime restores susceptibility against ceftazidime non-susceptible organisms.
- Active against multi-drug resistant (MDR) Gram negative organisms, including P. aeruginosa, ESBL GNB, and CRE.
- For complicated intra-abdominal infections (cIAI), caftazidime/avibactam must be used in combination with metronidazole.
- Infuse slowly over 2 hours.

Cerebrospinal Fluid Penetration: <10%

(also see ***Antibiotic Pearls & Pitfalls*** p. 530).

SELECTED REFERENCES:
Keepers TR, Gomez M, Celerl C, et al. Bactericidal activity, absence of serum effect, and time-kill kinetics of ceftazidime-avibactam against beta-lactamase-producing Enterobacteriaceae and Pseudomonas aeruginosa. Antimicrob Agents Chemother. 58:5297-5305, 2014. (PMID:24957838)

Lucasti C, Popescu I, Ramesh MK, et al. Comparative study of the efficacy and safety of ceftazidime/avibactam plus metronidazole versus meropenem in the treatment of complicated intra-abdominal infections in hospitalized adults: results of a randomized, double-blind, Phase II trial. J Antimicrob Chemother. 68:1183-1192, 2013. (PMID:23391714)

Mushtaq S, Warner M, Livermore DM. In vitro activity of ceftazidime+NXL 104 against Pseudomonas aeruginosa and other non-fermenters. J Antimicrob Chemother. 65:2376-2381,2010. (PMID:20801783)

Pogue JM, Bonomo RA, Kaye KS. Ceftazidime/Avibactam, Meropenem/Vaborbactam, or both? Clinical and formulary considerations. Clin Infect Dis. 68:519-524, 2019. (PMID: 30020449)

Tumbarello M, Trecarichi EM, Corona A, et al. Efficacy of Ceftazidime-Avibactam salvage therapy in patients with infections caused by Klebsiella pneumoniae carbapenemase producing K. pneumoniae. Clin Infect Dis. 68:355-364, 2019. (PMID: 29893802)

Vazquez JA, Gonzalez Patzan LD, Stricklin D, et al. Efficacy and safety of ceftazidime-avibactam versus imipenemcilastatin in the treatment of complicated urinary tract infections, including acute pyelonephritis, in hospitalized adults: results of a prospective, investigator-blinded, randomized study. Curr Med Res Opin. 28:1921-1931, 2012. (PMID:23145859)

Wagenlehner FM, Sobel JD, Newel R, et al. Ceftazidime-avibactam versus doripenem for the treatment of complicated urinary tract infections, including acute pyrlonephritis: Clin Infect Dis 63:754-762, 2016. (PMID:27313268)

Zhanel GG, Lawson CD, Adam H, et al. Ceftazidime-avibactam: a novel cephalosporin/beta-lactamase inhibitor combination. Drugs. 73:159-177, 2013. (PMID:23371303)

Ceftibuten (Cedax)

Drug Class: 3rd generation oral cephalosporin.
Usual Dose: 400 mg (PO) q24h.

Spectrum Synopsis*
Hits
Gram + : All non-enterococcal streptococci (except S. pneumoniae)
Gram – : Some GNB (including Klebsiella)
Problem pathogens: B. cepacia
Misses
Gram + : MSSA, MRSA, VSE, VRE, S. pneumoniae
Gram – : B. fragilis, most GNB (including P. aeruginosa)
Problem pathogens: Listeria, Nocardia, Acinetobacter, S. maltophilia

(Full **Susceptibility Profiles** p. 201).

Resistance Potential: Low
Pharmacokinetic Parameters:
Peak serum level: 18 mcg/mL
Bioavailability: 80%
Excreted unchanged: 56% (urine); 39% (fecal) Serum half-life (normal/ESRD): 2.4/22 hrs
Plasma protein binding: 65%
Volume of distribution (V_d): 0.2 L/kg
Primary Mode of Elimination: Renal
Dosage Adjustments*

CrCl 30–50 mL/min	200 mg (PO) q24h
CrCl < 30 mL/min	100 mg (PO) q24h

Post–HD dose	400 mg (PO)
Post–PD dose	200 mg (PO)
CVVH/CVVHD/ CVVHDF dose	200 mg (PO) q24h
Moderate hepatic insufficiency	No change
Severe hepatic insufficiency	No change

Drug Interactions: None.
Adverse Effects:
Uncommon
- Drug fever/rash
- Non-C. difficile diarrhea
- <u>C. difficile diarrhea/colitis</u>

Allergic Potential: High
Safety in Pregnancy: B

Additional Clinical Considerations:
• Little/no activity against S. aureus/S. pneumoniae.

Cerebrospinal Fluid Penetration: < 10%

(also see **Antibiotic Pearls & Pitfalls** p. 529).

SELECTED REFERENCES:
Andrews JW, Wise R, Baldwin DR, et al. Concentrations of ceftibuten in plasma and the respiratory tract following a single 400 mg oral dose. Int J Antimicrob Agents 5:141–144, 1995. (PMID:18611662)
Guay DR. Ceftibuten: A new expanded-spectrum oral cephalosporin. Ann Pharmacother 31:1022–33, 1997. (PMID:9296244)
Owens RC Jr, Nightingale CH, Nicolau DP. Ceftibuten: An overview. Pharmacother 17:707–20, 1997. (PMID:9250548)
Wiseman LR, Balfour JA. Ceftibuten: A review of its antibacterial activity, pharmacokinetic properties and clinical efficacy. Drugs 47:784–808, 1994. (PMID:7520858)
Website: www.pdr.net

―――― = serious side effect ▢ = black box warning. ND = no data. NR = not recommended. s = spectrum inadequate (at site). a = activity or experience inadequate. p = tissue penetration inadequate. *based on peak serum concentration after usual adult dose. †applicable to adult uncomplicated lower UTIs (CrCl > 30 mL/min).

Ceftizoxime (Cefizox)

Drug Class: 3rd generation cephalosporin.
Usual Dose: 2 gm (IV) q8h (see comments).

Spectrum Synopsis*

Hits

Gram + : All non-enterococcal streptococci, MSSA, some CoNS

Gram – : Most GNB, B. fragilis

Problem pathogens: Nocardia, B. cepacia

Misses

Gram + : MRSA, VSE, VRE

Gram – : P. aeruginosa

Problem pathogens: Listeria, Acinetobacter, S. maltophilia

Urine Spectrum

• Same as serum spectrum

(Full *Susceptibility Profiles* p. 201).

Resistance Potential: Low
Pharmacokinetic Parameters:

Peak serum level: 132 mcg/mL
Bioavailability: Not applicable
Excreted unchanged (urine): 90%
Serum half-life (normal/ESRD): 1.7/35 hrs
Plasma protein binding: 30%
Volume of distribution (V_d): 0.32 L/kg

Primary Mode of Elimination: Renal
Dosage Adjustments*

CrCl 50–80 mL/min	1 gm (IV) q8h
CrCl 10–50 mL/min	1 gm (IV) q12h
CrCl < 10 mL/min	1 gm (IV) q24h
Post–HD dose	1 gm (IV)

Post–PD dose	1 gm (IV)
CVVH/CVVHD/CVVHDF dose	1 gm (IV) q12h
Moderate hepatic insufficiency	No change
Severe hepatic insufficiency	No change

Drug Interactions: None.
Adverse Effects:

Common

• Drug fever/rash

Uncommon

• C. difficile diarrhea/colitis

• ↑ AST/ALT

Allergic Potential: High
Safety in Pregnancy: B

Additional Clinical Considerations:

• **PRNG dose:** 500 mg (IM) × 1 dose.

May increase LPS (endotoxin) release from GNB potentially increasing endotoxin mediated tissue damage.

Additional Pharmacokinetic Considerations*

Non-CSF	% of Serum Levels
Peritoneal fluid	<10%
Bile	50%
Synovial fluid	20%
Bone	<10%
Prostate	NR(p)
Urine	1500%
CSF	
Non-inflamed meninges	1%
Inflamed meninges (ABM)	10%

Meningeal dose = 3g (IV) q6h

(also see *Antibiotic Pearls & Pitfalls* p. 528).

—— = serious side effect ⬚ = black box warning. ND = no data. NR = not recommended. s = spectrum inadequate (at site). a = activity or experience inadequate. p = tissue penetration inadequate. *based on peak serum concentration after usual adult dose. †applicable to adult uncomplicated lower UTIs (CrCl > 30 mL/min).

SELECTED REFERENCES:
Klein NC, Cunha BA. Third-generation cephalo-
sporins. Med Clin North Am 79:705–19, 1995.
(PMID:7791418)
Donowitz GR, Mandell GL. Beta-lactam antibiotics.
N Engl J Med 318:419–26 and 318:490–500,
1993. (PMID:3277053)
Marshall WF, Blair JE. The cephalosporins. Mayo Clin
Proc 74:187–95, 1999. (PMID:10069359)
Website: www.pdr.net

Ceftolozane/Tazobactam (Zerbaxa)

Drug Class: Anti-pseudomonal cephalosporin/β-lactamase inhibitor.
Usual Dose: 1.5 gm (IV) q8h

Spectrum Synopsis*
Hits
> **Gram + :** Some viridans streptococci, C. perfringens
> **Gram – :** Most aerobic GNB (including ESBL + Klebsiella, Enterobacter, Serratia), P. aeruginosa, B. fragilis
> **Problem pathogens:**
> Acinetobacter, S. maltophilia, B. cepacia

Misses
> **Gram + :** VSE, VRE, MSSA, MRSA
> **Gram – :** Acinetobacter, S. maltophilia
> **Problem pathogens:**
> KPC, CRE

Urine Spectrum
- Same as serum spectrum
- Optimal urinary pH = 5–6
- Urine levels = 66/15 mcg/mL

(Full **Susceptibility Profiles** p. 201).

Resistance Potential: Low

Pharmacokinetic Parameters:
Peak serum level: 74.4/34 mcg/mL
Bioavailability: Not applicable
Excreted unchanged (urine): 95/80%
Serum half-life (normal/ESRD):
Plasma protein binding: 16-21%/30%
Volume of distribution (V_d): 0.21 L/kg
Primary Mode of Elimination: Renal
Dosage Adjustments:

CrCl 30–50 mL/min	750 mg (IV) q8h
CrCl 15–29 mL/min	375 mg (IV) q8h
HD dose	LD of 750 mg (IV) × 1 dose, 150 mg (IV) q8h give dose Post-HD
PD dose	ND
CVVH/CVVHD/ CVVHDF dose	ND
Moderate-severe hepatic insufficiency	No change

Drug Interactions: No significant interactions are anticipated between ceftolozane/tazobactam and substrates, inhibitors and inducers of cytochrome P450 enzymes

Adverse Effects:
Uncommon
- Headache
- Insomnia
- Nausea/diarrhea
- ↑ AST/ALT
- Constipation
- Hypotension

—— = serious side effect ☐ = black box warning. ND = no data. NR = not recommended. s = spectrum inadequate (at site). a = activity or experience inadequate. p = tissue penetration inadequate.
*based on peak serum concentration after usual adult dose. †applicable to adult uncomplicated lower UTIs (CrCl > 30 mL/min).

- Drug fever/rash
- Anemia

Rare

- C. difficile diarrhea/colitis
- Thrombocytosis

Allergic Potential:
Safety in Pregnancy: Category B

Additional Clinical Considerations:

- Useful for MDR Gram negative pathogens, including P. aeruginosa and ESBL producing GNB.
- *Ineffective against CRE.*
- *For treating cIAI, must add metronidazole 500 mg (IV) q8h.*

(also see *Antibiotic Pearls & Pitfalls* p. 530).

SELECTED REFERENCES:

Cho JA, Fiorenza MA, Estrada SJ. Ceftolozane/ Tazobactam: A novel cephalosporin/β-Lactamase Inhibitor combination. Pharmaco 35:701-715, 2015. (PMID:26133315)

Lucasti C, Hershberger E, Miller B, et al. Multicenter, double-blind, randomized, phase II trial to assess the safety and efficacy of ceftolozane/ tazobactam plus metronidazole compared with meropenem in adult patients with complicated intra abdominal infections. Antimicrob Agents and Chemotherapy. 58:5350-5357, 2014. (PMID:24982069)

Miller B, Hershberger E, Benziger D, et al. Pharmacokinetics and safety of intravenous ceftolozane/tazobactam in healthy adult subjects following single and multiple ascending doses. Antimicrob Agents Chemo 56:3086-3091, 2012. (PMID:22450972)

Sorbera M, Chung E, Ho CW, et al. Ceftolozane/ tazobactam: a new option in the treatment of complicated gram-negative infections. P & T 39:825-832, 2014. (PMID:25516692)

Zhanel GG, Chung P, Adam H, et al. Ceftolozane/ tazobactam: a novel cephalosprin/beta-lactamase inhibitor combination with activity against multidrug-resistant gram-negative bacilli. Drugs 74:31-51, 2014. (PMID:24352909)

Website: www.pdr.net

Ceftriaxone (Rocephin)

Drug Class: 3rd generation. cephalosporin.
Usual Dose: 1–2 gm (IV) q24h (see comments).

Spectrum Synopsis*
Hits
Gram + : All non-enterococcal streptococci, MSSA
Gram – : Most GNB
Problem pathogens: Nocardia
Misses
Gram + : MRSA, VSE, VRE
Gram – : P. aeruginosa, B. fragilis
Problem pathogens:
Listeria, Acinetobacter,
S. maltophilia, B. cepacia
Urine Spectrum
- Optimal urinary pH = 5–6.
- Same as serum spectrum
- Urine levels = 1000 mcg/mL

(Full *Susceptibility Profiles* p. 201).

Resistance Potential: Low
Pharmacokinetic Parameters:
Peak serum level: 151–257 mcg/mL
Bioavailability: Not applicable
Excreted unchanged (urine/feces): 33–67%
Serum half-life (normal/ESRD): 8/16 hrs
Plasma protein binding: 90%
Volume of distribution (V_d): 0.08–0.3 L/kg

——— = serious side effect ☐ = black box warning. ND = no data. NR = not recommended. s = spectrum inadequate (at site). a = activity or experience inadequate. p = tissue penetration inadequate. *based on peak serum concentration after usual adult dose. †applicable to adult uncomplicated lower UTIs (CrCl > 30 mL/min).

Primary Mode of Elimination: Renal/
Hepatic

Dosage Adjustments*

CrCl < 10 mL/min	No change
Post–HD dose	None
Post–HFHD dose	None
Post–PD dose	None
CVVH/CVVHD/ CVVHDF dose	No change
Moderate hepatic insufficiency	No change
Severe hepatic insufficiency	No change (max dose: 2 gm/d)

Drug Interactions: May cause intravascular precipitation with calcium containing solutions; lansoprazole (may ↑ QT$_c$ interval).

Adverse Effects:

Uncommon
- Drug fever/rash
- Non-C. difficile diarrhea
- <u>May interfere with platelet aggregation</u>
- Thrombocytosis
- ↑ AST/ALT

Rare
- Hemolytic anemia
- <u>Pseudobiliary lithiasis</u>

Allergic Potential: High

Safety in Pregnancy: *B. Avoid near term in 3rd trimester* (↑ incidence of kernicterus in newborns)

Additional Clinical Considerations:
- Except for ABM, the usual dose of ceftriaxone should be 1 gm (not 2 gm) q12-24h
- Hepatic penetration (vs. gallbadder bile) may require 2g (IV) q12-24h dosing

Additional Pharmacokinetic Considerations*

Non-CSF	% of Serum Levels
Peritoneal fluid	ND
Bile	>500%
Synovial fluid	10%
Bone	20%
Prostate	NR, ND
Urine†	60%
CSF	
Non-inflamed meninges	1%
Inflamed meninges (ABM)	10%

Meningeal dose = 2 gm (IV) q12h

(also see ***Antibiotic Pearls & Pitfalls*** p. 528).

SELECTED REFERENCES:
Borg R, Dotevall L, Hagberg L, et al. Intravenous ceftriaxone compared with oral doxycycline for the treatment of Lyme neuroborreliosis. Scand J Infect Dis 37:449–454, 2005. (PMID:16012005)

Carr DR, Stiefel U, Bonomo RA, et al. A comparison of Cefazolin versus Ceftriaxone for the treatment of methicillin-susceptible staphylococcus aureus bacteremia in a tertiary care VA medical center. Open forum infect dis. 5:1-5, 2018. (PMID: 30568987)

Feurle GE, Junga NS, Marth T. Efficacy of ceftriaxone or meropenem as initial therapies in Whipple's disease. Gastroenterology 138:478–486, 2010. (PMID: 19874276)

File TM Jr. Clinical implications and treatment of multiresistant Streptococcus pneumoniae pneumonia. Clin Microbiol Infect 12:31–41, 2006.

Freeman CD, Nightingale CH, Nicolau DP, et al. Serum bactericidal activity of ceftriaxone plus metronidazole against common intra-abdominal pathogens. Am J Hosp Pharm 51:1782–7, 1994. (PMID: 7942906)

Klein NC, Cunha BA. Third generation cephalosporins. Med Clin North Am 79:705–19, 1995. (PMID: 7791418)

Marshall WF, Blair JE. The cephalosporins. Mayo Clin Proc 74:187–95, 1999. (PMID:10069359)

Shelburne SA 3rd, Greenburg SB, Aslam S, et al. Successful ceftriaxone therapy of endocarditis

---

—— = serious side effect ☐ = black box warning. ND = no data. NR = not recommended. s = spectrum inadequate (at site). a = activity or experience inadequate. p = tissue penetration inadequate. *based on peak serum concentration after usual adult dose. †applicable to adult uncomplicated lower UTIs (CrCl > 30 mL/min)

due to penicillin non-susceptible viridans streptococci. J Infect 54:e108–e110, 2007. (PMID:16829611)

Website: www.pdr.net

Cefuroxime (Kefurox, Zinacef, Ceftin)

Drug Class: 2nd generation IV/oral cephalosporin.
Usual Dose: 1.5 gm (IV) q8h; 500 mg (PO) q12h (see comments).

Spectrum Synopsis*
Hits
Gram + : All non-enterococcal streptococci, MSSA, most CoNS
Gram – : Some GNB
Problem pathogens: None
Misses
Gram + : MRSA, VSE, VRE
Gram – : Serratia, P. aeruginosa, B. fragilis)
Problem pathogens: Listeria, Nocardia, Acinetobacter, S. maltophilia, B. cepacia

(Full *Susceptibility Profiles* p. 201).

Resistance Potential: Low
Pharmacokinetic Parameters:
Peak serum level: 100 (IV)/7 (PO) mcg/mL
Bioavailability: 52%
Excreted unchanged (urine): 89%
Serum half-life (normal/ESRD): 1.2/17 hrs
Plasma protein binding: 50%
Volume of distribution (V_d): 0.15 L/kg
Primary Mode of Elimination: Renal

Dosage Adjustments*

CrCl 20 –80 mL/min	No change
CrCl 10–20 mL/min	750 mg (IV) q12h 500 mg (PO) q12h
CrCl < 10 mL/min	750 mg (IV) q24h 250 mg (PO) q24h
Post–HD dose	750 mg (IV) 250 mg (PO)
Post–PD dose	750 mg (IV) 250 mg (PO)
CVVH/CVVHD/ CVVHDF dose	1 gm (IV) q12h 500 mg (PO) q12h
Moderate hepatic insufficiency	No change
Severe hepatic insufficiency	No change

Drug Interactions: None.
Adverse Effects:
Common
 • Non-C. difficile diarrhea
Uncommon
 • Drug fever/rash
 • Anemia
 • Eosinophilia
 • ↑ AST/ALT
Rare
 • C. difficile diarrhea/colitis
Allergic Potential: High
Safety in Pregnancy: B

Additional Clinical Considerations:
• Oral preparation penetrates oral/ respiratory secretions well.
• **PPNG dose:** 1 gm (IM) × 1 dose.
• **Ineffective for H. influenzae meningitis prophylaxis or therapy.**

—— = serious side effect ☐ = black box warning. ND = no data. NR = not recommended. s = spectrum inadequate (at site). a = activity or experience inadequate. p = tissue penetration inadequate. *based on peak serum concentration after usual adult dose. †applicable to adult uncomplicated lower UTIs (CrCl > 30 mL/min).

Additional Pharmacokinetic Considerations:	
Non-CSF	**% of Serum Levels**
Peritoneal fluid	30%
Bile	>100%
Synovial fluid	NR(s)
Bone	10%
Prostate	NR(p)
Urine	100%
CSF	
Non-inflamed meninges	<1%
Inflamed meninges (ABM)	<10%

(also see **Antibiotic Pearls & Pitfalls** p. 528).

SELECTED REFERENCES:

Gentry LO, Zeluff BJ, Cooley DA. Antibiotic prophylaxis in open-heart surgery: A comparison of cefamandole, cefuroxime, and cefazolin. Ann Thorac Surg 46:167–71, 1988. (PMID:3401076)

Marshall WF, Blair JE. The cephalosporins. Mayo Clin Proc 74:187–95, 1999. (PMID:10069359)

Perry Cm, Brogden RN. Cefuroxime axetil. A review of its antibacterial activity, pharmacokinetic properties, and therapeutic efficacy. Drugs 52:125–58, 1996. (PMID:8799689)

Website: www.pdr.net

Cephalexin (Keflex)

Drug Class: 1st generation oral cephalosporin.
Usual Dose: 500 mg – 1 gm (PO) q6h.

Spectrum Synopsis*
Hits
Gram + : All non-enterococcal streptococci, MSSA

Gram – : Some GNB (including Klebsiella)
Problem pathogens:
　None
Misses
　Gram + : MRSA, VSE, VRE
　Gram – : H. influenzae, most GNB
　　B. fragilis
　Problem pathogens:
　　Listeria, Nocardia, Acinetobacter,
　　S. maltophilia, B. cepacia
Urine Spectrum
　• Same as serum spectrum
　• Optimal urinary pH = 5–6
　• Urine levels = 1000 mcg/mL

(see **Susceptibility Profiles** p. 201).

Resistance Potential: Low
Pharmacokinetic Parameters:
Peak serum level: 18 mcg/mL
Bioavailability: 99%
Excreted unchanged (urine): > 90%
Serum half-life (normal/ESRD): 0.7/16 hrs
Plasma protein binding: 10%
Volume of distribution (V_d): 0.35 L/kg
Primary Mode of Elimination: Renal
Dosage Adjustments*

CrCl 10–50 mL/min	500 mg (PO) q12h
CrCl < 10 mL/min	500 mg (PO) q24h
Post–HD dose	500 mg (PO)
Post–PD dose	250 mg (PO)
CVVH/CVVHD/ CVVHDF dose	250 mg (PO) q8h

────── = serious side effect ☐ = black box warning. ND = no data. NR = not recommended. s = spectrum inadequate (at site). a = activity or experience inadequate. p = tissue penetration inadequate. *based on peak serum concentration after usual adult dose. †applicable to adult uncomplicated lower UTIs (CrCl > 30 mL/min).

Moderate hepatic insufficiency	No change
Severe hepatic insufficiency	No change

Drug Interactions: None.
Adverse Effects:
Common
- Nausea/Vomiting/diarrhea

Uncommon
- Drug fever/rash
- <u>C. difficile diarrhea/colitis</u>

Rare
- <u>Stevens-Johnson syndrome</u>
- <u>TEN</u>

Allergic Potential: High
Safety in Pregnancy: B

Additional Clinical Considerations:
- Highly active against S. aureus (MSSA) and Group A streptococci.
- *Limited activity against H. influenzae.*

Additional Pharmacokinetic Considerations:

Non-CSF	% of Serum Levels
Peritoneal fluid	NR(s)
Bile	>100%
Synovial fluid	ND
Bone	20%
Prostate	NR(p)
Urine†	>600%
CSF	
Non-inflamed meninges	<1%
Inflamed meninges (ABM)	<10%

(also see ***Antibiotic Pearls & Pitfalls*** p. 528).

SELECTED REFERENCES:
Chow M, Quintiliani R, Cunha BA, et al. Pharmacokinetics of high dose oral cephalosporins. J Pharmacol 19:185–194, 1979. (PMID:438352)
Cunha BA. Cephalexin remains the preferred antibiotic for uncomplicated cellulitis: revisited. J Chemo. 26:65-66, 2014. (PMID:24548092)
Cunha BA. Cephalexin remains preferred oral antibiotic therapy for uncomplicated cellulitis. Am J Med 121:e11–15, 2008. (PMID:18954824)
Cunha BA. Oral antibiotic therapy of serious systemic infections. Med Clin N Am 90:1197–1222, 2006. (PMID:17116444)
Marshall WF Blair JE. The cephalosporins. Mayo Clin Proc 74:187–95, 1999. (PMID:10069359)
Website: www.pdr.net

Chloramphenicol (Chloromycetin)

Drug Class: No specific class.
Usual Dose: 500 mg (IV/PO) q6h.

Spectrum Synopsis*
Hits
Gram + : All streptococci (including VSE, VRE), MSSA
Gram − : Most GNB (including Klebsiella), B. fragilis
Problem pathogens:
Listeria, S. maltophilia, B. cepacia
Misses
Gram + : MRSA
Gram − : Enterobacter, Serratia, P. aeruginosa
Problem pathogens:
Acinetobacter

(Full ***Susceptibility Profiles*** p. 196).

Resistance Potential: Low

—— = serious side effect ☐ = black box warning. ND = no data. NR = not recommended. s = spectrum inadequate (at site). a = activity or experience inadequate. p = tissue penetration inadequate. *based on peak serum concentration after usual adult dose. †applicable to adult uncomplicated lower UTIs (CrCl > 30 mL/min).

Pharmacokinetic Parameters:
Peak serum level: 9 mcg/mL
Bioavailability: 90%
Excreted unchanged (urine): 10%
Serum half-life (normal/ESRD): 2.5/3 hrs
Plasma protein binding: 50%
Volume of distribution (V_d): 1 L/kg

Primary Mode of Elimination: Hepatic

Dosage Adjustments*

CrCl < 50 mL/min	No change
Post–HD dose	500 mg (IV/PO)
Post–PD dose	None
CVVH/CVVHD/ CVVHDF dose	No change
Moderate— severe hepatic insufficiency	No change

Drug Interactions: Barbiturates ($\uparrow$ barbiturate effect, $\downarrow$ chloramphenicol effect); cyclophosphamide ($\uparrow$ cyclophosphamide toxicity); cyanocobalamin, iron ($\downarrow$ response to interacting drug); warfarin ($\uparrow$ INR); phenytoin ($\uparrow$ phenytoin toxicity); rifabutin, rifampin ($\downarrow$ chloramphenicol levels); sulfonylureas ($\uparrow$ sulfonylurea effect, hypoglycemia).

Adverse Effects:

Common
- Nausea/vomiting/diarrhea

Uncommon
- Dose dependent BM suppression ($\downarrow$WBC $\rightarrow$ RBC $\rightarrow$ platelets)

Rare
- Hepatotoxicity
- Optic neuritis
- Idiosyncratic aplastic anemia

Allergic Potential: Low
Safety in Pregnancy: A

Additional Clinical Considerations:
- Incompatible in solutions containing ampicillin, gentamicin, erythromycin, vancomycin.
- **Dose-related marrow suppression is common, and reversible.**
- Hepatic related to prolonged/high doses (> 4 gm/d).
- **Oral administration results in higher serum levels than IV administration.**
- Do not administer IM.
- Chloramphenicol is inactivated in bile.
- **Urinary concentrations are thera-peutically ineffective.**
- Chloramphenicol palmitate (PO) results in higher serum levels than with the same dose of chloramphenicol (IV) succinate preferentially excreted in the urine.
- Chloramphenicol palmitate penetrates well into WBCs.
- **Dose-related bone marrow suppression**
  Reversible bone marrow suppression. Aspirate shows vacuolated WBCs ("chloramphenicol effect", not toxicity). Does not precede aplastic anemia.
- **Idiosyncratic bone marrow toxicity**
  Irreversible aplastic anemia. May occur after only one dose; monitoring with serial CBCs is useless. Very rare. Usually associated with IM, intraocular, or oral administration. Rarely, if ever, with IV chloramphenicol.

—— = serious side effect ☐ = black box warning. ND = no data. NR = not recommended. s = spectrum inadequate (at site). a = activity or experience inadequate. p = tissue penetration inadequate. *based on peak serum concentration after usual adult dose. †applicable to adult uncomplicated lower UTIs (CrCl > 30 mL/min).

Additional Pharmacokinetic Considerations*

Non-CSF	% of Serum Levels
Peritoneal fluid	95%
Bile	NR(a)
Synovial fluid	ND
Bone	ND
Prostate	NR(a)
Urine	NR(a)
CSF	
Non-inflamed meninges	50%
Inflamed meninges (ABM)	90%

Meningeal dose = usual dose

(also see **Antibiotic Pearls & Pitfalls** p. 530).

SELECTED REFERENCES:

Ariyal A, Basnyat B, Koirala S, et al. Gatifloxacin versus chloramphenicol for uncomplicated enteric fever: an open-label, randomized, controlled trial. Lancet Infect Dis 11:445–454, 2011. (PMID:21531174)

Cunha BA. New uses of older antibiotics. Postgrad Med 100:68–88, 1997. (PMID:9126205)

Cunha BA. Oral antibiotic therapy of serious systemic infections. Med Clin N Am 90:1197–1222, 2006. (PMID:17116444)

Feder HM Jr, Osier C, Maderazo EG. Chloramphenicol: A review of its use in clinical practice. Rev Infect Dis 3:479–91, 1981. (PMID:6792681)

Kasten MJ. Clindamycin, metronidazole, and chloramphenicol. Mayo Clin Proc 74:825–33, 1999. (PMID:10473362)

Safdar A, Bryan CS, Stinson S, et al. Prosthetic valve endocarditis due to vancomycin-resistant Enterococcus faecium: treatment with chloramphenicol plus minocycline. Clin Infect Dis 34:61–3, 2002. (PMID:12015709)

Smilack JD, Wilson WE, Cocerill FR 3rd. Tetracycline, chloramphenicol, erythromycin, clindamycin, and metronidazole. Mayo Clin Proc 66:1270–80, 1991. (PMID:1749296)

Wareham DW, Wilson P. Chloramphenicol in the 21st century. Hosp Med 63:157–61, 2002. (PMID:11933819)
Website: www.pdr.net

Cidofovir (Vistide)

Drug class: Antiviral (HSV, CMV)
Usual dose: 5 mg/kg (IV) weekly for 2 weeks, then 5 mg/kg every 2 weeks
Pharmacokinetic Parameters:
Peak serum level: 19.6 mcg/mL
Bioavailability: not applicable
Excreted unchanged: 1%
Serum half-life (normal/ESRD): 2.2 h/ no data
Plasma protein binding: 6%
Volume of distribution (V_d): 0.54 L/kg
Primary Mode of Elimination: Renal
Dosage Adjustments*

Cr increase of 0.3–0.4 mg/dL above baseline	3 mg/kg (IV) (see usual dose for duration)
Cr increase of ≥ 0.5 mg/dL or + 3 proteinuria	Discontinue cidofovir
Moderate—severe hepatic insufficiency	No change

Drug Interactions: Amphotericin B, aminoglycosides, foscarnet, pentamidine, tenofovir, zidovudine (↑ nephrotoxicity).
Adverse Effects:
Common
- Nausea/vomiting
- Diarrhea

─── = serious side effect ▭ = black box warning. ND = no data. NR = not recommended. s = spectrum inadequate (at site). a = activity or experience inadequate. p = tissue penetration inadequate. *based on peak serum concentration after usual adult dose. †applicable to adult uncomplicated lower UTIs (CrCl > 30 mL/min).

- ↓ intraocular pressure
- Iritis/uveitis
- Creatinine
- ↑ serum
- Nephrotoxicity (normal saline prehydration and probenecid with each dose)
- Neutropenia

Uncommon
- Fanconi's syndrome

Rare
- Metabolic acidosis

Contraindications: If CrCl < 55 mL/min.

Allergic Potential: Low for cidofovir, high for probenecid.

Safety in Pregnancy: C

Additional Clinical Considerations:
- Patients should receive probenecid (2 g (PO) 3 hours before infusion start, then 1 g at 2 and again at 8 hours after completion of cidofovir infusion.
- Hydration with at least 1 L of normal saline with each dose of cidofovir (infuse over 1 hour)
- Contraindicated in severe hypersensitivity to probenecid or other sulfa drugs.
- CMV retinitis in HIV patients, patients must have all of the following: SrCr < 1.5 mg/dL, CrCl > 55 mL/min, urine protein < 100 mg/dL).

Highly active against CMV and HSV.
Some activity against BK virus, JC virus, VZV, and adenoviruses.
No activity against HHV-6, EBV, RSV, or influenza viruses.

Cerebrospinal Fluid Penetration: < 1%

SELECTED REFERENCES:

Ganguly N, Clough LA, Dubois LK, et al. Low-dose cidofovir in the treatment of symptomatic BK virus infection in patients undergoing allogenic hematopoietic stem cell transplantation: a retrospective analysis of an algorithmic approach. Transpl Infect Dis 12:406–411, 2010. (PMID:20487411)

Hua DK, Howard K, Craig JC, et al. Cost-effectiveness of cidofovir treatment of polyomavirus nephropathy in kidney transplant recipients. Transplantation 27:188–94, 2012. (PMID:22186937)

Lurrain NS, Chou S. Antiviral drug resistance of human cytomegalovirus, Clin Microbiol Rev 23:689–712, 2010. (PMID:20930070)

Pallet N, Burgard M, Quamouss O, et al. Cidofovir may be deleterious in BK virus-associated nephropathy. Transplantation 89:1542–1544, 2010. (PMID:20559110)

Website: www.pdr.net

Ciprofloxacin (Cipro)

Drug Class: Fluoroquinolone.

Usual Dose: 400 mg (IV) q12h; 500–750 mg (PO) q12h (see comments).

Spectrum Synopsis*

Hits

  Gram + : Some MSSA, non-enterococcal streptococci, most VSE

  Gram – : Most GNB (including P. aeruginosa)

  Problem pathogens: None

Misses

  Gram + : S. pneumoniae, most MSSA, MRSA, VRE

  Gram – : B. fragilis

───── = serious side effect ☐ = black box warning. ND = no data. NR = not recommended. s = spectrum inadequate (at site). a = activity or experience inadequate. p = tissue penetration inadequate. *based on peak serum concentration after usual adult dose. †applicable to adult uncomplicated lower UTIs (CrCl > 30 mL/min).

Problem pathogens:
Listeria, Nocardia,
Acinetobacter, S. maltophilia,
B. cepacia, CRE

Urine Spectrum
- Same as serum spectrum
- Optimal urinary pH = 6–7
- Urine levels = 300 mcg/mL

(see *Susceptibility Profiles* p. 208).

Resistance Potential: High
(S. pneumoniae, E. coli, P. aeruginosa;
↑ prevalence of MRSA)

Pharmacokinetic Parameters:
Peak serum level: 4.6 (IV)/2.9 (PO)
mcg/mL
Bioavailability: 70%
Excreted unchanged (urine): 70%
Serum half-life (normal/ESRD): 4/8 hrs
Plasma protein binding: 20–40%
Volume of distribution (V_d): 2.5 L/kg

Primary Mode of Elimination: Renal
Dosage Adjustments*

CrCl 30–50 mL/min	400 mg (IV) q12h 500 mg (PO) q12h
CrCl < 30 mL/min	400 mg (IV) q24h 500 mg (PO) q24h
Post–HD dose	200–400 mg (IV) 250–500 mg (PO)
Post–PD dose	200–400 mg (IV) 250–500 mg (PO)
CVVH/CVVHD/ CVVHDF dose	400 mg (IV) q12h 250 mg (PO) q12h
Moderate hepatic insufficiency	No change
Severe hepatic insufficiency	No change

Drug Interactions: Al++, Ca++, Fe++,
Mg++, Zn++ antacids, citrate/citric
acid, dairy products (↓ absorption of
ciprofloxacin only if taken together);
caffeine, cyclosporine, theophylline
(↑ interacting drug levels); cimetidine
(↑ ciprofloxacin levels); foscarnet (↑ risk
of seizures); oral hypoglycemics (slight ↑
or ↓ in blood glucose); NSAIDs (may ↑ risk
of seizures/CNS stimulation); phenytoin
(↑ or ↓ phenytoin levels); probenecid
(↑ ciprofloxacin levels); warfarin (↑ INR).

Adverse Effects:
Uncommon
- Nausea/vomiting
- Headache
- Dizziness
- Insomnia/delirium
- Malaise
- Encephalopathy
- <u>Seizures</u>
- Drug fever/rash
- Thrombocytopenia
- <u>C. difficile diarrhea/colitis</u> (↑ risk with PPIs)
- <u>Torsades de pointes</u>

Rare
- Tendinitis/tendon rupture

Allergic Potential: Low
Safety in Pregnancy: C

Additional Clinical Considerations:
- Enteral feeding decreases cipro floxacin absorption ≥ 30%.
- Use with caution in patients with severe renal insufficiency or seizure disorders.
- Administer 2 hours before or after H₂ antagonists, omeprazole, sucralfate,

---

—— = serious side effect ☐ = black box warning. ND = no data. NR = not recommended. s = spectrum inadequate (at site). a = activity or experience inadequate. p = tissue penetration inadequate. *based on peak serum concentration after usual adult dose. †applicable to adult uncomplicated lower UTIs (CrCl > 30 mL/min).

calcium, iron, zinc, multivitamins, or aluminum/magnesium containing medications.
- Administer ciprofloxacin (IV) as an intravenous infusion over 1 hour.
- **Nosocomial pneumonia dose:** 400 mg (IV) q8h.
- **↑ incidence of C. difficile diarrhea/ colitis with PPIs (for patients on PPIs during FQ therapy, D/C PPIs or switch to H₂ blocker for duration of FQ therapy).**

May inhibit antibiotic induced LPS (endotoxin) release from GNB potentially minimizing endotoxin mediated tissue damage.

Additional Pharmacokinetic Considerations:

Non-CSF	% of Serum Levels
Peritoneal fluid	95%
Bile	400%
Synovial fluid	20%
Bone	35%
Prostate	200%
Urine	4000%
CSF	
Non-inflamed meninges	10%
Inflamed meninges (ABM)	15%

Meningeal dose = 400 mg (IV) q8h

(also see ***Antibiotic Pearls & Pitfalls*** p. 533).

SELECTED REFERENCES:

Chou HW, Wang JL, Chang CH, et al. Risk of severe dysglycemia among diabetic patients receiving levofloxacin, ciprofloxacin, or moxifloxacin in Taiwan. Clin Infect Dis 57:971–980, 2013. (PMID:23948133)

Didier JP, Villet R, Huggler E, et al. Impact of ciprofloxacin exposure on Staphylococcus aureus genomic alterations linked with emergence of rifampin resistance. Antimicrob Agents Chemother 55:1946–1952, 2011. (PMID:21357297)

Fantin B, Duval X, Massias L, et al. Ciprofloxacin dosage and emergence of resistance in human commensal bacteria. Journal of Infect Dis 200: 390–398, 2009. (PMID:19563257)

Howell MD, Novack V, Grgurich P, et aJ. Iatrogenic gastric acid suppression and the risk of nosocomial Clostridium difficile infection. Arch Intern Med 170:784–790, 2010. (PMID:22458086)

Lewis GJ, Fang Z, Gooch M, et al. Decreased resistance of Pseudomonas aeruginosa with restriction of ciprofloxacin in a large teaching hospitals intensive care and intermediate care units. Infect Control Hosp Epidemiol 33:368–73, 2012. (PMID:23418632)

Linsky A, Gupta K, LawlerEV, et al. Proton pump inhibitors and risk for recurrent Clostridium difficile infection. Arch Intern Med 170:772–778, 2010. (PMID:20458084)

Masadeh MM, Mhaidat NM, Alzoubi KH, et al. Ciprofloxacin-induced antibacterial activity is reversed by vitamin E and vitamin C. Curr Microbiol 64:457–62, 2012. (PMID:22349957)

Miliani K, L'Heriteau, F, Lacave L, et al. Imipenem and ciprofloxacin consumption as factors associated with high incidence rates of resistance Pseudomonas aeruginosa in hospitals in northern France. J Hosp Infect 77:343–347, 2011. (PMID:21316805)

Sandberg T, Skoog G, Hermansson AB, et al. Ciprofloxacin for 7 days versus 14 days in women with acute pyelonephritis: a randomized, open-label and double-blind, placebo-controlled, non-inferiority trail. Lancet 4:484–90, 2012. (PMID:22726802)

Website: www.pdr.net

―――― = serious side effect ⬜ = black box warning. ND = no data. NR = not recommended. s = spectrum inadequate (at site). a = activity or experience inadequate. p = tissue penetration inadequate. *based on peak serum concentration after usual adult dose. †applicable to adult uncomplicated lower UTIs (CrCl > 30 mL/min).

Ciprofloxacin Extended-Release (Cipro XR)

Drug Class: Fluoroquinolone.
Usual Dose: 500 mg or 1000 mg (PO) q24h (see comments).

Spectrum Synopsis*
Hits
  Gram + : Some MSSA, most VSE
  Gram – : Most GNB (including
    P. aeruginosa)
  Problem pathogens:
    None
Misses
  Gram + : Many S. pneumoniae
  Gram – : B. fragilis, most MSSA, MRSA
  Problem pathogens:
    Listeria, Nocardia, Acineto-
    bacter, S. maltophilia, B. cepacia
Urine Spectrum
  • Same as serum spectrum

(see *Susceptibility Profiles* p. 208).

Resistance Potential: High
  (S. pneumoniae, E. coli, P. aeruginosa;
  ↑ prevalence of MRSA)
**Pharmacokinetic Parameters
(500/1000 mg):**
  Peak serum level: 1.59/3.11 mcg/mL
  Bioavailability: 70%
  Excreted unchanged (urine): 50–70%;
  22% excreted as active metabolite
  Serum half-life: 6.6/6.3 hrs
  Plasma protein binding: 20–40%
  Volume of distribution (V_d): 2.5 L/kg
Primary Mode of Elimination: Renal

Dosage Adjustments*

CrCl < 30 mL/min	No change for 500 mg dose; reduce 1000 mg dose to 500 mg (PO) q24h
Post–HD/PD dose	500 mg (PO)
CVVH/CVVHD/CVVHDF dose	same as for CrCl < 30 mL/min
Moderate—severe hepatic insufficiency	No change

Drug Interactions: Al++, Ca++, Fe++, Mg++, Zn++ antacids, citrate/citric acid, dairy products, didanosine (↓ absorption of ciprofloxacin only if taken together); caffeine, cyclosporine, theophylline (↑ interacting drug levels); cimetidine (↑ ciprofloxacin levels); foscarnet (↑ risk of seizures); insulin, oral hypoglycemics (slight ↑ or ↓ in blood glucose); NSAIDs (may ↑ risk of seizures/CNS stimulation); phenytoin (↑ or ↓ phenytoin levels); probenecid (↑ ciprofloxacin levels); warfarin (↑ INR).
Adverse Effects:
Uncommon
  • Drug fever/rash
  • C. difficile diarrhea/colitis
  • ↑ QTc
  • Torsades de pointes
  • Seizures
Rare
  • Tendinitis/tendon rupture
Allergic Potential: Low
Safety in Pregnancy: C

—— = serious side effect ☐ = black box warning. ND = no data. NR = not recommended. s = spectrum inadequate (at site). a = activity or experience inadequate. p = tissue penetration inadequate. *based on peak serum concentration after usual adult dose. †applicable to adult uncomplicated lower UTIs (CrCl > 30 mL/min).

Additional Clinical Considerations:
- **Uncomplicated UTI (acute cystitis) dose:** 500 mg (PO) q24h;
- **Complicated UTI/acute uncomplicated pyelonephritis dose:** 1000 mg (PO) q24h.
- Administer at least 2 hours before or 6 hours after H2 antagonists, omeprazole, sucralfate, calcium, iron, zinc, multivitamins, or aluminum/ magnesium containing medications.
- **↑ incidence of C. difficile diarrhea/ colitis with PPIs (for patients on PPIs during FQ therapy, D/C PPIs or switch to H2 blocker for duration of FQ therapy).**

(also see **Antibiotic Pearls & Pitfalls** p. 533).

SELECTED REFERENCE:
Website: www.pdr.net

Clarithromycin (Biaxin)

Drug Class: Macrolide.
Usual Dose: 500 mg (PO) q12h.

Spectrum Synopsis*
Hits
  Gram + : Some S. pneumoniae, VSE
  Gram − : B. fragilis
  Problem pathogens: Bordetella
Misses
  Gram + : Most GAS, most
    S. pneumoniae, most MSSA,
    MRSA, VRE
  Gram − : Most GNB, most H. influenzae
  Problem pathogens:
    Listeria, Nocardia, Acinetobacter,
    S. maltophilia, B. cepacia

(Full **Susceptibility Profiles** p. 196).

Resistance Potential: High
  (S. pneumoniae, GAS, MSSA)
Pharmacokinetic Parameters:
Peak serum level: 1–4 mcg/mL
Bioavailability: 50%
Excreted unchanged (urine): 20%
Serum half-life (normal/ESRD): 3–7/4 hrs
Plasma protein binding: 70%
Volume of distribution (V_d): 3 L/kg
Primary Mode of Elimination: Hepatic
Dosage Adjustments*

CrCl < 30 mL/min	250 mg (PO) q12h
Post–HD dose	500 mg (PO)
Post–PD dose	None
CVVH/CVVHD/ CVVHDF dose	No change
Moderate— severe hepatic insufficiency	No change

Drug Interactions: Amiodarone, procainamide, sotalol, astemizole, terfenadine, cisapride, pimozide (may ↑ QT interval, torsade de pointes); carbamazepine (↑ carbamazepine levels, nystagmus, nausea, vomiting, diarrhea); cimetidine, digoxin, ergot alkaloids, midazolam, triazolam, phenytoin, ritonavir, tacrolimus, valproic acid (↑ interacting drug levels); clozapine, corticosteroids (not studied); cyclosporine (↑ cyclosporine levels with toxicity); efavirenz (↓ clarithromycin levels); rifabutin, rifampin (↓ clarithromycin

———— = serious side effect ☐ = black box warning. ND = no data. NR = not recommended. s = spectrum inadequate (at site). a = activity or experience inadequate. p = tissue penetration inadequate. *based on peak serum concentration after usual adult dose. †applicable to adult uncomplicated lower UTIs (CrCl > 30 mL/min).

levels, ↑ interacting drug levels); statins (↑ risk of rhabdomyolysis); theophylline (↑ theophylline levels, nausea, vomiting, seizures, apnea); warfarin (↑ INR); zidovudine (↓ zidovudine levels).

Adverse Effects:

Uncommon

- Nausea/vomiting/diarrhea
- ↑ QTc

Rare

- C. difficile diarrhea/colitis

Allergic Potential: Low

Safety in Pregnancy: C

Additional Clinical Considerations:

- Peculiar "aluminum sand" taste sensation on swallowing.

(also see **Antibiotic Pearls & Pitfalls** p. 536).

SELECTED REFERENCES:

Alvarez-Elcoro S, Enzler MJ. The macrolides: Erythromycin, clarithromycin and azithromycin. Mayo Clin Proc 4:613–34, 1999. (PMID:10377939)

Bergman M, Huikko S, Huovinen P, et al. Macrolide and azithromycin use are linked to increased macrolide resistance in Streptococcus pneumoniae. Antimicrob Agents Chemother 50:3646–3650, 2006. (PMID:16940064)

Schlossberg D. Azithromycin and clarithromycin. Med Clin North Am 79:803–16, 1995. (PMID:7791424)

Website: www.pdr.net

Clarithromycin XL (Biaxin XL)

Drug Class: Macrolide.
Usual Dose: 1 gm (PO) q24h.

Spectrum Synopsis*

Hits

Gram + : Some S. pneumoniae, VSE

Gram − : B. fragilis

Problem pathogens:
  Bordetella

Misses

Gram + : Most GAS, most S. pneumoniae, most MSSA, MRSA, VRE

Gram − : Most GNB, most H. influenzae

Problem pathogens:
  Listeria, Nocardia, Acinetobacter, S. maltophilia, B. cepacia

---

(see **Susceptibility Profiles** p. 196).

Resistance Potential: High (S. pneumoniae, GAS, MSSA)

Pharmacokinetic Parameters:

Peak serum level: 3 mcg/mL
Bioavailability: 50%
Excreted unchanged (urine): 20%; 10–15%
excreted as active metabolite
Serum half-life (normal/ESRD): 4/4 hrs
Plasma protein binding: 70%
Volume of distribution (V_d): 3 L/kg

Primary Mode of Elimination: Hepatic

Dosage Adjustments*

CrCl < 30 mL/min	500 mg (PO) q24h
Post–HD dose	None
Post–PD dose	None
CVVH/CVVHD/ CVVHDF dose	No change

——— = serious side effect ▢ = black box warning. ND = no data. NR = not recommended. s = spectrum inadequate (at site). a = activity or experience inadequate. p = tissue penetration inadequate. *based on peak serum concentration after usual adult dose. †applicable to adult uncomplicated lower UTIs (CrCl > 30 mL/min).

| Moderate hepatic insufficiency | No change |
| Severe hepatic insufficiency | No change |

Drug Interactions: Amiodarone, procainamide, sotalol, astemizole, terfenadine, cisapride, pimozide (may ↑ QT interval, torsade de pointes); carbamazepine (↑ carbamazepine levels, nystagmus, nausea, vomiting, diarrhea); cimetidine, digoxin, ergot alkaloids, midazolam, triazolam, phenytoin, ritonavir, tacrolimus, valproic acid (↑ interacting drug levels); clozapine, corticosteroids (not studied); cyclosporine (↑ cyclosporine levels with toxicity); efavirenz (↓ clarithromycin levels); rifabutin, rifampin (↓ clarithromycin levels, ↑ interacting drug levels); statins (↑ risk of rhabdomyolysis); theophylline (↑ theophylline levels, nausea, vomiting, seizures, apnea); warfarin (↑ INR); zidovudine (↓ zidovudine levels).

Adverse Effects:
Uncommon
- Nausea/vomiting/diarrhea
- ↑ QTc

Rare
- C. difficile diarrhea/colitis

Allergic Potential: Low
Safety in Pregnancy: C

Additional Clinical Considerations:
- Two 500 mg tablets of XL preparation permits once daily dosing
- Decreased GI intolerance.

(also see **Antibiotic Pearls & Pitfalls** p. 536).

SELECTED REFERENCES:
Gotfried HM. Clarithromycin (Biaxin) extended-release tablet: a therapeutic review. Expert Rev Anti Infect Ther 1:9–20, 2003. (PMID:15482099)
Website: www.pdr.net

Clindamycin (Cleocin)

Drug Class: Lincosamide.
Usual Dose: 600 mg (IV) q8h; 150–300 mg (PO) q6h.

Spectrum Synopsis*
Hits
Gram + : All non-enterococcal streptococci, MSSA, some CA-MRSA
Gram – : B. fragilis
Problem pathogens: None
Misses
Gram + : All HA-MRSA, VSE, VRE
Gram – : All aerobic GNB
Problem pathogens: Listeria, Nocardia, Acinetobacter, S. maltophilia, B. cepacia

(Full **Susceptibility Profiles** p. 196).

Resistance Potential: Low
Pharmacokinetic Parameters:
Peak serum level: 2.5–10 mcg/mL
Bioavailability: 90%
Excreted unchanged (urine): 10%; 3.6% excreted as active metabolite
Serum half-life (normal/ESRD): 2.4/4 hrs

—— = serious side effect ☐ = black box warning. ND = no data. NR = not recommended. s = spectrum inadequate (at site). a = activity or experience inadequate. p = tissue penetration inadequate. *based on peak serum concentration after usual adult dose. †applicable to adult uncomplicated lower UTIs (CrCl > 30 mL/min).

Plasma protein binding: 90%
Volume of distribution (V_d): 1 L/kg
Primary Mode of Elimination: Hepatic
Dosage Adjustments*

CrCl < 10 mL/min	No change
Post–HD/PD dose	None
CVVH/CVVHD/CVVHDF dose	No change
Moderate—severe hepatic insufficiency	No change

Drug Interactions: Muscle relaxants, neuromuscular blockers (↑ apnea, respiratory paralysis); kaolin (↓ clindamycin absorption); theophylline (↑ theophylline levels, seizures).

Adverse Effects:
Common
- Nausea/vomiting/diarrhea

Uncommon
- Neuromuscular blockade
- Difficile diarrhea/colitis

Allergic Potential: Low
Safety in Pregnancy: B

Additional Clinical Considerations:
- ***Anti-spasmodics contraindicated in C. difficile diarrhea.***
- C. difficile diarrhea more common with PO vs. IV clindamycin.
- ***Clindamycin misses some Peptostreptococci, Fusobacteria, non-perfringens Clostridia, and Prevotella.***
- Penetrates well into PMNs.
- ***Dissolves biofilms/glycocalyx on plastic/metal devices***

Additional Pharmacokinetic Considerations*

Non-CSF	**% of Serum Levels**
Peritoneal fluid	75%
Bile	NR(s) 300%
Synovial fluid	30%
Bone	50%
Prostate	NR(s) 10%
Urine†	15%
CSF	
Non-inflamed meninges	1%
Inflamed meninges (ABM)	<10%

Meningeal dose = 600 mg (IV) q6h (for CNS toxoplasmosis only)

(also see ***Antibiotic Pearls & Pitfalls*** p. 531).

SELECTED REFERENCES:
Coyle EA, Cha R, Rybak MJ. Influences of linezolid, penicillin, and clindamycin, alone and in combination, on streptococcal pyrogenic exotoxin a release. Antimicrob Agents Chemother 47:1752–5, 2003. (PMID:12709354)
Czekaj J, Dinh A, Moldovan A, et al. Efficacy of a combined oral clindamycin-rifampicin regimen for therapy of staphylococcal osteoarticular infections. Scand J Infect Dis 43:962–967, 2011. (PMID:21916775)
Falagas ME, Gorbach SL. Clindamycin and metronidazole. Med Clin North Am 79:845–67, 1995. (PMID:7791427)
Lell B, Dremsner PG. Clindamycin as an antimalarial drug: review of clinical trials. Antimicrob Agents Chemother 46:2315–20, 2002. (PMID:12121896)
Website: www.pdr.net

Colistin (Coly-Mycin M)

Drug Class: Cell membrane antibiotic.
Usual Dose: 2.5 mg/kg (IV) q12h.
1 mg = 12,500 U. Colistin (Polymyxin E)

= serious side effect ☐ = black box warning. ND = no data. NR = not recommended. s = spectrum inadequate (at site). a = activity or experience inadequate. p = tissue penetration inadequate.
*based on peak serum concentration after usual adult dose. †applicable to adult uncomplicated lower UTIs (CrCl > 30 mL/min).

Spectrum Synopsis*

Hits
Gram + : None
Gram – : Aerobic GNB (including P. aeruginosa)
Problem pathogens:
ESBL + Klebsiella, Enterobacter, E. coli, S. maltophilia

Misses
Gram + : All
Gram – : Proteus, Serratia, B. fragilis
Problem pathogens:
Acinetobacter, B. cepacia

Urine Spectrum†
- Same as serum spectrum
- Optimal urinary pH = ND
- Urine levels = 100 mcg/mL

(Full *Susceptibility Profiles* p. 208).

Resistance Potential: Low
Pharmacokinetic Parameters:
Peak serum level: 5 mcg/mL
Bioavailability: Not applicable
Excreted unchanged (urine): 90%
Serum half-life (normal/ESRD): 9/13 hrs
Plasma protein binding: 50%
Volume of distribution (V_d): 0.09 L/kg
Primary Mode of Elimination: Renal
Dosage Adjustments*

CrCl 30–49 mL/min	3.5 mg/kg (IV) q24h
CrCl 10–29 mL/min	2.5 mg/kg (IV) q24h
CrCl < 10 mL/min	1.5 mg/kg (IV) q24h
Post–HD dose	None
Post–PD dose	None
CVVH/CVVHD/ CVVHDF dose	2.5 mg/kg (IV) q48h

Mild hepatic insufficiency	No change
Moderate— severe hepatic insufficience	No change

Drug Interactions: Neuromuscular blocking agents (↑ neuromuscular blockade); nephrotoxic drugs (↑ nephrotoxic potential).
Adverse Effects:
Common
- Nephrotoxicity (ATN)
Uncommon
- Dizziness
- Paresthesias
- Slurred speech
- Vertigo
- Blurry vision
- Drug rash/fever
- Respiratory arrest

Allergic Potential: Low
Safety in Pregnancy: C

Additional Clinical Considerations:
- ***Avoid loading dose to minimize nephrotoxicity.***
- **Useful for MDR P. aeruginosa and Acinetobacter species.**
- For P. aeruginosa or Acinetobacter meningitis also give amikacin 10–40 mg (IT) q24h or colistin 10 mg (IT) q24h.
- **As colistin is a prodrug, (delayed onset of antibacterial effect) *polymyxin preferred for sepsis***
- **Nebulizer dose:** 80 mg in saline q8h; for recurrent infection use 160 mg q8h.

———— = serious side effect ⬜ = black box warning. ND = no data. NR = not recommended. s = spectrum inadequate (at site). a = activity or experience inadequate. p = tissue penetration inadequate. *based on peak serum concentration after usual adult dose. †applicable to adult uncomplicated lower UTIs (CrCl > 30 mL/min).

- If possible, avoid aerosolized colistin, which may result in pulmonary/systemic toxicity due to the polymyxin E1 metabolite.
- **Continuous infusion dose:** give ½ of daily dose (IV) over 5–10 min, then give remaining ½ dose 1 hour after initial dose over next 24 hours.
- Acute renal toxicity ↑ with loading dose.

May inhibit antibiotic induced LPS (endotoxin) release from GNB *potentially minimizing endotoxin mediated tissue damage.*

Additional Pharmacokinetic Considerations:

Non-CSF	% of Serum Levels
Peritoneal fluid	ND
Bile	0%
Synovial fluid	ND
Bone	ND
Prostate	NR(p)
Urine†	70%
CSF	
Non-inflamed meninges	1%
Inflamed meninges (ABM)	25%
Meningeal (IT) dose:	
Intrathecal dose = 10 mg (IT) q24h	

(also see *Antibiotic Pearls & Pitfalls* p. 538).

SELECTED REFERENCES:

Bandali A, Bias TE. Efficacy and nephrotoxicity associated with various colistin dosing schemas for the treatment of multidrug resistant (MDR) infections. Infect Dis (Lond) 50:472-5, 2018. (PMID: 29228825)

Cascio A, Conti A, Sinardi L, et al. Post-neurosurgical multidrug-resistant Acinetobacter baumannii meningitis successfully treated with intrathecal colistin. A new case and a systematic review of the literature. Int J Infect Dis 14:e572–9, 2010. (PMID:19892577)

Cheng CY, Sheng WH, Wang JT, et al. Safety and efficacy of intravenous colistin (colistin methanesulphonate) for severe multidrug-resistant Gram-negative bacterial infections. Int J Antimicrob Agents 35:297–300, 2010. (PMID:20045293)

Couet W, Gregoire N, Marchan S, et al. Colistin pharmacokinetics: the fog is lifting. Clin Microbiol Infect 18: 30–39, 2012. (PMID:21988234)

Daikos GL, Skiada A, Pavleas J, et al. Serum bactericidal activity of three different dosing regimens of colistin with implications for optimum clinical use. J Chemother 22:175–178, 2010. (PMID:20566422)

Deryke CA, Crawford AJ, Uddin N, et al. Colistin dosing and nephrotoxicity in a large community teaching hospital. Antimicrob Agents Chemother 54:4503–4505, 2010. (PMID:20660694)

Falagas ME, Rafailidis PI. Nephrotoxicity of colistin: new insight into an old antibiotic. Clin Infect Dis 48:1729–1731, 2009. (PMID:19438398)

Falagas ME, Rafailidis PI, Ioannidou E, et al. Colistin therapy for microbiologically documented multi drug-resistant Gram-negative bacterial infections: a retrospective cohort study of 258 patients. Int J Antimicrob Agents 35:194–199, 2010. (PMID:20006471)

Gautam V, Shafiq N, Mouton JW, et al. Pharmacokinetics of colistin in patients with multidrug-resistant Gram-negative infections: A pilot study. Indian J Med Res 147:407-12, 2018. (PMID: 29998877)

Gauthier TP. Rifampicin plus colistin in the era of extensively drug-resistant Acinetobacter baumannii infections. Clin Infect Dis 57:359–362, 2013. (PMID:23616496)

Horton J, Pankey GA. Polymyxin B, colistin, and sodium colistimethate. Med Clin North Am 66:135–42, 1982. (PMID:6278236)

Kwa AL, Falagas ME, Michalopoulos A, et al. Benefits of aerosolized colistin for ventilator-associated pneumonia: absence of proof versus proof of absence? Clin Infect Dis 52:1278–1279, 2011. (PMID:21507926)

Linden PK, Kusne S, Coley K, et al. Use of parenteral colistin for the treatment of serious infection due to antimicrobial-resistant Pseudomonas aeruginosa. Clin Infect Dis 37:154–60, 2003. (PMID:14614688)

Markantonis SL, Markou N, Fousteri M, et al. Penetration of colistin into cerebrospinal fluid. Antimicrob Agents Chemother 53:4907–4910, 2009. (PMID:19704130)

Menna P, Salvatorelli E, Mattei A, et al. Modified Colistin Regimen for Critically ill patients with acute renal impairment and continuous renal replacement therapy. Chemotherapy 63:35-8, 2018. (PMID: 29334366)

Nation R, Gauonik S, Li J, et al. Updated US and European dose recommendations for Intravenous colistin: How do they perform? Clin Inf Dis 62:552-560, 2016. (PMID:26607424)

Paul M, Bishara J, Levcovich A, et al. Effectiveness and safety of colistin: prospective comparative cohort study. J Antimicrob Chemother 65:1019–1027, 2010. (PMID:20299494)

Plachouras D, Giamerllos-Bourboulis EJ, Kentepozidis N, et al. In vitro postantibiotic effect of colistin on multidrug-resistant Acinetobacter baumannii. Diagn Microbiol Infect Dis 57:419–422, 2007. (PMID:17188449)

Rigatto MH, Oliveira MS, Perdigao-Neto LV, et al. Multicenter prospective cohort study of renal failure in patients treated with colistin versus polymyxin B. Antimicrob Agents & Chemo 60:2443-2449, 2016. (PMID: 26856846)

Stein A, Raoult D. Colistin: an antimicrobial for the 21st century? Clin Infect Dis 35:901–2, 2002. (PMID:12228836)

Tarchini G. Nephrotoxicity associated with intravenous colistin. Clin Infect Dis 49:1773, 2009. (PMID:19891573)

Vardakas KZ, Mavroudis AD, Georgiou M, et al. Intravenous colistin combination antimicrobial treatment vs. monotherapy: a systematic review and meta-analysis. Int J Antimicrob Agents 51:535-47, 2018. (PMID: 29288723)

Wahby K, Chopra T, Chandrasekar P. Intravenous and Inhalational colistin-induced respiratory failure. Clin Infect Dis 50:e38–40, 2010. (PMID:20146630)

Yahav D, Farbman L, Leibovici L, et al. Colistin: New lessons on an old antibiotic. Clin Microbiol Infect 18:18–29, 2012. (PMID:22168320)

Website: www.pdr.net

Cycloserine (Seromycin)

Drug Class: TB drug.
Usual Dose: 250 mg (PO) q12h.
Pharmacokinetic Parameters:
   Peak serum level: 20 mcg/mL
   Bioavailability: 90%
   Excreted unchanged (urine): 65%
   Serum half-life (normal/ESRD): 10–25 hrs/ no data
   Plasma protein binding: No data
   Volume of distribution (V_d): 0.2 L/kg
Primary Mode of Elimination: Renal
Dosage Adjustments*

CrCl 10–50 mL/min	250 mg (PO) q12–24h
CrCl < 10 mL/min	250 mg (PO) q24h
Post–HD dose	None
Post–PD dose	250 mg (PO)

———— = serious side effect ☐ = black box warning. ND = no data. NR = not recommended. s = spectrum inadequate (at site). a = activity or experience inadequate. p = tissue penetration inadequate. *based on peak serum concentration after usual adult dose. †applicable to adult uncomplicated lower UTIs (CrCl > 30 mL/min).

CVVH/CVVHD/ CVVHDF dose	No change
Moderate— severe hepatic insufficiency	No change

Drug Interactions: Alcohol (seizures); ethambutol, ethionamide (drowsiness, dizziness); phenytoin (↑ phenytoin levels).

Adverse Effects:

Common
- Confusion
- Dizziness
- Headache
- Somnolence
- Psychosis

Uncommon
- Seizures

Allergic Potential: Low
Safety in Pregnancy: C

Additional Clinical Considerations:
- Avoid in patients with seizures.
- Ethambutol, ethionamide, or ethanol may increase CNS toxicity.

SELECTED REFERENCE:
Website: www.pdr.net

Dalbavancin (Dalvance)

Drug Class: Lipoglycopeptide
Usual Dose: Loading dose: 1500 mg (IV) × 1 dose or 1 gm (IV) × 1 dose, then
Maintenance dose: 500 mg (IV) 7 days later.

Spectrum Synopsis*

Hits
Gram + : All non-enterococcal streptococci, MSSA, MRSA, VISA, CoNS, VSE
Gram – : None
Problem pathogens: None

Misses
Gram + : VRSA, VRE
Gram – : All aerobic GNB, B. fragilis
Problem pathogens:
Listeria, Nocardia, Acinetobacter, S. maltophilia, B. cepacia

Resistance Potential: Low
Pharmacokinetic Parameters:
Peak serum level: 287 mcg/mL
Bioavailability not applicable
Excreted unchanged (urine/feces): 33%/20%
Serum half-life (nornal/ESRD): 346 h/376 h
Plasma protein binding: 93%
Volume of distribution (V_d): 0.1–0.19 L/kg
Primary Mode of Elimination: Renal
Dosage Adjustments*

CrCl < 30 mL/min	1125 mg (IV) × 1 dose or 750 mg (IV) then 325 mg (IV) 7 days later
Post–HD dose	No change
Post–PD dose	No change
CVVH dose	No change
Moderate severe hepatic insufficiency	No data

―――― = serious side effect ☐ = black box warning. ND = no data. NR = not recommended. s = spectrum inadequate (at site). a = activity or experience inadequate. p = tissue penetration inadequate. *based on peak serum concentration after usual adult dose. †applicable to adult uncomplicated lower UTIs (CrCl > 30 mL/min).

Drug Interactions: None
Adverse Effects:

Uncommon
- Headache
- GI upset
- ↑ AST/ALT
- Drug fever/rash
- Pruritus

Rare
- <u>C. difficile diarrhea/colitis</u>

Allergic Potential: Moderate
Safety in Pregnancy: C

Additional Clinical Considerations:
- Infuse slowly over 30 minutes to avoid "Red Man Syndrome"; hypersensitivity reactions
- Use with caution if patient had previous hypersensitivity reaction to other glycopeptides, e.g. vancomycin.

(also see ***Antibiotic Pearls & Pitfalls*** p. 537).

SELECTED REFERENCES:

Bailey J, Summers KM. Dalbavancin: a new lipoglycopeptide antibiotic. Am J Health Syst Pharm. 65:599-610, 2008. (PMID:18359966)

Boucher HW, Wilcox M, Talbot GH, et al. Once-weekly dalbavancin versus daily conventional therapy for skin infection. N Engl J Med. 370:2169-2179, 2014. (PMID:24897082)

Dunne M, Puttagunia S, Giodano, et al. A randomized clinical trial of single-dose versus weekly dalbavancin for treatment of acute bacterial skin and skin structure infection. Clin Inf Dis 62:545-546, 2016. (PMID:26611777)

Marbury T, Dowell JA, Seltzer E, et al. Pharmacokinetics of dalbavancin in patients with renal or hepatic impairment. J Clin Pharmacol. 49:465-476, 2009. (PMID:19368696)

Website: www.pdr.net

Dapsone

Drug Class: Antiparasitic, anti-leprosy, anti-PCP drug.
Usual Dose: 100 mg (PO) q24h (see comments).
Pharmacokinetic Parameters:
  Peak serum level: 1.8 mcg/mL
  Bioavailability: 85%
  Excreted unchanged (urine): 10%
  Serum half-life (normal/ESRD): 25/30 hrs
  Plasma protein binding: 80%
  Volume of distribution (V_d): 1.2 L/kg
Primary Mode of Elimination: Hepatic/Renal
Dosage Adjustments*

CrCl < 10 mL/min	No change
Post–HD dose	None
Post–PD dose	None
CVVH/CVVHD/CVVHDF dose	No change
Moderate hepatic insufficiency	No change
Severe hepatic insufficiency	No data

Drug Interactions: Didanosine (↓ dapsone absorption); oral contraceptives (↓ oral contraceptive effect); pyrimethamine, zidovudine (↑ bone marrow suppression); rifabutin, rifampin (↓ dapsone levels); trimethoprim (↑ dapsone and trimethoprim levels, methemoglobinemia).
Adverse Effects:
Common
- Hemolysis in G6PD deficiency
- Methemoglobinemia

───── = serious side effect ⬚ = black box warning. ND = no data. NR = not recommended. s = spectrum inadequate (at site). a = activity or experience inadequate. p = tissue penetration inadequate. *based on peak serum concentration after usual adult dose. †applicable to adult uncomplicated lower UTIs (CrCl > 30 mL/min).

Uncommon
- Nausea/vomiting
- Headache
- Drug fever/rash

Allergic Potential: High
Safety in Pregnancy: C

Additional Clinical Considerations:
- **Useful in sulfa (SMX) allergic patients.**
- Avoid, if possible, in G6PD deficiency or hemoglobin M deficiency.
- **PCP prophylaxis dose** = 100 mg (PO) q24h.
- **PCP therapy dose** = 100 mg (PO) q24h.

Cerebrospinal Fluid Penetration: < 50%

SELECTED REFERENCES:
East J, Blanton LS. Symptomatic hyperbilirubinemia secondary to dapsone-induced hemolysis and atazanavir therapy. Antimicrob Chemother 67:465–8, 2012. (PMID:22123706)
Website: www.pdr.net

Daptomycin (Cubicin)

Drug Class: Lipopeptide.
Usual Dose: <u>Complicated skin/skin structure</u> infections: 4 mg/kg (IV)* q24h. <u>Bacteremia, endocarditis</u>: 6 mg/kg (IV) q24h*. <u>Bacteremia, endocarditis</u> unresponsive to 6 mg/kg (IV) q24h × 3 days: 12 mg/kg (IV) q24h.

Spectrum Synopsis*
Hits
Gram + : MSSA, MRSA, CoNS, VSE, VRE
Gram – : None
Problem pathogens:
  None

Misses
Gram + : Corynebacterium JK
Gram – : All aerobic GNB, B. fragilis
Problem pathogens:
  Listeria, Nocardia

Urine Spectrum
- Same as serum spectrum

(see **Susceptibility Profiles** p. 208).

Resistance Potential: Low
Pharmacokinetic Parameters:
Peak serum level:
4 mg/kg = 58 mcg/mL; 6 mg/kg = 99 mcg/mL
Bioavailability: Not applicable
Excreted unchanged (urine): 80%
Serum half-life (normal/ESRD): 8.1/ 29.8 hrs
Plasma protein binding: 92%
Volume of distribution (V_d): 0.096 L/kg

Primary Mode of Elimination: Renal
Dosage Adjustments*

CrCl > 30 mL/min	No change
CrCl < 30 mL/min	4 mg/kg (IV) q48h or 6 mg/kg (IV) q48h or 12 mg/kg (IV) q48h
Post–HD dose	None
Post–PD dose	None
CVVH/CVVHD/ CVVHDF dose	8 mg/kg (IV) q48h
HD q 48–72h dose	10 mg/kg (IV) q HD*
Moderate— severe hepatic insufficiency	No change

*Give at end of HD.

---

* VSE/VRE MICs twice that of S. aureus i.e., enterococci require × 2 the dose used for MSSA/MRSA infections. For cSSSIs due to VSE/VRE, use 8 mg/kg (vs. 4 mg/kg for MSSA/MRSA). For VSE/VRE bacteremia/endocarditis, use 12 mg/kg (vs. 6 mg/kg for MSSA/MRSA).

Drug Interactions: Warfarin/statin (no significant interaction in small number of volunteers; consider temporary suspension of statins during daptomycin use).

Adverse Effects:

Common
- Non-C. difficile diarrhea

Uncommon
- Headache
- Insomnia
- Chest pain
- Hypertension
- CPK
- ↑ AST/ALT
- ↑ INR
- Eosinophilic pneumonia

Rare
- Peripheral neuropathy
- C. difficile diarrhea/colitis

Allergic Potential: No data

Safety in Pregnancy: B

Additional Clinical Considerations:
- Concentration-dependent killing
- Activity may be enhanced with an initial dose of gentamicin.
- Antecedent vancomycin (↑ cell wall thickness of staphylococci) predisposes to daptomycin resistance (penetration mediated resistance).
- ↑ daptomycin MICs with strains of S. aureus or VSE/VRE may be ↓ by adding a β-lactam to ↑ cell wall permeability to daptomycin; (for staphylococci add nafcillin for enterococci add ampicillin)
- **Prolonged high-dose daptomycin 12 mg/kg (IV) q24h has been used for MSSA/MRSA bacteremias/ABE unresponsive to lower doses or other anti-staphylococcal drugs without toxicity.**
- Post-antibiotic effect (PAE) up to 6 hours.
- Daptomycin may be given IV push over 5 minutes (500 mg dose given in 10 mL; 1 g dose given in 20 mL).

Additional Pharmacokinetic Considerations*

Non-CSF	% of Serum Levels
Peritoneal fluid	NR(s)
Bile	100%
Synovial fluid	ND
Bone	<10%
Prostate	NR(p)
Urine†	75%
CSF	
Non-inflamed meninges	2%
Inflamed meninges (ABM)	5%

Meningeal dose = NR(p)

*Daptomycin penetrates lung tissue well, but is inactivated by lung surfactant (organ specific antibiotic inhibition)

(also see **Antibiotic Pearls & Pitfalls** p. 535).

SELECTED REFERENCES:

Bassetti M, Nicco E, Ginocchio F, et al. High-dose daptomycin in documented Staphylococcus aureus infections. Int J Antimicrob Agents 36:459–461, 2010. (PMID:20846832)

Benevuto M, Benziger DP, Yankelev S, Vigliani G. Pharmacokinetics and tolerability of daptomycin at doses up to 12 milligrams per kilogram of body weight once daily in healthy volunteers.

─── = serious side effect ☐ = black box warning. ND = no data. NR = not recommended. s = spectrum inadequate (at site). a = activity or experience inadequate. p = tissue penetration inadequate. *based on peak serum concentration after usual adult dose. †applicable to adult uncomplicated lower UTIs (CrCl > 30 mL/min).

Antimicrobial Agents and Chemotherapy 50: 3245–49, 2006. (PMID:17005801)

Burkhardt O, Kielstein JT. A simplified three-times weekly daptomycin dosing regimen for chronic hemodialysis patients. Expert Rev Anti Infect Ther 8:11–14, 2010. (PMID:20014897)

Cantón R, Ruiz-Garbajosa P, Chaves RL, Johnson AP. A potential role for daptomycin in enterococcal infections: what is the evidence? J Antimicrob Chemother 65:1126–1136, 2010. (PMID:20363805)

Cervera C, Castaneda X, Pericas JM, et al. Clinical utility of daptomycin in infective endocarditis caused by Gram-positive cocci. Int J Antimicrob Agents 38:365–370, 2011. (PMID:21420835)

Crompton JA, North DS, McConnell SA, et al. Safety and efficacy of daptomycin in the treatment of osteomyelitis: results from the CORE Registry. J Chemother 21:414–420; 2009. (PMID:19622460)

Crompton JA, North DS, Yoon M, et al. Outcomes with daptomycin in the treatment of Staphylococcus aureus infections with a range of vancomycin MICs. J Antimicrob Chemother 65:1784–1791, 2010. (PMID:20554570)

Cunha BA, Mickail N, Eisenstein L. E. faecalis vancomycin sensitive enterococci (VSE) bacteremia unresponsive to vancomycin successfully treated with high dose daptomycin. Heart & Lung 36:456–461, 2007. (PMID:18005808)

Cunha BA, Eisenstein LE, Hamid NS. Pacemaker-induced Staphylococcus aureus mitral valve acute bacterial endocarditis complicated by persistent bacteremia from a coronary stent: Cure with prolonged/high-dose daptomycin without toxicity. Heart & Lung 35:207–11, 2006. (PMID:16701116)

Cunha BA, Hamid N, Kessler H, Parchuri S. Daptomycin cure after cefazolin treatment failure of methicillin-sensitive Staphylococcus aureus (MSSA) tricuspid valve acute bacterial endocarditis from a peripherally inserted central catheter (PICC) line. Heart & Lung 34:442–7, 2005. (PMID:16324966)

De Rosa FG, Mollaretti O, Cometto C, et al. Early experience with high dosage daptomycin for prosthetic infections. Clin Infect Dis 49:1772–1773, 2009. (PMID:19891570)

Dhand A, Bayer AS, Pogliano J, et al. Use of antistaphylococcal beta-lactams to increase daptomycin activity in eradicating persistent bacteremia due to methicillin-resistant Staphylococcus aureus: role of enhanced daptomycin binding. Clin Infec Dis 53:158–163, 2011. (PMID:21690622)

Doan TL, DePetrillo J, Singer C. Daptomycin-induced eosinophilia without pulmonary involvement. Am J Health Syst Pharm 67:2107–2109, 2010. (PMID:21116001)

Falagas ME, Giannopoulou KP, Ntziora F, et al. Daptomycin for endocarditis and/or bacteremia: a systematic review of the experimental and clinical evidence. J Antimicrob Chemother 60:7–19, 2007. (PMID:17550889)

Falcone M, Russo A, Venditti M, et al. Considerations for higher doses of daptomycin in critically ill patients with methicillin-resistant Staphylococcus aureus bacteremia. Clin Infect Dis 57:1568-1576, 2013. (PMID:2404629)

Figueroa DA, Mangini E, Amodio-Groton M, et al. Safety of high-dose intravenous daptomycin treatment: three-year cumulative experience in a clinical program. Clin Infect Dis 15;49:177–80, 2009. (PMID:19500039)

Hair PI, Keam SJ. Daptomycin: a review of its use in the management of complicated skin and soft-tissue infections and Staphylococcus aureus bacteraemia. Drugs 67:1483–1512, 2007. (PMID:17600394)

Hayes D Jr, Anstead MI, Kuhn RJ. Eosinophilic pneumonia induced by daptomycin. J Infect 54:e211–e213, 2007. (PMID:17207858)

Kanafani ZA, Boucher H, Fowler V, et al. Daptomycin compared to standard therapy for the treatment of native valve endocarditis. Enferm Infecc Microbiol Clin 28:498–503, 2010. (PMID:20188444)

King EA, McCoy J, Desai S, et al. Vancomycin-resistant enterococcal bacteraemia and daptomycin: J Antimicrob Chemother 66:2112–2118, 2011. (PMID:21697178)

Knol BM, Spieler PJ, et al. Neutropenia associated with prolonged daptomycin use. Clin Infect Dis 56:1353-1355, 2013. (PMID:23325425)

Kosmidis C, Levine DP. Daptomycin: pharmacology and clinical use. Expert Opin Pharmacother 11:615–625, 2010. (PMID:20163272)

Kullar R, Davis SL, Levine DP, et al. High-dose daptomycin for treatment of complicated gram-positive infections: a large, multicenter, retrospective study. Pharmacotherapy 31:527–536, 2011. (PMID:21923436)

Lichterfeld M, Ferraro MJ, Davis BT. High-dose daptomycin for the treatment of endocarditis caused by Staphylococcus aureus with intermediate susceptibility to glycopeptides. Int J Antimicrob Agents 35:96, 2010. (PMID:19896341)

Malizos K, Sarma J, Seaton RA, et al. Daptomycin for the treatment of osteomyelitis and orthopaedic device infections: real world clinical experience from a European registry. Eur J Clin Micro Inf Dis 35:111-118, 2016. (PMID:26563898)

Miller BA, Gray A, Leblanc TW, et al. Acute eosinophilic pneumonia secondary to daptomycin: a report of three cases. Clin Infect Dis 50:e63–68, 2010. (PMID:20420515)

Mohan S, McDermott BP, Cunha BA. Methicillin-resistant Staphylococcus aureus (MRSA) prosthetic valve endocarditis (PVE) with paravalvular abscess treated with daptomycin. Heart & Lung 34:69–71, 2005. (PMID:15647736)

Nguyen MH, Eels SJ, Tan J, et al. Pharmacokinetics of daptomycin during cardiopulmonary bypass surgery: A prospective, open-label investigation. Antimicrob Agents Chemother 55:2499–2505, 2011. (PMID:21444695)

Palavecino EI, Burnell JM. False daptomycin-nonsusceptible MIC results by microscan panel relative to Etest results for Staphylococcus aureus and enterococci. J Clin Micro. 51:281-283, 2013. (PMID:23077121)

Patel JB, Jevitt LA, Hageman J, et al. An association between reduced susceptibility to daptomycin and reduced susceptibility to vancomycin in Staphylococcus aureus. Clin Infect Dis 42:1652–3, 2006. (PMID:16652325)

Patel N, Cardone K, Grabe DW, et al. Use of pharmacokinetic and pharmacodynamic principles to determine optimal administration of daptomycin in patients receiving standardized thrice-weekly hemodialysis. Antimicrob Agents Chemother 55:1677–1683, 2011. (PMID:21282429)

Ritchie ND. Lovering AM, Seaton RA. Daptomycin in synovial fluid during treatment of methicillin-resistant Staphylococcus aureus septic arthritis. J Antimicrob Chemother 65:1314–1315, 2010. (PMID:2038272)

Stewart PS, Davison WM, Steenbergen JN. Daptomycin rapidly penetrates a Staphylococcus epidermidis biofilm. Antimicrob Agents Chemother 53:3505–3507, 2009. (PMID:19451285)

Tascini C, Congiorni C, Cori A, et al. Cardiovascular implantable electronic device endocarditis treated with daptomycin with or without transvenous removal. Heart & Lung 41:24–30, 2012. (PMID:2243696)

Traunmüller F, Schintler MV, Metzler J, et al. Soft tissue and bone penetration abilities of daptomycin in diabetic patients with bacterial foot infections. J Antimicrob Chemother 65:1252–1257, 2010. (PMID:20375031)

Van Hai SJ, Paterson DL, Gosbell IB. Emergence of daptomycin resistance following vancomycin-unresponsive Spaphylococcus aureus bacteraenia in daptomycin- native patient—a review of the literature. Eur J Clin Microbiol Infec Dis 30:603–610, 2011. (PMID:21191627)

Vilay AM, Grio M, Depestel DD, et al. Daptomycin pharmacokinetics in critically ill patients receiving continuous venovenous hemodialysis. Crit Care Med 39:19–25, 2011. (PMID:20890189)

Wu G, Abraham T, Rapp J, et al. Daptomycin: evaluation of a high-dose treatment strategy. Int J Antimicrob Agents 38:192–196, 2011. (PMID:2154959)

Website: www.pdr.net

——— = serious side effect ☐ = black box warning. ND = no data. NR = not recommended. s = spectrum inadequate (at site). a = activity or experience inadequate. p = tissue penetration inadequate. *based on peak serum concentration after usual adult dose. †applicable to adult uncomplicated lower UTIs (CrCl > 30 mL/min).

Darunavir (Prezista) DRV

Drug Class: HIV protease inhibitor.
Usual Dose: Treatment naive / treatment experienced with no darunavir resistance-associated substitutions: 800 mg (PO) q24h with ritonavir 100 mg (PO) q24h. Treatment experienced / genotyping not available: 600 mg (PO) q12h with ritonavir 100 mg (PO) q12h.

Pharmacokinetic Parameters:
  Peak serum level: 3.5 mcg/mL
  Bioavailability: 37% (alone) 82% (with ritonavir)
  Excreted unchanged: 41.2% (feces), 7.7% (urine)
  Serum half-life (normal/ESRD): 15/15 hrs
  Plasma protein binding: 95%
  Volume of distribution (V_d): ND

Primary Mode of Elimination: Fecal/Renal

Dosage Adjustments*

CrCl 10–50 mL/min	No change
CrCl < 10 mL/min	No data
Post–HD dose	No change
Post–PD dose	No change
CVVH/CVVHD/CVVHDF dose	No change
Mild—moderate hepatic insufficiency	No change
Severe hepatic insufficiency	Use with caution

Antiretroviral Dosage Adjustments

Efavirenz	No data
Nevirapine	No change

Didanosine	1 hour before or 1 hour after darunavir
Tenofovir	No change
Fosamprenavir	No change
Indinavir	No data
Lopinavir/ritonavir	Avoid
Saquinavir	Avoid
Rifabutin	150 mg (PO) qod

Drug Interactions: Indinavir, ketaconazole, nevirapine, tenofovir (↑ darunavir levels); lopinavir/ritonavir, saquinavir, efavirenz (↓ darunavir levels); concomitant administration of darunavir/ritonavir with agents highly-dependent on CYP3A for clearance, astemizole, cisapride, dihydroergotamine, ergonovine, ergotamine, methylergonovine, midazolam, pimozide, terfenadine, midazolam, triazolam (may ↓ darunavir levels and ↓ effectiveness); sildenafil, vardenafil, tadalafil (↑ PDE-5 inhibitors; sildenafil do not exceed 25 mg in 48 hrs, vardenafil do not exceed 2.5 mg in 72 hrs, or tadalafil do not exceed 10 mg in 72 hrs); clarithromycin (↑ QT_c).

Adverse Effects:
Common
- Diarrhea
- Nasopharyngitis
- Drug fever/rash
- Hyperglycemia
- Hyperlipidemia

Uncommon
- Headache
- ↑ AST/ALT

—— = serious side effect [____] = black box warning. ND = no data. NR = not recommended. s = spectrum inadequate (at site). a = activity or experience inadequate. p = tissue penetration inadequate. *based on peak serum concentration after usual adult dose. †applicable to adult uncomplicated lower UTIs (CrCl > 30 mL/min).

Rare

- <u>Immune reconstitution syndrome (IRIS)</u>

Contraindicated: lovastatin, simvastatin, atorvastatin (> 20 mg/day), rifapentine, boceprevir, telaprevir. Astemizole, terfenadine, ergot derivatives dihydroergotamine, ergonovine, ergotamine, methylergonovine, cisapride, pimozide, midazolam, triazolam.

Allergic Potential: High (see comments)
Safety in Pregnancy: C

Additional Clinical Considerations:

- Always take with food (increases AUC, Cmax by approximately 30%).
- Must be given with ritonavir to boost bioavailability.
- Darunavir contains a sulfonamide moiety (as do fosamprenavir and tipranavir); use with caution in patients with sulfonamide allergies.
- Phenobarbital, phenytoin, carbamazepine, or products containing St. John's wort, rifampin. Lovostatin and simvastatin may be taken with caution.

SELECTED REFERENCE
Website: www.pdr.net

Delafloxacin (Baxdela)

Drug Class: Fluoroquinolone.
Usual Dose: 300 mg (IV) q12h or 450 mg 450 mg (PO) q12h *(take without food)*

Spectrum Synopsis*

Hits

> **Gram + :** MSSA, MRSA, GAS, S. pneumoniae
> **Gram – :** Enterobacter, Pseudomonas aeruginosa
> **Problem pathogens:** Some Acinetobacter, Pseudomonas

Misses

> **Gram + :** VSE, VRE
> **Gram – :** B. fragilis, Klebsiella Serratia
> **Problem pathogens:** B. cepacia, S. maltophilia, Acinetobacter, Listeria, CRE

Urine Spectrum

- Optimal urinary pH = 5–6
- Same as serum spectrum
- Urine levels = 1000 mcg/mL

(Full *Susceptibility Profiles* p. 208).

Resistance Potential: Low
Pharmacokinetic Parameters:

> *Peak serum level: 8.37 mcg/mL*
> *Bioavailability: 59%*
> *Excreted unchanged: 58%*
> *Serum half-life (normal): 6 hrs*
> *Plasma protein binding: 84%*
> *Volume of distribution (V_d): 0.6 L/kg*

Primary Mode of Elimination: Hepatic
Dosage Adjustments*

	Oral	IV
CrCl 15–29 mL/min	450 mg (PO) q12h	200 mg (IV) q12h
CrCl < 15 mL/min	Avoid	Avoid

—— = serious side effect ☐ = black box warning. ND = no data. NR = not recommended. s = spectrum inadequate (at site). a = activity or experience inadequate. p = tissue penetration inadequate. *based on peak serum concentration after usual adult dose. †applicable to adult uncomplicated lower UTIs (CrCl > 30 mL/min).

Post-HD/Post-PD dose	Avoid	Avoid
CVVH dose	Avoid	Avoid
Hepatic insufficiency	No change	No change

Drug Interactions: Aluminum or magnesium-containing antacids, sucralfate, iron, MVI with iron or zinc, products with divalent or trivalent cations (eg DDI) should be given separately from oral delafloxacin. No drug interactions with IV delafloxacin. Steroids and other drugs that may (↑ risk of tendonitis/tendon rupture).

Adverse Effects:
Common
- Nausea/Vomiting
- Diarrha
- Headache
- ↑ AST/ALT

Uncommon
- C. difficile diarrhea/colitis
- Nervousness/agitation
- Insomnia
- Anxiety
- Nightmares
- Paranoia
- Dizziness
- Confusion
- Tremors
- Hallucinations
- Depression and suicidal thoughts
- Phebitis
- Hypoglycemia

Rare
- Tendonitis and tendon rupture
- Peripheral neuropathy
- Convulsions, ↑ ICP, toxic psychosis
- Worsening myasthenia gravis

- Rash
- Hypersensitivity reactions

Allergic Potential: Low

Additional Clinical Considerations:
- Take 2 hours before or 6 hours after aluminum or magnesium containing products or sucralfate.
- Administer without food.
- Infuse IV over 60 minutes
- No effect on QTc.

Additional Pharmacokinetic Considerations*

Non-CSF	% of Serum Levels
Peritoneal fluid	ND
Bile	ND
Synovial fluid	ND
Bone	ND
Prostate	ND
CSF	
Non-inflamed meninges	ND
Inflamed meninges (ABM)	ND
Meningeal dose	ND

(also see ***Antibiotic Pearls & Pitfalls*** p. 533).

SELECTED REFERENCES:
Nilius AM, et al. In vitro antibacterial potency and spectrum of ABT-492, a new fluoroquinolone. Antimicrob Agents Pharmacother 47:3260-69, 2003. (PMID: 14506039)
O'Riordan W, et al. A comparison of the safety and efficacy of intravenous followed by oral delafloxacin with vancomycin plus aztreonam for the treatment of acute bacterial skin and skin structure infections: a phase 3 multinational, double-blind, randomized study. Clin Infect Dis 67:657-66, 2018. (PMID: 29518178)
Pullman J, et al. Efficacy and safety of delafloxacin compared with vancomycin plus aztreonam for acute bacterial skin and skin structure infections: a Phase 3, double-blind, randomized study. J Antimicrob Chemother 72-3471-80. 2017, (PMID: 29029278)
Website: www.pdr.net.

―――― = serious side effect ☐ = black box warning. ND = no data. NR = not recommended. s = spectrum inadequate (at site). a = activity or experience inadequate. p = tissue penetration inadequate. *based on peak serum concentration after usual adult dose. †applicable to adult uncomplicated lower UTIs (CrCl > 30 mL/min).

Dolegravir (Tivicay) DTG

Drug class: HIV integrase strand transfer inhibitor (INSTI).

Usual dose: Treatment naïve or treatment experienced INSTI-naïve patients: 50 mg (PO) of q24h

Treatment naïve or treatment experienced INSTI naïve patients also on efavirenz, fosamprenavir/ritonavir, tipranavir/ritonavir, or rifampin: 50 mg (PO) of q12h

INSTI experienced with certain INSTI-associated resistance stitutions or clinically suspected INSTI resistance: 50 mg (PO) q12h

Pharmacokinetic Parameters:
Peak serum level: 3.6–4.1 mcg/L
Bioavailability: Not applicable
Excreted unchanged: 53% feces and 31% urine
Serum half-life (normal/ESRD): 14h/14h
Plasma protein binding: 98.9%
Volume of distribution (V_d): 17.4 L/kg
Primary Mode of Elimination: Hepatic
Dosage Adjustments*

CrCl <10 mL/min	No change
Post-HD dose	No data
Post-PO dose	No data
CVVH dose	No data
Moderate to severe hepatic insufficiency	Avoid (Child-Pugh C)

Drug Interactions: Should be taken 2 hours before or 6 hours after taking cation-containing antacids or laxatives, sucralfate, oral iron supplements, oral calcium supplements, or buffered medications; metabolized through UGT1A1 and to a lesser degree through CYP3A and also a substrate of UGT1A3, UGT1A9, BRCP and P-gp. Drugs that induce or inhibit these enzymes or transporters may affect dolutegravir levels; avoid concomitant oxcarbazepine, phenytoin, phenobarbital, carbamazepine, rifampin, St. John's wort; should not be used with etravirine without coadministration of atazanavir/ritonavir, darunavir/ritonavir, or lopinavir/ritonavir; coadministration with nevirapine should be avoided because there are insufficient data to make dosing recommendations; combinations of antiretrovirals that do not include metabolic inducers should be considered where possible for INSTI-experienced patients with certain INSTI-associated resistance substitutions or clinically suspected INSTI resistance.

Adverse Effects:
Common
- ↑ AST/ALT
- Hyperglycemia

Uncommon
- Insomnia
- Headache
- ↑ Bilirubin
- ↑ Lipase
- Diarrhea

Rare
- ↑ CPK

Allergic Potential: High.
Safety in Pregnancy: B

Additional Clinical Considerations:
- Coadministration with dufetilide in contraindicated; hypersensitivity reactions characterized by rash, constitutional findings, and sometimes organ dysfunction, including liver injury, discontinue dolutegravir if these occur; patients with underlying

---

———— = serious side effect ☐ = black box warning. ND = no data. NR = not recommended. s = spectrum inadequate (at site). a = activity or experience inadequate. p = tissue penetration inadequate. *based on peak serum concentration after usual adult dose. †applicable to adult uncomplicated lower UTIs (CrCl > 30 mL/min).

hepatitis B or C may be at increased risk for worsening or development of transaminase elevations; Safety not established in patients < 40 kg and < 12 yo.

SELECTED REFERENCES:
Cottrell ML, Hadzic T, Kashuba AD. Clinical pharmacokinetic, pharmacodynamic and drug-interaction profile of the integrase inhibitor dolutegravir. Clin Pharmacokinet 52:981–994, 2013. (PMID:23824675)
Website: www.pdr.net

Doripenem (Doribax)

Drug Class: Carbapenem.
Usual Dose: 1 gm (IV) q8h.

Spectrum Synopsis*
Hits
   Gram + : All non-enterococcal streptococci, CoNS, MSSA, VSE
   Gram – : All aerobic GNB (including P. aeruginosa), B. fragilis
   Problem pathogens:
      Acinetobacter, ESBL +
      Klebsiella, Enterobacter,
      E. coli, Meropenem
      resistant P. aeruginosa
Misses
   Gram + : MRSA, VRE
   Gram – : None
   Problem pathogens:
      Listeria, Nocardia,
      S. maltophilia, B. cepacia, CRE
Urine Spectrum
   • Same as serum spectrum

(see **Susceptibility Profiles** p. 208).

Resistance Potential: Low
Pharmacokinetic Parameters:

Peak serum level: 23 mcg/mL
Bioavailability: Not applicable
Excreted unchanged (urine): 40%
Serum half-life (normal/ESRD): 1/6.20 hrs
Plasma protein binding: 8.1%
Volume of distribution (V_d): 16.8 L/kg
Primary Mode of Elimination: Renal
Dosage Adjustments*

CrCl 30–50 mL/min	1 gm (IV) q12h
CrCl 10–30 mL/min	500 mg (IV) q12h
CrCl < 10 mL/min	500 mg (IV) q24h
Post–HD dose	250 mg (IV)
Post–HFHD dose	500 mg (IV)
Post–PD dose	500 mg (IV)
CVVH/CVVHD/ CVVHDF dose	500 mg (IV) q12h[†]
Moderate hepatic insufficiency	No change
Severe hepatic insufficiency	No change

Drug Interactions: Valproic acid (↓ valproic acid levels).
Adverse Effects:
Common
   • Headache
   • Nausea
   • Non-C. difficile diarrhea
Uncommon
   • Pruritus
   • Rash
   • Phlebitis
   • ↑ AST/ALT
   • Oral candidiasis
Rare
   • Pneumonitis (if administered by inhalation)

――― = serious side effect ☐ = black box warning. ND = no data. NR = not recommended. s = spectrum inadequate (at site). a = activity or experience inadequate. p = tissue penetration inadequate.
*based on peak serum concentration after usual adult dose. †applicable to adult uncomplicated lower UTIs (CrCl > 30 mL/min).

Allergic Potential: Anaphylaxis (rare)
Safety in Pregnancy: B

Additional Clinical Considerations:
- **cSSSIs, cIAIs, or UTIs dose:**
  500 mg (IV) q8h. Infuse over 1 hour.
- **_MDR P. aeruginosa, MDR Acinetobacter baumannii/noso-comial pneumonia dose:_** 1 gm (IV) q8h.
- **For NP/VAP, infuse IV over 4 hours.**
- **Unlike meropenem, doripenem should not be used for meningitis.**

May inhibit antibiotic induced LPS (endotoxin) release from GNB *potentially minimizing endotoxin mediated tissue damage.*

Additional Pharmacokinetic Considerations*

Non-CSF	% of Serum Levels
Peritoneal fluid	15%
Bile	117%
Synovial fluid	ND
Bone	ND
Prostate	NR(p)
Urine[†]	70%
CSF	
Non-inflamed meninges	0%
Inflamed meninges (ABM)	<1%

(also see **Antibiotic Pearls & Pitfalls** p. 529).

SELECTED REFERENCES:
Anderson DL. Doripenem. Drugs for Today 42:399–404, 2006. (PMID:16845443)
Hellwig TR, Onisk ML, Chapman BA. Potential interaction between valproic acid and doripenem. Curr Drug Saf 6:54–58, 2011. (PMID:21241241)
Lister PD. Carbapenems in the USA: focus on doripenem. Expert Rev Anti Infect Ther 5:793–809, 2007. (PMID:17914914)
Pankuch GA, Seifert H, Appelbaum PC. Activity of doripenem with and without levofloxacin, amikacin, and colistin against Pseudomonas aeruginosa and Acinetobacter baumannii. Diagn Microbiol Infect Dis 67:191–197, 2010. (PMID:20388710)
Paterson DL, DePestel DD. Doripenem. Clin Infect Dis 49:291–298, 2009. (PMID:19527173)
Wall GC, Nayima VA, Neumeister KM. Assessment of hypersensitivity reactions in patients receiving carbapenem antibiotics who report antibiotics a history of penicillin. J Chemo. 26:150-153, 2014. (PMID:24090971)
Website: www.pdr.net

Doxycycline (Vibramycin, Vibra-tabs)

Drug Class: 2nd generation tetracycline.
Usual Dose: 100 mg (IV/PO) q12h or 200 mg (IV/PO) q24h (PI dose). For **serious systemic infections**, begin with a **Loading Regimen:** 200 mg (IV/PO) q12h × 3 days **(PK dose)**, then continue at same dose or decrease to the usual **Maintenance dose:** 100 mg (IV/PO) q12h to complete therapy.

Spectrum Synopsis*
Hits
  Gram + : Most S. pneumoniae VRE, Some CA-MRSA
  Gram – : GC, E. coli, B. fragilis
  Problem pathogens: Atypical CAP pathogens, anthrax, plague, Listeria, Nocardia, Acinetobacter, Oral anerobes

---

———— = serious side effect [⬚] = black box warning. ND = no data. NR = not recommended. s = spectrum inadequate (at site). a = activity or experience inadequate. p = tissue penetration inadequate. *based on peak serum concentration after usual adult dose. †applicable to adult uncomplicated lower UTIs (CrCl > 30 mL/min).

Misses
   Gram + : VSE, GAS, GBS
   Gram – : Most GNB
   Problem pathogens:
       HA-MRSA plus ESBL + E. coli,
       Klebsiella, Enterobacter,
       P. aeruginosa, CRE
Urine Spectrum†
• Same as serum spectrum *plus*
   Klebsiella, P. aeruginosa
• Optimal urinary pH = 5–6
• Urine levels = 300 mcg/mL

(see **Susceptibility Profiles** p. 196).

Resistance Potential: Low
Pharmacokinetic Parameters:
   *Peak serum level: 100/200 mg =
   4/8 mcg/mL*
   Bioavailability: 93%
   Excreted unchanged (urine): 40%
   *Serum half-life (normal/ESRD): 18–22
   hrs/18–22 hrs*
   Plasma protein binding: 82%
   Volume of distribution (V_d): 0.75 L/kg
Primary Mode of Elimination: Hepatic
Dosage Adjustments*

CrCl < 10 mL/min	No change
Post–HD or PD dose	None
CVVH/CVVHD/CVVHDF dose	No change
Moderate—severe hepatic insufficiency	No change

Drug Interactions: Antacids,
Al^{++}, Ca^{++}, Fe^{++}, Mg^{++}, Zn^{++},
multivitamins, sucralfate (minimal ↓
doxycycline absorption); barbiturates,
carbamazepine, phenytoin

(↓ doxycycline half-life); bicarbonate
(↓ doxycycline absorption,
↑ doxycycline clearance); warfarin
(↑ INR).
Adverse Effects:
Common
• Nausea/vomiting
• Non-C. difficile diarrhea
Uncommon
• Drug rash
• ↑ BUN
Rare
• Photosensitivity
• Stevens-Johnson syndrome
• Toxic epidermal necrolysis (TEN)
Allergic Potential: Low
Safety in Pregnancy: D

Additional Clinical Considerations:
• *Tetracycline susceptibilities do not
   predict doxycycline effectiveness
   against S. pneumoniae, MSSA, MRSA.*
• **Due to high urinary concentrations
   doxycycline IV/PO effective in
   treating lower UTIs due to GNBs,
   e.g. resistant P. aeruginosa
   (susceptibility testing related to
   achievable serum concentrations).**
• Doxycycline susceptibilities are not the
   same as tigecycline susceptibilities.
• **Protective against C. difficile.**
• *Does not ↑ AST/ALT.*
• *Serum half life increases with multiple
   doses.*
• **For MRSA (regardless of
   doxycycline susceptibilities), *use
   minocycline instead of doxycycline.***

―――― = serious side effect ☐ = black box warning. ND = no data. NR = not recommended. s = spectrum inadequate (at site). a = activity or experience inadequate. p = tissue penetration inadequate. *based on peak serum concentration after usual adult dose. †applicable to adult uncomplicated lower UTIs (CrCl > 30 mL/min).

May inhibit antibiotic induced LPS (endotoxin) release from GNB potentially minimizing endotoxin mediated tissue damage.

Additional Pharmacokinetic Considerations*	
Non-CSF	**% of Serum Levels**
Peritoneal fluid	ND
Bile	300%
Synovial fluid	ND
Bone	85%
Prostate	NR$_{(P)}$
Urine†	300%
CSF	
Non-inflamed meninges	25%
Inflamed meninges (ABM)	25%
Meningeal dose = 200 mg (IV) q12h	

(also see **Antibiotic Pearls & Pitfalls** p. 530).

SELECTED REFERENCES:

Borg R, Dotevall L, Hagberg L, et al. Intravenous ceftriaxone compared with oral doxycycline for the treatment of Lyme neuroborreliosis. Scand J Infect Dis 37:449–454, 2005. (PMID:16012005)

Cunha BA, Baron J, Cunha CB. Similarities and differences between doxycycline and minocycline: clinical and antimicrobial stewardship considerations. Eur J Clin Microbiol Infect Dis 37:15-20, 2018. (PMID: 28819873)

Cunha BA, Cunha CB, Pharmacokinetic Considerations in antibiotic selection for the optimal therapy of mycoplasma pneumoniae encephalitis. European Journal of Medical Microbiology and Infectious Disease 38: (In press) 2019. (PMID: 30680554)

Cunha BA, Elyasi M, Singh P, Jimada I. Lyme Carditis with Isolated left bundle branch block and myocarditis successfully treated with oral doxycycline. ID cases 11:48-50, 2018. (PMID: 29326870)

Cunha BA. Gran A, Raza M. Persistent extended-spectrum B-lactamase-positive Escherichia coli chronic prostatitis successfully treated with a combination of fosfomycin and doxycycline. Int. J Antimicrob Agents. 45:427-429, 2015. (PMID:25662814)

Cunha BA. Minocycline is a reliable and effective oral option to treat methicillin-resistant-resistant Staphylococcus aureus skin and soft-tissue infections, including doxycycline treatment failures. Int J Antimicrob Agents. 43:386-387, 2014. (PMID:24559866)

Cunha BA, Minocycline versus doxycycline for methicillin-resistant Staphylococcus aureus (MRSA): in vitro susceptibility versus in vivo effectiveness. Int J Antimicrob Agents 35:517–8, 2012. (PMID:20202796)

Cunha BA. Oral doxycycline for non-systemic urinary tract infections (UTIs) due to P. aeruginosa and other Gram negative uropathogens. Eur J Clin Microbiol Infect Dis 31:2865–8, 2012. (PMID:22767268)

Cunha BA. Doxycycline for nursing home acquired pneumonia (NHAP). Scandinavian Journal of Infectious Disease 41:77–78, 2009. (PMID:18821134)

Cunha BA. New uses for older antibiotics: nitrofurantoin, amikacin, colistin, polymyxin B, doxycycline, and minocycline revisited. Med Clin North Am 90:1089–1107, 2006. (PMID:17116438)

Cunha BA. Oral antibiotic therapy of serious systemic infections. Med Clin N Am 90:1197–1222, 2006. (PMID:17116444)

Cunha BA. Doxycycline for community-acquired pneumonia. Clin Infect Dis 37:870, 2003. (PMID:12955665)

Cunha BA, Domenico PD, Cunha CB. Pharmacodynamics of doxycycline. Clin Micro Infect 6:270–3, 2000. (PMID:11168126)

Cunha BA. Doxycycline re-revisited. Arch Intern Med 159:1006–7, 1999. (PMID:10326943)

Doernberg SB, Winston LG, Deck LH, et al. Does Doxycycline protect against development of Clostridium difficile infection? Clin Infect Dis 55:615–20, 2012. (PMID:22563022)

Johnson JR. Doxycycline for treatment of community-acquired pneumonia. Clin Infect Dis 35:632, 2002. (PMID:12173142)

Jones RN, Sader HS, Fritsche TR. Doxycycline use for community-acquired pneumonia: contemporary in vitro spectrum of activity against Streptococcus

---

—— = serious side effect ▭ = black box warning. ND = no data. NR = not recommended. s = spectrum inadequate (at site). a = activity or experience inadequate. p = tissue penetration inadequate. *based on peak serum concentration after usual adult dose. †applicable to adult uncomplicated lower UTIs (CrCl > 30 mL/min).

pneumoniae. Diagn Microbiol Infect Dis 49:147–9, 2004. (PMID:15183865)

Karkkonen K, Stiernstedt SH, Karisson M. Follow-up of patients treated with oral doxycycline for Lyme neuroborreliosis. Scand J Infect Dis 33:259–262, 2001. (PMID:11345216)

Psomas KC, Brun M, Causse A, et al. Efficacy of a ceftriaxone and doxycycline in the treatment of early syphilis. Magn Reson Imaging 30:271–82, 2012. (PMID:22119040)

Raoult D. Doxycycline for Mansonella perstans Infection. N Engl J Med 362:272–273, 2010. (PMID:20089982)

Schwartz BS, Graber CJ, Diep BA, et al. Doxycycline, not minocycline, induces its own resistance in multidrug-resistant community-associated methicillin-resistant Staphylococcus aureus clone USA300. Clin Infect Dis 48:1483–1484, 2009. (PMID:19374563)

Shea KW, Ueno Y, Abumustafa F, Cunha BA. Doxycycline activity against Streptococcus pneumoniae. Chest 107:1775–6, 1995. (PMID:7497817)

Tan KR, Magill AJ, Parise ME, et al. Doxycycline for malaria chemoprophylaxis and treatment: report from the CDC expert meeting on malaria chemoprophylaxis. Am J Trop Med Hyg 84:517–531, 2011. (PMID:21460003)

Teh B, Grayson ML, Johnson PD, et al. Doxycycline vs. macrolides in combination therapy for treatment of community-acquired pneumonia. Clin Microbiol Infect 18:71–3, 2012. (PMID:22284533)

Turner JD, Mand S, Debrah AY, et al. A randomized, double-blind clinical trial of a 3-week course of doxycycline plus albendazole and ivermectin for the treatment of Wuchereria bancrofti infection. Clin Infect Dis 42:1081–9, 2006. (PMID:16575724)

Wormser GP, Wormser RP, Cunha BA, et al. How safe is doxycycline for young children or for pregnant or breast feeding women? Diagnostic microbiology infectious disease 93:238-242, 2019. (PMID: 30442509)

Website: www.pdr.net

Efavirenz (Sustiva) EFV

Drug Class: HIV NNRTI (non-nucleoside reverse transcriptase inhibitor).
Usual Dose: 600 mg (PO) q24h.
Pharmacokinetic Parameters:
Peak serum level: 12.9 mcg/mL
Bioavailability: Increased with food
Excreted unchanged (urine): 14–34%
Serum half-life (normal/ESRD): 40–55 hrs/ no data
Plasma protein binding: 99%
Volume of distribution (V_d): ND
Primary Mode of Elimination: Hepatic
Dosage Adjustments*

CrCl < 60 mL/min	No change
Post–HD or PD dose	None
CVVH/CVVHD/ CVVHDF dose	No change
Moderate—severe hepatic insufficiency	No change

Antiretroviral Dosage Adjustments

Delavirdine	No data
Indinavir	Indinavir 1000 mg q8h
Lopinavir/ritonavir (l/r)	Consider l/r 533/133 mg q12h in PI-experienced patients
Nelfinavir	No change
Nevirapine	No data
Ritonavir	Ritonavir 600 mg q12h (500 mg q12h for intolerance)
Saquinavir	Avoid use as sole PI

—— = serious side effect ☐ = black box warning. ND = no data. NR = not recommended. s = spectrum inadequate (at site). a = activity or experience inadequate. p = tissue penetration inadequate. *based on peak serum concentration after usual adult dose. †applicable to adult uncomplicated lower UTIs (CrCl > 30 mL/min).

Rifampin	No change
Rifabutin	Rifabutin 450–600 mg q24h or 600 mg 2–3x/ week if not on protease inhibitor
Telaprevir increase telaprevie 1125 mg q7–9h	
Voriconazole: give efavirenz 300 mg q24h, voriconazole 400 mg q12h	

Drug Interactions: Antiretrovirals, rifabutin, rifampin (see dose adjustment grid, above); astemizole, terfenadine, cisapride, ergotamine, midazolam, carbamazepine, phenobarbital, phenytoin (monitor anticonvulsant levels; use with caution); verapamil, diltiazem (↓ calcium channel blocker levels) caspofungin, itraconazole, posaconazole (↓ anti fungal levels); methadone, clarithromycin (↓ interacting drug levels; titrate methadone dose to effect; consider using azithromycin instead of clarithromycin).

Contraindications: Triazolam, rifapentine, boceprevir.

Adverse Effects:

Common
- Bad dreams
- Dizziness
- Neuropsychiatric symptoms, difficulty concentrating, somnolence
- Drug fever/rash

Uncommon
- ↑ AST/ALT

Rare
- E. multiforme/Stevens-Johnson syndrome

Allergic Potential: High

Safety in Pregnancy: D

Additional Clinical Considerations:
- Rash/CNS symptoms usually resolve spontaneously over 2–4 weeks.
- Take at bedtime.
- Avoid taking after high fat meals (levels ↑ 50%).

Cerebrospinal Fluid Penetration: 1%

SELECTED REFERENCE:
Website: www.pdr.net

Efavirenz + Emtricitabine + Tenofovir disoproxil fumarate (Atripla) EFV/FTC/TDF

Drug Class: HIV

Usual Dose: 1 tablet (efavirenz 600 mg/ emtricitabine 200 mg/tenofovir 300 mg) (PO) q24h (*take without food*).

Pharmacokinetic Parameters:
Peak serum level: 4.0/1.8 mcg/mL/ 296 ng/mL
Bioavailability: NR/93%/25%
Excreted unchanged: < 1% unchanged and 14–30% as metabolites/86%/32%
Serum half-life (normal/ESRD): (40–55 hrs/~10 hrs on hemodialysis)/(10 hrs/ extended)/(17 hrs/no data)
Plasma protein binding: 99/< 4/< 0.7%
Volume of distribution (V_d): NR/NR/1.2 L/kg

—— = serious side effect ☐ = black box warning. ND = no data. NR = not recommended. s = spectrum inadequate (at site). a = activity or experience inadequate. p = tissue penetration inadequate. *based on peak serum concentration after usual adult dose. †applicable to adult uncomplicated lower UTIs (CrCl > 30 mL/min).

Primary Mode of Elimination: Hepatic/
Renal/Renal
Dosage Adjustments*

CrCl 50–80 mL/min	No change
CrCl 10–50 mL/min	Avoid
CrCl < 10 mL/min	Avoid
Post–HD dose	Avoid
Post–PD dose	Avoid
CVVH/CVVHD/ CVVHDF dose	Avoid
Mild hepatic insufficiency	No data
Moderate— severe hepatic insufficiency	No data

Antiretroviral Dosage Adjustments

Fosamprenavir/ ritonavir	An additional 100 mg/ day (300 mg total) of ritonavir is recommended when ATRIPLA is administered with fosamprenavir/ ritonavir q24h. No change in ritonaviir dose when ATRIPLA is administered with fosamprenavir/ritonavir q12h
Atazanavir	Atazanavir 300 mq q24h Ritonavir 100 mg q12h
Indinavir	Indinavir 1000 mg q8h
Lopinavir/ ritonavir	Increase lopinavir/ ritonavir to 600/150 mg (3 tablets) q12h

Ritonavir	No data
Saquinavir	Avoid
Didanosine	Avoid
Rifabutin	Rifabutin 450–600 mg q24h or 600 mg 2–3x/ week if not on protease inhibitor
Rifampin	No data

Drug Interactions: Antiretrovirals, rifabutin (see dose adjustment grid above); astemizole, cisapride, ergotamine, methylergonovine, midazolam, triazolam, St John's Wort ($\downarrow$ efavirenz levels), voriconazole ($\downarrow$ voriconazole levels; avoid); caspofungin ($\downarrow$ caspofungin levels); carbamazepine, phenytoin, phenobarbital (monitor anticonvulsant levels; use with caution; potential for $\downarrow$ efavirenz levels); statins (may $\downarrow$ statin levels); methadone, ($\downarrow$ methadone levels); clarithromycin (may $\downarrow$ clarithromycin effectiveness, consider using azithromycin). Should not be administered concurrently with astemizole, cisapride, midazolam, triazolam, or ergot derivatives. Significantly reduces voriconazole drug levels.

Adverse Effects:
Common
- Dizziness
- Insomnia/bad dreams
- Impaired concentration
- Confusion
- Agitation
- Hallucinations

——— = serious side effect ☐ = black box warning. ND = no data. NR = not recommended. s = spectrum inadequate (at site). a = activity or experience inadequate. p = tissue penetration inadequate. *based on peak serum concentration after usual adult dose. †applicable to adult uncomplicated lower UTIs (CrCl > 30 mL/min).

- Somnolence
- *Psychiatric symptoms* (depression, suicidal ideation, paranoid reactions)
- Hyperlipidemia

Uncommon

- Amnesia
- Euphoria
- Drug fever/rash
- Redistribution of body fat

Rare

- Stevens-Johnson Syndrome
- Pancreatitis
- Immune reconstitution syndrome (IRIS)

Allergic Potential: High
Safety in Pregnancy: D

Additional Clinical Considerations:
- Rash/CNS effects usually resolve in a few weeks.
- Take at bedtime on empty stomach.
- High fat meals can ↑ efavirenz by 50%.
- Use with caution in patients with history of seizures (↑ risk of convulsions).

Cerebrospinal Fluid Penetration: 1%

SELECTED REFERENCE:
Website: www.pdr.net

Elviteglavir/Cobicistat/ Emtricitabine/Tenofivir alafenamide (Genvoya)

Drug class: INSTI/CYP3A inhibitor/2 NRTIs.

Usual dose: 1 tablet q24h with food (contains 150 mg elvitegravir, 150 mg of cobicistat, 200 mg emtricitabine, 10 mg tenofovir alafenamide)

Pharmacokinetic Parameters:
Peak serum level: 2/1.5/2/0.16 mcg/mL
Bioavailability: unknown/unknown/92%/ unknown
Excreted unchanged: 7/8/70/1%
Serum half-life (normal): 13/3/10/0.5h
Plasma protein binding: 99/98/4/80%
Volume of distribution (V_d): ND

Primary Mode of Elimination: Hepatic/ Hepatic/Renal/Hepatic

Dosage Adjustments*

CrCl < 30 mL/min	Avoid
Post-HD dose	No data
Post-PD dose	No data
CVVH dose	No data
Mild to moderate hepatic insufficiency	No change
Severe hepatic insufficiency	Avoid

Drug Interactions: Contraindicated with drugs that strongly induce CYP3A. Do not use with other antiretrovirals, cobicistat inhibits CYP3A, CYP2D6 and P-gp. Do not administer with other NNRTI's. Antacid and H2 blockers should be separated. Any drug that induces or inhibits CYP3A has the potential to increase or decrease

---

rilpivirine levels and should only be used if benefit outweighs risk.

Adverse Effects:

Common

- Lactic acidosis, severe hepatomegaly
- Nausea
- Diarrhea
- Headache
- Fatigue

Uncommon

- Redistribution/accumulation body fat
- Immune reconstitution syndrome (IRIS)
- Renal insufficiency
- Bone loss and mineralization defects

Allergic Potential: Low

Safety in Pregnancy: B

Additional Clinical Considerations:

- Not indicated for treatment of acute hepatitis B.
- Test patients for hepatitis B prior to treatment, contraindicated with drugs highly dependent on CYP3A.
- Separate antacids from Genvoya by at least 2 hours.

SELECTED REFERENCE:
www.pdr.net

Elvitegravir + Cobicistat + Emtricitabine + Tenofovir disoproxil fumarate (Stribild) EVG/COBI/FTC/TDF

Drug class Antiretroviral agent: HIV Integrase strand transfer inhibitor. (elvitagravir 150 mg), pharmacokinetic enhancer (cobicistat 150 mg), and 2 nucleos(t)ide analog HIV-1 reverse transcriptase inhibitors (emtricitabine 200 mg and tenofovir disoproxil fumarate 300 mg)

Usual dose: 1 tablet q24h with food

Pharmacokinetic Parameters:

Peak serum level: 1.7/1.1/1.9/0.45 mcg/mL
Bioavailability: Increased with food
Excreted unchanged: minimal for elvitegravir and cobicistat, ↑ 100% for emtricitabine and tenofovir disoproxil fumarate
Serum half-life (normal/ESRD): 9/3/12/11 (not recommended in renal failure)
Plasma protein binding: 98/98/4/0.7%
Volume of distribution (V_d): ND

Primary Mode of Elimination: Hepatic (elvitegravir and cobicistat); Renal (emtricitabine and tenofovir disoproxil fumarate)

Dosage Adjustments*

CrCl < 50 mL/min	Avoid
Post-HD dose	Avoid
Post-PD dose	Avoid
CVVH dose	Avoid
Severe hepatic insufficiency	Avoid

Drug Interactions: Inhibitor of CYP3A, CYP2D6 and CYP2C9; and p-glycoprotein; metabolized by CYP3A and CYP2D6; antacids (may ↓ elvitegravir absorption).

Contraindications: Nephrotoxic drugs

——— = serious side effect ☐ = black box warning. ND = no data. NR = not recommended. s = spectrum inadequate (at site). a = activity or experience inadequate. p = tissue penetration inadequate. *based on peak serum concentration after usual adult dose. †applicable to adult uncomplicated lower UTIs (CrCl > 30 mL/min).

Adverse Effects:
Common
- Nausea
- Diarrhea
- Redistribution of body fat

Uncommon
- Renal insufficiency
- Decreased bone density

Rare
- Immune reconstitution syndrome (IRIS)
- Lactic acidosis and massive hepatomegaly with steatosis

Allergic Potential: Not available
Safety in Pregnancy: B

Additional Clinical Considerations:
- *Not approved for HIV patients co-infected with HBV*

SELECTED REFERENCES:
Desimmie BA, Schrijvers R, Debyser Z. Elvitegravir: a once daily alternative to raltegravir. Lancet Infect Dis 12:3–5, 2012. (PMID:220150178)
Sax PE, DeJesus E, Mills A, et al. Co-formulated elvitegravir, cobicistat, emtricitabine, and tenofovir versus co-formulated efavirenz, emtricitabine, and tenofovir for initial treatment of HIV-1 infection: a randomised, double-blind, phase 3 trial, analysis of results after 48 weeks. Lancet 379:2439–48, 2012. (PMID:22748591)
Website: www.pdr.net

Emtricitabine (Emtriva) FTC

Drug Class: HIV NRTI (nucleoside reverse transcriptase inhibitor).
Usual Dose: 200 mg (PO) q24h.
Pharmacokinetic Parameters:
Peak serum level: 1.8 mcg/mL
Bioavailability: 93%
Excreted unchanged (urine): 86%
Serum half-life (normal/ESRD): 10 hrs/ extended
Plasma protein binding: 4%
Primary Mode of Elimination: Renal
Dosage Adjustments*

CrCl ≥ 50 mL/min	200 mg (PO) q24h
CrCl 30–49 mL/min	200 mg (PO) q48h
CrCl 15–29 mL/min	200 mg (PO) q72h
CrCl < 15 mL/min	200 mg (PO) q96h
Post–HD dose	200 mg (PO)
Post–PD dose	200 mg (PO)
CVVH/CVVHD/ CVVHDF dose	200 mg (PO) q72h
Moderate— severe hepatic insufficiency	No change

Drug Interactions: No significant interactions with indinavir, stavudine, zidovudine, famciclovir, tenofovir.
Adverse Effects:
Common
- Dizziness
- Headache
- Nausea/diarrhea
- Drug fever/rash
- Abdominal pain

Uncommon
- Bad dreams
- Fatigue

—— = serious side effect ☐ = black box warning. ND = no data. NR = not recommended. s = spectrum inadequate (at site). a = activity or experience inadequate. p = tissue penetration inadequate. *based on peak serum concentration after usual adult dose. †applicable to adult uncomplicated lower UTIs (CrCl > 30 mL/min).

Rare

- Skin hyperpigmentation on palms and soles
- <u>Immune reconstitution syndrome (IRIS)</u>
- Lactic acidosis and hepatomegaly
- Post-treatment exacerbation of HBV hepatitis.

Allergic Potential: Low

Safety in Pregnancy: B

Additional Clinical Considerations:

- May be taken with or without food.
- Does not inhibit CYP450 enzymes.
- Mean intracellular half-live of 39 h.
- Potential cross-resistance to lamivudine and zalcitabine.
- Should not be coadministered with drugs containing lamivudine.

Cerebrospinal Fluid Penetration: No data

SELECTED REFERENCES:

Dando TM, Wagstaff AJ. Emtricitabine/tenofovir disoproxil fumarate. Drugs 64:2075–82, 2004. (PMID:15341498)

Saag MS. Emtricitabine, a new antiretroviral agent with activity against HIV and hepatitis B virus. Clin Infect Dis 42:128–31, 2006. (PMID:16323102)

Sax PE, Tierney C, Collier AC, et al. Abacavir/lamivudine versus tenofovir DF/emtricitabine as part of combination regimens for initial treatment of HIV: final results. J Infect Dis 204:1191–201, 2011. (PMID:21917892)

Website: www.pdr.net

Emtricitabine + Tenofovir disoproxil fumarate (Truvada) FTC/TDF

Drug Class: HIV NRTI (nucleoside reverse transcriptase inhibitor) + nucleotide analogue.

Usual Dose: One tablet (PO) q24h (each tablet contains 200 mg of emtricitabine + 300 mg of tenofovir).

Pharmacokinetic Parameters:

Peak serum level: 1.8/0.3 mcg/mL
Bioavailability: 93%/27% if fasting (39% with high fat meal)
Excreted unchanged (urine): 86/32%
Serum half-life (normal/ESRD): (10 hrs/ extended)/(17 hrs/ND)
Plasma protein binding: 4/0.7–7.2%
Volume of distribution (V_d): ND/ 1.3 L/kg

Primary Mode of Elimination: Renal

Dosage Adjustments*

CrCl ≥ 50 mL/min	No change
CrCl 30–49 mL/min	One capsule (PO) q48h
CrCl 15–29 mL/min	Avoid
CrCl < 15 mL/min	Avoid
Post–HD dose	Avoid
Post–PD dose	Avoid
CVVH/CVVHD/ CVVHDF dose	Avoid
Moderate— severe hepatic insufficiency	No change

— = serious side effect ☐ = black box warning. ND = no data. NR = not recommended. s = spectrum inadequate (at site). a = activity or experience inadequate. p = tissue penetration inadequate. *based on peak serum concentration after usual adult dose. †applicable to adult uncomplicated lower UTIs (CrCl > 30 mL/min).

Drug Interactions: No significant interactions with indinavir, stavudine, zidovudine, famciclovir, lamivudine, lopinavir/ritonavir, efavirenz, methadone, oral contraceptives. Tenofovir ↑ didanosine levels which may result in severe pancreatitis. Tenofovir reduces systemic exposure to atazanavir; whenever the two are co-administered, the recommended dose of atazanavir is 300 mg once daily with ritonavir 100 mg once daily. Atazanavir may increase tenofovir levels. Avoid coadministration with didanosine.

Adverse Effects:

Common

- Headache
- Nausea/vomiting/diarrhea
- GI upset
- Drug fever/rash

Rare

- Immune reconstitution syndrome (IRIS)
- Redistribution/accumulation of body fat
- ↓ bone density
- Renal insufficiency renal failures
- Lactic acidosis and hepatomegaly
- Post-treatment exacerbation of HBV

Allergic Potential: Low
Safety in Pregnancy: B

Additional Clinical Considerations:

- May be taken with or without food.
- Does not inhibit CYP450 enzymes.
- Mean intracellular half-life with emtricitabine is 39 hours.
- Potential cross-resistance to lamivudine, zalcitabine, abacavir, didanosine.

Cerebrospinal Fluid Penetration: No data

SELECTED REFERENCES:

Dando TM, Wagstaff AJ. Emtricitabine/tenofovir disoproxil fumarate. Drugs 64:2075–82, 2004. (PMID:15341497)

Thompson MA, Aberg JA, Cahn P, et al. Antiretroviral treatment of adult HIV infection: 2012 recommendations of the International Antiviral Society — USA panel. JAMA 308:387–402, 2012. (PMID:22820792)

Website: www.pdr.net

Emtricitabine/Rilpivirine/ Tenofovir (Complera) FTC/RPV/TDF

Drug Class: HIV 2 NRTI/1 NNRTI.

Usual Dose: 1 tablet (PO) q24h (contains 200 mg emtricitabine, 25 mg rilpivirine, 300 mg tenofovir).

Pharmacokinetic Parameters:

Peak serum level: 1.8/1/0.3 mcg/mL
Bioavailability: 93/ND/25%
Excreted unchanged: 86/1/75%
Serum half-life (normal): 10/50/17 hrs
Plasma protein binding: unknown/99/1%
Volume of distribution (V_d): ND

Primary Mode of Elimination: Renal/ Hepatic/Renal

Dosage Adjustments*

CrCl < 50 mL/min	Avoid
Post-HD dose	Avoid
Post-PD dose	Avoid

—— = serious side effect ☐ = black box warning. ND = no data. NR = not recommended. s = spectrum inadequate (at site). a = activity or experience inadequate. p = tissue penetration inadequate. *based on peak serum concentration after usual adult dose. †applicable to adult uncomplicated lower UTIs (CrCl > 30 mL/min).

CVVH/CVVHD/CVVHDF dose	Avoid
Mild—moderate hepatic insufficiency	No change
Severe hepatic insufficiency	No data

Drug Interactions: Do not administer with other NNRTIs. Antacid and H2 blockers should be separated. Any drug that induces or inhibits CYP3A has the potential to increase or decrease rilpivirine levels and should only be used if benefit outweighs risk, clarithromycin (↓ clarithromycin levels).

Contraindications: carbamazepine, oxycarbazepine, phenobarbital, phenytoin, rifabutin, rifampin, rifapentine, proton pump inhibitors, dexamethasone (except single dose), **St. John's Wort.**

Adverse Effects:

Common
- Nausea/vomiting/diarrhea
- Fatigue
- Dizziness
- Drug fever/rash

Uncommon
- Headache
- Depression
- Insomnia
- Bad dreams

Rare
- <u>Immune reconstitution syndrome (IRIS)</u>
- <u>Redistribution/accumulation of body fat</u>
- Lactic acidosis and severe hepatomegaly with steatosis

- Post-treatment exacerbation of HBV hepatitis

Allergic Potential: Low
Safety in Pregnancy: B

Additional Clinical Considerations:
- Monitor BMD in patients at risk for pathological fractures.
- *Not approved for HIV patients co-infected with HBV.*

Cerebrospinal Fluid Penetration: *ND*

SELECTED REFERENCE:
Website: www.pdr.net

Entecavir (Baraclude)

Drug Class: Antiviral (HBV).
Usual Dose: 0.5 mg (PO) q24h; 1 mg (PO) q24h for lamivudine-refractory patients or with decompensated liver disease. (*take without food*)

Pharmacokinetic Parameters:
Peak serum level: 4.2 ng/mL (for 0.5 mg dose)
Bioavailability: Similar for tablet and oral solution
Excreted unchanged (urine): 62–73%
Serum half-life (normal/ESRD): 128–139 hrs
Plasma protein binding: No information
Volume of distribution (V_d): ND

Primary Mode of Elimination: Renal
Dosage Adjustments* (based on 0.5 mg dose)

CrCl > 50 mL/min	No change
CrCl 30–50 mL/min	0.25 mg (PO) q24h

───── = serious side effect ☐ = black box warning. ND = no data. NR = not recommended. s = spectrum inadequate (at site). a = activity or experience inadequate. p = tissue penetration inadequate. *based on peak serum concentration after usual adult dose. †applicable to adult uncomplicated lower UTIs (CrCl > 30 mL/min).

CrCl 10–30 mL/min	0.15 mg (PO) q24h
CrCl < 10 mL/min	0.05 mg (PO) q24h
Post-HD	0.05 mg (PO or 0.5 mg (PO) q week)
Post–PD	0.05 mg (PO)
Moderate—severe hepatic insufficiency	No change

Drug Interactions: Cyclosporin, tacrolimus (may ↑ entecavir levels).
Adverse Effects:
Common
• Drug fever
• ↑ AST/ALT
• ↑ Creatinine
Uncommon
• Fatigue
• Headache
• Nausea
• Cough
• Upper abdominal pain
• Upper respiratory tract infection
Rare
• Severe acute exacerbations of HBV hepatitis
• Resistance to HIV nucleoside reverse transcriptase inhibitors
• Lactic acidosis and severe hepato-megaly with steatosis

Allergic Potential: No information
Safety in Pregnancy: C

Additional Clinical Considerations:
• Effective in lamivudine resistant patients.
• Available as tablets and oral solution.

SELECTED REFERENCES:
Honkoop P, De Man RA. Entecavir: a potent new antiviral drug for hepatitis B. Expert Opin Investig Drugs 12:683–8, 2003. (PMID:12665423)

Keating GM. Entecavir: a review of its use in the treatment of chronic hepatitis B in patients with decompensated liver disease. Drugs 24:2511–29, 2011. (PMID:22141390)

Petersen J, Ratziu V, Buti M, et al. Entecavir plus tenofovir combination as recurrent therapy in pre-treated chronic hepatitis B patients: an international multicenter cohort study. J Hepatol 56:520–6, 2012. (PMID:22037226)

Pol S, Lampertico, P. First-line treatment of chronic hepatitis B with entecavir or tenofovir in 'Real-life' setting; from clinical trials to clinical practice. J Viral Hepat 19:377–86, 2012. (PMID:22571899)

Rivkin A. A review of entecavir in the treatment of chronic hepatitis B infection. Curr Med Res Opin 21:1845–56, 2005. (PMID:16307706)

Scotto G, D'Addiego G, Giammario A, et al. Tenofovir plus entecavir as rescue therapy for multidrug-resistant chronic hepatitis B. Liver Int 32:171–2, 2012. (PMID:22098064)

Tsai Mc, Lee CM, Chiu KW, et al. A comparison of telbivudine and entecavir for chronic hepatitis B in real-world clinical practice. J Antimicrob Chemother 67:696–9, 2012. (PMID:22174039)

Website: www.pdr.net

Ertapenem (Invanz)

Drug Class: Carbapenem.
Usual Dose: 1 gm (IV/IM) q24h.

Spectrum Synopsis*
Hits
Gram + : All non-enterococcal streptococci, MSSA
Gram – : Most aerobic GNB, B. fragilis
Problem pathogens: Acinetobacter, ESBL + Klebsiella, Enterobacter, E. coli
Misses
Gram + : MRSA, VSE, VRE
Gram – : P. aeruginosa
Problem pathogens: Listeria Nocardia, S. maltophilia, B. cepacia, CRE

———— = serious side effect [   ] = black box warning. ND = no data. NR = not recommended. s = spectrum inadequate (at site). a = activity or experience inadequate. p = tissue penetration inadequate. *based on peak serum concentration after usual adult dose. †applicable to adult uncomplicated lower UTIs (CrCl > 30 mL/min).

Urine Spectrum
- Same as serum spectrum
- Optimal urinary pH = 5–6
- Urine levels = 1000 mcg/mL

(Full *Susceptibility Profiles* p. 208).

Resistance Potential: Low
Pharmacokinetic Parameters:
Peak serum level: 150 mcg/mL
Bioavailability: 90% (IM)
*Excreted unchanged (urine): 40%; 40%
excreted as active metabolite*
Serum half-life (normal/ESRD): 4/14 hrs
Plasma protein binding: 95%
Volume of distribution (V_d): 0.12 L/kg
Primary Mode of Elimination: Renal
Dosage Adjustments*

CrCl 30–80 mL/min	No change
CrCl < 30 mL/min	500 mg (IV) q24h
Post–HD dose	If dosed < 6 h prior to HD, give 150 mg (IV)
Post–PD dose	No information
CVVH/CVVHD/ CVVHDF dose	500 mg (IV) q24h
Moderate – Severe hepatic insufficiency	No change

* If dosed > 6 h prior to HD, no Post–HD needed.

Drug Interactions: Not a substrate/inhibitor of cytochrome P 450 enzymes; probenecid (↓ clearance of ertapenem). Valproic acid (↓ seizure threshold).
Adverse Effects:
Common
- Nausea/vomiting/diarrhea
Uncommon
- Headache

- ↑ AST/ALT
- Injection site reactions
Rare
- C. difficile diarrhea/colitis
Allergic Potential: Low
Safety in Pregnancy: B

Additional Clinical Considerations:
- May be given by IV push
- Compared to imipenem or meropenem, **ertapenem has little activity against VSE, Acinetobacter, or P. aeruginosa.**
- **Safe to use in penicillin allergic patients.**

*May inhibit antibiotic induced LPS
(endotoxin) release from GNB potentially minimizing endotoxin mediated
tissue damage.*

Additional Pharmacokinetic Considerations*

Non-CSF	% of Serum Levels
Peritoneal fluid	ND
Bile	10%
Synovial fluid	ND
Bone	ND
Prostate	NR(p)
Urine	600%
CSF	
Non-inflamed meninges	1%
Inflamed meninges (ABM)	5–20%

(also see *Antibiotic Pearls & Pitfalls* p. 529).

SELECTED REFERENCES:
Beovic B, Kreft S, Seme K, et al. Does ertapenem
    alter the susceptibility of Pseudomonas
    aeruginosa to carbapenems? J Chemother
    23:216–220, 2011. (PMID:21803699)

——— = serious side effect ☐ = black box warning. ND = no data. NR = not recommended. s = spectrum inadequate (at site). a = activity or experience inadequate. p = tissue penetration inadequate. *based on peak serum concentration after usual adult dose. †applicable to adult uncomplicated lower UTIs (CrCl > 30 mL/min).

Boselli E, Breilh D, Djabarouti S, et al. Diffusion of
ertapenem into bone and synovial tissues.
J Antimicrob Chemother 60:893–896, 2007.
(PMID:17704514)

Collins VL, Marchaim D, Pogue JM, et al. Efficacy
of ertapenem for treatment of bloodstream
infections caused by extended-spectrum-B-
lactamase-producing Enterobacteriaceae.
Antimicrob Agents Chemother 56:2173–7, 2012.
(PMID:22290982)

Congeni BL. Ertapenem. Expert Opin Pharmacother
11:669–672, 2010. (PMID:20163277)

Cunha BA, Guiga J, Gerson S. Predictors of ertapenem
therapeutic efficacy in the treatment of urinary
tract infections (UTIs) in hospitalized adults: the
importance of renal insufficiency and urinary pH.
Eur J Clin Microbiol Infect Dis 35:673-679, 2016.
(PMID:26873378)

Cunha BA. No need for an initial test dose of
meropenem or ertapenem in patients reporting
anaphylactic reactions to penicillins. J Chemo
27:317-318, 2015. (PMID:25566799)

Cunha BA, Jose A, Hage J. Ertapenem: Lack of allergic
reactions in hospitalized adults reporting a history
of penicillin allergy. Int J Antimicrob Agents
42:585–586, 2013. (PMID:24139887)

Cunha BA, Lenopoli S, Hage JE. Klebsiella
pneumoniae septic wrist arthritis successfully
treated with ertapenem and levofloxacin. J
Chemother 23:376–7, 2011. (PMID:22233826)

Cunha BA, Ertapenem. A review of its microbiologic,
pharmacokinetic and clinical aspects. Drugs Today
(Barc). 38:195–213, 2002. (PMID:12532175)

Fong JJ, Rose L, Radigan EA. Clinical outcomes
with ertapenem as a first-line treatment option
of infections caused by extended-spectrum
b-lactamase producing gram-negative
bacteria. Ann Pharmacother 46:347–52, 2012.
(PMID:22395259)

Graham DR, Lucasti C, Malafaia O, et al. Ertapenem
once daily versus piperacillin-tazobactam 4
times per day for treatment of complicated skin
and skin-structure infections in adults: results
of a prospective, randomized, double-blind
multicenter study. Clin Infect Dis 34:1460–8, 2002.
(PMID:12015692)

Itani KMF, Wilson SE, Awad SS, et al. Ertapenem
versus cefotetan prophylaxis in elective
colorectal surgery. N Engl J Med 355:2640–51,
2006. (PMID:18182989)

Liao FF, Huang YB, Chen CY. Decrease in serum
valproic acid levels during treatment with

ertapenem. Am J Health Syst Pharm 67:1260–
1264, 2010. (PMID:20651316)

Lauf L, Ozsvar Z, Mitha I, et al. Phase 3 study
comparing tigecycline and ertapenem in patients
with diabetic foot injections with and without
osteomyelitis. Diagn Microbiol Infect Dis. 78:469-
480, 2014. (PMID:24439136)

Verdier MC, Seguin P, Le Touvet B, et al. Ertapenem
in plasma and peritoneal fluid from patients
with severe intra-abdominal infections. J
Antimicrob Chemother 66:1934–1936, 2011.
(PMID:21632578)

Wall GC, Nayima VA, Neumeister KM. Assessment
of hypersensitivity reactions in patients receiving
carbapenem antibiotics who report antibiotics a
history of penicillin. J Chemo. 26:150-153, 2014.
(PMID:24090971)

Wiskirchen DE, Housman ST, Quintiliani R,
et al. Comparative pharmacokinetics,
pharmacodynamics and tolerability of ertapenem
1 gram/day administered as a rapid 5 minute
infusion versus the standard 30 minute infusion
in healthy adult volunteers. Pharmacotherapy
33:266-74, 2013. (PMID: 23400916)

Website: www.pdr.net

Erythromycin (various)

Drug Class: Macrolide.
Usual Dose: 1 gm (IV) q6h; 500 mg (PO) q6h (*take without food*).

Spectrum Synopsis*
Hits
Gram + : VSE, some GAS, some MSSA
Gram – : Oral anaerobes
Problem pathogens: Bordetella
Misses
Gram + : Most GAS, most S. pneumoniae, most MSSA, MRSA, VRE
Gram – : Most aerobic GNB, most H. influenzae, B. fragilis
Problem pathogens: Nocardia,

------ = serious side effect ☐ = black box warning. ND = no data. NR = not recommended. s = spectrum inadequate (at site). a = activity or experience inadequate. p = tissue penetration inadequate. *based on peak serum concentration after usual adult dose. †applicable to adult uncomplicated lower UTIs (CrCl > 30 mL/min).

Urine Spectrum[†]

- VSE
- Many GNB uropathogens with urinary alkaline pH
- Optimal urinary pH = 6–7
- Urine levels = 30 mcg/mL

(Full *Susceptibility Profiles* p. 196).

Resistance Potential: High
(S. pneumoniae, GAS, MSSA)

Pharmacokinetic Parameters:
Peak serum level: 12 (IV);1.2 (PO) mcg/mL
Bioavailability: 50%
Excreted unchanged (urine): 5%; 5%
exerted as active metabolite
Serum half-life (normal/ESRD): 1.4/5.4 hrs
Plasma protein binding: 80%
Volume of distribution (V_d): 0.5 L/kg

Primary Mode of Elimination: Hepatic
Dosage Adjustments*

CrCl < 10 mL/min	No change
Post–HD/PD dose	None
CVVH/CVVHD/CVVHDF dose	No change
Moderate—severe hepatic insufficiency	No change

Drug Interactions: Amiodarone, procainamide, sotalol, astemizole, terfenadine, cisapride, pimozide (↑ QTc); carbamazepine (↑ carbamazepine levels, nystagmus, nausea, vomiting, diarrhea; avoid combination); cimetidine, digoxin, ergot alkaloids, felodipine, midazolam, triazolam, phenytoin, ritonavir, tacrolimus, valproic acid (↑ interacting drug levels); clozapine (↑ clozapine levels; CNS toxicity); corticosteroids (↑ corticosteroid effect); cyclosporine (↑ cyclosporine levels with toxicity); efavirenz (↓ erythromycin levels); rifabutin, rifampin (↓ erythromycin levels, ↑ interacting drug levels); statins (↑ risk of rhabdomyolysis); theophylline (↑ theophylline levels, nausea, vomiting, seizures, apnea); warfarin (↑ INR); zidovudine (↓ zidovudine levels).

Adverse Effects:

Common

- Nausea/vomiting
- Abdominal pain
- Non-C. difficile diarrhea

Uncommon

- Injection site phlebitis

Rare

- ↑ QTc
- Torsade de pointes

Allergic Potential: Low
Safety in Pregnancy: B

Additional Clinical Considerations:

- GAS and MSSA resistance
- ↑ **prevalence of S. pneumoniae resistance.**

Additional Pharmacokinetic Considerations:	
Non-CSF	**% of Serum Levels**
Peritoneal fluid	NR(s)
Bile	400%
Synovial fluid	NR(p)
Bone	NR(s)
Prostate	100%
Urine[†]	15%

—— = serious side effect ☐ = black box warning. ND = no data. NR = not recommended. s = spectrum inadequate (at site). a = activity or experience inadequate. p = tissue penetration inadequate.
*based on peak serum concentration after usual adult dose. †applicable to adult uncomplicated lower UTIs (CrCl > 30 mL/min).

CSF

Non-inflamed meninges	<1%
Inflamed meninges (ABM)	<10%

(also see ***Antibiotic Pearls & Pitfalls***
p. 536).

SELECTED REFERENCES:

Amsden GW. Erythromycin, clarithromycin, and azithromycin: Are the differences real? Clinical Therapeutics 18:572, 1996. (PMID:8851453)

Bergman M, Huikko S, Huovinen P, et al. Macrolide and azithromycin use are linked to increased macrolide resistance in Streptococcus pneumoniae. Antimicrob Agents Chemother 50:3646–3650, 2006. (PMID:16940064)

Daneman N, McGeer A, Green K, et al. Macrolide resistance in bacteremic pneumococcal disease.: Implications for patient management. Clin Infect Dis 43:432–438, 2006. (PMID:16838231)

Jain R, Danzinger LH. The macrolide antibiotics: a pharmacokinetic and pharmacodynamic overview. Curr Pharm Des 10:3045–53, 2004. (PMID:15544496)

Jenkins SG, Farrell DJ. Increase in pneumococcus macrolide resistance, United States. Emerging Infect Dis 15:1260–1264, 2009. (PMID:19751588)

Suzuki S, Yamazaki T, Narita M. Clinical evaluation of macrolide-resistant Mycoplasma pneumoniae. Antimicrobial Agents and Chemotherapy 50:709–12, 2006. (PMID:16436730)

Website: www.pdr.net

Ethambutol (Myambutol) EMB

Drug Class: TB drug.
Usual Dose: 15 mg/kg (PO) q24h (see comments).
Pharmacokinetic Parameters:
Peak serum level: 2–5 mcg/mL
Bioavailability: 80%
Excreted unchanged (urine): 50%
Serum half-life (normal/ESRD): 4/10 hrs
Plasma protein binding: 20%
Volume of distribution (V_d): 2 L/kg
Primary Mode of Elimination: Renal/ Hepatic
Dosage Adjustments*

CrCl < 30 mL/min	15 mg/kg (PO) 3×/ week
CrCl 15–30 mL/min	15 mg/kg (PO) q36h
Post-HD/PD dose	None
CVVH/CVVHD/ CVVHDF dose	15 mg/kg (PO) q36h
Moderate— severe hepatic insufficiency	No change

Drug Interactions: Aluminum salts, didanosine buffer (↓ ethambutol and interacting drug absorption).
Adverse Effects:
Common
- Nausea/vomiting
- ↑ Uric acid

Uncommon
- Metallic taste
- Leukopenia
- Thrombocytopenia
- Drug fever/rash
- Peripheral neuropathy
- ↓ Visual acuity
- Color blindness (red-green)
- Optic neuritis

Allergic Potential: Low
Safety in Pregnancy: C

—— = serious side effect ☐ = black box warning. ND = no data. NR = not recommended. s = spectrum inadequate (at site). a = activity or experience inadequate. p = tissue penetration inadequate. *based on peak serum concentration after usual adult dose. †applicable to adult uncomplicated lower UTIs (CrCl > 30 mL/min).

Additional Clinical Considerations:
- Optic neuritis may occur with high doses (≥ 15 mg/kg/day).
- **TB D.O.T. dose:** 4 gm (PO) 2 × /week or 3 gm (PO) 3 × /week.
- **MAI dose:** 15 mg/kg (PO) q24 (with azithromycin 500 mg [PO] q24).

Cerebrospinal Fluid Penetration:
Non-Inflamed meninges: 1%
Inflamed meninges: 40%

Meningeal dose = 25 mg/kg (PO) q24h.

SELECTED REFERENCES:

McIllerson H, Wash P, Burger A, et al. Determinants of rifampin, isoniazid, pyrazinamide and ethambutol pharmacokinetics in a cohort of tuberculosis patients. Antimicrob Agents Chemother 50:1170–77, 2006. (PMID:16569826)

Van Scoy RE, Wilkowske CJ. Antituberculous agents. Mayo Clin Proc 67:179–87, 1992. (PMID:1347579)

Website: www.pdr.net

Ethionamide (Trecator)

Drug Class: TB drug.
Usual Dose: 500 mg (PO) q12h.
Pharmacokinetic Parameters:
Peak serum level: 5 mcg/mL
Bioavailability: 99%
Excreted unchanged (urine): 1%
Serum half-life (normal/ESRD): 2/9 hrs
Plasma protein binding: 30%
Volume of distribution (V_d): No data

Primary Mode of Elimination: Renal/Hepatic
Dosage Adjustments*

CrCl < 40 mL/min	No change
Post-HD/PD dose	No information
CVVH/CVVHD/CVVHDF dose	No information
Moderate hepatic insufficiency	No change
Severe hepatic insufficiency	500 mg (PO) q24h

Drug Interactions: Cycloserine (↑ neurologic toxicity); ethambutol (↑ GI distress, neuritis, hepatotoxicity); INH (peripheral neuritis, hepatotoxicity); pyrazinamide, rifampin (hepatotoxicity).

Adverse Effects:
Common
- Headache
- Metallic taste
- Nausea/vomiting/diarrhea

Uncommon
- Tremor
- Olfactory disturbances
- Psychotic disturbances
- Central/peripheral neuropathy
- Alopecia
- Impotence
- Gynecomastia
- Hypoglycemia
- ↑ AST/ALT

Rare
- Optic neuritis

Allergic Potential: Low
Safety in Pregnancy: C

─────── = serious side effect ☐ = black box warning. ND = no data. NR = not recommended. s = spectrum inadequate (at site). a = activity or experience inadequate. p = tissue penetration inadequate. *based on peak serum concentration after usual adult dose. †applicable to adult uncomplicated lower UTIs (CrCl > 30 mL/min).

Additional Clinical Considerations:
- Additive toxicity with thiacetazone

Cerebrospinal Fluid Penetration: 100%

Meningeal dose = usual dose.

SELECTED REFERENCE:
Website: www.pdr.net

Eravacycline (Xerava)

Drug Class: Fluorocycline tetracycline.
Usual Dose: 1 mg/kg (IV) q12h

Spectrum Synopsis*
Hits
  Gram + : VSE, VRE, MSSA, MRSA,
    S. pneumoniae
  Gram – : S. maltophilia, B. fragilis
  Problem pathogens: Atypical CAP
    pathogens, Acinetobacter,
    M. abscessus, CRE
Misses
  Gram + : None
  Gram – : P. aeruginosa
  Problem pathogens: B. capacia

(See **Susceptibility Profiles** p. 196).

Resistance Potential: Low
Pharmacokinetic Parameters:
Peak serum level: 2.12 mcg/mL
Bioavailability: Not applicable
Excreted unchanged: 34%
Serum half-life (normal): 20 hrs
Plasma protein binding: 79–90%
Volume of distribution (V_d): 5 L/kg
Primary Mode of Elimination: Hepatic
Dosage Adjustments*

CrCl < 5 mL/min	No change
Post-HD/Post-PD dose	No change
CVVH dose	No change
Mild-to-moderate hepatic insufficiency	No change
Severe hepatic insufficiency	1 mg/kg (IV) q12h, then 1 mg/kg (IV) q24h

Drug Interactions: Increase dose when used with strong CYP3A inducers.
Adverse Effects:
Common
- Nausea/Vomiting
- Non-C. difficile diarrhea

Uncommon
- <u>C. difficile diarrhea/colitis</u>
- Hypotension
- <u>Wound dehiscence</u>
- ↑ AST/ALT
- ↓ Prothrombin

Rare
- Drug fever/rash

Additional Clinical Considerations:
- Compatible with 0.9% NaCl
- Administer over 60 minutes.

Additional Pharmacokinetic Considerations:*	
Non-CSF	**% of Serum Levels**
Peritoneal fluid	ND
Bile	>500%
Synovial fluid	ND
Bone	ND
Prostate	ND
Urine†	60%

―――― = serious side effect ☐ = black box warning. ND = no data. NR = not recommended. s = spectrum inadequate (at site). a = activity or experience inadequate. p = tissue penetration inadequate. *based on peak serum concentration after usual adult dose. †applicable to adult uncomplicated lower UTIs (CrCl > 30 mL/min).

CSF	
Non-inflamed meninges	1%
Inflamed meninges (ABM)	10%

(also see **Antibiotic Pearls & Pitfalls** p. 530).

SELECTED REFERENCES:

Livermore DM, et al. In vitro activity of eravacycline against carbapenem-resistant. Enterobacteriaceae and Acinetobacter baumanii. Antimicrob Agents Chemother 60:3840-44, 2016. (PMID: 27044556)

Newman JV, et al. Randomized, double-blind, placebo-controlled studies of the safety and pharmacokinetics of single and multiple ascending doses of eravacycline, Antimicrob agents chemother 62: 2018. (PMID: 30150464)

Solomkin J, et al. Assessing the efficacy and eafety of eravacycline vs ertapenem in complicated intra-abdominal infections in the investigating Gram-Negative infections treated with eravacycline (IGNITE 1) Trial. JAMA 152:224-232, 2017. (PMID: 27851857)

Sutcliffe JA, et al. Antibacterial activity of eravacycline (TP-434), a novel fluorocycline against hospital and community pathogens. Antimicrob agents chemother 57:5548-58, 2013. (PMID: 23979750)

Thakare R, et al. Eravacycline for the treatment of patients with bacterial infections. Drugs today 54:245-54, 2018. (PMID: 29869646)
Xerava Prescribing information.

Zhanel GG, Lawrence CK, Adam H, et al. Review of eravacycline, a novel fluorocycline antibacterial agent. Drugs 76:567-88, 2016. (PMID: 26863149)
Website: www.pdr.net.

Famciclovir (Famvir)

Drug Class: Antiviral (HSV, VZV, HHV-6)
Usual Dose:
HSV-1/2: <u>Herpes labialis:</u> 500 mg (PO) q12h × 7 days.
<u>Genital herpes:</u> *Initial therapy*: 1 g (PO) q12h × 1 day. *Recurrent/intermittent*

therapy (< 6 episodes/year): normal host: 125 mg (PO) q12h × 5 days; HIV-positive: 500 mg (PO) q12h × 7 days. *Chronic suppressive therapy* (> 6 episodes/year): 250 mg (PO) q12h × 1 year.
<u>Meningitis/encephalitis:</u> 500 mg (PO) q8h × 10 days.
VZV: <u>Chickenpox:</u> 500 mg (PO) q8h × 5 days.

<u>Herpes zoster</u> (shingles) (dermatomal/disseminated): 500 mg (PO) q8h × 7–10 days.
<u>VZV Pneumonia:</u> 500 mg (PO) q8h ×7–10 days.
Pharmacokinetic Parameters:
Peak serum level: 3.3 mcg/mL
Bioavailability: 77%
Excreted unchanged (urine): 60%
Serum half-life (normal/ESRD): 2.5/13 hrs
Plasma protein binding: 20%
Volume of distribution (V_d): 1.1 L/kg
Primary Mode of Elimination: Renal
Dosage Adjustments for HSV/VZV* (based on 250 mg [PO] q8h/500 mg [PO] q8h)

CrCl 40–60 mL/min	No change/500 mg (PO) q12h
CrCl 20–40 mL/min	125 mg (PO) q24h/ 500 mg (PO) q24h
CrCl < 20 mL/min	125 mg (PO) q24h/ 250 mg (PO) q24h
Post–HD dose	125 mg (PO)/ 250 mg (PO)
Post–PD dose	None
CVVH/CVVHD/ CVVHDF dose	125 mg (PO) q24h/ 500 mg (PO) q24h

------ = serious side effect [_____] = black box warning. ND = no data. NR = not recommended. s = spectrum inadequate (at site). a = activity or experience inadequate. p = tissue penetration inadequate. *based on peak serum concentration after usual adult dose. †applicable to adult uncomplicated lower UTIs (CrCl > 30 mL/min).

| Moderate hepatic insufficiency | No change |
| Severe hepatic insufficiency | Use with caution |

Drug Interactions: Digoxin ($\uparrow$ digoxin levels).

Adverse Effects:

Common
- Headache
- Nausea/vomiting/diarrhea

Uncommon
- Dysmenorrhea
- Neutropenia
- $\uparrow$ AST/ALT

Rare
- Renal insufficiency (dose related)
- Seizures/tremors (dose related)

Allergic Potential: Low
Safety in Pregnancy: B

Additional Clinical Considerations:
- 99% converted to penciclovir in liver/GI tract.

Highly active against HSV, VZV, and HHV-6.
Some activity against CMV.
No activity against EBV, RSV, or adenoviruses.
Cerebrospinal Fluid Penetration: 50%
Meningeal dose = VZV dose.

SELECTED REFERENCES:

Luber AD, Flaherty JF Jr. Famciclovir for treatment of herpesvirus infections. Ann Pharmacother 30:978–85, 1996. (PMID:8876860)

Website: www.pdr.net

Fluconazole (Diflucan)

Drug Class: Azole antifungal.
Usual Dose: *Loading Dose* **(LD)** = **twice the maintenance dose × 1 dose,** then *Maintenance Dose* **(MD)** q24h

Candidemia:
    LD = 800 mg (IV/PO) × 1 then
    MD = 400 mg (IV/PO) q24h

Mucocutaneous candidiasis:
    LD = 400 mg (IV/PO) × 1 then
    MD = 200 mg (IV/PO) q24h

Candida esophagitis:
    LD = 200 mg (IV/PO) × 1 then
    MD = 100 mg (IV/PO) q24h

Candiduria:
    LD = 200 mg (IV/PO) × 1 then
    MD = 100 mg (IV/PO) q24h

Pharmacokinetic Parameters:
Peak serum level: 6.7 mcg/mL
Bioavailability: 90%
Excreted unchanged (urine): 80%; 11% excreted as active metabolite
Serum half-life (normal/ESRD): 27/100 hrs
Plasma protein binding: 12%
Volume of distribution (V_d): 0.7 L/kg

Primary Mode of Elimination: Renal
Dosage Adjustments*

CrCl < 50 mL/min	100 mg (IV/PO) q24h
Post–HD dose	200 mg (IV/PO)
Post–PD dose	200 mg (IV/PO)
CVVH/CVVHD/ CVVHDF dose	200–400 mg (IV/PO) q24h

= serious side effect ☐ = black box warning. ND = no data. NR = not recommended. s = spectrum inadequate (at site). a = activity or experience inadequate. p = tissue penetration inadequate. *based on peak serum concentration after usual adult dose. †applicable to adult uncomplicated lower UTIs (CrCl > 30 mL/min).

| Moderate hepatic insufficiency | No change |
| Severe hepatic insufficiency | No change |

Drug Interactions: Astemizole, cisapride, terfenadine, amiodarone (may ↑ QT interval, torsades de pointes); cyclosporine, oral hypoglycemics, tacrolimus, theophylline, zidovudine (↑ interacting drug levels with possible toxicity); hydrochlorothiazide (↑ fluconazole levels); phenytoin, rifabutin, rifampin (↓ fluconazole levels, ↑ interacting drug levels); warfarin (↑ INR).

Adverse Effects:

Uncommon

- Nausea/vomiting/diarrhea
- Abdominal pain

Rare

- Hypokalemia
- Angioedema
- Anaphylactic reactions
- ↑ QTc
- Torsade de pointes

Allergic Potential: Low

Safety in Pregnancy: D

Additional Clinical Considerations:

- Not effective against most non-albicans Candida.

Highly active against C. albicans, C. tropicalis, C. parasilosis, and C. lusitaniae.

Moderately active against Cryptococcus, Histoplasmosis, Blastomycosis, Sporotrichosis, Penicillum marneffei, Paracoccidiomycosis and Coccidiomycosis.

Some (dose dependent) activity against C. glabrata.

No activity against C. krusei, C. guilliermondii, C. rugosa, Mucor, Fusarium, Pseudallescheria Scedosporium, Trichosporon, Malassezia, Hansenula, Geotrichum, Rhodotorula, or Aspergillus.

Cerebrospinal Fluid Penetration:
Non-Inflamed meninges: 50–90%
Inflamed meninges: 50–90%

Meningeal dose = 400 mg (IV/PO) q24h.

SELECTED REFERENCES:

Cha R, Sobel JD. Fluconazole for the treatment of candidiasis: 15 years experience. Expert Rev Anti Infect Ther 2:357–66, 2004. (PMID:15482201)

Kowalsky SF, Dixon DM. Fluconazole: A new antifungal agent. Clin Pharmacol 10:179–94, 1991. (PMID:2040125)

Nussbaum JC, Jackson A, Namarika D, et al. Combination flucytosine and high-dose fluconazole compared with fluconazole monotherapy for the treatment of Cryptococcal meningitis: a randomized trial in Malawi. Clin Infect Dis 50:338–344, 2010. (PMID:20038244)

Smego RA jr, Ahmad H. The role of fluconazole in the treatment of Candida endocarditis: a meta-analysis. Medicine 90:237–249, 2011. (PMID:21694646)

Sousa AQ, Frutuoo MS, Moraes EA, et al. High-dose oral fluconazole therapy effective for cutaneous leishmaniasis due to Leishmania (Vianna) braziliensis. Clin Infect Dis 53:693–695, 2011. (PMID:21890773)

Terrell CL. Antifungal agents: Part II The azoles. Mayo Clin Proc 74:78–100, 1999. (PMID:9987539)

Zhai B, Zhou H, Yang L, et al. Polymyxin B, in combination with fluconazole, exerts a potent fungicidal effect. J Antimicrob Chemother 65:931–938, 2010. (PMID:20167587)

Website: www.pdr.net

—— = serious side effect [___] = black box warning. ND = no data. NR = not recommended. s = spectrum inadequate (at site). a = activity or experience inadequate. p = tissue penetration inadequate. *based on peak serum concentration after usual adult dose. †applicable to adult uncomplicated lower UTIs (CrCl > 30 mL/min).

Flucytosine (Ancobon) 5-FC

Drug Class: Antifungal.
Usual Dose: 25 mg/kg (PO) q6h.
Pharmacokinetic Parameters:
Peak serum level: 3.5 mcg/mL
Bioavailability: 80%
Excreted unchanged (urine): 90%
Serum half-life (normal/ESRD): 4/85 hrs
Plasma protein binding: 4%
Volume of distribution (V_d): 0.6 L/kg

Primary Mode of Elimination: Renal
Dosage Adjustments*

CrCl 20–40 mL/min	37.5 mg/kg (PO) q12h
CrCl 10–20 mL/min	37.5 mg/kg (PO) q18h
CrCl < 10 mL/min	37.5 mg/kg (PO) q24h
Post–HD dose	37.5 mg/kg (PO)
Post–PD dose	1 gm (PO)
CVVH/CVVHD/ CVVHDF dose	37.5 mg/kg (PO) q18h
Moderate—severe insufficiency	No change

Drug Interactions: Cytarabine
(↓ flucytosine effect); zidovudine
(neutropenia).
Adverse Effects:
Common
• Concusion

• Headache
• Hallucinations
• Nausea/vomiting/diarrhea
• Abdominal pain
Uncommon
• Drug fever/rash
• Leukopenia
• Anemia
• Thrombocytopenia
• ↑ AST/ALT
Rare
• Caution in renal unsufficiency
Allergic Potential: High
Safety in Pregnancy: C

Additional Clinical Considerations:
• **Always use in combination with amphotericin B** for cryptococcal meningitis.
Highly active against Cryptococcus neoformans.
Some activity against C. albicans.
No activity against other yeasts/fungi.
Cerebrospinal Fluid Penetration:
Non-Inflamed meninges: 100%
Inflamed meninges: 100%
Meningeal dose = usual dose.

SELECTED REFERENCE:
Website: www.pdr.net

────── = serious side effect ☐ = black box warning. ND = no data. NR = not recommended. s = spectrum inadequate (at site). a = activity or experience inadequate. p = tissue penetration inadequate. *based on peak serum concentration after usual adult dose. †applicable to adult uncomplicated lower UTIs (CrCl > 30 mL/min).

Foscarnet (Foscavir)

Drug Class: Antiviral (CMV, HHV-6).
Usual Dose: <u>HSV:</u> 40 mg/kg (IV) q12h ×
2–3 weeks; <u>CMV:</u> *Induction Dose:* 90 mg/kg
(IV) q12h × 2 weeks, then *Maintenance Dose:*
90–120 mg/kg (IV) q24h until cured. *Relapse/
Reinduction Dose:* 120 mg/kg (IV) q24h × 2
weeks.

Pharmacokinetic Parameters:
Peak serum level: 150 mcg/mL
Bioavailability: Not applicable
Excreted unchanged (urine): 85%
Serum half-life (normal/ESRD): 2–4/25 hrs
Plasma protein binding: 17%
Volume of distribution (V_d): 0.5 L/kg
Primary Mode of Elimination: Renal/
Hepatic

Dosage Adjustments*

Induction	
CrCl 50–80 mL/min	40–50 mg/kg (IV) q8h
CrCl 20–50 mL/min	20–30 mg/kg (IV) q8h
CrCl < 20 mL/min	Avoid
Maintenance	
CrCl 50–80 mL/min	60–70 mg/kg (IV) q24h
CrCl 20–50 mL/min	65–80 mg/kg (IV) q48h
CrCl < 20 mL/min	Avoid
Post–HD dose	60 mg/kg (IV)
Post–HF HD dose	60 mg/kg (IV)

Post–PD dose	None
CVVH/CVVHD/ CVVHDF dose	Induction: 20–30 mg/kg (IV) q8h; maintenance: 65–80 mg/kg (IV) q48h
Mod. hepatic insufficiency	No change
Severe hepatic insufficiency	No change

Infusion pump must be used. Adequate hydration is recommended to prevent renal toxicity
† Higher doses may be considered for early
reinduction due to progression of CMV
retinitis, and for patients showing excellent
tolerance.

Drug Interactions: Ciprofloxacin (↑ risk of
seizures); amphotericin B, aminoglycosides,
cis-platinum, cyclosporine, ritonavir, saquinavir (↑ nephrotoxicity); pentamidine IV
(severe hypocalcemia); zidovudine (↑ inci-
dence/severity of anemia).

Adverse Effects:
Common
- Drug fever/rash
- Headache
- Nausea/vomiting/diarrhea
- Anemia
- Hypokalemia
- Hypocalcemia,
- Hypomagnesemia
- Hypophosphatemia
- Renal insufficiency

——— = serious side effect ⬜ = black box warning. ND = no data. NR = not recommended. s = spectrum inadequate (at site). a = activity or experience inadequate. p = tissue penetration inadequate.
*based on peak serum concentration after usual adult dose. †applicable to adult uncomplicated lower UTIs
(CrCl > 30 mL/min).

Uncommon
- Oral/genital ulcers
- Bone marrow suppression
- Peripheral neuropathy
- Hallucinations
- Tremors
- Seizures

Rare
- Nephrogenic diabetes insipidus

Allergic Potential: Low
Safety in Pregnancy: C

Additional Clinical Considerations:
- Renal failure minimized by adequate hydration. Dilute with 150 cc normal saline per 1 gm foscarnet. Do not mix with other types of solutions. Administer by IV slow infusion ≤ 1 mg/kg/min using an infusion pump.

Highly active against CMV and HHV-6.

Some activity against EBV, HSV and VZV.

No activity against RSV or adenoviruses.

Cerebrospinal Fluid Penetration:
  Non-Inflamed meninges: 90%
  Inflamed meninges: 100%

Meningeal dose = usual dose.

SELECTED REFERENCE:
Website: www.pdr.net

Fosfomycin disodium IV (Contempo, Fomicyt)

Drug Class: epoxide antibiotic.
Usual Dose: 6 gm (IV) q8h

Spectrum Synopsis*
Hits
  Gram + : MSSA, MRSA, VSE, VRE
  Gram − : Pseudomonas aeruginosa
  Problem pathogens: S. maltophilia
    B. cepacia, Acinetobacter
Misses
  Gram + : GBS
  Gram − : Morganella morganii,
    B. fragilis
  Problem pathogens:
    Listeria, CRE

Urine Spectrum†
- Same as urinary spectrum
- Optimal urinary pH = 6
- Urine levels

(Full **Susceptibility Profiles** p. 208).

Resistance Potential: Low
Pharmacokinetic Parameters:
  Peak serum level: 200 mcg/mL
  Bioavailability: Not applicable
  Excreted unchanged: 74–80%
  Serum half-life (normal): 2.8 hrs
  Plasma protein binding: 3%
  Volume of distribution (V_d): 0.45 L/kg

Primary Mode of Elimination: Renal
Dosage Adjustments*

CrCl 31–50 mL/min	No change
CrCl 11–30 mL/min	↓ dose by 50%
CrCl < 15 mL/min	↓ dose by 80%
Post–HD dose	2 gm Post-HD
Post–PD dose	2 gm Post-PD
CVVH dose	8 gm (IV) q8h
Mild to moderate—hepatic insufficiency	No change
Severe hepatic insufficiency	No change

────── = serious side effect ☐ = black box warning. ND = no data. NR = not recommended. s = spectrum inadequate (at site). a = activity or experience inadequate. p = tissue penetration inadequate. *based on peak serum concentration after usual adult dose. †applicable to adult uncomplicated lower UTIs (CrCl > 30 mL/min).

Drug Interactions: None
Adverse Effects:
Common
- Headache
- Bradycardia
- Hypernatremia
- Hypokalemia
- Phebitis

Uncommon
- Nausea/vomiting
- Non-C. difficile diarrhea
- ↑AST/ALT

Rare
- C. difficile diarrhea/colitis
- Fatty liver

Allergic Potential: Low

Additional Clinical Considerations:

Indication	Daily dose
Osteomyelitis	12–24 gm* in 2–3 divided doses 6 gm (IV) q12h— 8 gm (IV) q8h
Complicated urinary tract infection (UTI)	12–16 gm* in 2–3 divided doses 4 gm (IV) q8h or 8 gm (IV) q12h
Nosocomial pneumonia (NP)	12–24 gm* in 2–3 divided doses 6 gm (IV) q12h— 8 gm (IV) q8h
Acute bacterial meningitis (ABM)	16–24 gm* in 3–4 divided doses 6 gm (IV) q8h

*The high-dose regimen in 3 divided doses should be used in severe infections expected or known to be caused by less susceptible bacteria. Individual doses should not equal 8 gm.

Additional Pharmacokinetic Considerations*

Non-CSF	% of Serum Levels
Lung	44–54%
Bone	50%
Fluid	10-15%
CSF	
Non-inflamed meninges	10%
Inflamed meninges	15%

Meningeal dose = 6 gm (IV) q8h

(see **Antibiotic Pearls & Pitfalls.** p. 537).

SELECTED REFERENCES:
Dimopoulos G, Koulenti D, Parker SL, et al. Intravenous fosfomycin for the treatment of multidrug resistant pathogens: what is the evidence on dosing regimens? Expert Rev Anti Infect Ther doi: 10.1080/14787240.2019.1573669, 2019. (PMID: 30668931)

Pfeifer G, Frenkel C, Entzian W. Pharmacokinetic aspects of cerebrospinal fluid penetration of fosfomycin. Int J Clin Pharmacol Res 5:171-174, 1985. (PMID: 4018950)

Zhanel GG, Zhanel MA, Karlowsky JA. Intravenous fosfomycin: an assessment of its potential for use in the treatment of systemic infections in Canada. Can J Infect Dis 2018. (PMID: 30046362)

Website:www.pdr.net

Fosfomycin tromethamine PO (Monurol)

Drug Class: Urinary antibiotic.
Usual Dose: 3 gm (PO) q24h (*take without food*)

Spectrum Synopsis*
Hits
  Gram + : VSE, VRE
  Gram – : All GNB (including Serratia, Proteus, P. aeruginosa)

―――― = serious side effect ☐ = black box warning. ND = no data. NR = not recommended. s = spectrum inadequate (at site). a = activity or experience inadequate. p = tissue penetration inadequate. *based on peak serum concentration after usual adult dose. †applicable to adult uncomplicated lower UTIs (CrCl > 30 mL/min).

Problem pathogens:
ESBL + Klebsiella, Enterobacter, E. coli, Acinetobacter, CRE
Misses
Gram + : GBS
Gram − : Few aerobic GNB, B. fragilis
Problem pathogens:
S. maltophilia, B. cepacia
Urine Spectrum†
* Same as urinary spectrum
* Optimal urinary pH = 5–6
* Urine levels = 1000 mcg/mL

(Full **Susceptibility Profiles** p. 208).
Resistance Potential: Low
Pharmacokinetic Parameters:
Peak serum level: 26 mcg/mL
Bioavailability: 37%
Excreted unchanged (urine): 60%; 40% excreted as active metabolite
Serum half-life (normal/ESRD): 5.7/50 hrs
Plasma protein binding: 3%
Volume of distribution (V_d): 2 L/kg
Primary Mode of Elimination: Renal
Dosage Adjustments*

CrCl 10–50 mL/min	No change
CrCl < 10 mL/min	Use with caution
Post–HD dose	3 gm (PO)
Post–PD dose	1 gm (PO)
CVVH/CVVHD/CVVHDF dose	No change
Moderate—severe hepatic insufficiency	No change

Drug Interactions: Antacids, metoclopramide (↓ fosfomycin effect).

Adverse Effects:
Common
* Headache
* Nausea/vomiting/diarrhea
Uncommon
* ↑ AST/ALT
* Hypoglycemia
Rare
* Thrombocytosis
Allergic Potential: Low
Safety in Pregnancy: B

Additional Clinical Considerations:
* **Useful for GNB or VSE/VRE cystitis/ CAB.**
* Treat cystitis as *single dose* in females.
* **One of the few oral antibiotics active against most strains of MDR P. aeruginosa, MDR Klebsiella pneumoniae, and MDR Acinetobacter baumanii in urine** (*cystitis/CAB*).
* Treatment of MDR GNB cystitis/ CAB (*change Foley before beginning therapy.* Use 3 g (PO) q 3 days × 2–3 doses).
* Urine levels > 128 mcg/mL at 36–48 h.
* **For prostatitis due to MDR GNB, use fosfomycin 3 g (PO) q3 days × 3 weeks.**
* Fosfomycin (concentration dependent PK/PD) successful when given q3 days due to its long PAE with GNB.

——— = serious side effect ⬜ = black box warning. ND = no data. NR = not recommended. s = spectrum inadequate (at site). a = activity or experience inadequate. p = tissue penetration inadequate. *based on peak serum concentration after usual adult dose. †applicable to adult uncomplicated lower UTIs (CrCl > 30 mL/min).

Additional Pharmacokinetic Considerations*

Non-CSF	% of Serum Levels
Peritoneal fluid	ND
Bile	ND
Synovial fluid	ND
Bone	25%
Prostate	25%
CSF	
Non-inflamed meninges	NR(p)
Inflamed meninges (ABM)	NR(p)

(see **Antibiotic Pearls & Pitfalls.** p. 537).

SELECTED REFERENCES:

Auer S, Wojna A, Hell M. Oral treatment options for ambulatory patients with urinary tract infections caused by extended-spectrum-beta-lactamase-producing Escherichia coli. Antimicrob Agents Chemother 54:4006–4008, 2010. (PMID:20585127)

Cunha BA, Gran A, Raza M. Persistent extended-spectrum B-lactamase-positive Escherichia coli chronic prostatitis successfully treated with a combination of fosfomycin and doxycycline. Int J Antimicrob Agents 45:427-429, 2015. (PMID:25662814)

Dinh A, Salomon J, Bru JP, et al. Fosfomycin: efficacy against infections caused by multidrug-resistant bacteria. Scand J infect Dis 44:182–9, 2012. (PMID:22176655)

Falagas ME, Kastoris AC, Kapaskelis AM, et al. Fosfomycin for the treatment of multidrug-resistant, including extended-spectrum β-lactamase producing, Enterobacteriaceae infections: a systematic review. Lancet Infect Dis 10:43–50, 2010. (PMID:20129548)

Gardiner BJ, Mahony AA, Ellis AG. Is fosfomycin a potential treatment alternative for multidrug-resistant gram-negative prostatitis? Clin Infect Dis 58:e101-105, 2014. (PMID:24170195)

Liu HY, Lin HC, Lin YC, et al. Antimicrobial susceptibilities of urinary extended-spectrum beta-lactamase-producing Escherichia coli and Klebsiella pneumoniae to fosfomycin and nitrofurantoin in a teaching hospital in Taiwan. J Microbiol Immunol Infect 44:364–368, 2011. (PMID:21524974)

Livermore DM, Warner M, Mushtaq S, et al. What remains against carbapenem-resistant Enterbacteriaceae? Evaluation of chloramphenicol, ciprofloxacin, colistin, fosfomycin, minocycline, nitrofurantoin, temocillin and tigecycline. In J Antimicrob Agents 37:415–419, 2011. (PMID:21429716)

Pontikis K, Karaiskos I, Bastani S, et al. Outcomes of critically ill intensive care unit patients treated with fosfomycin for infections due to pandrug-resistant and extensively drug-resistant carbapenemase-producing Gram-negative bacteria. Int J Antimicrob Agents 43:52-59, 2014. (PMID:24183799)

Website: www.pdr.net

Ganciclovir (Cytovene)

Drug Class: Antiviral (CMV, HSV, HHV-6) (see comments).

Usual Dose: *Induction Dose:* 5 mg/kg (IV) q12h × 2 weeks; *Maintenance Dose:* 5 mg/kg (IV) q24h or 1 gm (PO) q8h.

Pharmacokinetic Parameters:

Peak serum level: 8.3 (IV)/1.2 (PO) mcg/mL
Bioavailability: 5%
Excreted unchanged (urine): 90%
Serum half-life (normal/ESRD): 3.6/28 hrs
Plasma protein binding: 1%
Volume of distribution (V_d): 0.74 L/kg

Primary Mode of Elimination: Renal

———— = serious side effect ☐ = black box warning. ND = no data. NR = not recommended. s = spectrum inadequate (at site). a = activity or experience inadequate. p = tissue penetration inadequate. *based on peak serum concentration after usual adult dose. †applicable to adult uncomplicated lower UTIs (CrCl > 30 mL/min).

Dosage Adjustments*

CrCl 50–70 mL/min	2.5 mg/kg (IV) q12h (induction); 2.5 mg/kg (IV) q24h (maintenance); 500 mg (PO) q8h
CrCl 25–50 mL/min	2.5 mg/kg (IV) q24h (induction); 1.25 mg/kg (IV) q24h (maintenance); 500 mg (PO) q12h
CrCl 10–25 mL/min	1.25 mg/kg (IV) q24h (induction); 0.625 mg/kg (IV) q24h (maintenance); 500 mg (PO) q24h
CrCl < 10 mL/min	1.25 mg/kg (IV) 3x/week (induction); 0.625 mg/kg (IV) 3x/week (maintenance); 500 mg (PO) 3x/week
Post–HD dose	1.25 mg/kg (IV) (induction); 0.625 mg/kg (IV) (maintenance); 500 mg (PO)
Post–PD dose	Same dose as Post–HD
CVVH/CVVHD/CVVHDF dose	Same dose as CrCl 50–70 mL/min
Moderate hepatic insufficiency	No change
Severe hepatic insufficiency	No change

Drug Interactions: Cytotoxic drugs (may produce additive toxicity: stomatitis, bone marrow depression, alopecia); imipenem (↑ risk of seizures); probenecid (↑ ganciclovir levels); zidovudine (↓ ganciclovir levels, ↑ zidovudine levels, possible neutropenia); didanosine (↑ didanosine levels); cyclosporine, amphotericin, (↑ nephrotoxicity); mycophenolate mofetil (↑ mycophenolate mofetil and ganciclovir levels in renal insufficiency); tenofovir (↑ tenofovir, ganciclovir levels).

Adverse Effects:

Common
- Drug fever/rash
- Nausea/vomiting/diarrhea
- Retinal detachment
- ↑ Creatinine
- Leukopenia, anemia and thrombocytopenia

Uncommon
- Headache

Rare
- Hallucinations
- Ventricular arrhythmias (VT/torsades de pointes)
- Seizures/tremors (dose related)
- Aspermatogenesis, carcinogenic, teratogenic

Allergic Potential: High

Safety in Pregnancy: C

—— = serious side effect ⬚ = black box warning. ND = no data. NR = not recommended. s = spectrum inadequate (at site). a = activity or experience inadequate. p = tissue penetration inadequate. *based on peak serum concentration after usual adult dose. †applicable to adult uncomplicated lower UTIs (CrCl > 30 mL/min).

Additional Clinical Considerations:
- **Induction dose** usually given IV.
- **Maintenance dose** may be given IV or PO.
- For PO therapy use valganciclovir (not PO ganciclovir).
- Reduce dose with neutropenia/ thrombocytopenia.
- Bioavailability increased with food: 5% fasting; 6–9% with food; 28–31% with fatty food.

***Highly active* against CMV, HHV-6, and HSV.**

***Some activity* against VZV, EBV, and adenoviruses.**

***No activity* against RSV**

Cerebrospinal Fluid Penetration: 70%

Meningeal dose = usual dose.

SELECTED REFERENCES:

Jacobsen T, Sipointis N. Drug interactions and toxicities associated with the antiviral management of cytomegalovirus infection. Am J Health Syst Pharm 67:1417–1425, 2010. (PMID:20720240)

Matthews T, Boehme R. Antiviral activity and mechanism of action of ganciclovir. Rev Infect Dis 10:490–4, 1988. (PMID:2847285)

Website: www.pdr.net

Gentamicin (Garamycin)

Drug Class: Aminoglycoside.
Usual Dose: 240 mg or 5 mg/kg (IV) q24h (preferred over q8h dosing) (see comments).

Spectrum Synopsis*
Hits
  Gram + : MSSA, VSE (with ampicillin)
  Gram − : Most aerobic GNB (some P. aeruginosa)
  Problem pathogens:
    Listeria, Acinectobacter
Misses
  Gram + : MRSA, VRE
  Gram − : Many P. aeruginosa, B. fragilis
  Problem pathogens:
    Nocardia, S. maltophilia, B. cepacia
Urine Spectrum†
- Same as serum spectrum
- Optimal urinary pH = 6–7
- Urine levels = 400 mcg/mL

(Full **Susceptibility Profiles** p. 208).

Resistance Potential: High
(P. aeruginosa)

Pharmacokinetic Parameters:
Peak serum levels: 4–8 mcg/mL (q8h dosing); 16–24 mcg/mL (q24h dosing)
Bioavailability: Not applicable
Excreted unchanged (urine): 95%
Serum half-life (normal/ESRD): 2.5/48 hrs
Plasma protein binding: < 5%
Volume of distribution (V_d): 0.3 L/kg
Primary Mode of Elimination: Renal
Dosage Adjustments*

CrCl 50–80 mL/min	120 mg (IV) q24h or 2.5 mg/kg (IV) q24h
CrCl 10–50 mL/min	120 mg (IV) q48h or 2.5 mg/kg (IV) q48h

———— = serious side effect [＿＿] = black box warning. ND = no data. NR = not recommended. s = spectrum inadequate (at site). a = activity or experience inadequate. p = tissue penetration inadequate. *based on peak serum concentration after usual adult dose. †applicable to adult uncomplicated lower UTIs (CrCl > 30 mL/min).

CrCl < 10 mL/min	80 mg (IV) q48h or 1.25 mg/kg (IV) q48h
Post–HD dose	80 mg (IV) or 1 mg/kg (IV)
Post–PD dose	40 mg (IV) or 0.5 mg/kg (IV)
Post–HFHD dose	120 mg (IV) or 2.5 mg/kg
Post-dose	120 mg (IV) or 2.5 mg/kg (IV)
CVVH/CVVHD/CVVHDF dose	120 mg (IV) q48h or 2.5 mg/kg (IV)
Moderate hepatic insufficiency	No change
Severe hepatic insufficiency	No change

Drug Interactions: Amphotericin B, cephalothin, cyclosporine, enflurane, methoxyflurane, NSAIDs, polymyxin B, radiographic contrast, vancomycin (↑ nephrotoxicity); cis-platinum (↑ nephrotoxicity, ↑ ototoxicity); loop diuretics (↑ ototoxicity); neuromuscular blocking agents, magnesium sulfate (↑ apnea, prolonged paralysis); non-polarizing muscle relaxants (↑ apnea).
Adverse Effects:
Uncommon
- Neuromuscular blockade with rapid infusion/absorption (long/peritoneum)
- Reversible non-oilguric renal failure (ATM) prolonged/extremely high serum trough levels
- Ototoxicity only with prolonged/

extremely high peak serum levels (usually irreversible), Cochilear toxicity (1/3 of ototoxicity) manifests as ↓ high frequency hearing (deafness is unusual)
- Vestibular toxicity (2/3 of ototoxicity) develops before ototoxicity (typically manifests as tinnitus)
Safety in Pregnancy: D

Additional Clinical Considerations:
- **Synergy dose:** 2.5 mg/kg (IV) q24h or 120 mg (IV) q24h.
- **Single daily dosing virtually eliminates nephrotoxic/ototoxic potential.**
- IV infusion should be given slowly over 1 hour.
- **May be given IM.**
- **Avoid intraperitoneal infusion due to risk of neuromuscular blockade.**
- Avoid intratracheal/aerosolized intrapulmonary instillation, which predisposes to antibiotic resistance.
- Vd ↑ with edema/ascites, trauma, burns, cystic fibrosis (may require ↑ dose).
- Vd ↓ with dehydration, obesity (may require ↑ dose).
- **Renal cast counts are the best indicator of aminoglycoside nephrotoxicity, not serum creatinine.**
- Dialysis removes ~ 1/3 of gentamicin from serum.
- **CAPD dose:** 2–4 mg/L dialysate (IP) with each exchange.
- **Therapeutic Serum Concentrations** (for therapeutic efficacy, *not* toxicity):
  Peak (q24h/q8h dosing) = 16–24/8–10 mcg/mL

———— = serious side effect ☐ = black box warning. ND = no data. NR = not recommended. s = spectrum inadequate (at site). a = activity or experience inadequate. p = tissue penetration inadequate. *based on peak serum concentration after usual adult dose. †applicable to adult uncomplicated lower UTIs (CrCl > 30 mL/min).

Trough (q24h/q8h dosing)
= 0/1–2 mcg/mL
May inhibit antibiotic induced
LPS (endotoxin) release from GNB
potentially minimizing endotoxin
mediated tissue damage.

Additional Pharmacokinetic Considerations:

Non-CSF	% of Serum Levels
Peritoneal fluid	40%
Bile	30%
Synovial fluid	NR(a)
Bone	ND
Prostate	NR(p)
CSF	
Non-inflamed meninges	<1%
Inflamed meninges (ABM)	20%

Meningeal dose = 5 mg (IT) q24h
(always give with systemic IV therapy.

(also see ***Antibiotic Pearls & Pitfalls***
p. 531).

SELECTED REFERENCES:

Bruss JB. Lack of evidence associating nephrotoxicity with low-dose gentamicin for Staphylococcus aureus bacteremia and endocarditis. Clin Infect Dis 49:806, 2009. (PMID:19653850)

Cosgrove SE, Vigliani GA, Campion M, et al. Initial low-dose gentamicin for Staphylococcus aureus bacteremia and endocarditis is nephrotoxic. Clin Infect Dis 48:713–721, 2009. (PMID:19207079)

Cunha BA. Aminoglycosides: Current role in antimicrobial therapy. Pharmacotherapy 8:334–50, 1988. (PMID:3146747)

Edson RS, Terrell CL. The aminoglycosides. Mayo Clin Proc 74:519–28, 1999. (PMID:10319086)

Freeman CD, Nicolau DP, Belliveau PP, et al. Once-daily dosing of aminoglycosides: Review and recommendations for clinical practice.

J Antimicrob Chemother 39:677–86, 1997. (PMID:9222035)

Munita JM, Arias CA, Murray BE. Enterococcus faecalis infective endocarditis: Is it time to abandon aminoglycosides? Clin Infect Dis 56:1269-1272, 2013. (PMID:23392395)

Snydman, DR, McDermott LA, Jacobus NV. Evaluation of in vitro interaction of daptomycin with gentamicin or beta-lactam antibiotics against Staphylococcus aureus and Enterococci by FIC index and timed-kill curves. J Chemother 17:614–21, 2005. (PMID:16433191)

Website: www.pdr.net

Griseofulvin (Fulvicin, Grifulvin, Ultra, Gris-PEG, Grisactin)

Drug Class: Antifungal.
Usual Dose: 500 mg-1 gm (PO) q24h (microsize); 330–375 mg (PO) q24h (ultramicrosize).
Pharmacokinetic Parameters:
Peak serum level: 1–2 mcg/mL
Bioavailability: 50%
Excreted unchanged (urine): 1%
Serum half-life (normal/ESRD): 9/22 hrs
Plasma protein binding: 84%
Volume of distribution (V_d): No data
Primary Mode of Elimination: Hepatic
Dosage Adjustments*

CrCl < 10 mL/min	No change
Post–HD or PD dose	None
CVVH/CVVHD/ CVVHDF dose	No change
Moderate hepatic insufficiency	No change
Severe hepatic insufficiency	Use with caution

——— = serious side effect ⬛ = black box warning. ND = no data. NR = not recommended. s = spectrum inadequate (at site). a = activity or experience inadequate. p = tissue penetration inadequate. *based on peak serum concentration after usual adult dose. †applicable to adult uncomplicated lower UTIs (CrCl > 30 mL/min).

Drug Interactions: Alcohol (↑ griseofulvin toxicity); barbiturates (↓ griseofulvin levels); oral contraceptives, warfarin (↓ interacting drug levels).
Adverse Effects:
Common
- Headache
- Nausea/vomiting/diarrhea
- Photosensitivity
- Drug fever/rash

Uncommon
- Angular stomatits
- Glossitis
- Leukopenia

Allergic Potential: Moderate
Safety in Pregnancy: C

Additional Clinical Considerations:
- May exacerbate SLE/acute intermittent porphyria.
- Take microsize griseofulvin with fatty meal to ↑ absorption to ~ 70%.
- Ultramicrosize griseofulvin is absorbed 1.5 times better than microsize griseofulvin.

SELECTED REFERENCE:
Website: www.pdr.net

Imipenem/Cilastatin (Primaxin)

Drug Class: Carbapenem.
Usual Dose: 1 gm (IV) q6h (see comments).

Spectrum Synopsis*
Hits
   Gram + : All non-enterococcal streptococci, MSSA, CoNS, VSE
   Gram – : All GNB (most P. aeruginosa), B. fragilis
   Problem pathogens: None

Misses
   Gram + : MRSA, VRE
   Gram – : Some P. aeruginosa
   Problem pathogens:
      S. maltophilia, B. cepacia, ESBL + Klebsiella, Enterobacter, E. coli, CRE
Urine Spectrum†
- Same as serum spectrum
- Optimal urinary pH = ND
- Urine levels = 300 mcg/mL

(Full *Susceptibility Profiles* p. 208).

Resistance Potential: High (P. aeruginosa, ↑ prevalence of MRSA)
Pharmacokinetic Parameters:
Peak serum level: 42–116 mcg/mL
Bioavailability: Not applicable
Excreted unchanged (urine): 70%
Serum half-life (normal/ESRD): 1/4 hrs
Plasma protein binding: 20% / 40% (cilastatin)
Volume of distribution (V_d): 0.2 L/kg
Primary Mode of Elimination: Renal
Dosage Adjustments*

CrCl 40–70 mL/min	500 mg (IV) q6h
CrCl 20–40 mL/min	250 mg (IV) q8h
CrCl < 20 mL/min†	250 mg (IV) q12h
Post–HD dose	250 mg (IV)
Post–PD dose	250 mg (IV)
CVVH/CVVHD/ CVVHDF dose	500 mg (IV) q8h
Moderate hepatic insufficiency	No change
Severe hepatic insufficiency	No change

† Avoid if CrCl ≤ 5 mL/min unless dialysis is instituted within 48 hours.

——— = serious side effect ☐ = black box warning. ND = no data. NR = not recommended. s = spectrum inadequate (at site). a = activity or experience inadequate. p = tissue penetration inadequate. *based on peak serum concentration after usual adult dose. †applicable to adult uncomplicated lower UTIs (CrCl > 30 mL/min).

Drug Interactions: Cyclosporine
($\uparrow$ cyclosporine levels); ganciclovir
($\uparrow$ risk of seizures); probenecid
($\uparrow$ imipenem levels); valproic acid
($\downarrow$ seizure threshold).

Adverse Effects:

Uncommon
- Phlebitis
- Drug fever/rash
- Nausea/vomiting/diarrhea
- Seizures

Rare
- C. difficile diarrhea/colitis

Allergic Potential: Low
Safety in Pregnancy: C

Additional Clinical Considerations:
- Imipenem:cilastatin (1:1). Infuse 1 gm (IV) over 40–60 minutes.
- Imipenem is renally metabolized by dehydropeptidase I; cilastatin is an inhibitor of this enzyme, effectively preventing the metabolism of imipenem.
- Imipenem/cilastatin can be given IM (IM absorption: imipenem 75%; cilastatin 100%).
- *Fully susceptible organisms dose: 500 mg (IV) q6h;*
- *Less susceptible organisms (e.g., P. aeruginosa) dose: 1 gm (IV) q6–8h.*
- *Seizures more likely in renal insufficiency/high doses (> 2 gm/d).*
- **Low incidence of cross reactions with β-lactams.**

May inhibit antibiotic induced LPS (endotoxin) release from GNB potentially minimizing endotoxin mediated tissue damage.

Additional Pharmacokinetic Considerations*

Non-CSF	% of Serum Levels
Peritoneal fluid	70%
Bile	30%
Synovial fluid	30%
Bone	20%
Prostate	NR(p)
CSF	
Non-inflamed meninges	1%
Inflamed meninges (ABM)	30%

(also see ***Antibiotic Pearls & Pitfalls*** p. 529).

SELECTED REFERENCES:

Balfour JA, Bryson HM, Brogden RN. Imipenem/cilastatin: An update of its antibacterial activity, pharmacokinetics, and therapeutic efficacy in the treatment of serious infections. Drugs 51:99–136, 1996. (PMID:8741235)

Barza M. Imipenem: First of a new class of beta-lactam antibiotics. Ann Intern Med 103:552–60, 1985. (PMID:3898954)

Helinger WC, Brewer NS. Carbapenems and monobactams: Imipenem, meropenem, and aztreonam. Mayo Clin Proc 74:420–34, 1999. (PMID:10221472)

Lamoth F, Erard V, Asner S, et al. High imipenem blood concentrations associated with toxic encephalopathy in a patient with mild renal dysfunction. Int J Antimicrob Agents 34:386–388, 2009. (PMID:19596561)

Lautenbach E, Weiner MG, Nachamkin I, et al. Imipenem resistance among Pseudomonas aeruginosa Isolates: risk factors for infection and impact of resistance on clinical and economic outcomes. Infection Control and Hosp Epidemiol 27:893–900, 2006. (PMID:16941312)

Maravi-Poma E, Gener J, Alvarez-Lerma F, et al. Spanish group for the study of septic complications in severe acute pancreatitis. Early antibiotic treatment (prophylaxis) of septic complications in severe acute necrotizing pancreatitis: a prospective, randomized, multicenter study comparing two regimens with imipenem-cilastatin. Intensive Care Med 29:1974–80, 2003. (PMID:14551680)

—— = serious side effect [ ] = black box warning. ND = no data. NR = not recommended. s = spectrum inadequate (at site). a = activity or experience inadequate. p = tissue penetration inadequate. *based on peak serum concentration after usual adult dose. †applicable to adult uncomplicated lower UTIs (CrCl > 30 mL/min).

Miliani K, L'Heriteau F, Lacave L, et al. Imipenem and ciprofloxacin consumption as factors associated with high incidence rates of resistance Pseudomonas aeruginosa in hospitals in northern France. J Hosp Infect 77:343–347, 2011. (PMID:21316805)

Saltoglu N, Dalkiran A, Tetiker T, et al. Piperacillin/tazobactam versus imipenem/cilastatin for severe diabetic foot infections: a prospective, randomized clinical trial in a university hospital. Clin Microbiol Infect 16:1252–1257, 2010. (PMID:19832720)

Website: www.pdr.net

Imipenem/Cilastatin/Relebactam (Recarbrio)

Drug Class: Carbapenem/β-lactamase inhibitor
Usual Dose: 1.25 gm (IV) (500 mg/500 mg/250 mg) q6h

Spectrum Synopsis*
Hits
   Gram + : VSE, MSSA
   Gram – : Most GNBs, B. fragilis
   Problem pathogens: P. aeruginosa, Acinetobacter, CRE
Misses
   Gram + : VRE, MRSA
   Gram – : S. maltophilia, B. cepacia
   Problem pathogens:
Urine Spectrum:
   • Same as serum spectrum
   • Urine levels = ND

(Full *Susceptibility Profiles* p. 208).

Resistance Potential: Low
Pharmacokinetic Parameters:
   Peak serum level: 16.7 mcg/mL
   Bioavailability: Not applicable
   Excreted unchanged (urine): 95-100%

Serum half-life (normal): 1.35-1.8 hrs
Plasma protein binding: ND
Volume of distribution (V_d): 0.29 L/kg
Primary Mode of Elimination: Renal
Dosage Adjustments*

CrCl 60–89 mL/min	1 gm (IV) q6h
CrCl 30–59 mL/min	750 mg (IV) q6h
CrCl 15-29 mL/min	500 mg (IV) q6h
CrCl < 15 mL/min	Avoid
Post-HD dose	500 mg (IV)
Post-PD dose	500 mg (IV)
CVVH dose	No data
Mild hepatic insufficiency	No change
Moderate hepatic insufficiency	No change
Severe hepatic insufficiency	No change

Drug Interactions: None
Adverse Effects:
Uncommon
   • Somnolence
   • Headache
   • Parasthesias
   • Phebitis
   • Nausea
   • Diarrhea
   • Abdominal distension
   • Erythema
Uncommon
   • Drug fever/rash
Rare
   • C. difficile diarrhea/colitis

——— = serious side effect ☐ = black box warning. ND = no data. NR = not recommended. s = spectrum inadequate (at site). a = activity or experience inadequate. p = tissue penetration inadequate. *based on peak serum concentration after usual adult dose. †applicable to adult uncomplicated lower UTIs (CrCl > 30 mL/min).

Allergic Potential: Low
Safety in Pregnancy: Unknown

Additional Clinical Considerations:
• None

Additional Pharmacokinetic Considerations:	
Non-CSF	**% of Serum Levels**
Peritoneal fluid	70%
Bile	30%
Synovial fluid	30%
Bone	20%
Prostate	NR(p)
CSF	
Non-inflamed meninges	1%
Inflamed meninges	30%

(also see *Antibiotic Pearls & Pitfalls* p. 530).

SELECTED REFERENCES:
Karlowsky JA, Lob SH, Young K, et al. Activity of imipenem/relebactam against Pseudomonas aeruginosa with antimicrobial-resistant phenotypes from seven global regions: SMART 2015-2016. J Global antimicrob resist 15:140-47, 2018. (PMID: 30071354)
Petty LA, Henig O, Patel TS, et al. Overview of meropenem-vaborbactam and newer antimicrobial agents for the treatment of carbapenem-resistant Enterobacteriaceae. Infection Drug Resist 11:1461-72, 2018. (PMID: 30254477)
Rhee EG, Rizk ML, Calder N, et al. Pharmacokinetics, safety and tolerability of single ad multiple doses of relebactam, a β-lactamase inhibitor, in combination with imipenem and cilastatin in healthy participants. Antimicrob Agents Chemother 62:1-16, 2018. (PMID: 29914955)
Zhanel GG, Lawrence CK, Adma H, et al. Imipenem-relebactam and meropenem-varbpbactam: two novel carbapenem-β-lactamase inhibitor combinations. Drugs 78:65-98, 2018. (PMID: 29230684)
Website: www.pdr.net

Isavuconazole (Cresemba)

Drug Class: Azole antifungal.
Usual Dose: Loading dose: 200 mg (IV) q8h × 48 hrs, then **Maintenance dose:** 200 mg (IV/PO) q24h.
Pharmacokinetic Parameters:
Peak serum level: 1.85 – 2.56 mcg/mL
Bioavailability (IV/PO): 98%
Excreted unchanged: no data
Serum half-life (normal/ESRD): IV $t_{1/2}$ = 76–104 hrs; PO $t_{1/2}$ = 56–77 hrs/ND
Plasma protein binding: 98%
Volume of distribution (V_d): 4.4–7.7 L/kg
Primary Mode of Elimination: Hepatic
Dosage Adjustments*

CrCl < 30 mL/min	No change
Post–HD dose	No change
Post–PD dose	No change
CVVH dose	No change
Mild/Moderate Hepatic insufficiency	200 mg (IV) q8h × 48 hrs, then 100 mg (IV/PO) q24h
Severe hepatic insufficiency	Avoid use

Drug Interactions: CYP3A4 substrate; Concomitant use of CYP3A4 inhibitors and inducers is not recommended. No clinically relevant interactions with warfarin or cyclosporine.
Adverse Effects:
Common
• Peripheral edema
• Headache

―――― = serious side effect ☐ = black box warning. ND = no data. NR = not recommended. s = spectrum inadequate (at site). a = activity or experience inadequate. p = tissue penetration inadequate. *based on peak serum concentration after usual adult dose. †applicable to adult uncomplicated lower UTIs (CrCl > 30 mL/min).

- Fatigue
- Nausea/vomiting/diarrhea
- Abdominal pain
- Constipation
- Dyspnea
- Cough
- Hypokalemia
- ↑ AST/ALT

Uncommon
- Drug fever/rash
- <u>Hypersensitivity reactions</u>
- Infusion related reactions
- Shortened QTc
- <u>Febrile neutropenia</u>

Allergic Potential: Low (potential anaphylaxis/severe cutaneous reactions 1.9%)

Safety in Pregnancy: Unknown

Additional Clinical Considerations:
- Water soluble azole, which does not require cyclodextrin for IV solubility.
- Isavuconazonium, is a prodrug (water soluble) that is rapidly hydrolyzed in the blood, to the active moiety, isavuconazole (lipid soluble).
- Available as both IV and PO formulations.
- Only azole that does not prolong the QT interval.
- Following reconstitution, IV isavuconazonium may spontaneously hydrolyze and precipitate as insoluble isavuconazole (an inline filter is recommended to remove precipitates).

***Highly active* against Candida albicans; non-albicans Candida, Cryptococcus, Aspergillus, Mucor; *No activity* against Pseudallescheria/Scedosporium, Fusaria.**

Bile Penetration: Good

Cerebrospinal Fluid Penetration: < 10%

SELECTED REFERENCES:

Faici DR, Pasqualotto AC. Profile of isavuconazole and its potential in the treatment of severe invasive fungal infections. Infection and Drug Resistance. 6:163-174, 2013. (PMID:24187505)

Gregson L, Goodwin J, Johnson A, et al. In vitro susceptibility of Aspergillus fumigatus to isavuconazole: correlation with itraconazole, voriconazole, and posaconazole. Antimicrobl Agents Chemo. 57:5778-5780, 2013. (PMID:24041890)

Livermore J, Hope W. Evaluation of the pharmacokinetics and clinical utility of isavuconazole for treatment of invasive fungal infections. Expert Opinion on Drug Metab & Tox. 8:759-765, 2012. (PMID:22530880)

Seyedmousavi S, Venweij PE, Mouton JW. Isavuconazole, a broad-spectrum triazole for the treatment of systemic fungal diseases. Expert Review Anti-infective Therapy. 13:9-27, 2015. (PMID:25488140)

Thompson GR, 3rd, Wederhold NP. Isavuconazole: a comprehensive review of spectrum of activity of a new triazole. Mycopathologia. 170:291-313, 2010. (PMID:20524153)

Website: www.pdr.net

Isoniazid (INH)

Drug Class: TB drug.

Usual Dose: 300 mg (PO) q24h or 5 mg/kg (see comments).

Pharmacokinetic Parameters:
Peak serum level: 7 mcg/mL
Bioavailability: 90%

_____ = serious side effect [_____] = black box warning. ND = no data. NR = not recommended. s = spectrum inadequate (at site). a = activity or experience inadequate. p = tissue penetration inadequate. *based on peak serum concentration after usual adult dose. †applicable to adult uncomplicated lower UTIs (CrCl > 30 mL/min).

Excreted unchanged (urine): 50–70%
Serum half-life (normal/ESRD): 1/1 hr
Plasma protein binding: 15%
Volume of distribution (V_d): 0.75 L/kg
Primary Mode of Elimination: Hepatic
Dosage Adjustments*

CrCl < 10 mL/min	No change
Post–HD dose	300 mg
Post–PD dose	300 mg
CVVH/CVVHD/CVVHDF dose	None
Moderate hepatic insufficiency	No change
Severe hepatic insufficiency	Use with caution

Drug Interactions: Alcohol, rifampin
(↑ risk of ↑ AST/ALT); alfentanil
(↑ duration of alfentanil effect);
aluminum salts (↓ isoniazid absorption);
carbamazepine, phenytoin (↑ interacting
drug levels); itraconazole (↓ itraconazole
levels); warfarin (↑ INR).
Adverse Effects:
Common
• Peripheral neuropathy
• Neurotoxicity
• ↑ AST/ALT
Uncommon
• Drug fever/rash
• Drug induced ANA/SLE
• Hemolytic anemia
Rare
• Severe hepatitis and sometimes fulminant hepatic failure

Allergic Potential: Low
Safety in Pregnancy: C

Additional Clinical Considerations:
• Administer with 50 mg of pyridoxine daily to prevent peripheral neuropathy.

• Increased blood pressure/rash with tyramine–containing products, e.g., cheese/wine.
• ↑ Hepatotoxicity in slow acetylators.
• **Slow acetylator dose:** 150 mg (PO) q24h.
• **TB D.O.T. dose:** 15 mg/kg or 900 mg (PO) 3x/week.

Cerebrospinal Fluid Penetration:
Non-Inflamed meninges: 90%
Inflamed meninges: 90%
Meningeal dose = usual dose.

SELECTED REFERENCES:
CDC. Severe Isoniazid-associated liver injuries among persons being treated for latent tuberculosis infection. MMWR 59:224–229, 2010. (PMID:20203555)
McIllerson H, Wash P, Burger A, et al. Determinants of rifampin, isoniazid, pyrazinamide and ethambutol pharmacokinetics in a cohort of tuberculosis patients. Antimicrob Agents Chemother 50:1170–77, 2006. (PMID:16569826)
Pina JM, Clotel L, Ferrer A, et al. Cost-effectiveness of rifampin for 4 months and isoniazid for 9 months in the treatment of tuberculosis infection. Eur J Clin Microbiol Inf Dis 32:647-655,2013. (PMID:23238684)
Van Scoy RE, Wilkowske CJ. Antituberculous agents. Mayo Clin Proc 67:179–87, 1992. (PMID:1347579)
Website: www.pdr.net

Itraconazole (Sporanox)

Drug Class: Azole antifungal.
Usual Dose: 200 mg (PO, capsules or solution, solution produces better absorption) q12h or q24h (*take without food*). Depending on disease severity, **Loading dose:** IV therapy 200 mg IV q12h × 2 days, then **Maintenance dose:** IV only 200 mg (IV) q24h; PO follow-up to

—— = serious side effect ☐ = black box warning. ND = no data. NR = not recommended. s = spectrum inadequate (at site). a = activity or experience inadequate. p = tissue penetration inadequate. *based on peak serum concentration after usual adult dose. †applicable to adult uncomplicated lower UTIs (CrCl > 30 mL/min).

IV therapy for serious infection is 200 mg PO q12h.

Pharmacokinetic Parameters:
Peak serum level: 2.8 mcg/mL
Bioavailability: 55% (capsules)/90% (solution)
Excreted unchanged (urine): 1%
Serum half-life (normal/ESRD): 21–64/ 35 hrs
Plasma protein binding: 99.8%
Volume of distribution (V_d): 10 L/kg

Primary Mode of Elimination: Hepatic; metabolized predominantly by the cytochrome P450 isoenzyme system (CYP3A4)

Dosage Adjustments*

CrCl > 30 mL/min	No change
CrCl < 30 mL/min	No change for (PO); avoid (IV) due to ↑ cyclodextrin
Post–HD dose	100 mg (IV/PO)
Post–PD dose	None
CVVH/CVVHD/ CVVHDF dose	No change
Moderate hepatic insufficiency	No change†
Severe hepatic insufficiency	Use with caution

† ↑ $t_{1/2}$ of itraconazole in patients with hepatic insufficiency should be considered when given with medications metabolized by P450 isoenzymes. Also see Adverse Effects for information regarding patients who develop liver dysfunction.

Drug Interactions: *Itraconazole may ↑ plasma levels of:* alfentanil, buspirone, busulfan, carbamazepine, cisapride, cyclosporine, digoxin, dihydropyridines, docetaxel, dofetilide, methylprednisolone, oral hypoglycemics (↑ risk of hypoglycemia), pimozide, quinidine, rifabutin, saquinavir, sirolimus, tacrolimus, trimetrexate, verapamil, vinca alkaloids, warfarin; alprazolam, diazepam, midazolam, triazolam (↑ sedative/ hypnotic effects); atorvastatin, lovastatin, simvastatin (↑ risk of rhabdomyolysis); indinavir, ritonavir, saquinavir; coadministration of oral midazolam, triazolam, lovastatin, or simvastatin with itraconazole is contraindicated; coadministration of cisapride, pimozide, quinidine, amiodarone, or dofetilide with itraconazole is contraindicated due to the risk of ↑ QT_c/life-threatening ventricular arrhythmias. *Decreased itraconazole levels may occur with:* antacids, carbamazepine, H_2-receptor antagonists, isoniazid, nevirapine, phenobarbital, phenytoin, proton pump inhibitors, rifabutin, rifampin; coadministration of rifampin with itraconazole is not recommended. *Increased itraconazole levels may occur with:* clarithromycin, erythromycin, indinavir, ritonavir.

Adverse Effects:
Common
• Nausea/vomiting/diarrhea
Uncommon
• Headache
• Abdominal pain
• Drug rash
• ↑ AST/ALT
• Hypertriglyceridemia
• Hypokalemia
Rare
• Cardiac arrhythmias
• Congestive heart failure

——— = serious side effect ☐ = black box warning. ND = no data. NR = not recommended. s = spectrum inadequate (at site). a = activity or experience inadequate. p = tissue penetration inadequate. *based on peak serum concentration after usual adult dose. †applicable to adult uncomplicated lower UTIs (CrCl > 30 mL/min).

- Do not use for the treatment of onychomycosis with CHF, or history of CHF

Allergic Potential: Low
Safety in Pregnancy: C

Additional Clinical Considerations:
- **Oral itraconazole:** Requires gastric acidity for absorption. When antacids are required, administer ≥ 1 hour before or 2 hours after itraconazole capsules.
- Oral solution is better absorbed without food (capsules are better absorbed with food).
- Capsule bioavailability is food dependent (40% fasting/90% post-prandial).
- For oral therapy, bioavailability of 10 mL of solution without food = 100 mg capsule with food.
- Administer with a cola beverage in patients with achlorhydria or taking H2-receptor antagonists/other gastric acid suppressors.
- Oral solution produces more reliable blood levels and is preferred for oral/esophageal candidiasis.
- **IV itraconazole:** Hydroxypropyl-b-cyclodextrin stabilizer in IV formulation accumulates in renal failure.
- IV itraconazole should not be used in patients with CrCl < 30 mL/min; (if possible, use the oral preparation).

Highly active against C. albicans, non-albicans Candida, Cryptococcus, Histoplasmosis, Blastomycosis, Paracoccidiomycosis, Sporotrichosis.

Active against dermatophytes.
No activity against Pseudallescheria/ Scedosporium, Fusaria or Mucor.

Bile Penetration: 3–18%
Cerebrospinal Fluid Penetration: < 10%

SELECTED REFERENCES:

Boogaerts M, Winston DJ, Bow EJ, et al. Intravenous and oral itraconazole versus intravenous amphotericin B deoxycholate as empirical antifungal therapy for persistent fever in neutropenic patients with cancer who are receiving broad-spectrum antibacterial therapy. A randomized controlled trial. Ann Intern Med 135:412–22, 2001. (PMID:11560454)

Bruggemann RJM, Alffenaar JWC, Blijlevens NMA, et al. Clinical relevance of the pharmoacokinetic interactions of azole antifungal drugs with coadministered agents. Clin Infect Dis 48:1441–1458, 2009. (PMID:19361301)

Calvopina M, Guevara AG, Armijos RX, et al. Itraconazole in the treatment of New World mucocutaneous leishmaniasis. Int J Dermatol 43:659–63, 2004. (PMID:15357745)

Caputo R. Itraconazole (Sporanox) in superficial and systemic fungal infections. Expert Rev Anti Infect Ther 1:531–42, 2004. (PMID:15482150)

Conte JE Jr, Golden JA, Kipps J, et al. Intrapulmonary pharmacokinetics and pharmacodynamics of itraconazole and 14-hydroxyitraconazol steady state. Antimicrob Agents Chemother 48:3823–7, 2004. (PMID:15388441)

Horousseau JL, Dekker AW, et al. Itraconazole oral solution for primary prophylaxis of fungal infections in patients with hematological malignancy and profound neutropenia: a randomized, double-blind, double-placebo, multicenter trial comparing itraconazole and amphotericin B. Antimicrob Agents Chemother 44:1887–93, 2000. (PMID:10858349)

——— = serious side effect ⬜ = black box warning. ND = no data. NR = not recommended. s = spectrum inadequate (at site). a = activity or experience inadequate. p = tissue penetration inadequate. *based on peak serum concentration after usual adult dose. †applicable to adult uncomplicated lower UTIs (CrCl > 30 mL/min).

Marks DI, Pagliuca A, Kibbler CC, et al. Voriconazole versus itraconazole for antifungal prophylaxis following allogeneic haematopoietic stem cell transplantation. Br J Haematol 155:318–327, 2011. (PMID:21880032)

Urunsak M, Ilkit M, Evruke C, et al. Clinical and mycological efficacy of single-day oral treatment with itraconazole (400 mg) in acute vulvovaginal candidosis. Mycoses 47:422–7, 2004. (PMID:15504127)

Website: www.pdr.net

Ketoconazole (Nizoral)

Drug Class: Azole antifungal.
Usual Dose: 200 mg (PO) q24h.
Pharmacokinetic Parameters:
Peak serum level: 3.5 mcg/mL
Bioavailability: 82%
Excreted unchanged (urine): 2–4%
Serum half-life (normal/ESRD): 6/20 hrs
Plasma protein binding: 99%
Volume of distribution (V_d): 2 L/kg
Primary Mode of Elimination: Hepatic
Dosage Adjustments*

CrCl < 40 mL/min	No change
Post–HD dose	None
Post–PD dose	None
CVVH/CVVHD/CVVHDF dose	No change
Moderate hepatic insufficiency	Use with caution
Severe hepatic insufficiency	Avoid

Drug Interactions: Astemizole, cisapride, terfenadine, amiodarone (may ↑ QT interval, torsades de pointes); carbamazepine, INH (↓ ketoconazole levels); cimetidine, famotidine, nizatidine, ranitidine, omeprazole, INH (↓ ketoconazole absorption); cyclosporine, digoxin, loratadine, tacrolimus (↑ interacting drug levels with possible toxicity); didanosine (↓ ketoconazole levels); midazolam, triazolam (↑ interacting drug levels, ↑ sedative effects); oral hypoglycemics (severe hypoglycemia); phenytoin, rifabutin, rifampin (↓ ketoconazole levels, ↑ interacting drug); statins (↑ statin levels; rhabdomyolysis reported); warfarin (↑ INR).
Adverse Effects:
Common
• Nausea/vomiting/diarrhea
Uncommon
• Abdominal pain
• Pruritus
Rare
• ↑ QTc
• Torsades de pointes
• Anaphylaxis
Contraindications:
• Serious hepatotoxicity, including fulminant hepatic failure
• Contraindicated with dofetilide, quinidine, pimozide, and cisapride
Allergic Potential: Low
Safety in Pregnancy: C

Additional Clinical Considerations:
• Dose-dependent reduction in gonadal (androgenic) function.
• Decreased cortisol production with doses ≥ 800 mg/day, but **does not result in adrenal insufficiency**.
• Give oral doses with citric juices.

───── = serious side effect ☐ = black box warning. ND = no data. NR = not recommended. s = spectrum inadequate (at site). a = activity or experience inadequate. p = tissue penetration inadequate. *based on peak serum concentration after usual adult dose. †applicable to adult uncomplicated lower UTIs (CrCl > 30 mL/min).

***Highly active** against dermatophytes, Malassezia, Candida albicans.*
***Some activity** against Aspergillus, Coccidiomycosis, Paracoccidio mycosis, Histoplasmosis.*
***No activity** against Pseudallescheria/ Scedosporium, Fusaria or Mucor.*

Cerebrospinal Fluid Penetration: < 10%

SUGGESTED REFERENCES:

Kaur IP, Kakkar S. Topical delivery of antifungal agents. Expert Opin Drug Deliv 7:1303–1327, 2010. (PMID:20961206)

Terrell CL. Antifungal agents: Part II. The azoles. Mayo Clin Proc 74:78–100, 1999. (PMID:9987539)

Zhao Y, Li L, Wang JJ, et al. Cutaneous malasseziasls: dermititis and omychomycosis caused by Malassezia. Int J Dermatol 49:141–145, 2010. (PMID:20465637)

Website: www.pdr.net

Lamivudine (Epivir) 3TC

Drug Class: HIV NRTI (nucleoside reverse transcriptase inhibitor); antiviral HBV.
Usual Dose: 150 mg (PO) q12h or 300 mg (PO) q24h (HIV); 100 mg (PO) q24h (HBV).
Pharmacokinetic Parameters:
Peak serum level: 1.5 mcg/mL
Bioavailability: 86%
Excreted unchanged (urine): 71%
Serum half-life (normal/ESRD): 5–7/20 hrs
Plasma protein binding: 36%
Volume of distribution (V_d): 1.3 L/kg
Primary Mode of Elimination: Renal
Dosage Adjustments* (HIV/HBV dose)

CrCl 30–50 mL/min	150 mg (PO) q24h /100 mg (PO), then 50 mg (PO) q24h
CrCl 15–30 mL/min	100 mg (PO) q24h /100 mg (PO), then 25 mg (PO) q24h
CrCl 5–15 mL/min	50 mg (PO) q24h /35 mg (PO), then 15 mg (PO) q24h
CrCl < 5 mL/min	25 mg (PO) q24h /35 mg (PO), then 10 mg (PO) q24h
Post–HD dose	25 mg (PO)/10 mg (PO)
Post–PD dose	None
CVVH/CVVHD/ CVVHDF dose	100 mg (PO) q24h /100 mg (PO), then 25 mg (PO) q24h
Moderate hepatic insufficiency	No change
Severe hepatic insufficiency	Use with caution

Drug Interactions: Didanosine, zalcitabine (↑ risk of pancreatitis); TMP–SMX (↑ lamivudine levels); zidovudine + lamivudine not recommended.
Adverse Effects:
Common
- Headache
- Nausea
- Nasal congestion
- Cough
- Malaise
- Neuropathy

───── = serious side effect ☐ = black box warning. ND = no data. NR = not recommended. s = spectrum inadequate (at site). a = activity or experience inadequate. p = tissue penetration inadequate. *based on peak serum concentration after usual adult dose. †applicable to adult uncomplicated lower UTIs (CrCl > 30 mL/min).

Uncommon
- Dizziness
- Drug rash
- Pancreatitis
- Leukopenia

Rare
- <u>Immune reconstitution syndrome (IRIS)</u>
- Lactic acidosis with hepatic steatosis
- Lamivudine to treat HIV contains a higher dose of lamivudine than Epivir-HB® used to treat chronic HBV. Severe acute exacerbations of HBV may occur in patients co-infected with HBV and HIV after discontinuing lamivudine.

Allergic Potential: Low
Safety in Pregnancy: C

Additional Clinical Considerations:
- Prevents development of AZT resistance and restores AZT susceptibility.
- May be taken with or without food.

Cerebrospinal Fluid Penetration: 15%

SELECTED REFERENCES:

Diaz-Brito V, Leon A, Knobel H, et al. Post-exposure prophylaxis for HIV-infection: a clinical trail comparing lopinavir/ritonavir versus atazanavir each with zidovudine/lamivudine. Antivir Ther 17:337–46, 2012. (PMID:22293542)

Liaw YF, Sung JY, Chow WC, et al. Lamivudine for patients with chronic hepatitis B and advanced liver disease. N Engl J Med 351:1521–31, 2004. (PMID:15470215)

Perry CM, Faulds D. Lamivudine. A review of its antiviral activity, pharmacokinetic properties and therapeutic efficacy in the management of HIV infection. Drugs 53:657–80, 1997. (PMID:9098665)

Sax PE, Tierney C, Collier AC, et al. Abacavir/lamivudine versus tenofovir DF/emtricitabine as part of combination regimens for initial treatment of HIV: final results. J Infect Dis 204:1191–201, 2011. (PMID:21917892)

Sheng YJ, Liu JY, Tong SW, et al. Lamivudine plus adefovir combination therapy versus entecavir monotherapy for lamivudine-resistant chronic hepatitis B: a systematic review and meta-analysis. Virol J. 8:393, 2011. (PMID:21824397)

Website: www.pdr.net

Lamivudine + Zidovudine (Combivir) 3TC/ZDV

Drug Class: HIV NRTIs combination.
Usual Dose: Combivir tablet = 150 mg lamivudine + 300 mg zidovudine. Usual dose = 1 tablet (PO) q12h.

Pharmacokinetic Parameters:
Peak serum level: 2.6/1.2 mcg/mL
Bioavailability: 82/60%
Excreted unchanged (urine): 86/64%
Serum half-life (normal/ESRD): [6/1.1]/[20/2.2] hrs
Plasma protein binding: <36/<38%
Volume of distribution (V_d): 1.3/1.6 L/kg

Primary Mode of Elimination: Renal

Dosage Adjustments*

CrCl 50–80 mL/min	No change
CrCl 10–50 mL/min	Avoid
CrCl < 10 mL/min	Avoid
Post–HD dose	Avoid
Post–PD dose	Avoid
CVVH/CVVHD/CVVHDF dose	Avoid
Moderate hepatic insufficiency	Avoid
Severe hepatic insufficiency	Avoid

―――― = serious side effect ☐ = black box warning. ND = no data. NR = not recommended. s = spectrum inadequate (at site). a = activity or experience inadequate. p = tissue penetration inadequate. *based on peak serum concentration after usual adult dose. †applicable to adult uncomplicated lower UTIs (CrCl > 30 mL/min).

Drug Interactions: Atovaquone (↑ zidovudine levels); stavudine (antagonist to stavudine; avoid combination); ganciclovir, doxorubicin (neutropenia); tipranavir (↓ zidovudine levels); TMP–SMX (↑ lamivudine and zidovudine levels); vinca alkaloids (neutropenia).

Adverse Effects:

Common
- Nausea/vomiting/diarrhea
- Anorexia
- Headache
- Malaise/fatigue
- Fever/chills

Uncommon
- Insomnia
- Peripheral neuropathy
- Pancreatitis

Rare
- Immune reconstitution syndrome (IRIS)
- Fat redistribution/accumulation
- Lactic acidosis with hepatic steatosis
- Zidovudine has been associated with hematologic toxicity including neutropenia and severe anemia. Prolonged used of zidovudine has been associated with symptomatic myopathy. Lactic acidosis and severe hepatomegaly with steatosis, including fatal cases. Severe acute exacerbations of HBV have been reported in patients co-infected with HBV after discontinuing lamivudine.

Allergic Potential: Low
Safety in Pregnancy: C.

Cerebrospinal Fluid Penetration:
Lamivudine = 12%; Zidovudine = 60%

SELECTED REFERENCE:
Website: www.pdr.net

Leflunomide (Arava)

Drug Class: Antiviral (CMV).
Usual Dose: 100 mg/day (PO) × 3 days, then 20 mg (PO) q24h.

Pharmacokinetic Parameters:
Peak serum level: 8 mcg/mL
Bioavailability: 80%
Excreted unchanged: 0%
Serum half-life (normal/ESRD): 14 days/ no data
Plasma protein binding: 99%
Volume of distribution (V_d): 0.13 L/kg

Primary Mode of Elimination: Hepatic/ Renal

Dosage Adjustments*

CrCl 15–30 mL/min	Use with caution
CrCl < 15 mL/min	Use with caution
Post–HD dose	Use with caution
Post–PD dose	Use with caution
CVVH/CVVHD/ CVVHDF dose	Use with caution
Moderate— severe hepatic insufficiency	Avoid if ↑ SGOT/ SGPT > 2 × n or pre-existing liver disease

Drug Interactions: May inhibit CYP 2C9; rifampin (↑ levels of active metabolite, M1); hepatotoxic drugs.

Adverse Effects:

Common
- Headache

—— = serious side effect ⬜ = black box warning. ND = no data. NR = not recommended. s = spectrum inadequate (at site). a = activity or experience inadequate. p = tissue penetration inadequate. *based on peak serum concentration after usual adult dose. †applicable to adult uncomplicated lower UTIs (CrCl > 30 mL/min).

- Nausea/diarrhea
- Alopecia
- Rash
- Respiratory tract infections

Uncommon
- Hypertension
- Hypersensitivity reactions
- Abdominal and back pain
- ↑ AST/ALT
- Severe liver injury including fulminant hepatotoxicity

Rare
- Interstitial lung disease
- Stevens-Johnson syndrome
- TEN
- Teratogenicity and embryolethality

Allergic Potential: Low
Safety in Pregnancy: X

Additional Clinical Considerations:
- Alternate therapy of CMV after 1st line therapies fail.
- Do not use with pre-existing liver disease; metabolized to active metabolite (M1).
- Not recommended in patients with severe, uncontrolled infections, bone marrow dysplasia or severe immunodeficiency.
- Prolonged administration leads to significant accumulation.
- Screen for TB before starting leflunomide.
- Avoid live vaccinations while on leflunomide.
- *Discontinue if ↑ AST/ALT > 3 × n.*

SELECTED REFERENCES:
Avery RK, et al. Utility of leflunomide in the treatment of complex cytomegalovirus syndromes. Transplantation 90:419–26, 2010. (PMID:20683281)
Chacko B, John GT. Leflunomide for cytomegalovirus: bench to bedside. Transpl Infest Dis 14:111–20, 2012. (PMID:22093814)
Website: www.pdr.net

Levofloxacin (Levaquin)

Drug Class: Respiratory quinolone.
Usual Dose: 500–750 mg (IV/PO) q24h.

Spectrum Synopsis*
Hits
  Gram + : Non-enterococcal streptococci, most MSSA, most VSE
  Gram – : Most GNB (including P. aeruginosa)
  Problem pathogens: Some Acinetobacter
Misses
  Gram + : MRSA, VRE
  Gram – : B. fragilis
  Problem pathogens: Listeria, Nocardia Most Acinetobacter, S. maltophilia, B. cepacia
Urine Spectrum[+]:
- Same as serum spectrum
- Optimal urinary pH = 6–7
- Urine levels = 300 mcg/mL

(Full **Susceptibility Profiles** p. 208).

Resistance Potential: Low
Pharmacokinetic Parameters:
  Peak serum level: 5–8 mcg/mL

= serious side effect [ ] = black box warning. ND = no data. NR = not recommended. s = spectrum inadequate (at site). a = activity or experience inadequate. p = tissue penetration inadequate. *based on peak serum concentration after usual adult dose. [+]applicable to adult uncomplicated lower UTIs (CrCl > 30 mL/min).

Bioavailability: 99%
Excreted unchanged (urine): 87%
Serum half-life (normal/ESRD): 7 hrs/40 hrs
Plasma protein binding: 30%
Volume of distribution (V_d): 1.3 L/kg

Primary Mode of Elimination: Renal

Dosage Adjustments* (based on 750 mg/500 mg (V/PO) q24h

CrCl > 50 mL/min	No change
CrCl 20–50 mL/min	750 mg (IV/PO) q48h/500 mg (IV/PO), then 250 mg (IV/PO) q24h
CrCl < 20 mL/min	750 mg (IV/PO) then 500 mg (IV/PO), q48h/500 mg (IV/PO), then 250 mg (IV/PO) q48h
HD/CAPD dose	500 mg (IV/PO) q48h
Post-HD dose	None
Post-HFHD dose	250 mg (IV/PO)
Post-PD dose	250 mg (IV/PO)
CVVH/CVVHD/CVVHDF dose	500 mg (IV/PO) q48h/250 mg (IV/PO) q24h
HD q48-72h dose	500 mg (IV/PO) q HD*
Moderate hepatic insufficiency	No change
Severe hepatic insufficiency	No change

*Give at end of HD.

Drug Interactions: Al^{++}, Fe^{++}, Mg^{++}, Zn^{++} antacids (↓ absorption of levofloxacin if taken together); NSAIDs (CNS stimulation); probenecid (↑levofloxacin levels); warfarin (↑ INR).

Adverse Effects:

Uncommon
- Headache
- Insomnia
- AGEP (acute generalized exanthematous pustulosis)

Rare
- ↑ QTc
- Peripheral neuropathy
- Delirium
- Tendinitis and tendon rupture
- C. difficile diarrhea/colitis (↑ risk with PPIs)

Allergic Potential: Low
Safety in Pregnancy: C

Additional Clinical Considerations:
- Take 2 hours before or after aluminum/magnesium-containing antacids.
- Does not increase digoxin concentrations.
- May ↑ QTc interval, particularly in patients with predisposing conditions or medications e.g., amiodarone
- **Acute bacterial sinusitis dose:** 750 mg (PO) q24h × 5 days.
- **CAP dose:** 750 mg (IV/PO) q24h × 5 days.
- **Nosocomial pneumonia dose:** 750 mg (IV/PO) q24h × 7–14 days.
- **cSSSI dose:** 750 mg (IV/PO) q24h × 7-14 days.
- **TB dose (alternate drug in MDR TB regimen):** 500 mg (PO) q24h.

—— = serious side effect ☐ = black box warning. ND = no data. NR = not recommended. s = spectrum inadequate (at site). a = activity or experience inadequate. p = tissue penetration inadequate. *based on peak serum concentration after usual adult dose. †applicable to adult uncomplicated lower UTIs (CrCl > 30 mL/min).

- **Complicated UTI/acute pylonephritis dose:** 750 mg (IV/PO) q24h × 5 days.
- **↑ incidence of C. difficile diarrhea/colitis with PPIs (for patients on PPIs during FQ therapy, D/C PPIs or switch to H2 blocker for duration of FQ therapy).**
- Effective against oral anaerobes/above the waist but not anaerobes below the waist e.g. B. fragilis.

May inhibit antibiotic induced LPS (endotoxin) release from GNB potentially minimizing endotoxin mediated tissue damage.

Additional Pharmacokinetic Considerations*

Non-CSF	% of Serum Levels
Peritoneal fluid	100%
Bile	100%
Synovial fluid	100%
Bone	100%
Prostate	100%
CSF	
Non-inflamed meninges	<1%
Inflamed meninges (ABM)	15%

(also see **Antibiotic Pearls & Pitfalls** p. 533).

SELECTED REFERENCES:

Alvarez-Lerma F, Grau S, Alvarez-Beltran. Levofloxacin in the treatment of ventilator-associated pneumonia. Clin Microbiol Infect 12:81–92, 2006. (PMID:16669931)

Bucaneve G, Micozzi A, Menichetti F, et al. Levofloxacin to prevent bacterial infection in patients with cancer and neutropenia. N Engl J Med 353:977–87, 2005. (PMID:16148283)

Chou HW, Wang JL, Chang CH, et al. Risk of severe dysglycemia among diabetic patients receiving levofloxacin, ciprofloxacin, or moxifloxacin in Taiwan. Clin Infect Dis 57:971-980, 2013. (PMID:23948133)

File TM Jr, Milkovich G, Tennenberg AM, et al. Clinical implications of 750 mg, 5-day levofloxacin for the treatment of community-acquired pneumonia. Curr Med Res Opin 20:1473–81, 2004. (PMID:15383197)

Garcia-Vazquez E, Mensa J, Sarasa M, et al. Penetration of levofloxacin into the anterior chamber (aqueous humour) of the human eye after intravenous administration. Eur J Clin Microbiol Infect Dis 26:137–140, 2007. (PMID:17216423)

Gergs U, Ihlefeld D, Clauss T, et al. Population Pharmacokinetics of Levofloxacin in Plasma and Bone of Patients Undergoing Hip or Knee Surgery. Clin Pharmacol Drug Dev 7:692-698, 2018. (PMID: 29251833)

Heffernan AJ, Sime FB, Lipman J, et al. Intrapulmonary pharmacokinetics of antibiotics used to treat nosocomial pneumonia caused by gram-negative bacilli: a systematic review. Int J Antimicrob Agents. [Epub ahead of print]. 2018. (PMID: 30472292)

Klausner HA, Brown P, Peterson J, et al. Double-blind, randomized comparison of levofloxacin 750 mg once daily for 5 days versus ciprofloxin for 10 days in the treatment of acute pyelonephritis. Curr Med Res Opin 23:2637–2645, 2007. (PMID:17880755)

Kuriyama T, Williams DW, Yanagisawa M, et al. Antimicrobial susceptibility of 800 anaerobic isolates from patients with dentoalveolar infection to 13 oral antibiotics. Oral Microbiol Immunol 22:285–288, 2007. (PMID:1760050)

Lee CK, Boyle MP, Diener-West M, et al. Levofloxacin pharmacokinetics in adult cystic fibrosis. Chest 131:796–802, 2007. (PMID:17356095)

Marchetti F, Viale P. Current and future perspectives for levofloxacin in severe Pseudomonas aeruginosa infections. J Chemotherapy 15:315–322, 2003. (PMID:12962358)

Maurin M, Raoult D. Bacteriostatic and bactericidal activity of levofloxacin against Rickettsia rickettsii, Rickettsia conorii, 'Israel spotted fever group rickettsii' and Coxiella burnetii. Journal of Antimicrobial Chemotherapy 39:725–30, 1997. (PMID:9222041)

——— = serious side effect ☐ = black box warning. ND = no data. NR = not recommended. s = spectrum inadequate (at site). a = activity or experience inadequate. p = tissue penetration inadequate. *based on peak serum concentration after usual adult dose. †applicable to adult uncomplicated lower UTIs (CrCl > 30 mL/min).

Nightingale CH, Grant EM, Quintiliani R. Pharmacodynamics and pharmacokinetics of levofloxacin. Chemotherapy 46:6–14, 2000. (PMID:10810208)

Nista EC, Candelli M, Zocco, MA, et al. Levofloxacin-based triple therapy in first-line treatment for Helicobacter pylori eradication. Am J Gastroenterol 101:1985–90, 2006. (PMID:16968503)

Pankey GA, Ashcraft DS. In vitro synergistic/additive activity of levofloxacin with meropenem against Stenotrophomonas maltophilia. Diagn Microbiol Infect Dis 67:297–300, 2010. (PMID:20542209)

Pugh RJ, Cooke RPD, Dempsey G. Short course antibiotic therapy for Gram-negative hospital-acquired pneumonia in the critically ill. J of Hosp Infect 74:337–343, 2010. (PMID:20202717)

Website: www.pdr.net

Linezolid (Zyvox)

Drug Class: Oxazolidinone.
Usual Dose: 600 mg (IV/PO) q12h.

Spectrum Synopsis*
Hits
Gram + : All streptococci, MSSA, MRSA, Most CoNS, VSE, VRE
Gram – : None
Problem pathogens: Corynebacterium JK, Listeria, Nocardia, M. abscessus
Misses
Gram + : Misses ~25% of CoNS, "tolerant" strains of MSSA, MRSA, Group D enterococci
Gram – : B. fragilis
Problem pathogens: Listeria, Nocardia, Acinetobacter, S. maltophilia, B. cepacia

(Full *Susceptibility Profiles* p. 208).

Resistance Potential: Low
Pharmacokinetic Parameters:
 Peak serum level: 15–21 mcg/mL
 Bioavailability: 100% (IV and PO)
 Excreted unchanged (urine): 30%
 Serum half-life (normal/ESRD): 6.4/7.1 hrs
 Plasma protein binding: 31%
 Volume of distribution (V_d): 0.64 L/kg
Primary Mode of Elimination: Hepatic/ Metabolized
Dosage Adjustments*

CrCl < 10 mL/min	No change
Post–HD dose	600 mg (IV/PO)
Post–PD dose	None
CVVH/CVVHD/CVVHDF dose	No change
Moderate hepatic insufficiency	No change
Severe hepatic insufficiency	Use with caution

Drug Interactions: Pseudoephedrine, tyramine-containing foods (↑ risk of hypertensive crisis); Serotonin syndrome: fever, delerium, hypertension, tremor/ clonus, hyperreflexia. Serotonergic agents, e.g., SSRIs, MAOIs, St. John's wort, ritonavir (↑ risk of serotonin syndrome).
Adverse Effects:
Common
- Headache
- Nausea/vomiting/diarrhea
- Mild/reversible thrombocytopenia
- Leukopenia

───── = serious side effect ☐ = black box warning. ND = no data. NR = not recommended. s = spectrum inadequate (at site). a = activity or experience inadequate. p = tissue penetration inadequate. *based on peak serum concentration after usual adult dose. †applicable to adult uncomplicated lower UTIs (CrCl > 30 mL/min).

Uncommon
- ↑ AST/ALT
- ↑ Bilirubin
- <u>Myelosuppression (usually reversible after 2 weeks)</u>

Rare
- <u>Lactic acidosis</u>
- Hypoglycemia
- <u>Optic neuritis</u>
- <u>Peripheral neuropathy</u>

Allergic Potential: Low
Safety in Pregnancy: C

Additional Clinical Considerations:
- ***Ideal for IV-to-PO switch programs.***
- Unlike vancomycin, ***linezolid use does not increase VRE prevalence.***
- Unlike quinupristin/dalfopristin, linezolid is active against E. faecalis (VSE).
- **Effective oral therapy for MRSA, MRSE, and E. faecium (VRE) infections.**
- *Alternate therapy for Nocardia and Listeria infections.*
- Protective against C. difficile.

Additional Pharmacokinetic Considerations*

Non-CSF	% of Serum Levels
Peritoneal fluid	NR(s)
Bile	200%
Synovial fluid	25%
Bone	50%
Prostate	NR(s)
CSF	
Non-inflamed meninges	ND
Inflamed meninges (ABM)	70%

Meningeal dose:
 Meningeal dose = usual dose

(also see ***Antibiotic Pearls & Pitfalls*** p. 535).

SELECTED REFERENCES:

Aeziokoro CO, Cannon JP, Pachucki CT, et al. The effectiveness and safety of oral linezolid for the primary and secondary treatment of osteomyelitis. J Chemother 17:643–50, 2005. (PMID:16433195)

Bassetti M, Bagueid M, Bouza E, et al. European perspective and update on the management of complicated skin and soft tissue infections due to methicillin-resistant Staphylococcus aureus after more than 10 years of experience with linezolid. Clin Microb Infect. 4:3-18, 2014. (PMID:24580738)

Bassetti M, Vitale F, Melica G, et al. Linezolid in the treatment of gram-positive prosthetic joint infections. J Antimicrob Chemother 55:387–390, 2005. (PMID:15705640)

Castro P, Soriano A, Escrich C, Villalba G, et al. Linezolid treatment of ventriculoperitoneal shunt infection without implant removal. Eur J Clin Microbiol Infect Dis 24:603–606, 2005. (PMID:16187055)

Chang KC, Leung CC, Daley CL. Linezolid for multidrug-resistant tuberculosis. Lancet Infect Dis 12:502–3, 2012. (PMID:22742623)

Colli A, Compodonico R, Gherli T. Early switch from vancomycin to oral linezolid for treatment of gram-positive heart valve endocarditis. Ann Thorac Surg 84:87–91, 2007. (PMID:17588391)

Conte JE Jr, Golden JA, Dipps J, et al. Intrapulmonary pharmacokinetics of linezolid. Antimicrob Agents Chemother 46:1475–1480, 2002. (PMID:11959585)

Cunha BA, Jaber N, Blum S. Antibiotic Stewardship Implications of Empiric Vancomycin or Linezolid for Ventilator Associated Pneumonia: MRSA Coverage has no effect on outcomes.

Cunha BA. Antimicrobial therapy of multidrug-resistant Streptococccus pneumoniae, vancomycin-resistant enterococci, and methicillin-resistant Staphyloccus aureus. Med Clin N Am 90:1165–82, 2006. (PMID:17116442)

—— = serious side effect ☐ = black box warning. ND = no data. NR = not recommended. s = spectrum inadequate (at site). a = activity or experience inadequate. p = tissue penetration inadequate. *based on peak serum concentration after usual adult dose. †applicable to adult uncomplicated lower UTIs (CrCl > 30 mL/min).

International Journal Of Antimicrobial Agents 13:27-28, 2018. (PMID: 29909171)

Cunha BA. Oral antibiotic therapy of serious systemic infections. Med Clin N Am 90:1197–1222, 2006. (PMID:17116444)

Estes KS, Derendorf H. Comparison of the pharmacokinetic properties of vancomycin, linezolid, tigecycline, and daptomycin. Eur J. Med Res 15:533–543, 2010. (PMID:21163728)

Falagas ME, Manta KG, Ntziora F, et al. Linezolid for the treatment of patients with endocarditis: a systematic review of published evidence. J Antimicrob Chemother 58:273–280, 2006. (PMID:16735427)

Hill EE, Herijgers P, Herregods MC, Peetermans WE. Infective endocarditis treated with linezolid: case report and literature review. Eur J Clin Microbiol Infect Dis 25:202–4, 2006. (PMID:1652577)

Hoyo I, Martinez-Pastor J, Garcia-Ramiro S, et al. Decreased serum linezolid concentrations in two patients receiving linezolid and rifampicin due to bone infections. Scand J Infect Dis 44:548–50, 2012. (PMID:2238532)

Joson J, Grover C, Downer C, et al. Successful treatment of methicillin-resistant Staphylococcus aureus mitral valve endocarditis with sequential linezolid and telavancin monotherapy following daptomycin failure. J Antimicrob Chemother 66:2186–2188, 2011. (PMID:21653600)

Johnson JR. Linezolid versus vancomycin for methicillin-resistant Staphylococcus aureus infections. Clin Infect Dis 36:236–7, 2003. (PMID:12522761)

Kruse AJ, Peederman SM, Bet PM, Debets-Oseenkopp YJ. Successful treatment with linezolid of meningitis due to methicillin-resistant Staphylococcus epidermidis refractory to vancomycin treatment. Eur J Clin Microb Infect 215:135–7, 2006. (PMID:16474940)

Kutscha-Lissberg F, Hebler U, Muhr G, et al. Linezolid penetration into bone and joint tissues infected with methicillin-resistant staphylococci. Antimicrob Agents Chemother 47:3964–6, 2003. (PMID:14638510)

Lauridsen TK, Bruun LE, Rasmussen RV, et al. Linezolid as rescue treatment for left-sided infective endocarditis: an observational, retrospective, multicenter study. Eur J Clin Microbiol Infect Dis 31:2567–2574, 2012. (PMID:22431272)

Lawrence KR, Adra M, Gillman PK. Serotonin toxicity associated with the use of linezolid: a review of postmarketing data. Clin Infect Dis 42:1578–83, 2006. (PMID:16652315)

Mikamo H, Takesue Y, Iwamoto Y, et al. Efficacy, safety and pharmacokinetics of tedizolid versus linezolid in patients with skin and soft tissue infections in Japan - Results of a randomized, multicentre phase 3 study. J infect chemother 24:434-42, 2018. (PMID: 29530544)

Moreillon P, Wilson WR, Leclercq R, et al. Single-dose oral amoxicillin or linezolid for prophylaxis of experimental endocarditis due to vancomycin-susceptible and vancomycin-resistant Enterococcus faecalis. Antimicrob Agents Chemother 51:1661–1665, 2007. (PMID:17353251)

Myrianthefs P, Markantonis SL, Vlachos K, et al. Serum and cerebrospinal fluid concentrations of linezolid in neurosurgical patients. Antimicrob Agents Chemother 50:3971–76, 2006. (PMID:16982782)

Ravindran V, John J, Kaye GC, et al. Successful use of oral linezolid as a single active agent in endocarditis unresponsive to conventional antibiotic therapy. J Infect 47:164–6, 2003. (PMID:12860152)

Rao N, Ziran BH, Hall RA, et al. Successful treatment of chronic bone and joint infections with oral linezolid. Clin Orthop 427:67–71, 2004. (PMID:15552139)

Schecter GF, Scott C, True L, et al. Linezolid in the treatment of multidrug-resistant tuberculosis. Clin Infect Dis 50:49–55, 2010. (PMID:19947856)

Siegel RE. Linezolid to decrease length of stay in the hospital for patients with methicillin-resistant Staphylococcus aureus infection. Clin Infect Dis 36:124–5, 2003. (PMID:12491215)

Souli M, Pontikis K, Chryssouli Z, et al. Successful treatment of right-sided prosthetic valve endocarditis due to methicillin-resistant teicoplanin-heteroresistant Staphylococcus

---

= serious side effect [_____] = black box warning. ND = no data. NR = not recommended. s = spectrum inadequate (at site). a = activity or experience inadequate. p = tissue penetration inadequate. *based on peak serum concentration after usual adult dose. †applicable to adult uncomplicated lower UTIs (CrCl > 30 mL/min).

aureus with linezolid. Eur J Clin Microbiol Infect Dis 24:760–762, 2005. (PMID:16283218)

Stein GE, Schooley SL, Havlichek DH, et al. Outpatient intravenous antibiotic therapy compared with oral linezolid in patients with skin and soft tissue infections: a pharmacoeconomic analysis. Infectious Dis in Clin Practice 16:235–240, 2008. (PMID:20055750)

Stevens DL, Herr D, Lampiris H, et al. Linezolid versus vancomycin for the treatment of methicillin-resistant Staphylococcus aureus infections. Clin Infect Dis 34:1481–90, 2002. (PMID:12015695)

Valerio M, Pedromingo M, Munoz P, et al. Potential protective role of linezolid against Clostridium difficile infection. Int J Antimicrob Agents 39:414–9, 2012. (PMID:22445203)

Villani P, Pegazzi MB, Marubbi F, et al. Cerebrospinal fluid linezolid concentrations in postneurosurgical central nervous system infections. Antimicrob Agents Chemother 46:936–7, 2002. 11850294)

Viswanathan P, Iarikov D, Wassel R, Davidson A, Nambiar S. Hypoglycemia in patients treated with linezolid. Clin Infect Dis 59:634-635, 2014. (PMID:2496534)

Zhang L, Pang Y, Yu X, et al. Linezolid in the treatment of extensively drug-resistant tuberculosis. Infection. 42:705-711, 2014. (PMID:24902521)

Website: www.pdr.net

Lopinavir + Ritonavir (Kaletra) LPV/RTV

Drug Class: HIV protease inhibitor combination.

Usual Dose: Therapy-naive: 400/100 mg q12h or 800/200 mg q24h (if <3 lopinavir resistance—associated substitutions).

Pharmacokinetic Parameters:
Peak serum level: 9.6/≤ 1 mcg/mL
Bioavailability: No data
Excreted unchanged (urine): 3%
Serum half-life (normal/ESRD): 5–6/ 5–6 hrs
Plasma protein binding: 99%
Volume of distribution (V_d): No data/ 0.44 L/kg

Primary Mode of Elimination: Hepatic

Dosage Adjustments*

CrCl < 10 mL/min	No change
Post–HD dose	None
Post–PD dose	None
CVVH/CVVHD/ CVVHDF dose	No change
Moderate hepatic insufficiency	No change
Severe hepatic insufficiency	Avoid

Antiretroviral Dosage Adjustments

Fosamprenavir	Avoid
Delavirdine	No data
Efavirenz	Consider lopinavir/ ritonavir 500/125 mg q12h
Indinavir	Indinavir 600 mg q12h
Nelfinavir	Same as for efavirenz
Nevirapine	Same as for efavirenz
Rifabutin	Max. dose of rifa-butin 150 mg qod or 3 times per week
Saquinavir	Saquinavir 1000 mg q12h

Drug Interactions: Antiretrovirals, rifabutin, (see dose adjustment grid, above); Rifampin may reduce lopinavir levels leading to drug failure and should be avoided. Sidenafil, tadalafil, and virdenafil levels will be greatly increased and their dosage must be decreased. Antiarhythmics such as amiodarone, bepredil, lidocaine and quinidine may increase levels. Once daily dosing not recommended in pregnancy or for patients receiving efavirenz, nevirapine, fosamprenavir, nelfinavir, carbamazepine, phenytoin, or phenobarbital. Tacrolimus, cyclosporine and rapamycin levels can be altered leading to increased toxicity. Methadone levels may be decreased leading to withdrawal reactions. Fluticasone levels may increase leading to Cushing like syndrome, astemizole, terfenadine, benzodiazepines, cisapride, ergotamine, flecainide, pimozide, propafenone, rifampin, statins, tenofovir ($\downarrow$ lopinavir levels, $\uparrow$ tenofovir levels). $\downarrow$ effectiveness of oral contraceptives. Insufficient data on other drug interactions listed for ritonavir alone. At end of drug interaction add lopinavir/ resolution contains alcohol and can lead to a disulfram reaction when administered with metronidazole clarithromycin ($\uparrow$ QT$_c$).
Contraindications: St. John's wort, boceprevir, telaprevir, rifapentine.
Adverse Effects:
Common
- Diarrhea
- Nausea/vomiting
- $\uparrow$ AST/ALT
- Abdominal pain

- Hyperlipidemia
- <u>Fat redistribution/accumulation</u>
Uncommon
- Headache
- Paresthesias
- Asthenia
- Hepatotoxicity
- Hyperglycemia
- $\uparrow$ Uric acid
- $\uparrow$ CPK
- Pancreatitis
Rare
- <u>Immune reconstitution syndrome (IRIS)</u>
Allergic Potential: Low
Safety in Pregnancy: C

Additional Clinical Considerations:
- Tablet may be taken with or without food.
- With oral solution, Lopinavir serum concentrations increased 54% with moderately fatty meals.

SELECTED REFERENCE:
Website: www.pdr.net

Loracarbef (Lorabid)

Drug Class: 2nd generation oral cephalosporin.
Usual Dose: 400 mg (PO) q12h (*take without food*).

Spectrum Synopsis*
Hits
  Gram + : All non-enterococcal streptococci (including S. pneumoniae)

—— = serious side effect ☐ = black box warning. ND = no data. NR = not recommended. s = spectrum inadequate (at site). a = activity or experience inadequate. p = tissue penetration inadequate. *based on peak serum concentration after usual adult dose. †applicable to adult uncomplicated lower UTIs (CrCl > 30 mL/min).

Gram – : Some GNB (including
Klebsiella, H. influenzae)
Problem pathogens:
None
Misses
Gram + : MSSA, MRSA, VSE, VRE
Gram – : Most GNB (including
Proteus, P. aeruginosa), B. fragilis
Problem pathogens:
Listeria, Nocardia, Acinetobacter,
S. maltophilia, B. cepacia

(Full *Susceptibility Profiles* p. 201).

Resistance Potential: Low
Pharmacokinetic Parameters:
Peak serum level: 14 mcg/mL
Bioavailability: 90%
Excreted unchanged (urine): 90%
Serum half-life (normal/ESRD): 1.2/32 hrs
Plasma protein binding: 25%
Volume of distribution (V_d): 0.35 L/kg
Primary Mode of Elimination: Renal
Dosage Adjustments*

CrCl 10–50 mL/min	200 mg (PO) q24h
CrCl < 10 mL/min	200 mg (PO) q72h
Post–HD dose	400 mg (PO)
Post–PD dose	200 mg (PO)
CVVH/CVVHD/ CVVHDF dose	200 mg (PO) q12h
Moderate hepatic insufficiency	No change
Severe hepatic insufficiency	No change

Drug Interactions: None.
Adverse Effects:
Common
• Drug fever/rash
Uncommon
• ↑ AST/ALT
Rare
• C. difficile diarrhea/colitis
Allergic Potential: Low
Safety in Pregnancy: B

Additional Clinical Considerations:
• **CAP dose:** 400 mg (PO) q12h.
• **Sinusitis/tonsillitis dose:** 200 mg
(PO) q12h.

Cerebrospinal Fluid Penetration: < 10%

(also see *Antibiotic Pearls & Pitfalls*
p. 528).

SELECTED REFERENCE:
Website: www.pdr.net

Meropenem (Merrem/ Meronem)

Drug Class: Carbapenem.
Usual Dose: 1 gm (IV) q8h

Spectrum Synopsis*
Hits
Gram + : Non-enterococcal
streptococci, CoNS, MSSA, VSE
Gram – : Most aerobic GNB,
P. aeruginosa, B. fragilis
Problem pathogens:
Some Acinetobacter, Klebsiella,
Enterobacter, Serratia

_____ = serious side effect [⬜] = black box warning. ND = no data. NR = not recommended. s = spectrum inadequate (at site). a = activity or experience inadequate. p = tissue penetration inadequate.
*based on peak serum concentration after usual adult dose. †applicable to adult uncomplicated lower UTIs
(CrCl > 30 mL/min).

Misses
   Gram + : MRSA, VRE
   Gram − : Some MDR P. aeruginosa
   Problem pathogens:
      S. maltophilia, CRE
Urine Spectrum†
* Same as serum spectrum
* Optimal urinary pH = unaffected by urine pH
* Urine levels = 1000 mcg/mL

(Full *Susceptibility Profiles* p. 208).

Resistance Potential: Low
Pharmacokinetic Parameters:
   Peak serum level: 49 mcg/mL
   Bioavailability: Not applicable
   Excreted unchanged (urine): 70%
   Serum half-life (normal/ESRD): 1/7 hrs
   Plasma protein binding: 2%
   Volume of distribution (V_d): 0.35 L/kg
Primary Mode of Elimination: Renal
Dosage Adjustments* (based on 1 gm dose; for 500 mg dosing use half of dose shown in grid)

CrCl 25–50 mL/min	1 gm (IV) q12h
CrCl 10–25 mL/min	500 mg (IV) q12h
CrCl < 10 mL/min	500 mg (IV) q24h
Post–HD dose	500 mg (IV)
Post–HFHD dose	500 mg (IV)
Post–PD dose	500 mg (IV)
CVVH/CVVHD/CVVHDF dose	1 gm (IV) q12h

HD q 48–72h dose	2 gm (IV) q HD*
Moderate hepatic insufficiency	No change
Severe hepatic insufficiency	No change

*Give at end of HD.

Drug Interactions: Probenecid (↑ meropenem half-life by 40%), valproic acid (↓ seizure threshold).

Adverse Effects:
Uncommon
* Headache
Rare
* C. difficile diarrhea/colitis Meningeal meropenem (↓ voriconazole levels)
Allergic Potential: Low
Safety in Pregnancy: B

Additional Clinical Considerations:
* *MDR GNBs, cystic fibrosis/ meningitis dose:* 2 gm (IV) q8h
* *uSSSIs/UTIs dose:* 500 mg (IV) q8h.
* **Meropenem is the *only carbapenem that may be given by IV bolus injection***

   May inhibit antibiotic induced LPS (endotoxin) release from GNB potentially minimizing endotoxin mediated tissue damage.

Additional Pharmacokinetic Considerations*

Non-CSF	% of Serum Levels
Peritoneal fluid	100%
Bile	75%§

──── = serious side effect ☐ = black box warning. ND = no data. NR = not recommended. s = spectrum inadequate (at site). a = activity or experience inadequate. p = tissue penetration inadequate. *based on peak serum concentration after usual adult dose. †applicable to adult uncomplicated lower UTIs (CrCl > 30 mL/min).

Synovial fluid	40%
Bone	15%
Prostate	NR 15%
CSF	
Non-inflamed meninges	10%
Inflamed meninges (ABM)	15%
Meningeal Dose = 2 gm (IV) q8h	
§ with obstruction = 40%	

(also see **Antibiotic Pearls & Pitfalls** p. 529).

SELECTED REFERENCES:

Berman SJ, Fogarty CM, Fabian T, et al. Meropenem monotherapy for the treatment of hospital-acquired pneumonia: results of a multicenter trial. J Chemother 16:362–71, 2004. (PMID:15332712)

Cheng AC, Fisher DA, Anstey NM, et al. Outcomes of patients with melioidosis treated with meropenem. Antimicrob Agents Chemother 48:1763–5, 2004. (PMID:15105132)

Conte JE Jr, Golden JA, Kelley MG, Zurlinden E. Intrapulmonary pharmacokinetics and pharmacodynamics of meropenem. Int J Antimicrob Agents 26:449–56, 2005. (PMID:16280244)

Cunha BA. No need for an initial test dose of meropenem or ertapenem in patients reporting anaphylactic reactions to penicillins. J. Chemo 27:317-318, 2015. (PMID:25566799)

Cunha BA. Meropenem: lack of cross reactivity in penicillin allergic patients. Journal of Chemotherapy 20:233–237, 2008. (PMID:18467251)

Cunha BA. The safety of meropenem in elderly and renally impaired patients. Intern J Antimicrob Ther 11:167–179, 1999. (PMID:10221422)

Doh K, Woo H, Hur J, et al. Population pharmacokinetics of meropenem in burn patients. J Antimicrob Chemother 65:2428–2435, 2010. (PMID:20817742)

Louie A, Grasso C, Bahniuk N, et al. The combination of meropenem and levofloxacin is synergistic with respect to both Pseudomonas aeruginosa kill rate and resistance suppression. Antimicrob Agents Chemother 54:2646–2654, 2010. (PMID:20368395)

Pankey GA, Ashcraft DS. In vitro synergistic/additive activity of levofloxacin with meropenem against Stenotrophomonas maltophilia. Diagn Microbiol Infect Dis 67:297–300, 2010. (PMID:20542209)

Romano A, Viola M, Gueant-Rodriguez R, et al. Tolerability of meropenem in patients with IgE-mediated hypersensitivity of penicillins. Ann Intern Med 146:266–69, 2007. (PMID:17310050)

Taccone FS, Cotton F, Roisin S, et al. Optimal meropenem concentrations to treat multidrug-resistant Pseudomonas aeruginosa septic shock. Antimicrob Agents Chemother 56:2129–31, 2012. (PMID:22290984)

Yamada Y, Ikawa K, Nakamura K, et al. Prostatic penetration of meropenem after intravenous administration in patients undergoing transurethral resection fo the prostate. J Chemother 23:179–180, 2011. (PMID:21742590)

Website: www.pdr.net

Meropenem/Vaborbactam (Vabomere, Melinta) MER/VAB

Drug Class: Carbapemen/β-lactamase inhibitor.
Usual Dose: 4 gm (IV) q8h

Spectrum Synopsis*
Hits
  Gram + : MSSA, VSE
  Gram – : Most GNBs, Pseudomonas aeruginosa
  Problem pathogens: B. capacia, CRE
Misses
  Gram + : MRSA, VRE
  Gram – : S. maltophilia, Acinetobacter
  Problem pathogens:
    Some MBL CRE

―――― = serious side effect ⬜ = black box warning. ND = no data. NR = not recommended. s = spectrum inadequate (at site). a = activity or experience inadequate. p = tissue penetration inadequate. *based on peak serum concentration after usual adult dose. †applicable to adult uncomplicated lower UTIs (CrCl > 30 mL/min).

(Full *Susceptibility Profiles* p. 208).
Resistance Potential: Low ↑
Pharmacokinetic Parameters:
*Peak serum level: Meropenem: 43–57
mcg/mL/Vaborbactam: 5–71 mcg/mL
Bioavailability: Not applicable
Excreted unchanged: Meropenem:
40–60%/Vaborbactam: 75–95%
Serum half-life (normal): Meropenem
1.2–2.3 hrs/Vaborbactam 1.68–2.25 hrs
Plasma protein binding: Meropenem:
2%/Vaborbactam: 33%
Volume of distribution (V_d): Meropenem:
0.29 L/kg/Vaborbactam: 0.27 L/kg*
Primary Mode of Elimination: Renal
Dosage Adjustments*

CrCl 30–49 mL/min	2 g (IV) q8h
CrCl 15–29	2 g (IV) q12h
CrCl < 15 mL/min	1 g (IV) q12h
Post–HD dose	Post-HD
Post–PD dose	Post-PD
CVVH dose	2 gm (IV) q12h
Mild to moderate hepatic insufficiency	No change
Severe hepatic insufficiency	Avoid

Drug Interactions: Meropenem valproic
acid and divalproex levels, probenecid ↑
MER/VAB levels)

Adverse Effects:
Common
- Phlebitis

- Nausea
- Diarrhea
- Headache
- ↑AST/ALT
- Hypokalemia
Uncommon
- C. difficile diarrhea/colitis
Rare
- Drug fever
- Thrombocytopenia
- Neuromotor impairment
Allergic Potential: Low
Safety in Pregnancy: Infuse B

Additional Clinical Considerations:
- *Infuse dose over 3 hours*
- Only compatible with 0.9% NaCl

(also see *Antibiotic Pearls & Pitfalls*
p. 530).

SELECTED REFERENCES:
Castanheria M, et al. Meropenem-vaborbactam
tested against contemporary gram-negative
isolates collected worldwide during 2014,
including carbapenem-resistant, KPC-producing,
multidrug-resistant, and extensively drug-
resistant Enterobacteriaceas. Antimicrob Agents
Chemother. 61. (PMID: 28652234)
Kaye KS, et al. Effect of meropenem-vaborbactam
vs piperacillin-tazobactam on clinical cure or
improvement and microbial eradication in
complicated urinary tract infection: the TANGO
I randomized clinical trial. JAMA: 319:788-99,
2018. (PMID: 29486041)
Pogue JM, Bonomo RA, Kaye KS. Ceftazidime/
Avibactam, Meropenem/Vaborbactam, or both?
Clinical and formulary considerations. Clin Infect
Dis 68:519-524, 2019 (PMID: 30020449)

"Usual dose" assumes normal renal/hepatic function. * For renal insufficiency, give usual dose × 1 followed by maintenance dose per CrCl. For dialysis patients, dose the same as for CrCl < 10 mL/min and give supplemental (post-HD/PD dose) immediately after dialysis. CrCl = creatinine clearance; CVVH = continuous veno-venous hemofiltration; HD/PD = hemo-dialysis/peritoneal dialysis.

Zhanel GG. Imipenem-relebactam and meropenem-varbobactam: two novel carbapenem-b-lactamase inhibitor combinations. Drugs 78:65–98, 2018. (PMID:29230684)

Methenamine hippurate (Hiprex, Urex) Methenamine mandelate (Mandelamine)

Drug Class: Urinary antibiotic.
Usual Dose: 1 gm (PO) q6h (hippurate); 1 gm (PO) q6h (mandelate).
Spectrum: All Gram + and Gram – uropathogens.
Resistance Potential: None
  Pharmacokinetic Parameters:
  Peak serum level: Not applicable
  Bioavailability: 90%
  Excreted unchanged (urine): 90%
  Serum half-life (normal/ESRD): 4 hrs/ND
  Plasma protein binding: Not applicable
  Volume of distribution (V_d): Not applicable
Primary Mode of Elimination: Renal
Dosage Adjustments*

CrCl 50–80 mL/min	Avoid
CrCl 10–50 mL/min	Avoid
CrCl < 10 mL/min	Avoid
Post–HD dose	Avoid
Post–PD dose	Avoid
CVVH/CVVHD/CVVHDF dose	Avoid
Moderate hepatic insufficiency	No change
Severe hepatic insufficiency	Avoid

Drug Interactions: Acetazolamide, sodium bicarbonate, thiazide diuretics ($\downarrow$ antibacterial effect if $\uparrow$ urinary pH $\geq$ 5.5).
Adverse Effects:
Uncommon
  • Nausea/vomiting
  • Drug fever/rash
  • $\uparrow$ AST/ALT
Allergic Potential: Low
Safety in Pregnancy: C

Additional Clinical Considerations:
  • Effectiveness depends on maintaining an acid urine (pH $\leq$ 5.5) with acidifying agents (e.g., ascorbic acid).
  • **Useful only for catheter-associated bacteriuria (CAB)**, not UTIs.
  • **Forms formaldehyde in acid urine (resistance does not develop).**
  • Requires 4–5 hours in an acid urine pH $\leq$ 5.5 to generate effective form-aldehyde levels.

SELECTED REFERENCES:
Cunha BA, Comer JB, Pharmacokinetic considerations in the treatment of urinary tract infections. Conn Med 43:347–53, 1979. (PMID:467046)
Klinge D, Mannisto P, Mantyla R, et al. Pharmacokinetics of methenamine in healthy volunteers. J Antimicrob Chemother 9:209–16, 1982. (PMID:7076604)
Musher DM, Griffith DP. Generation of formaldehyde from methenamine: Effect of pH and concentration, and antibacterial effect. Antimicrob Agents Chemother 6:708–11, 1974. (PMID:4451344)
Website: www.pdr.net

Metronidazole (Flagyl)

Drug Class: Nitroimidazole antiparasitic/antibiotic.
Usual Dose: 1 gm (IV) q24h **(PK dose)**, 500 mg (IV/PO) q6–8h **(PI dose)** (see comments).

———— = serious side effect ⬜ = black box warning. ND = no data. NR = not recommended. s = spectrum inadequate (at site). a = activity or experience inadequate. p = tissue penetration inadequate. *based on peak serum concentration after usual adult dose. †applicable to adult uncomplicated lower UTIs (CrCl > 30 mL/min).

Spectrum Synopsis*
Hits
  Gram + : None
  Gram – : B. fragilis
  Problem pathogens: C. difficile
Misses
  Gram + : All
  Gram – : All aerobic GNB
  Problem pathogens:
    Some non-B. fragilis anerobes

(Full *Susceptibility Profiles* p. 196).

Resistance Potential: Low
  (H. pylori, Gardnerella, Prevotella)
Pharmacokinetic Parameters:
  Peak serum level: 26 (IV)/12 (PO) mcg/mL
  Bioavailability: 100%
  Excreted unchanged (urine): 20%
  Serum half-life (normal/ESRD): 8/14 hrs
  Plasma protein binding: 20%
  Volume of distribution (V_d): 0.25–0.85 L/kg
Primary Mode of Elimination: Hepatic
Dosage Adjustments*

CrCl 10–50 mL/min	No change
CrCl < 10 mL/min	500 mg (IV) q24h/ 250 mg (PO) q12h
Post–HD dose	1 gm (IV) 500 mg (PO)
Post–PD dose	1 gm (IV) 500 mg (PO)
CVVH/CVVHD/ CVVHDF dose	No change
Mild-moderate hepatic insufficiency	No change
Severe hepatic insufficiency	500 mg (IV/PO) q24h

Drug Interactions: Alcohol (disulfiram-like reaction); disulfiram (acute toxic psychosis); warfarin ($\uparrow$ INR); phenobarbital, phenytoin ($\uparrow$ metronidazole metabolism).
Adverse Effects:
Common
- Headache
- Metallic taste
- Nausea/vomiting/diarrhea
Uncommon
- Peripheral neuropathy
- Disulfiram-like reactions (with EtOH)
Rare
- Encephalopathy
- Seizures
- Aseptic meningitis
- Carcinogenic in animals
Allergic Potential: Low
Safety in Pregnancy: B (avoid in 1st trimester)

Additional Clinical Considerations:
- For intra-abdominal/pelvic sepsis **(plus anti-aerobic GNB drug).** Q24h dosing is preferred to q6h/ q8h dosing because of long half-life ($t_{1/2}$ = 8 h).
- **C. difficile diarrhea dose:** 250 mg (PO) q6h.
- **C. difficile colitis dose:** 500 mg (IV/ PO) q6-8h or 1 gm (IV) q24h.
- **For severe C. difficile colitis, add anti-GNB coverage,** e.g., ertapenem or meropenem (for microscopic/ macroscopic perforation/peritonitis).
- **Use increases VRE prevalence.** *Metronidazole misses some anerobes eg, Propionibacteria, Actinobacillus, Eikinella, and limited activity against*

——— = serious side effect [   ] = black box warning. ND = no data. NR = not recommended. s = spectrum inadequate (at site). a = activity or experience inadequate. p = tissue penetration inadequate.
*based on peak serum concentration after usual adult dose. †applicable to adult uncomplicated lower UTIs (CrCl > 30 mL/min).

Actinomyces, Mobiluncus and Clostridium ramosum.

Additional Pharmacokinetic Considerations*

Non-CSF	% of Serum Levels
Peritoneal fluid	25%
Bile	100%§
Synovial fluid	35%
Bone	100%
Prostate	NR(s)
CSF:	
Non-inflamed meninges	30%
Inflamed meninges (ABM)	100%

Meningeal dose = usual dose

(also see **Antibiotic Pearls & Pitfalls** p. 536).

SELECTED REFERENCES:
Bouza E, Burillo A, Munoz P, Antimicrobial therapy of Clostridium difficile-associated diarrhea. Med Clin N Am 90:1141–63, 2006. (PMID:17116441)
Desai JA, Dobson J, Melanson M, et al. Metronidazole-induced encephalopathy: case report and review of MRI findings. Can J Neurol Sci 38:512–513, 2011. (PMID:21515514)
Falagas ME, Gorbach SL. Clindamycin and metronidazole. Med Clin North Am 79:845–67, 1995. (PMID:7791427)
Freeman CD, Klutman NE. Metronidazole: A therapeutic review and update. Drugs 54:679–708, 1997. (PMID:9360057)
Freeman CD, Nightingale CH, Nicolau DP, et al. Serum bactericidal activity of ceftriaxone plus metronidazole against common intra-abdominal pathogens. Am J Hosp Pharm 51:1782–7, 1994. (PMID:7942906)
Ishikawa T, Okamura S, Oshimoto H, et al. Metronidazole plus ciprofloxacin therapy for active Crohn's disease. Intern Med 42:318–21, 2003. (PMID:12729319)
Musher DM, Aslam S, Logan N, et al. Relatively poor outcome after treatment of Clostridium difficile colitis with metronidazole. Clinical Infectious Disease 40:1586–90, 2005. (PMID:15889354)
Vasa CV, Glatt AE. Effectiveness and appropriateness of empiric metronidazole for Clostridium difficile diarrhea. Am J Gastroenterol 98:354–8, 2003. (PMID:12591054)
Wang S, Cunha BA, Hamid NS, et al. Intravenous metronidazole: once daily vs. multiple dosing in intra-abdominal infections. Journal of Chemotherapy 19:410–416, 2007. (PMID:17855185)
Website: www.pdr.net

Mezlocillin (Mezlin)

Drug Class: Anti-pseudomonal penicillin.
Usual Dose: 3 gm (IV) q6h.

Spectrum Synopsis*
Hits
 Gram + : All non-enterococcal streptococci, VSE
 Gram – : Most GNB aerobic, P. aeruginosa, B. fragilis
 Problem pathogens: None
Misses
 Gram + : MRSA, VRE
 Gram – : Some aerobic GNB
 Problem pathogens: Listeria, Nocardia, Acinetobacter, S. maltophilia, B. cepacia

Urine Spectrum†
• Same as serum spectrum
• Optimal urinary pH = ND

Resistance Potential: Low
Pharmacokinetic Parameters:
 Peak serum level: 300 mcg/mL
 Bioavailability: Not applicable
 Excreted unchanged (urine): 65%
 Serum half-life (normal/ESRD): 1.1/4 hrs

———— = serious side effect ☐ = black box warning. ND = no data. NR = not recommended. s = spectrum inadequate (at site). a = activity or experience inadequate. p = tissue penetration inadequate. *based on peak serum concentration after usual adult dose. †applicable to adult uncomplicated lower UTIs (CrCl > 30 mL/min).

Plasma protein binding: 30%
Volume of distribution (V_d): 0.18 L/kg
Primary Mode of Elimination: Renal
Dosage Adjustments*

CrCl > 30 mL/min	No change
CrCl 10–30 mL/min	3 gm (IV) q8h
CrCl < 10 mL/min	2 gm (IV) q8h
Post–HD dose	3 gm (IV)
Post–PD dose	None
CVVH/CVVHD/ CVVHDF dose	3 gm (IV) q8h
Moderate hepatic insufficiency	No change
Severe hepatic insufficiency	3 gm (IV) q12h

Drug Interactions: Aminoglycosides (inactivation of mezlocillin in renal failure); warfarin (↑ INR); oral contraceptives (↓ oral contraceptive effect); cefoxitin (↓ mezlocillin effect).
Adverse Effects:
Common
• Diarrhea
Uncommon
• Drug fever/rash
• ↓ Platelet aggregation (dose dependent)
Rare
• C. difficile diarrhea/colitis
• Serum sickness
• Stevens-Johnson Syndrome
• Anaphylactic reactions
Allergic Potential: Low
Safety in Pregnancy: B

Additional Clinical Considerations:
• Dose-dependent half-life ($t_{1/2}$).

May increase LPS (endotoxin) release from GNB *potentially increasing endotoxin mediated tissue damage*

Additional Pharmacokinetic Considerations:

Non-CSF	% of Serum Levels
Peritoneal fluid	ND
Bile	3000%
Synovial fluid	ND
Bone	6%
Prostate	NR(p)
CSF	
Non-inflamed meninges	<10%
Inflamed meninges (ABM)	30%

SELECTED REFERENCE:
Website: www.pdr.net

Micafungin (Mycamine)

Drug Class: Echinocandin antifungal.
Usual Dose:
Candidemia:
    100 mg (IV) q24h.
Esophageal candidiasis:
    150 mg (IV) q24h.
Prophylaxis of candidal infections in stem cell transplants:
    50 mg (IV) q24h.
Pharmacokinetic Parameters:
Peak serum level: 5.1 mcg/mL (50 mg);
11.2 mcg/mL (100 mg); 16.4 mcg/mL
(150 mg)
Bioavailability: Not applicable
Excreted unchanged (urine): 11%
Serum half-life (normal/ESRD): 10–15 hrs/no change
Plasma protein binding: > 99%
Volume of distribution (V_d): 0.39 L/kg

––––––– = serious side effect ☐ = black box warning. ND = no data. NR = not recommended. s = spectrum inadequate (at site). a = activity or experience inadequate. p = tissue penetration inadequate. *based on peak serum concentration after usual adult dose. †applicable to adult uncomplicated lower UTIs (CrCl > 30 mL/min).

Primary Mode of Elimination: Hepatic

Dosage Adjustments

CrCl < 10 mL/min	No change
Post–HD dose	None
Post–PD dose	None
CVVH/CVVHD/CVVHDF dose	No change
Mild or Moderate hepatic insufficiency	No change
Severe hepatic insufficiency	Use with caution

Drug Interactions: Sirolimus AUC ↑ by 21% with no change in Cmax (monitor for sirolimus toxicity), nifedipine AUC, and Cmax ↑ by 18% and 42%, respectively (monitor for nifedipine toxicity).

Adverse Effects:

Common

- Nausea/vomiting/diarrhea
- Abdominal pain
- Drug rash
- Neutropenia
- Anemia
- Thrombocytopenia
- ↑ AST/ALT
- Hypokalemia
- Hypomagnesemia

Uncommon

- Electrolyte abnormalities: hypocalcemia, hypoglycemia, hyperglycemia, hypernatremia, hyperkalemia

Allergic Potential: Low

Safety in Pregnancy: C

Additional Clinical Considerations:

- Administer by IV infusion over one hour infusions may result in more frequent histamine mediated reactions.

- Most cost effective parenteral antifungal for *empiric therapy* of systemic Candida/Aspergillus infections

Highly active against Candida albicans and non-albicans Candida (↓ susceptibility to *C. parasilosis*)***, and Hansenula. Some activity against Aspergillus. No activity against Cryptococcus, Fusarium, Pseudallescheria/ Scedosporium, Trichosporon, Rhodotorula or Mucor.***

Cerebrospinal Fluid Penetration: < 1%

SELECTED REFERENCES:

Andes D, Safdar N. Efficacy of micafungin for the treatment of candidemia. Eur J Clin Microbiol Infect Dis 24:662–664, 2005. (PMID:16247615)

Chandraseka PH, Sobel JD. Micafungin: A New Echinocandin. Clin Infect Dis 42:1171–78, 2006. (PMID:16575738)

Cornely OA, Marty FM, Stucker F, et al. Efficacy and safety of micafungin for treatment of serious Candida infections in patients with or without malignant disease. Mycoses 54:838–47, 2011. (PMID:21668522)

Higashiyama Y, Kohno S. Micafungin: a therapeutic review. Expert Rev Anti Infect Ther 2:345–55, 2004. (PMID:15482206)

Isumikawa K, Ohtsu Y, Kawabata M, et al. Clinical efficacy of micafungin for chronic pulmonary aspergillosis. Med Mycol 45:273–278, 2007. (PMID:17464848)

Kohno S, Izumikawa K, Ogawa K, et al. Intravenous micafungin versus voriconazole for chronic pulmonary aspergillosis. J Infect 61:410–418, 2011. (PMID:20797407)

Pappas PG, Rotstein CM, Betts RF, et al. Micafungin versus caspofungin for treatment of candidemia and other forms of invasive candidiasis. Clin Infect Dis 45:883–893, 2007. (PMID:17806055)

Toubai T, Tanaka J, Ota S, et al. Efficacy and safety of micafungin in febrile neutropenic patients treated for hematological malignancies. Intern Med 46:3–9, 2007. (PMID:17202726)

Wiederhold NP, Lewis JS 2nd. The echinocandin micafungin: a review of the pharmacology,

---

= serious side effect ☐ = black box warning. ND = no data. NR = not recommended. s = spectrum inadequate (at site). a = activity or experience inadequate. p = tissue penetration inadequate. *based on peak serum concentration after usual adult dose. †applicable to adult uncomplicated lower UTIs (CrCl > 30 mL/min).

spectrum of activity, clinical efficacy and safety. Expert Opin Pharmacother 8:1155–1166, 2007. (PMID:17516879)

Yamaguchi M, Kurokawa T, Ishiyama K, et al. Efficacy and safety of micafungin as an empirical therapy for invasive fungal infections in patients with hematologic disorders: a multicenter, prospective study. Ann Hematol 90:1209–17, 2011. (PMID:21695388)

Yoshida M, Tamura K, Imamura M, et al. Efficacy and safety of micafungin as an empirical antifungal therapy fir suspected fungal infection in neutropenic patients with hematological disorders. Ann Hematol 91:449–57, 2012. (PMID:21894476)

Website: www.pdr.net

Minocycline (Minocin)

Drug Class: 2nd generation tetracycline.
Usual Dose: Loading dose: 200 mg (IV/PO) × 1 dose, then **Maintenance dose:** 100 mg (IV/PO) q12h.

Spectrum Synopsis*
Hits
Gram + : MRSA (CA-MRSA, HA-MRSA), MRSA, VRE
Gram – : Most aerobic GNB, B. fragilis
Problem pathogens:
Listeria, Nocardia, Acinetobacter, S. maltophilia, B. cepacia, CRE
Misses
Gram + : GAS, VSE
Gram – : Some GNB
Problem pathogens:
P. aeruginosa
Urine Spectrum[†]
• Same as serum spectrum
• Optimal urinary pH = 5.6
• Urine levels = 300 mcg/mL

(see **Susceptibility Profiles** p. 196).

Resistance Potential: Low
Pharmacokinetic Parameters:

Peak serum level: 4 mcg/mL
Bioavailability: 95%
Excreted unchanged (urine): 10%
Serum half-life (normal/ESRD): 15–23/18–69 hrs
Plasma protein binding: 75%
Volume of distribution (V_d): 1.5 L/kg
Primary Mode of Elimination: Hepatic
Dosage Adjustments*

CrCl < 10 mL/min	No change
Post–HD/PD dose	None
CVVH/CVVHD/CVVHDF dose	No change
Moderate hepatic insufficiency	No change
Severe hepatic insufficiency	100 mg (IV/PO) q24h

Drug Interactions: Antacids, Al^{++}, Ca^{++}, Fe^{++}, Mg^{++}, Zn^{++}, multivitamins, sucralfate ($\downarrow$ minocycline absorption); isotretinoin (pseudotumor cerebri); warfarin ($\uparrow$ INR).
Adverse Effects:
Common
• Nausea/vomiting/diarrhea
• Headache
• Dizziness (vestibular)
Uncommon
• Drug induced SLE
• Skin hyperpigmentation (with long-term therapy)
Rare
• Stevens-Johnson Syndrome
Allergic Potential: Low
Safety in Pregnancy: D

Additional Clinical Considerations:
• ***Eeffective against Nocardia.***
Effective IV/PO against serious systemic MSSA/MRSA infections, e.g., MSSA/MRSA ABE, osteomyelitis, or meningitis. Tetracycline susceptibilities do not

—— = serious side effect ☐ = black box warning. ND = no data. NR = not recommended. s = spectrum inadequate (at site). a = activity or experience inadequate. p = tissue penetration inadequate. *based on peak serum concentration after usual adult dose. †applicable to adult uncomplicated lower UTIs (CrCl > 30 mL/min).

predict minocycline effectiveness against MSSA, MRSA, and Acinetobacter sp. *Even if MSSA/MRSA susceptible to doxycycline, minocycline more reliably effective.* For neuroborreliosis minocycline may be preferable to doxycycline

May inhibit antibiotic induced LPS (endotoxin) release from GNB *potentially minimizing endotoxin mediated tissue damage.*

Additional Pharmacokinetic Considerations*

Non-CSF	% of Serum Levels
Peritoneal fluid	ND
Bile	600%
Synovial fluid	ND
Bone	90%
Prostate	100%
CSF	
Non-inflamed meninges	50%
Inflamed meninges (ABM)	50%
Meningeal dose = usual dose	

(also see ***Antibiotic Pearls & Pitfalls*** p. 530).

SELECTED REFERENCES:

Bouza E. New therapeutic choices for infections caused by methicillin-resistant Staphylococcus aureus. Clin Microbiol Infect Dis 15:44–52, 2009. (PMID:19951334)

Copeland KFT, Brooks JI. A Novel use for an old drug: the potential for minocycline as anti-HIV adjuvant therapy. J Infect Dis 201:1115–1117, 2010. (PMID:20205572)

Cunha BA, Baron J, Cunha CB. Doxycycline vs. Minocycline Similarities and Differences: Clinical and Antimicrobial Stewardship Considerations. European Journal of Clinical Microbiology & Infectious Disease 37:15-20, 2018. (PMID: 28819873)

Cunha BA. Minocycline is a reliable and effective oral option to treat methicillin-resistant Staphylococcus aureus skin and soft-tissue infections, including doxycycline treatment failures. Int J Antimicrob Agents. 43:386–387, 2014. (PMID:24559866)

Cunha BA. Pharmacoeconomic advantages of oral minocycline for the therapy of methicillin-resistant Staphylococcus aureus (MRSA) Skin and Soft Tissue Infections (SSTIs). Euro Clin Microb & Infect Dis. 33:1869-1871, 2014. (PMID:24838676)

Cunha BA. Minocycline, often forgotten but preferred to trimethoprim-sulfamethoxazole or doxycycline for the treatment of community-acquired methicillin-resistant Staphylococcus aureus skin and soft-tissue infections. Int J Antimicrob Agents 42:497-499, 2013. (PMID:24126085)

Cunha BA. Minocycline versus doxycycline for methicillin-resistant Staphylococcus aureus (MRSA): in vitro susceptibility versus in vivo effectiveness. Int J Antimicrob Agents 35:517–8, 2012. (PMID:20202796)

Cunha BA. Minocycline versus doxycycline for CA-MRSA: in vitro versus in vivo differences. International Journal of Antimicrobial Agents 35:517–518, 2010. (PMID:20202796)

Cunha BA. Minocycline vs. doxycycline for the antimicrobial therapy of lyme neuroborreliosis. Clin Infect Dis 30:237–238, 2000. (PMID:10619782)

Elkayam O, Yaron M, Caspi D. Minocycline-induced autoimmune syndromes: an overview. Semin Arthritis Rheum 28:392–397, 1999. (PMID:10406406)

Ritchie DJ, Garavaglia-Wilson A. A Review of Intravenous Minocycline for Treatment of Multidrug-Resistant Acinetobacter Infections. Clin Infect Dis 59:S374-S380, 2014. (PMID:25371513)

Schwartz BS, Graber CJ, Diep BA, et al. Doxycycline, not minocycline, induces Its own resistance in multidrug-resistant community-associated methicillin-resistant Staphylococcus aureus clone USA300. Clin Infect Dis 48:1483–1484, 2009. (PMID:19374563)

Website: www.pdr.net

────── = serious side effect ⬜ = black box warning. ND = no data. NR = not recommended. s = spectrum inadequate (at site). a = activity or experience inadequate. p = tissue penetration inadequate. *based on peak serum concentration after usual adult dose. †applicable to adult uncomplicated lower UTIs (CrCl > 30 mL/min).

Moxifloxacin (Avelox)

Drug Class: Respiratory quinolone.
Usual Dose: 400 mg (IV/PO) q24h.

CVVH/CVVHD/CVVHDF dose	No change
Moderate hepatic insufficiency	No change
Severe hepatic insufficiency	No change

Spectrum Synopsis*
Hits
　Gram + : Some MSSA, VSE
　Gram – : Most GNB (including B. fragilis
　Problem pathogens:
　　Acinetobacter, B. cepacia, S. maltophilia
Misses
　Gram + : VRE, most streptococci, MRSA
　Gram – : P. aeruginosa
　Problem pathogens:
　　Listeria, Nocardia
Urine Spectrum†
　• Same as serum spectrum
　• Optimal urinary pH = 6–7
　• Urine levels = 10 mcg/mL

(Full **Susceptibility Profiles** p. 208).
Resistance Potential: Low
Pharmacokinetic Parameters:
Peak serum level: 4.4 (IV)/4.5 (PO) mcg/ mL
Bioavailability: 90%
Excreted unchanged (urine): 20%
Serum half-life (normal/ESRD): 12/12 hrs
Plasma protein binding: 50%
Volume of distribution (V_d): 2.2 L/kg
Primary Mode of Elimination: Hepatic
Dosage Adjustments*

CrCl < 10 mL/min	No change
Post–HD dose	None
Post–PD dose	None

Drug Interactions: Al^{++}, Fe^{++}, Mg^{++}, Zn^{++} antacids, citrate/citric acid, dairy products (↓ absorption of fluoroquinolones only if taken together); amiodarone, procainamide, sotalol (may ↑ QT_c interval, torsade de pointes), rifampicin (↓ moxifloxacin levels).

Adverse Effects:
Uncommon
　• Headache
　• Insomnia
　• Nausea/vomiting
　• Non-C. difficile diarrhea
Rare
　• Peripheral neuropathy
　• ↑ QTc
　• Tendinitis and tendon rupture
　• C. difficile diarrhea/colitis (↑ risk with PPIs)

Allergic Potential: Low
Safety in Pregnancy: C

Additional Clinical Considerations:
　• **Only quinolone with anti–B. fragilis activity.**
　• **FQ with the highest activity against S. pneumoniae, VSE, and MSSA.**
　• Metabolized to microbiologically-inactive glucuronide (M1)/sulfate (M2) conjugates.
　• Take 4 hours before or 8 hours after calcium or magnesium containing antacids
　• C8-methoxy group increases activity and decreases resistance potential.

——— = serious side effect ⬜ = black box warning. ND = no data. NR = not recommended. s = spectrum inadequate (at site). a = activity or experience inadequate. p = tissue penetration inadequate. *based on peak serum concentration after usual adult dose. †applicable to adult uncomplicated lower UTIs (CrCl > 30 mL/min).

- **TB dose** *(alternate drug in MDR TB drug regimens)*: 400 mg (PO) q24h or 800 mg (PO) q24h if also on RIF.
- **↑ Incidence of C. difficile diarrhea/ colitis with PPIs (for patients on PPIs during FQ therapy, D/C PPIs or switch to H2 blocker for duration of FQ therapy).**

May inhibit antibiotic induced LPS (endotoxin) release from GNB potentially minimizing endotoxin mediated tissue damage.

Additional Pharmacokinetic Considerations*

Non-CSF	% of Serum Levels
Peritoneal fluid	75%
Bile	93%[§]
Synovial fluid	75%
Bone	60%
Prostate	>200%
CSF	
Non-inflamed meninges	<1%
Inflamed meninges (ABM)	<10%

Meningeal dose = 400–800 mg (IV/PO) q24h

(also see **Antibiotic Pearls & Pitfalls** p. 533).

SELECTED REFERENCES:

Balfour JA, Wiseman LR. Moxifloxacin. Drugs 57:363–73, 1999. (PMID:10193688)

Cheadle W, Lee JT, Napolitano LM, et al. Clinical update on the use of moxifloxacin in the treatment of community-acquired complicated intra-abdominal infections. Surg Infect 11:487–494, 2010. (PMID:20583956)

Chou HW, Wang JL, Chang CH, et al. Risk of severe dysglycemia among diabetic patients receiving levofloxacin, ciprofloxacin, or moxifloxacin in Taiwan. Clin Infect Dis 57:971-980, 2013. (PMID:23948133)

Cox H, Ford N, Keshavjee S, et al. Rational use of moxifloxacin for tuberculosis treatment. Lancet Infect Dis 11: 259–260, 2011. (PMID:21453864)

Ewig S, Hecker H, Suttorp N, et al. Moxifloxacin monotherapy versus B-lactam mono or combination therapy in hospitalized patients with community-acquired pneumonia. J Infect 62: 218–225, 2011. (PMID:21276814)

Gillespie SH, Crook AM, McHugh TD, et al. Four-month moxifloxacin-based regimens for drug-sensitive tuberculosis. NEJM 371:1577-1587, 2014. (PMID:25196020)

Jindani A, Harrison TS, Nunn AJ, et al. High-dose rifapentine with moxifloxacin for pulmonary tuberculosis. NEJM 371:1599-1608, 2014. (PMID:25337749)

Lapi F, Wilchesky M, Abbas K, et al. Fluoroquinolones and the risk of serious arrhythmia: A population-based study. Clin Infect Dis 55:1457–65, 2012. (PMID:22865870)

Lobera T, Audicana MT, Alarcon E, et al. Allergy to quinolones: low cross-reactivity to levofloxacin. J Investig Allergol Clin Immunol 20: 607–611, 2010. (PMID:21314003)

Malincarne L, Ghebtegzabher M, Moretti MV, et al. Penetration of moxifloxacin into bone in patients undergoing total knee arthroplasty. J Antimicrob Chemother 57:950–4, 2006. (PMID:16551691)

Malingoni MA, Song J, Herrington J, et al. Randomized controlled trial of moxifloxacin compared with piperacillin-tazobactam and amoxicillin-clavulanate for the treatment of complicated intra-abdominal infections. Ann Surg 244:204–11, 2006. (PMID:16858182)

—— = serious side effect ☐ = black box warning. ND = no data. NR = not recommended. s = spectrum inadequate (at site). a = activity or experience inadequate. p = tissue penetration inadequate. *based on peak serum concentration after usual adult dose. [†]applicable to adult uncomplicated lower UTIs (CrCl > 30 mL/min).

Mendel C, Springsklee M. Moxifloxacin for tuberculosis. Lancet Infect Dis 176–17, 2012. (PMID:22361419)

Mu YP, Liu RL, Wang LQ, et al. Moxifloxacin monotherapy for treatment of complicated intro-abdominal infections: a meta-analysis of randomized controlled trials. Int J Clin 66:210–7, 2012. (PMID:22257046)

Pranger AD, Van Altena R, Aarnoutse RE, et al. Evaluation of moxifloxacin for the treatment of tuberculosis: 3 years of experience. Eur Respir J. 38: 884–894, 2011. (PMID:21310881)

Rijnders BJ. Moxifloxacin for community-acquired pneumonia. Antimicrob Agents Chemother 47:444–445, 2003. (PMID:12499236)

Schulze MH, Keller C, Müller A, et al. Rickettsia ryphi infection with interstitial pneumonia in a traveler treated with moxifloxacin. J Clin Microb 49: 741–743, 2011. (PMID:21123528)

Sionidou M, Manika K, Pitsiou G, et al. Moxifloxacin in COPD: pharmacokinetics and penetration into bronchial secretions in ward and ICU patients. Antimicrob Agents Chemother. [Epub ahead of print]. 2019. (PMID: 30642928)

Stass, H, Rink AD, Delesen H, et al. Pharmacokinetics and peritoneal penetration of moxifloxacin in peritonitis. J Antimicrob Chemother 58:693–6, 2006. (PMID:16895940)

Torres A, Muir JF, Corris P, et al. Effectiveness of oral moxifloxacin in standard first-line therapy in community-acquired pneumonia. Eur Respir J 21:135–43, 2003. (PMID:12570122)

Website: www.pdr.net

Nafcillin (Unipen)

Drug Class: Anti-staphylococcal (MSSA) penicillin.
Usual Dose: 2 gm (IV) q4h.

Spectrum Synopsis*
Hits
  Gram + : GAS, MSSA
  Gram – : None
  Problem pathogens: None
Misses
  Gram + : MRSA, VSE, VRE
  Gram – : All GNB, B. fragilis
  Problem pathogens:
    Listeria, Nocardia, Acineto-
    bacter, S. maltophilia, B. cepacia

Resistance Potential: Low
Pharmacokinetic Parameters:
  Peak serum level: 80 mcg/mL
  Bioavailability: Not applicable
  Excreted unchanged (urine): 10–30%
  Serum half-life (normal/ESRD): 0.5/4 hrs
  Plasma protein binding: 90%
  Volume of distribution (V_d): 0.24 L/kg
Primary Mode of Elimination: Hepatic
Dosage Adjustments*

CrCl < 10 mL/min	No change
Post–HD/PD dose	None
CVVH/CVVHD/ CVVHDF dose	No change
Moderate— severe hepatic insufficiency	No change

Drug Interactions: Cyclosporine (↓ cyclosporine levels); nifedipine, warfarin (↓ interacting drug effect).
Adverse Effects:
Uncommon
  • Drug fever/rash

―――― = serious side effect ☐ = black box warning. ND = no data. NR = not recommended. s = spectrum inadequate (at site). a = activity or experience inadequate. p = tissue penetration inadequate. *based on peak serum concentration after usual adult dose. †applicable to adult uncomplicated lower UTIs (CrCl > 30 mL/min).

- Injection site reactions
- Leukopenia

Rare
- Interstitial nephritis
- <u>C. difficile diarrhea/colitis</u>

Allergic Potential: High
Safety in Pregnancy: B

Additional Clinical Considerations:
- **Avoid oral formulation** (not well absorbed/erratic serum levels).

Additional Pharmacokinetic Considerations*

Non-CSF	% of Serum Levels
Peritoneal fluid	NR(s)
Bile	20%
Synovial fluid	ND
Bone	ND
Prostate	NR(p)
CSF	
Non-inflamed meninges	1%
Inflamed meninges (ABM)	20%

Meningeal dose = 2 gm (IV) q4h

SELECTED REFERENCES:
Youngster I, Shenoy ES, Hooper D, et al.
Comparative evaluation of the tolerability of cefazolin and nafcillin for treatment of methicillin-susceptible staphlococcus aureus infections in the outpatient setting. Clin Infect Dis 59:369-375, 2014. (PMID:24785233)
Website: www.pdr.net

Nevirapine (Viramune) NVP

Drug Class: HIV NNRTI (non-nucleoside reverse transcriptase inhibitor).
Usual Dose: 200 mg (PO) q24h × 2 weeks, then 200 mg (PO) q12h.

Pharmacokinetic Parameters:
Peak serum level: 0.9–3.6 mcg/mL
Bioavailability: 90%
Excreted unchanged (urine): 5%
Serum half-life (normal/ESRD): 40 hrs/ no data
Plasma protein binding: 60%
Volume of distribution (V_d): 1.4 L/kg
Primary Mode of Elimination: Hepatic
Dosage Adjustments*

CrCl 10–50 mL/min	No change
CrCl < 20 mL/min	Use with caution
Post–HD dose	200 mg (PO)
Post–PD dose	None
CVVH/CVVHD/ CVVHDF dose	No change
Moderate hepatic insufficiency	Use with caution
Severe hepatic insufficiency	Avoid

Antiretroviral Dosage Adjustments

Delavirdine	No data
Efavirenz	No data
Indinavir	Indinavir 1000 mg q8h
Lopinavir/ ritonavir (l/r)	Consider l/r 600/150 mg q12h in PI-experienced patients
Nelfinavir	No data
Ritonavir	No change
Saquinavir	No data
Rifampin	Avoid
Rifabutin	Use with caution

—— = serious side effect ☐ = black box warning. ND = no data. NR = not recommended. s = spectrum inadequate (at site). a = activity or experience inadequate. p = tissue penetration inadequate. *based on peak serum concentration after usual adult dose. †applicable to adult uncomplicated lower UTIs (CrCl > 30 mL/min).

Drug Interactions: Antiretrovirals, rifabutin, rifampin (see dose adjustment grid, above); carbamazepine, phenobarbital, phenytoin (monitor anticonvulsant levels); caspofungin ($\downarrow$ caspofungin levels), itraconazole ($\downarrow$ itraconazole/$\uparrow$ nevirapine levels), voriconazole ($\uparrow$ nevirapine levels); ethinyl estradiol ($\downarrow$ ethinyl estradiol levels; use additional/alternative method); methadone ($\downarrow$ methadone levels; titrate methadone dose to effect); tacrolimus ($\downarrow$ tacrolimus levels) clarithromycin ($\downarrow$ clarithromycin levels), rifapentine (avoid).

Adverse Effects:
Fulminant hepatic failure often associated with rash. Hepatotoxicity can occur in 68th gender, all CD_4 counts and at any time during treatment.

Common
- Drug rash
- Hyperlipidemia
- $\uparrow$ AST/ALT

Uncommon
- Headache
- Nausea
- Fatigue

Rare
- Stevens-Johnson Syndrome
- TEN
- Vigilance is warranted during the first 6 weeks of therapy, which is the period of greatest risk of these events

Allergic Potential: High
Safety in Pregnancy: B

Additional Clinical Considerations:
- Absorption not affected by food.
- Not to be used for post-exposure prophylaxis (potential for fatal hepatitis).

- Do not start nevirapine following severe hepatic, skin or hypersensitivity reactions.

Cerebrospinal Fluid Penetration: 45%

SELECTED REFERENCE:
Website: www.pdr.net

Nitazoxanide (Alinia)

Drug Class: Antiprotozoal; anti-C. diffcile antibiotic.
Usual Dose: 500 mg (PO) q12h.
Pharmacokinetic Parameters:
Peak serum level: 9.1–10.6 mcg/mL; tizoxanile/tizoxanile glucuronide (metabolites)
Bioavailability: ND
Excreted unchanged (urine): < 10%
Serum half-life (normal/ESRD): ND
Plasma protein binding: 99%
Volume of distribution (V_d): ND
Primary Mode of Elimination: Hepatic (66%); Renal (34%)
Dosage Adjustments*

CrCl 50–80 mL/min	No change
CrCl 10–50 mL/min	250 mg (PO) q12h
CrCl < 10 mL/min	Use with caution
Post–HD dose	None
Post–PD dose	None
CVVH/CVVHD/CVVHDF dose	No change
Mild/moderate	No change
Mild hepatic insufficiency	No change
Moderate—severe hepatic insufficiency	Use with caution

——— = serious side effect ☐ = black box warning. ND = no data. NR = not recommended. s = spectrum inadequate (at site). a = activity or experience inadequate. p = tissue penetration inadequate. *based on peak serum concentration after usual adult dose. †applicable to adult uncomplicated lower UTIs (CrCl > 30 mL/min).

Drug Interactions: Avoid in patients with hypersensitivity to salicylates.
Adverse Effects:
Uncommon
- Headache
- Nausea/vomiting/diarrhea
- Abdominal pain

Rare
- Dizziness
- Flu-like syndrome
- Yellow discoloration of sclera/urine

Allergic Potential: Low
Safety in Pregnancy: B

> **Additional Clinical Considerations:**
> *Effective for C. difficile diarrhea/colitis (including metronidazole /vancomycin failures).*
> Synergistic with oseltamisir against influenza.
> Nitazoxanide concentrates in GI tract but is not present in serum. Absorption greatly increased with food.
> ($\uparrow$ plasma levels of metabolites ~ 50%).
> **Preferred therapy for *Cryptosporidia* and giardiasis. Also effective against *Cyclospora* and *Iospora. H. pylori, B. hominis, rotavirus,* and *norovirus.***
> Nitazoxanide also has activity against influenza, RSV, HPIV, coronavirus, HBV, HCV, HIV, dengue, JE, and SARS-CoV-2.

(also see *Antibiotic Pearls & Pitfalls* p. 538).

SELECTED REFERENCES:
Basu PP, Rayapudi K, Pacana T, et al. A randomized study comparing levofloxacin, omeprazole, nitazoxanide, and doxycycline versus triple therapy for the eradication of Helicobacter pylori. Am J Gastroroent 106:1970–5, 2011. (PMID:21989146)

Bouza E, Burillo A, Munoz P. Antimicrobial therapy of Clostridium difficile-associated diarrhea. Med Clin N Am 90:1141–63, 2006. (PMID:17116441)

Freeman J, Baines SD, Todhunter SL, et al. Nitazoxanide is active against Clostridium difficile strains with reduced susceptibility to metronidazole. J Antimicrob Chemother 66:1407–1408, 2011. (PMID:21393199)

Gilles HM, et al. Treatment of intestinal parasitic infections: a review of nitazoxanide. Trends in Parasitology 18:95–7, 2002. (PMID:11854075)

Gurgen D, Hogan D, Grace E, et al. Nitazoxanide in the treatment of chronic cutaneous leishmaniasis resistant to traditional sodium stidogluconate. J Am Acad Dermatol 64: 202–203, 2011. (PMID:21167419)

Haffizulla J, Hartman A, Hoppers M, et al. Effect of nitazoxanide in adults and adolescents with acute uncompoicated influenza: a double-blind, randomized, placebo-controlled, phase 2b/3 trial. Lanect Infect Dis 14:609–618, 2014. (PMID:24852376)

Musher DM, Logan N, Hamill RJ, et al. Nitazoxanide for the treatment of Clostridium difficile colitis. Clin Infect. Dis 43:421–30, 2006. (PMID:16838229)

Rossingnol JF, Elfert A, Keeffe EB. Treatment of chronic hepatitis C using a 4-week lead-in with nitazoxanide before peginterferon plus nitazoxanide. J Clin Gastroenterol 44:504–509, 2010. (PMID:20048684)

Rossingnol JF. Nitazoxanide: a first-in-class broad-spectrum antiviral agent. Antiviral Rsch 110:94–103,2014. (PMID:25108173)

Website: www.pdr.net

Nitrofurantoin (Macrodantin, Macrobid)

Drug Class: Urinary antibiotic.
Usual Dose: 100 mg (PO) q12h.

> **Urine Spectrum:**
> **Hits**
>   Gram + : VSE, VRE
>   Gram – : Most GNB
>   **Problem pathogens:**
>   ESBL + Klebsiella, Entero-
>   bacter, E. coli, CRE, most
>   metallo-beta-lactamases (NDM-1)

——— = serious side effect ☐ = black box warning. ND = no data. NR = not recommended. s = spectrum inadequate (at site). a = activity or experience inadequate. p = tissue penetration inadequate. *based on peak serum concentration after usual adult dose. †applicable to adult uncomplicated lower UTIs (CrCl > 30 mL/min).

Misses

  Gram + : GBS

  Gram – : Proteus, Serratia,
    P. aeruginosa

  Problem pathogens:
    Acinetobacter, S. maltophilia,
    B. cepacia

- Optimal urinary pH = 5–6
- Urine levels = 100 mcg/mL

(Full *Susceptibility Profiles* p. 208).

Resistance Potential: Low

Pharmacokinetic Parameters:

  Peak serum level: 1 mcg/mL
  Bioavailability: 80%
  Excreted unchanged (urine): 25%
  Serum half-life (normal/ESRD): 0.5/1 hrs
  Plasma protein binding: 40%
  Volume of distribution (V_d): 0.8 L/kg

Primary Mode of Elimination: Renal

Dosage Adjustments*

CrCl 50–80 mL/min	100 mg (PO) q12h
CrCl 30–50 mL/min	100 mg (PO) q24h
CrCl < 30 mL/min	Avoid
Post–HD dose	Avoid
Post–PD dose	Avoid
CVVH/CVVHD/CVVHDF dose	Avoid
Moderate hepatic insufficiency	No change
Severe hepatic insufficiency	No change

Drug Interactions: Antacids, magnesium ($\downarrow$ nitrofurantoin absorption); probenecid ($\uparrow$ nitrofurantoin levels).

Adverse Effects:

Common
- Nausea
- Headache

Uncommon
- Urine discoloration
- Pneumonitis (acute)
- AIHA

Rare
- <u>Chronic hepatitis*</u>
- <u>Peripheral neuropathy*</u>
- <u>Pneumonitis (chronic interstitial)*</u>
- <u>Pulmonary fibrosis*</u>

Allergic Potential: Moderate

Safety in Pregnancy: B

Additional Clinical Considerations:
- **For CAB/lower UTIs only. Useful for asymptomatic bacteriuria of pregnancy.** No transplacental transfer.
- Chronic toxicities associated with prolonged use/renal insufficiency.
- Optimal effectiveness if CrCl > 60 mL/min. Usually effective if CrCl > 30 mL/min. **Avoid if CrCl < 30 mL/min.**
- Effective for VSE/VRE catheter associated bacteriuria (CAB)/lower UTIs.

Nitrofurantoin: Effects of Urinary pH on Urinary Tract Concentrations and Antimicrobial Antibiotic Activity

	Renal concentration	Urine concentration	Antimicrobial activity†
Alkaline urine (pH > 6)	+	+++	++
Acidic urine (pH = 5-6)	+++	+	++++

†against susceptible uropathogens

———— = serious side effect ☐ = black box warning. ND = no data. NR = not recommended. s = spectrum inadequate (at site). a = activity or experience inadequate. p = tissue penetration inadequate. *based on peak serum concentration after usual adult dose. †applicable to adult uncomplicated lower UTIs (CrCl > 30 mL/min).

(also see *Antibiotic Pearls & Pitfalls*
p. 534).

SELECTED REFERENCES:
Auer S, Wojna A, Hell M. Oral treatment options
    for ambulatory patients with urinary tract
    infections caused by extended-spectrum-beta-
    lactamase-producing Escherichia coli. Antimicrob
    Agents Chemother 54:4006–4008, 2010.
    (PMID:20585127)
Cunha BA, Cunha CB, Lam B, et al. Nitrofurantoin
    Safety and Effectiveness in Treating Acute
    Uncomplicated Cystitis (AUC) in Hospitalized
    Adults with Renal Insufficiency: Antibiotic
    Stewardship Implications. European Journal of
    Clinical Microbiology and Infectious Disease 36:
    1213-1216, 2017. (PMID: 28155015)
Cunha BA. Prophylaxis for recurrent urinary tract
    infections: nitrofurantoin, not trimethoprim-
    sulfamethoxazole or cranberry juice. Arch Intern
    Med 172:82–3, 2012. (PMID:22232158)
Cunha BA, Schoch P, Hage JE. Oral therapy of
    catheter-associated bacteriuria (CAB) in the ear
    of antibiotic resistance: nitrofurantoin revisited. J
    Chemother 24:122–4, 2012. (PMID:22546769)
Cunha BA, Schoch PE, Hage JR. Nitrofurantoin:
    preferred empiric therapy for community-
    acquired-lower urinary tract infections. Mayo Clin
    Proc 86:1243–4, 2011. (PMID:22134943)
Cunha BA. Nitrofurantoin: An update. OB/GYN
    44:399–406, 1989. (PMID:2659522)
Livermore DM, Warner M, Mushtaq S, et
    al. What remains against carbapenem-
    resistant Enterobacteriaceae? Evaluation
    of chloramphenicol, ciprofloxacin, colistin,
    fosfomycin, minocycline, nitrofurantoin,
    temocillin and tigecycline. Int J Antimicrob
    Agents 37:415–9, 2011. (PMID:21429716)
McKinnel JA, Stollenwerk NS, Jung CW, et
    al. Nitrofurantoin compares favorably to
    recommended agents as empirical treatment
    of uncomplicated urinary tract infections in
    a decision and cost analysis. Mayo Clin Proc
    86:480–8, 2011. (PMID:21576512)
Mendoza-Valdes A, Rosete A, Rios Bueno E, Frentzel A,
    et al. Antimicrobial and clinical efficacy of
    nitrofurantoin in the treatment of acute lower
    urinary tract infections in adults. Med Klin 105:
    698–704, 2010. (PMID:20981588)
Website: www.pdr.net

Ofloxacin (Oflox)

Drug Class: Quinolone.
Usual Dose: 400 mg (IV/PO) q12h (see
comments).

Spectrum Synopsis*
Hits
  Gram + : Non-enterococcal
    streptococci,
    Most MSSA, most VSE
  Gram – : Most GNB (including
    P. aeruginosa)
  Problem pathogens:
    Some Acinetobacter,
    S. maltophilia, B. cepacia
Misses
  Gram + : MRSA, VRE
  Gram – : B. fragilis
  Problem pathogens:
    Listeria Nocardia,
    Most Acinetobacter,
    S. maltophilia, B. cepacia

Urine Spectrum†
  • Same as serum spectrum
  • Optimal urinary pH = 6–7

(Full *Susceptibility Profiles* p. 208).

Resistance Potential: Low
Pharmacokinetic Parameters:
  Peak serum level: 5.5–7.2 mcg/mL
  Bioavailability: 95%
  Excreted unchanged (urine): 90%
  Serum half-life (normal/ESRD): 6/40 hrs
  Plasma protein binding: 32%
  Volume of distribution (V_d): 2 L/kg
Primary Mode of Elimination: Renal
Dosage Adjustments*

―――― = serious side effect 〔――〕 = black box warning. ND = no data. NR = not recommended. s = spectrum inadequate (at site). a = activity or experience inadequate. p = tissue penetration inadequate.
*based on peak serum concentration after usual adult dose. †applicable to adult uncomplicated lower UTIs
(CrCl > 30 mL/min).

CrCl 20–50 mL/min	400 mg (IV/PO) q24h
CrCl < 20 mL/min	200 mg (IV/PO) q24
Post–HD dose	200 mg (IV/PO)
Post–PD dose	200 mg (IV/PO)
CVVH/CVVHD/ CVVHDF dose	300 mg (IV/PO) q24h
Mild-moderate hepatic insufficiency	No change
Severe hepatic insufficiency	400 mg (IV/PO) q24h

Drug Interactions: Al^{++}, Ca^{++}, Fe^{++}, Mg^{++}, Zn^{++} antacids, citrate/citric acid, dairy products (↓ absorption of ofloxacin only if taken together); cimetidine (↑ ofloxacin levels); cyclosporine (↑ cyclosporine levels); NSAIDs (CNS stimulation); probenecid (↑ ofloxacin levels); warfarin (↑ INR).

Adverse Effects:
Uncommon
- Headache
- Insomnia
- Blurred vision
- Nausea/vomiting/diarrhea
- Drug/fever rash
- Mild neuroexcitatory symptoms

Rare
- C. difficile diarrhea/colitis
- ↑ QTc
- TEN
- Stevens-Johnson syndrome
- Tendinitis and tendon rupture

Allergic Potential: Low
Safety in Pregnancy: C

Additional Clinical Considerations:
- H_2 antagonist increases half-life by ~ 30%.
- Take ofloxacin 2 hours before or after calcium/magnesium containing antacids.
- **PPNG dose:** 400 mg (PO) × 1 dose.
- **NGU/cervicitis dose:** 300 mg (PO) q12h × 1 week.

Bile Penetration: 1500%
Cerebrospinal Fluid Penetration: <10%

(also see ***Antibiotic Pearls & Pitfalls*** p. 533).

SELECTED REFERENCE:
Website: www.pdr.net

Omadacycline (Nuzyra)

Drug Class: Tetracycline
Usual Dose:
CABP: Loading dose: 200 mg (IV) × 1 dose or 100 mg (IV) q12h, then
Maintenance dose: 100 mg (IV) q24h or 300 mg (PO) q24h
ABSSSIs: As above or days 1 and 2,
Loading dose: 450 mg (PO) q24h then
Maintenance dose: 300 mg (PO) q24h

Spectrum Synopsis*
Hits
  Gram + : VSE, VRE, MSSA, MRSA
  Gram – : B. fragilis
  Problem pathogens: PRSP, Acinetobacter
Misses
  Gram + : Listeria
  Gram – : P. aeruginosa
  Problem pathogens: B. cepacia, S. maltophilia, CRE

(Full ***Susceptibility Profiles*** p. 208)

—— = serious side effect ☐ = black box warning. ND = no data. NR = not recommended. s = spectrum inadequate (at site). a = activity or experience inadequate. p = tissue penetration inadequate. *based on peak serum concentration after usual adult dose. †applicable to adult uncomplicated lower UTIs (CrCl > 30 mL/min).

Resistance Potential: Low

Pharmacokinetic Parameters:

Peak serum level: 3.4 mcg/mL
Bioavailability: 34.5%
Excreted unchanged: 21%
Serum half-life (normal/ESRD): 16/18 hrs
Plasma protein binding: 20%
Volume of distribution (Vd): 2.7 L/kg

Primary Mode of Elimination: Biliary 70%, Renal (30%)

Dosage Adjustments*

	Oral	IV
CrCl < 15 mLmin	No change	No change
Post-HD/ Post-PD dose	No change	No change
CVVH dose	No change	No change
Mild to moderate hepatic insufficiency	No change	No change
Severe hepatic insufficiency	No change	No change

Drug Interactions: Avoid antacids containing aluminum, calcium, or magnesium, bismuth subsalicylate and iron containing preparations. Monitor and/or adjust dose of anticoagulant due to effect on prothrombin.

Adverse Effects:

Common

- Headache
- Nausea/vomiting
- Constipation
- Phlebitis
- ↑AST/ALT

Uncommon

- Diarrhea
- C. difficile colitis
- Nervousness/Anxiety
- Agitation
- Tremors
- Nightmares/Insomnia
- Paranoia
- Dizziness
- Confusion
- Hallucinations
- Depression and suicidal thoughts or acts
- Hypoglycemia

Rare

- Drug fever/rash

Allergic Potential: Low

Additional Clinical Considerations:
- Avoid in 2nd and 3rd trimester of pregnancy, during breastfeeding, and in children due to effect on tooth development and inhibition of bone growth.
- Without food

(also see **Antibiotic Pearls & Pitfalls** p. 530)

SELECTED REFERENCES:

Carvalhaes CG, et al. Antimicrobial activity of omadacycline tested against clinical bacterial isolates from hospitals in China (including Hong Kong) and Taiwan: results from the Sentry antimicrobial surveillance program (2013-2016). Antimicrob Agents Chemother pii: AAC.02262-18. doi: 10.1128/AAC. 022262-18, 2019. (PMID: 30617092)

Noe GJ, et al. A randomized, evaluator-blind, phase 2 study comparing the safety and efficacy of omadacycline to those of linezolid for the treatment of complicated skin and skin strucutre

—— = serious side effect ☐ = black box warning. ND = no data. NR = not recommended. s = spectrum inadequate (at site). a = activity or experience inadequate. p = tissue penetration inadequate. *based on peak serum concentration after usual adult dose. †applicable to adult uncomplicated lower UTIs (CrCl > 30 mL/min).

infections. Antimicrob Agents Chemother 56:5650-54, 2012. (PMID: 22908151).

Pfaller MA, et al. Surveillance of omadacycline activity tested against clinical isolates from the United States and Europe as part of the 2016 SENTRY antimicrobial surveillance program. Antimicrob Agents Chemother 62: pii: e02327-17. doi: 10.1128/AAC.02327-17, 2018. (PMID: 29378719).

Website:www.pdr.net

Oritavancin (Orbactiv)

Drug Class: Lipoglycopeptide
Usual Dose: 1200 mg (IV) x 1 dose

Spectrum Synopsis*
Hits
  Gram + : MSSA, MRSA, VISA, CoNS, VSE
  Gram – : None
  Problem pathogens: None
Misses
  Gram + : VRSA, VRE
  Gram – : All GNB, B. fragilis
  Problem pathogens:
    Listeria Nocardia, Acinetobacter, S. maltophilia, B. cepacia

Resistance Potential: Low
Pharmacokinetic Parameters:
Peak serum level: 138 mcg/mL
Bioavailability: Not applicable
Excreted unchanged (urine/feces): < 5%/< 1%
Serum half-life (normal/ESRD): 245 hr/ No data
Plasma protein binding: 85%
Volume of distribution (Vd): 1.25 L/kg
Primary Mode of Elimination: renal

Dosage Adjustments*

CrCl < 30 mL/min	No change (use with caution)
Post–HD dose	No change (use with caution)
Post–PD dose	No change (use with caution)
CVVH dose	No data
Hepatic insufficiency	No change

Drug Interactions: ↑ warfarin levels, monitor INR. Oritavancin is a weak inhibitor of CYP2C19 & CYP2C9; it is a weak inducer of CYP3A4.
Adverse Effects:
Common
• Nausea/vomiting/diarrhea
Uncommon
• Headache/dizziness
• Skin abscesses
• ↑ AST/ALT
• Phlebitis
• Hypersensitivity reactions
Rare
• C. difficile diarrhea/colitis
Allergic Potential: Low
Safety in Pregnancy: C

Additional Clinical Considerations:
Oritavancin artificially prolongs coagulation tests: activated clotting time (ACT); artificial effects last for 48 hours for PTT, 24 hours for PT and 24 hours for INR. Oritavancin is not removed during hemodialysis. Useful for VRE infections. Infuse slowly over 3 hours; if infusion reaction develops, slow the

---

⎯⎯⎯ = serious side effect ☐ = black box warning. ND = no data. NR = not recommended. s = spectrum inadequate (at site). a = activity or experience inadequate. p = tissue penetration inadequate. *based on peak serum concentration after usual adult dose. †applicable to adult uncomplicated lower UTIs (CrCl > 30 mL/min).

rate or interrupt infusion and then resume infusion upon resolution. Use of unfractionated heparin is contraindicated for 48 hours after oritavancin administration. ↑ incidence of osteomyelitis vs. vancomycin; institute alternate therapy if osteomyelitis is known or suspected osteomyelitis. Oritavancin may adhere to C. difficile spores, potentially preventing early inhibition of germinated cells; this may reduce the risk of recurrent C. difficile.

Cerebrospinal Fluid Penetration:

Non-inflamed meninges: 1%

Inflamed meninges: 10%

(also see ***Antibiotic Pearls & Pitfalls*** p. 537)

SELECTED REFERENCES:

Belley A, Arhin FF, Sarmiento I, et al. Pharmacodynamics of a simulated single 1,200-milligram dose of oritavancin in an in vitro pharmacokinetic/pharmacodynamic model of methicillin-resistant staphylococcus aureus infection. Antimicrob Agents Chemother. 57:205-211, 2013. (PMID:23089749)

Chilton CH, Freeman J, Baines SO, et al. Evaluation of the effect of oritavancin on Clostridium difficile spore germination, outgrowth and recovery. J Antimicrob Chemother. 68:2078-2082, 2013. (PMID:23759507)

Corey GR, Good S, Jiang H, et al. Single-Dose Oritavancin Versus 7-10 Days of Vancomycin in the Treatment of Gram-Positive Acute Bacterial Skin and Skin Structure Infections: The SOLO II Noninferiority Study. Clin Infect Dis. 60:254-262, 2015. (PMID:25294250)

Corey GR, Kabler H, Mehra P, et al. Single-dose oritavancin in the treatment of acute bacterial skin infections. N Engl J Med. 370:2180-2190, 2014. (PMID:24897083)

Kumar A, Mann HJ, Keshtgarpour M, et al. In vitro characterization of oritavancin clearance from human blood by low-flux, high-flux, and continuous renal replacement therapy dialyzers. Int J Artif Organs. 34:1067-1074, 2011. (PMID:22183520)

Mendes RE, Farrell OJ, Sader HS, et al. Activity of oritavancin against Gram-positive clinical isolates responsible for documented skin and soft-tissue infections in European and US hospitals (2010-13). J Antimicrob Chemother. 70:498-504, 2015. (PMID:25362568)

Tice A. Oritavancin: a new opportunity for outpatient therapy of serious infections. Clin Infect Dis. 54 Suppl 3:S239-243, 2012. (PMID:22431855)

Website: www.pdr.net

Oseltamavir (Tamiflu)

Drug class: Antiviral (influenza A+B).

Usual dose: <u>Treatment:</u> 75 mg (PO) q12h × 5 days; <u>Prophylaxis:</u> 75 mg (PO) q24h × 10 days.

Pharmacokinetic Parameters:

Peak serum level: 65.2 mcg/L

Bioavailability: 75%

Excreted unchanged: 1%

Serum half-life (normal/ESRD): 1–3 hours/ ND

Plasma protein binding: 42%

Volume of distribution (V_d): 23–26 L/kg

Primary Mode of Elimination: Renal (oseltamivir carboxylate)

Dosage Adjustments*

CrCl > 60 mL/min	No adjustment
CrCl 30–60 mL/min	30 mg (PO) q12h (treatment) 30 mg (PO) q24h (prophylaxis)
CrCl 10–30 mL/min	30 mg (PO) q24h
Post-HD dose	30 mg (PO)
Post-PD dose	30 mg (PO)

——— = serious side effect ☐ = black box warning. ND = no data. NR = not recommended. s = spectrum inadequate (at site). a = activity or experience inadequate. p = tissue penetration inadequate. *based on peak serum concentration after usual adult dose. [†]applicable to adult uncomplicated lower UTIs (CrCl > 30 mL/min).

CVVH/CVVHD/ CVVHDF dose	30 mg (PO) q24h (treatment) 30 mg (PO) q24h (prophylaxis)
Moderate— severe hepatic insufficiency	Use with caution

Drug Interactions: Live attenuated influenza vaccine 2 weeks before or 2 days after oseltamivir.
Adverse Effects:
Common
- Nauses/vomiting/diarrhea
Rare
- Epistaxis
Allergic Potential: Low
Safety in Pregnancy: C
Additional Clinical Considerations:
- Optimally begin prophylaxis within 3 days of exposure.

SELECTED REFERENCE:
Website: www.pdr.net

Oxacillin (Prostaphlin)

Drug Class: Anti-staphylococcal (MSSA) penicillin.
Usual Dose: 1–2 gm (IV) q4h.

Spectrum Synopsis*
Hits
  Gram + : GAS, MSSA
  Gram – : None
  Problem pathogens:
    None
Misses
  Gram + : MRSA, VSE, VRE
  Gram – : B. fragilis
  Problem pathogens: All

Resistance Potential: Low
Pharmacokinetic Parameters:
  Peak serum level: 43 mcg/mL
  Bioavailability: Not applicable
  Excreted unchanged (urine): 39–66%
  Serum half-life (normal/ESRD): 0.5/1 hrs
  Plasma protein binding: 94%
  Volume of distribution (V_d): 0.2 L/kg
Primary Mode of Elimination: Renal
Dosage Adjustments* (based on 2 gm q4h)

CrCl 10–80 mL/min	No change
CrCl < 10 mL/min	No change
Post–HD dose	None
Post–PD dose	None
CVVH/CVVHD/ CVVHDF dose	No change
Moderate hepatic insufficiency	No change
Severe hepatic insufficiency	No change

Drug Interactions: Cyclosporine ($\downarrow$ cyclosporine levels); nifedipine, warfarin ($\downarrow$ interacting drug effect).
Adverse Effects:
Common
- Nausea/vomiting/diarrhea
Uncommon
- Drug fever/rash
- Leukopenia
Rare
- Hepatitis
Allergic Potential: High
Safety in Pregnancy: B

—— = serious side effect ☐ = black box warning. ND = no data. NR = not recommended. s = spectrum inadequate (at site). a = activity or experience inadequate. p = tissue penetration inadequate. *based on peak serum concentration after usual adult dose. †applicable to adult uncomplicated lower UTIs (CrCl > 30 mL/min).

Additional Clinical Considerations:
- **Avoid oral formulation** (not well absorbed/erratic serum levels).

Cerebrospinal Fluid Penetration:
Non-inflamed meninges: 1%
Inflamed meninges: 10%

Meningeal dose = 2 gm (IV) q4h.

SELECTED REFERENCE:
Website: www.pdr.net

Penicillin G (various)

Drug Class: Natural penicillin.
Usual Dose: 2–4 mu (IV) q4h (see comments).

Spectrum Synopsis*
Hits
  Gram + : GAS, GBS
  Gram − : Some GNB
  Problem pathogens:
    Oral anaerobes
Misses
  Gram + : MSSA, MRSA, VSE, VRE
  Gram − : Most GNB (including H. influenzae), B. fragilis
  Problem pathogens:
    Listeria, Nocardia, B. cepacia
    Acinetobacter, S. maltophilia,
Urine Spectrum†
- Same as serum spectrum
- Optimal urinary pH = 5–6
- Urine levels = 100 mcg/mL

(Full **Susceptibility Profiles** p. 196).

Resistance Potential: Low
Pharmacokinetic Parameters:
Peak serum level: 20–40 mcg/mL

Bioavailability: Not applicable
Excreted unchanged (urine): 80%
Serum half-life (normal/ESRD): 0.5/5.1 hrs
Plasma protein binding: 60%
Volume of distribution (V_d): 0.3 L/kg
Primary Mode of Elimination: Renal
Dosage Adjustments*

CrCl 50–80 mL/min	2–4 mu (IV) q4h
CrCl 10–50 mL/min	1–2 mu (IV) q4h
CrCl < 10 mL/min	1 mu (IV) q8h
Post–HD dose	2 mu (IV)
Post–PD dose	0.5 mu (IV)
CVVH/CVVHD/ CVVHDF dose	2 mu (IV) q6h
Moderate hepatic insufficiency	No change
Severe hepatic insufficiency	No change

Drug Interactions: Probenecid
($\uparrow$ penicillin G levels).
Adverse Effects:
Common
- Nausea/vomiting
Uncommon
- Drug fever/rash
- Jarisch-Herxheimer reactions
- Anaphylactic reactions
Rare
- Serum sickness
- Erythema multiforme/ Stevens-Johnson Syndrome

Allergic Potential: High
Safety in Pregnancy: B

——— = serious side effect ☐ = black box warning. ND = no data. NR = not recommended. s = spectrum inadequate (at site). a = activity or experience inadequate. p = tissue penetration inadequate. *based on peak serum concentration after usual adult dose. †applicable to adult uncomplicated lower UTIs (CrCl > 30 mL/min).

Additional Clinical Considerations:
- **1°, 2°, early latent syphilis dose:** PCN benzathine 2.4 mu (IM) × 1 dose.
- **Late latent syphilis dose:** PCN benzathine 2.4 mu (IM) q8h once weekly × 3.
- **Neurosyphilis dose:** PCN G 4 mu (IV) q4h × 2 weeks.

Bile Penetration: 500%
Cerebrospinal Fluid Penetration:
Non-inflamed meninges: 1%
Inflamed meninges: 5%
Meningeal dose = 4 mu (IV) q4h.

(also see **Antibiotic Pearls & Pitfalls** p. 526).

SELECTED REFERENCE:
Website: www.pdr.net

Penicillin V (various)

Drug Class: Natural penicillin.
Usual Dose: 500 mg (PO) q6h.
(Take without food).

Spectrum Synopsis*
Hits
  Gram + : GAS, GBS
  Gram − : Some GNB
  Problem pathogens:
    Oral anaerobes
Misses
  Gram + : MSSA, MRSA, VSE, VRE
  Gram − : Most GNB (including H. influenzae), B. fragilis
  Problem pathogens:
    Listeria, Nocardia, B. cepacia
    Acinetobacter, S. maltophilia,

Urine Spectrum†
- Same as serum spectrum
- Optimal urinary pH = 5–6

(Full **Susceptibility Profiles** p. 196).

Resistance Potential: Low
Pharmacokinetic Parameters:
  Peak serum level: 5 mcg/mL
  Bioavailability: 60%
  Excreted unchanged (urine): 80%
  Serum half-life (normal/ESRD): 0.5/8 hrs
  Plasma protein binding: 70%
  Volume of distribution (V_d): 0.5 L/kg
Primary Mode of Elimination: Renal
Dosage Adjustments*

CrCl 10–50 mL/min	No change
CrCl < 10 mL/min	250–500 mg (PO) q6h
Post–HD dose	250 mg (PO)
Post–PD dose	250 mg (PO)
CVVH/CVVHD/CVVHDF dose	500 mg (PO) q6h
Moderate hepatic insufficiency	No change
Severe hepatic insufficiency	No change

Drug Interactions: Probenecid (↑ penicillin V levels).
Adverse Effects:
Common
- Nausea/vomiting/diarrhea
Uncommon
- Drug fever/rash
- <u>Anaphylactic reactions</u>
Rare

——— = serious side effect ☐ = black box warning. ND = no data. NR = not recommended. s = spectrum inadequate (at site). a = activity or experience inadequate. p = tissue penetration inadequate. *based on peak serum concentration after usual adult dose. †applicable to adult uncomplicated lower UTIs (CrCl > 30 mL/min).

- Serum sickness
- Erythema multiforme/
  Stevens-Johnson Syndrome
- C. difficile diarrhea/colitis

Allergic Potential: High
Safety in Pregnancy: B

Additional Clinical Considerations:
- Jarisch–Herxheimer reactions may occur when treating spirochetal infections, e.g., Lyme disease, syphilis, yaws.

Cerebrospinal Fluid Penetration: <10%

(also see **Antibiotic Pearls & Pitfalls** p. 526).

SELECTED REFERENCE:
Website: www.pdr.net

Pentamidine (Pentam 300, NebuPent)

Drug Class: Antiparasitic.
Usual Dose: 4 mg/kg (IV) q24h (see comments).
Pharmacokinetic Parameters:
  Peak serum level: 0.6–1.5 mcg/mL
  Bioavailability: Not applicable
  Excreted unchanged (urine): 50%
  Serum half-life (normal/ESRD): 6.4/90 hrs
  Plasma protein binding: 69%
  Volume of distribution (V_d): 5 L/kg
Primary Mode of Elimination: Metabolized
Dosage Adjustments*

CrCl < 10 mL/min	No change
Post–HD dose	None
Post–PD dose	None
CVVH/CVVHD/CVVHDF dose	No change
Moderate—severe hepatic insufficiency	No change

Drug Interactions: Alcohol, valproic acid, didanosine, (↑ risk of pancreatitis); foscarnet (severe hypocalcemia reported; do not combine); amphotericin B, aminoglycosides, capreomycin, cis-platinum, colistin, methoxyflurane, polymyxin B, vancomycin, other nephrotoxic drugs (↑ nephrotoxicity).
Adverse Effects:
Common
- Injection site reactions
- Renal insufficiency

Uncommon
- Hypoglycemia
- Hypotension
- Leukopenia
- Anemia
- Thrombocytopenia
- ↑ AST/ALT
- ↑ BUN

Rare
- Pancreatitis
- Torsades de pointes

Allergic Potential: High
Safety in Pregnancy: C

——— = serious side effect [____] = black box warning. ND = no data. NR = not recommended. s = spectrum inadequate (at site). a = activity or experience inadequate. p = tissue penetration inadequate. *based on peak serum concentration after usual adult dose. †applicable to adult uncomplicated lower UTIs (CrCl > 30 mL/min).

Additional Clinical Considerations:

- **Well absorbed IM, but painful.**
- May be used at a dose of 300 mg via aerosol q month to prevent pentamidine.
- Caution should be used with inhalent pentamidine especially around pregnant employees (may induce spontaneous abortion)
- Careful attention should be made to the proper aerosolization of medication so that it is distributed evenly through the lung.
- Adverse effects with aerosolized pentamidine include chest pain, arrhythmias, dizziness, wheezing, coughing, dyspnea, headache, anorexia, nausea, diarrhea, rash, pharyngitis.
- **If PCP patient also has pulmonary TB, aerosolized pentamidine treatments may expose medical personnel to TB via droplet inhalation.**
- **Nebulizer dose:** Inhaled pentamidine isethionate (NebuPent) 300 mg monthly (via Respirgard II nebulizer) can be used for PCP prophylaxis
- **Nebulized pentamidine less effective than IV/IM pentamidine and is not effective against extrapulmonary PCP.**
- Use with caution in renal disease.

Cerebrospinal Fluid Penetration: <10%

SELECTED REFERENCES:

Goa KL, Campoli-Richards DM. Pentamidine isethionate: A review of its antiprotozoal activity, pharmacokinetic properties and therapeutic use in Pneumocystis carinii pneumonia. Drugs 33:242–58, 1987. (PMID:3552596)

Monk JP, Benfield P. Inhaled pentamidine: An overview of its pharmacological properties and a review of its therapeutic use in Pneumocystis carinii pneumonia. Drugs 39:741–56, 1990. (PMID:2191850)

Sattler FR, Cowam R. Nielsen DM, et al. Trimethoprim-sulfamethoxazole compared with pentamidine for treatment of Pneumocystis carinii pneumonia in the acquired immunodeficiency syndrome. Ann Intern Med 109:280–7, 1988. (PMID:3260759)

Website: www.pdr.net

Peramivir (Rapivab)

Drug Class: Antiviral (influenza A+B).
Usual Dose: 600 mg (IV) × 1 dose.
Pharmacokinetic Parameters:
Peak serum level: 46 mcg/mL
Bioavailability: not applicable
Excreted unchanged: ND
Serum half-life (normal/ESRD): 7–20 hrs/ND
Plasma protein binding: ND
Volume of distribution (V_d): ND
Primary Mode of Elimination: Renal
Dosage Adjustments*
Drug Interactions: *ND.*
Adverse Effects:
Uncommon
- Diarrhea
- Neutropenia

—— = serious side effect ☐ = black box warning. ND = no data. NR = not recommended. s = spectrum inadequate (at site). a = activity or experience inadequate. p = tissue penetration inadequate. *based on peak serum concentration after usual adult dose. †applicable to adult uncomplicated lower UTIs (CrCl > 30 mL/min).

- ↑ AST/ALT
- ↑ CPK

Rare
- Abnormal behavior/hallucinations
- Delirium
- Drug fever/rash
- Erythema multiforme

Allergic Potential: Low (do not use if severely allergic to other neuroaminidase inhibitors)

Safety in Pregnancy: C

Additional Clinical Considerations:
- For single dose treatment of adult and pediatric patients with influenza A.
- **For patients not responding to either oral or inhaled antiviral therapy or when drug delivery not possible or suboptimal by another route.**
- For optimal effectiveness give within 2 days of influenza onset.

***Highly active** against influenza A*.

Cerebrospinal Fluid Penetration: No data

SELECTED REFERENCES:

Castillo R, Holland LE, Bolz DA. Peramivir and its use in H1N1 influenza. Drugs Today (Barc) 46:399–408 2010. (PMID:20571608)

Kohno S, Kida H, Mizuguchi M, et al. Efficacy and safety of intravenous peramivir for treatment of seasonal influenza virus infection. Antimicrob Agents Chemother 54:4568–4574, 2010. (PMID:20713668)

Kohno S, Kida H, Mizuguchi M, et al. Intravenous peramivir for treatment of influenza A and B virus infection in high-risk patients. Antimicrob Agents Chemother 55:2803–2812, 2011. (PMID:21464252)

Moss RB, Davey RT, Steigbigel RT, et al. Targeting pandemic influenza: a primer on influenza antivirals and drug resistance. J Antimicrob Chemother 65:1086–1093, 2010. (PMID:20375034)

Thomas B, Hollister AS, Muczynski KA. Peramivir clearance in continuous renal replacement therapy. Hemodial Int 14:339–340, 2010. (PMID:20491974)

Website: www.pdr.net

Piperacillin (Pipracil)

Drug Class: Anti-pseudomonal penicillin.
Usual Dose: 3 gm (IV) q4-6h (see comments).

Spectrum Synopsis*
Hits
  Gram + : GAS, VSE MSSA
  Gram – : Most GNB, (including P. aeruginosa), B. fragilis
  Problem pathogens: Animal bite pathogens
Misses
  Gram + : MRSA, VRE
  Gram – : Some GNB
  Problem pathogens: Listeria, Nocardia, Acinetobacter, S. maltophilia, B. cepacia
Urine Spectrum†
- Same as serum spectrum
- Optimal urinary pH = 5–6
- Urine levels = 100 mcg/mL

(Full ***Susceptibility Profiles*** p. 196).

Resistance Potential: Low
  Pharmacokinetic Parameters:
  Peak serum level: 412 mcg/mL
  Bioavailability: Not applicable

——— = serious side effect ⬜ = black box warning. ND = no data. NR = not recommended. s = spectrum inadequate (at site). a = activity or experience inadequate. p = tissue penetration inadequate. *based on peak serum concentration after usual adult dose. †applicable to adult uncomplicated lower UTIs (CrCl > 30 mL/min).

Excreted unchanged (urine): 50–70%
Serum half-life (normal/ESRD): 1/3 hrs
Plasma protein binding: 16%
Volume of distribution (V_d): 0.24 L/kg
Primary Mode of Elimination: Renal

Dosage Adjustments* (based on 4 gm q8h)

CrCl 20–50 mL/min	3 gm (IV) q8h
CrCl < 20 mL/min	3 gm (IV) q12h
Post–HD dose	1 gm (IV)
Post–PD dose	2 gm (IV)
CVVH/CVVHD/ CVVHDF dose	3 gm (IV) q8h
Moderate or severe hepatic insufficiency	No change

Drug Interactions: Aminoglycosides (inactivation of piperacillin in renal failure); warfarin (↑ INR); oral contraceptives (↓ oral contraceptive effect); cefoxitin (↓ piperacillin effect).

Adverse Effects:
Uncommon
- Drug fever/rash
- Leukopenia
- Hemolytic anemia
- Thrombocytopenia
- Jarisch-Herxheimer reaction
- Anaphylactic reactions

Rare
- Serum sickness
- Erythema multiforme/Stevens-Johnson Syndrome
- C. difficile diarrhea/colitis

Allergic Potential: High
Safety in Pregnancy: B

Additional Clinical Considerations:
- **Most active anti-pseudomonal penicillin against P. aeruginosa.**
- **Nosocomial pneumonia/ P. aeruginosa dose:** 3 gm (IV) q4h.

Meningeal dose = usual dose.

May increase LPS (endotoxin) release from GNB *potentially increasing endotoxin mediated tissue damage.*

Additional Pharmacokinetic Considerations*

Non-CSF	% of Serum Levels
Peritoneal fluid	ND
Bile	1000%
Synovial fluid	ND
Bone	20%
Prostate	NR(p)
CSF	
Non-inflamed meninges	1%
Inflamed meninges (ABM)	30%

Meningeal dose = 3 gm (IV) q4h

SELECTED REFERENCES:

Tan JS, File TM, Jr. Antipseudomonal penicillins. Med Clin North Am 79:679–93, 1995. (PMID:7791416)
Website: www.pdr.net

Piperacillin/Tazobactam (Zosyn, Tazocin)

Drug Class: Anti-pseudomonal penicillin/β-lactamase inhibitor.

—— = serious side effect ☐ = black box warning. ND = no data. NR = not recommended. s = spectrum inadequate (at site). a = activity or experience inadequate. p = tissue penetration inadequate. *based on peak serum concentration after usual adult dose. †applicable to adult uncomplicated lower UTIs (CrCl > 30 mL/min).

Usual Dose: 3.375 gm (IV) q6h
(PI dose) or 4.5 gm (IV) q8h **(PK dose)**
(see comments).

Spectrum Synopsis*
Hits
  Gram + : GAS, MSSA, VSE
  Gram – : Most GNB (including
    P. aeruginosa), B. fragilis
  Problem pathogens:
    Animal bite pathogens
Misses
  Gram + : MRSA, VRE
  Gram – : Some GNB
  Problem pathogens:
    Listeria, Nocardia, B. cepacia
    Acinetobacter, S. maltophilia
Urine Spectrum†
- Same as serum spectrum
- Optimal urinary pH = 5–6
- Urine levels = 100 mcg/mL

(Full **Susceptibility Profiles** p. 196).

Resistance Potential: Low
Pharmacokinetic Parameters:
  Peak serum level: 298/34 mcg/mL
  Bioavailability: Not applicable
  Excreted unchanged (urine): 60/80%
  *Serum half-life (normal/ESRD): [1.5/8] /
  [1/7] hrs*
  Plasma protein binding: 30/30%
  Volume of distribution (V_d): 0.3/0.21 L/kg
Primary Mode of Elimination: Renal
Dosage Adjustments* (also see
comments)

CrCl 20–40 mL/min	2.25 gm (IV) q6h 3.375 gm (IV) q6h for NP
CrCl < 20 mL/min	2.25 gm (IV) q8h 2.25 (IV) q6h for NP

CrCl < 10 mL/min	2.25 gm (IV) q8h
Post–HD dose	0.75 gm (IV)
Post–PD dose	None
CVVH/CVVHD/CVVHDF dose	3.375 gm (IV) q6h
Moderate—severe hepatic insufficiency	No change

Drug Interactions: Aminoglycosides
($\downarrow$ aminoglycoside levels); vecuronium
($\uparrow$ vecuronium effect); probenecid
($\uparrow$ piperacillin/tazobactam levels);
methotrexate ($\uparrow$ methotrexate levels).
Adverse Effects:
Common
- Nausea/vomiting
- <u>C. difficile diarrhea/colitis</u>
Uncommon
- Insomnia
- Headache
- Constipation
- Drug fever/rash
- Hypertension
- Eosinophilia
- Leukopenia (with prolonged use
  > 21 days)
- Thrombocytopenia
- Thrombocytosis
- $\uparrow$ AST/ALT
- $\uparrow$ PT/PTT
- Hyperglycemia
Rare
- Hemolytic anemia
Allergic Potential: High
Safety in Pregnancy: B

Additional Clinical Considerations:
- Only modest P. aeruginosa activity.

───── = serious side effect ☐ = black box warning. ND = no data. NR = not recommended. s = spectrum inadequate (at site). a = activity or experience inadequate. p = tissue penetration inadequate. *based on peak serum concentration after usual adult dose. †applicable to adult uncomplicated lower UTIs (CrCl > 30 mL/min).

- For more P. aeruginosa activity must use high dose 4.5 g (IV) q6h *plus* amikacin
- **For P. aeruginosa/nosocomial pneumonia (normal CrCl) use 4.5 g (IV) q6h *plus* amikacin 1 g (IV) q24h.**
- **P. aeruginosa/nosocomial pneumonia dosing with ↑ CrCl:**
  CrCl > 40 mL/min: 4.5 gm (IV) q6h.
  CrCl 20–40 mL/min: 3.375 gm (IV) q6h.
  CrCl < 20 mL/min: 2.25 gm (IV) q6h.
  Hemodialysis (HD) doses: 2.25 gm (IV) q8h; give 0.75 gm (IV) post–HD on HD days.

Additional Pharmacokinetic Considerations	
Non-CSF	**% of Serum Levels**
Peritoneal fluid	50%
Bile	6000%
Synovial fluid	50%
Bone	25%
Prostate	NR(p)
CSF	
Non-inflamed meninges	1%
Inflamed meninges (ABM)	30%

(also see ***Antibiotic Pearls & Pitfalls*** p. 530).

SELECTED REFERENCES:
Bauer SR, Salem C, Connor MJ Jr, et al. Pharmacokinetics and pharmacodynamics of piperacillin-tazobactam in 42 patients treated with concomitant CRRT. Clin J Am Soc Nephrol 7:452–457, 2012. (PMID:22282479)
Gin A, Dilay L, Karlowsky JA, et al. Piperacillin-tazobactam: a beta-lactam/beta-lactamase inhibitor combination. Expert Rev Anti Infect Ther 5:365–383, 2007. (PMID:57547502)
Hayashi Y, Roberts JA, Paterson DL, et al. Pharmacokinetic evaluation of piperacillin-tazobactam. Expert Opin Drug Metab Toxicol 6:1017–1031, 2010. (PMID:20636224)
Mikulska M, Furfaro E, Del Bono V, et al. Piperacillin/tazobactam seems to be no longer responsible for false-positive results of the galactomannan assay. J Antimicrob Chemother 67:1746–1748, 2012. (PMID:22499998)
Mattoes HM, Capitano B, Kim MK, et al. Comparative pharmacokinetic and pharmacodynamic profile of piperacillin/tazobactam 3.375 G Q4H and 4.5 G Q6H. Chemotherapy 458:59–63, 2002. (PMID:12011536)
Saltoglu N, Dalkiran A, Tetiker T, et al. Piperacillin/tazobactam versus imipenem/cilastatin for severe diabetic foot infections: a prospective, randomized clinical trial in a university hospital. Clin Microbiol Infect 16:1252–1257, 2010. (PMID:19832720)
Website: www.pdr.net

Plazomycin (Zemdri)

Drug Class: Aminoglycoside.
Usual Dose: 15 mg/kg (IV) q12h

Spectrum Synopsis*
Hits
Gram + : None
Gram – : Most GNB
Problem pathogens:
Acinetobacter, P. aeruginosa, CRE
Misses
Gram + : VSE, VRE, MSSA, MRSA
Gram – : B. fragilis
Problem pathogens:
S. maltophilia, B. cepacia
Urine Spectrum†
• Same as serum spectrum
• Optimal urinary pH : *ND*
• Urinary levels = 805 mcg/mL

(Full ***Susceptibility Profiles*** p. 208).

———— = serious side effect ☐ = black box warning. ND = no data. NR = not recommended. s = spectrum inadequate (at site). a = activity or experience inadequate. p = tissue penetration inadequate. *based on peak serum concentration after usual adult dose. †applicable to adult uncomplicated lower UTIs (CrCl > 30 mL/min).

Resistance Potential: Low to moderate

Pharmacokinetic Parameters:
Peak serum level: 51 mcg/mL
Bioavailability: Not applicable
Excreted unchanged: 97.5%
Serum half-life (normal): 3.5 hrs
Plasma protein binding: 20%
Volume of distribution (V_d): 0.44 L/kg

Primary Mode of Elimination: Renal

Dosage Adjustments*

CrCl 60–90 mL/min	15 mg/kg (IV) q24h
CrCl 30–59 mL/min	10 mg/kg (IV) q24h
CrCl 15–30 mL/min	10 mg/kg (IV) q48h
CrCl < 15 mL/min	Avoid
Post-HD dose	*ND*
Post-PD dose	*ND*
CVVH dose	*ND*
Mild to moderate hepatic insufficiency	No change
Severe hepatic insufficiency	No change

Drug Interactions: None
Adverse Effects:
Common
• ↑ Creatinine
• Diarrhea
• Hypertension
Uncommon
• Nephrotoxicity

• Ototoxocity
• Neuromuscular blockade
• Potential Fetal harm
• Headache
• Nausea/vomiting
• Hypotension
Rare:
• Dyspnea
• Constipation
• ↑AST/ALT
• Hypokalemia
Allergic Potential: Low

Additional Clinical Considerations:
• Monitor creatinine clearance.
• For adult complicated urinary tract infections
• Monitor serum levels to maintain trough below 3 mcg/mL, monitor at second dose. Extend dose interval by 1.5 fold if trough is above 3 mcg/mL
• Do not administer if patient has history of hypersensitivity to aminoglycosides
• Avoid in pregnancy.

Additional Pharmacokinetic Considerations*

Non-CSF	% of Serum Levels
No Data	
CSF	
No Data	

Meningeal dose: *ND*

(also see ***Antibiotic Pearls & Pitfalls*** p. 531).

――― = serious side effect ☐ = black box warning. ND = no data. NR = not recommended. s = spectrum inadequate (at site). a = activity or experience inadequate. p = tissue penetration inadequate. *based on peak serum concentration after usual adult dose. †applicable to adult uncomplicated lower UTIs (CrCl > 30 mL/min).

SELECTED REFERENCES:
Cass RT, et al. Pharmacokinetics and safety of single and multiple doses of ACHN-490 injection administered intravenously in healthy subjects. Antimicrob Agents Chemother 55:5874-80, 2011. (PMID: 21911572)

Castanheria M. et al. In vitro activity of plazomicin against Enterobacteriaceae isolates carrying genes encoding aminoglycoside-modifying enzymes most common in US Census divisions. Diagn Microbial Infect Dis; pii: S0732-8893(18)30316-X. doi: 10.1016/j.diagmicrobio.2018.10.023. [Epub ahead of print], 2018. (PMID: 30661726)

Karasikos I, et al. Novel β-lactam-β-lactamase inhibitor combinations: expectations for the treatment of carbapenem-resistant Gram-negative pathogens. Expert Opin Drug Metab Toxicol; 10:1-17, 2019. (PMID: 30626244)

Martins AF, et al. Antimicrobial activity of plazomicin against Enterobacteriaceae-producing carbapenemases from 50 Brazilian medical centers. Diagn Microbial Infect Dis; 90:228-32, 2018. (PMID: 29223516)

Shaeer KM, et al. Plazomicin: a next generation aminoglycoside. Pharmacotherapy, 2018. (PMID: 30511766)

Website:www.pdr.net

Polymyxin B

Drug Class: Cell membrane antibiotic.
Usual Dose: 1–1.25 mg/kg (IV) q12h (1 mg = 10,000 units) (see comments).

Spectrum Synopsis*
Hits
  Gram + : None
  Gram – : Most GNB, (including P. aeruginosa)
  Problem pathogens:
    S. maltophilia, ESBL + Klebsiella,
    Enterobacter, E. coli, CRE
Misses
  Gram + : All streptococci, MSSA, MRSA, VSE, VRE

Gram – : Proteus, Serratia, B. fragilis
Problem pathogens:
  Listeria, Nocardia,
  Acinetobacter, B. cepacia
Urine Spectrum[†]
- Same as serum spectrum
- Ineffective for AUC/CAB due to subtherapeutic urine levels

(Full **Susceptibility Profiles** p. 208).

Pharmacokinetic Parameters:
  Peak serum level: 8 mcg/mL
  Bioavailability: Not applicable
  Excreted unchanged (urine): 60%
  Serum half-life (normal/ESRD): 6/48 hrs
  Plasma protein binding: < 10%
  Volume of distribution (V_d): ND
Primary Mode of Elimination: Renal
Dosage Adjustments*

CrCl < 5 mL/min	0.5 mg/kg (IV) q12h
Post–HD/PD dose	No information
CVVH/CVVHD/ CVVHDF dose	0.5 mg/kg (IV) q12h
Moderate— severe hepatic insufficiency	No change

Drug Interactions: Amphotericin B, amikacin, gentamicin, tobramycin, vancomycin (↑ nephrotoxicity).
Adverse Effects:
Uncommon
- Nephrotoxicity
- Neuromuscular blockade (respiratory paralysis)

Resistance Potential: Low
Allergic Potential: Low
Safety in Pregnancy: B

------ = serious side effect ⬜ = black box warning. ND = no data. NR = not recommended. s = spectrum inadequate (at site). a = activity or experience inadequate. p = tissue penetration inadequate. *based on peak serum concentration after usual adult dose. †applicable to adult uncomplicated lower UTIs (CrCl > 30 mL/min).

Additional Clinical Considerations:
- Less potential nephrotoxicity compared to colistin.
- Avoid intraperitoneal infusion due to risk of neuromuscular blockade.
- Increased risk of reversible non-oliguric renal failure (ATN) when used with other nephrotoxic drugs. No ototoxic potential.
- **Nebulizer dose for multidrug resistant P. aeruginosa in cystic fibrosis/bronchiectasis:** 80 mg in saline via aerosol/nebulizer q8h (for recurrent infection use 160 mg).
- Dissolve 50 mg (500,000 u) into 10 mL for IT administration.

May inhibit antibiotic induced LPS (endotoxin) release from GNB potentially minimizing endotoxin mediated tissue damage.

Additional Pharmacokinetic Considerations*

Non-CSF	% of Serum Levels
Peritoneal fluid	NR(s)
Bile	NR(p)
Synovial fluid	*ND*
Bone	*ND*
Prostate	NR(p)
CSF	
Non-inflamed meninges	<1%
Inflamed meninges (ABM)	<10%

Meningeal dose:
- **Intrathecal (IT) polymyxin B dose:** 5 mg (50,000 u) q24h × 3 days, then q48h × 2 weeks give with IV therapy.

(also see ***Antibiotic Pearls & Pitfalls*** p. 538).

SELECTED REFERENCES:
Cavaillon JM. Polymyxin B for endotoxin removal in sepsis. Lancet Infect Dis 11:426–7, 2011. (PMID:21616454)
Falagas ME, Kasiakou SK. Colistin: the revival of polymyxins for the management of multidrug-resistant gram-negative bacterial infections. Clin Infect Dis 40:1333–41, 2005. (PMID:15825037)
Kassamali Z, Rotschafer JC, Jones RN, et al. Polymyxins: wisdom does not always come with age. Clin Infect Dis 57:877-884, 2013. (PMID:23738146)
Kunin CM. The Pharmacokinetics of Polymyxin B are Dependent on Binding and Release from Deep-Tissue Compartments. Clin Infect Dis 48:842–844, 2009. (PMID:19220156)
Parchuri S, Mohan S, Young S, Cunha BA. Chronic ambulatory peritoneal dialysis associated peritonitis ESBL producing Klebsiella pneumoniae successfully treated with polymyxin B. Heart & Lung 34:360, 2005. (PMID:16157192)
Rigatoo MH, Oliveira MS, Perdigao-Neto LV, et al. Multicenter prospective cohort study of renal failure in patients treated with colistin versus polymyxin B. Antimicrob Agents & Chemo 60:2443-2449, 2016. (PMID: 26856846)
Website: www.pdr.net

Posaconazole (Noxafil)

Drug Class: Triazole antifungal.
Usual Dose: <u>Prophylaxis of invasive Aspergillus and Candida infections in high-risk patients:</u>[†] **Loading dose:** 300 mg (PO) q12h × 1 day, then **Maintenance dose:** 300 mg (PO) q12h × 1 day, then 300 mg (PO) q24h (DRTs) <u>Oropharyngeal candidiasis:</u> **Loading dose:** 100 mg (PO) q12h × 1 day, then **Maintenance dose:** 100 mg (PO) q24h (oral suspension) × 13 days; <u>Fluconazole and/or itraconazole-resistant strains:</u> use 400 mg (PO) q12h duration based on clinical response.
Pharmacokinetic Parameters:
Peak serum level: 3 mcg/mL
Bioavailability: Absorption is ↑ 2–6-fold with a high fat meal

---

= serious side effect ☐ = black box warning. ND = no data. NR = not recommended. s = spectrum inadequate (at site). a = activity or experience inadequate. p = tissue penetration inadequate. *based on peak serum concentration after usual adult dose. †applicable to adult uncomplicated lower UTIs (CrCl > 30 mL/min). DRT = delayed release tablets.

Excreted unchanged (urine): < 1%
Excreted unchanged (feces): 66%
Serum half-life (normal/ESRD): 35/35 hrs
Plasma protein binding: 98.2%
Volume of distribution (V_d): 1774 L

Primary Mode of Elimination: Hepatic

Dosage Adjustments*

CrCl < 50 mL/min	No change
Post–HD dose	Use IV with caution (PO dose same)
Post–PD dose	Use IV with caution (PO dose same)
CVVH/CVVHD/CVVHDF dose	Use IV with caution (PO dose same)
Moderate—severe hepatic insufficiency	No change

Drug Interactions: Posaconazole is metabolized by hepatic glucuronidation. Inducers (e.g., rifampin, phenytoin) may alter disposition. Amiodarone, rifabutin, phenytoin, cimetidine ($\downarrow$ posaconazole levels 50%). Posaconazole inhibits hepatic CYP3A4 and can increase levels of drugs metabolized by this enzyme. QT prolonging drugs terfenadine, astemizole, cisapride, pimozide, halofantrine, quinidine ($\uparrow$ interacting drug levels, $\uparrow$ risk of cardiac arrhythmias); ergot ($\uparrow$ ergot levels); statins ($\uparrow$ statin levels and risk of rhabdomyolysis); vinca alkaloids ($\uparrow$ vinca alkaloid levels and risk of neurotoxicity); cyclosporine, tacrolimus, sirolimus, midazolam and other benzodiazepines metabolized by CYP3A4, calcium channel blockers metabolized by

CYP3A4 (diltiazem, verapamil, nifedipine, nisoldipine); digoxin, sulfonylureas, ritonavir, indinavir ($\uparrow$ interacting drug levels); rifampin, omperazole ($\downarrow$ posaconazole levels).

Adverse Effects:

Common

- Headache/cough
- Nausea/vomiting/diarrhea
- Abdominal pain
- Neutropenia
- Hypokalemia
- Hypomagnesemia
- $\uparrow$ AST/ALT

Uncommon

- Torsades de pointes

Allergic Potential: Low

Safety in Pregnancy: C

Additional Clinical Considerations:

- Take with a high fat meal.
- Doses not interchangeable between oral suspension, delayed release tablets (DRTs).
- IV dose = DRT dose.

***Highly active* against Candida albicans, most non-albicans Candida, Aspergillus, Crypotococcus, Histoplasmosis, Blastomycocis, Sporotrichosis, Paracoccidiomycosis.**

***Some activity* against Coccidiomycosis, Fusarium, C. glabrata, and Mucor.**

***No activity* against Pseudallescheria/ Scedosporium.**

Cerebrospinal Fluid Penetration: >10%

SELECTED REFERENCES:

Bruggemann RJM, Alffenaar JWC, Blijlevens NMA, et al. Clinical relevance of the pharmacokinetic interactions of azole antifungal drugs with coadministered agents. Clin Infect Dis 48:1441–1458, 2009. (PMID:19361301)

Cornely OA Helfgott D, Langston A, et al. Pharmacokinetics of different dosing strategies of oral posaconazole in patients with compromised gastrointestinal function and who are at high risk for invasive fungal infection. Antimicrob Agents Chemother 56:2652–8, 2012. (PMID:22290953)

Cornely OA, Maertens J, Winston DJ, et al. Posaconazole vs. fluconazole or itraconazole prophylaxis in patients with neutropenia. N Engl J Med 356:348–59, 2007. (PMID:17251531)

Dekkers BGJ, Bakker M, van der Elst KCM, et al. Therapeutic Drug Monitoring of Posaconazole: an update. Curr Fungal Infect Rep 10:51–61, 2016. (PMID: 27358662)

Dodds Ashley ES, Alexander BD. Posaconazole. Drugs Today 41:393–400, 2005. (PMID:16110346)

Felton TW, Baxter C, Moore CB, et al. Efficacy and safety of posaconazole for chronic pulmonary aspergillosis. Clin Infect Dis 51:1383–1391, 2010. (PMID:2105417)

Girmenia C, Frustaci AM, Gentile G, et al. Posaconazole prophylaxis during front-line chemotherapy of acute myeloid leukemia: a single-center real-life experience. Haematologica 97:560–7, 2012. (PMID:22102702)

Green MR, Woolery JE. Optimising absorption of posaconazole. Mycoses 54:775–779, 2011. (PMID:21615538)

Greenberg RN, Mullane K, van Burik JA, et al. Posaconazole as salvage therapy for zygomycosis. Antimicrob Agents Chemother 50:126–33, 2006. (PMID:16377677)

Hoenigl M, Raggam RB, Salzer HJ, et al. Posaconazole plasma concentrations and invasive mould infections in patients with haematological malignancies. Int J Antimicrob Agents 39:510–3, 2012. (PMID:22481057)

Howard SJ, Lestner JM, Sharp A, et al. Pharmacokinetics and pharmacodynamics of posaconazole for invasive pulmonary aspergillosis: clinical implications for antifungal therapy. J Infect Dis 203:1324–1332, 2011. (PMID:21357943)

Keating GM, Posaconazole. Drugs 65:1553–69, 2005. (PMID:16033292)

Kim MM, Vikram HR, Kusne S, et al. Treatment of refractory coccidioidomycosis with voriconazole or posaconazole. Clin Infect Dis, 53:1060–6, 2011. (PMID:22045955)

Lipp HP. Posaconazole: clinical pharmacokinetics and drug interactions. Mycoses 54:32–38, 2011. (PMID:21126270)

Raad II, Hachem RY, Herbrecht R, et al. Posaconazole as salvage treatment for invasive fusariosis in patients with underlying hematologic malignancy and other conditions. Clin Infect Dis 42:1398–403, 2006. (PMID:16619151)

Restrepo A, Tobon A, Clark B, et al. Salvage treatment of histoplasmosis with posaconazole. Salvage treatment of histoplasmosis with posaconazole. J Infect 54:319–327, 2007. (PMID:16824608)

Ullmann AJ, Cornely OA, Burchardt A, et al. Pharmacokinetics, safety, and efficacy of posaconazole in patients with persistent febrile neutropenia or refractory invasive fungal infection. Antimicrob Agents Chemother 50:658–66, 2006. (PMID:16436724)

SELECTED REFERENCE:

Website: www.pdr.net

Primaquine

Drug Class: Antimalarial, Anti-PCP.

Usual Dose: Antimalarial Dose: 15 mg (base 26.3 mg) (PO) q24h. **PCP Dose:** 15–30 mg (PO) q24h plus clindamycin 600 mg (IV) or 300 mg (PO) q6h.

Pharmacokinetic Parameters:

Peak serum level: 30–100 mcg/mL
Bioavailability: 90%
Excreted unchanged (urine): 3.6%
Serum half-life (normal/ESRD): 3.7–9.6/ 3.7–9.6 hrs

———— = serious side effect [   ] = black box warning. ND = no data. NR = not recommended. s = spectrum inadequate (at site). a = activity or experience inadequate. p = tissue penetration inadequate. *based on peak serum concentration after usual adult dose. †applicable to adult uncomplicated lower UTIs (CrCl > 30 mL/min).

Plasma protein binding: 75%
Volume of distribution (V_d): ND
Primary Mode of Elimination: Hepatic
Dosage Adjustments*

CrCl < 80 mL/min	No change
Post–HD/Post–PD dose	None
CVVH/CVVHD/CVVHDF dose	No change
Hepatic insufficiency	No change

Drug Interactions: Avoid in patients receiving bone marrow suppressive drugs (↑ risk of agranulocytosis), alcohol (↑ GI side effects), quinacrine (↑ primaquine levels/toxicity).
Adverse Effects:
Common
- Headache
- Nausea/vomiting
- Abdominal pain

Uncommon
- Hemolytic anemia with G6PD deficiency
- Leukopenia (dose dependent)
- Methemoglobinemia in NADH-methemoglobin reductase-deficiency

Allergic Potential: Low
Safety in Pregnancy: D

Additional Clinical Considerations:
- Take with food to ↓ GI side effects.
- Use with caution in G6PD deficiency.
- Use with caution in NADH reductase deficiency.

Cerebrospinal Fluid Penetration: No data

SELECTED REFERENCE:
Website: www.pdr.net

Pyrazinamide (PZA)

Drug Class: TB drug.
Usual Dose: 25 mg/kg (PO) q24h (max. 2 gm) (see comments).
Pharmacokinetic Parameters:
Peak serum level: 30–50 mcg/mL
Bioavailability: 90%
Excreted unchanged (urine): 10%
Serum half-life (normal/ESRD): 9/26 hrs
Plasma protein binding: 10%
Volume of distribution (V_d): 0.9 L/kg
Primary Mode of Elimination: Hepatic
Dosage Adjustments*

CrCl < 30 mL/min	25 mg/kg (PO) 3×/week
Post–HD dose	25 mg/kg (PO) or 1 gm (PO)
Post–PD dose	None
CVVH/CVVHD/CVVHDF dose	25 mg/kg (PO) 3×/week
Moderate hepatic insufficiency	Use with caution
Severe hepatic insufficiency	Avoid

Drug Interactions: INH, rifabutin, rifampin (may ↑ risk of hepatoxicity).
Adverse Effects:
Uncommon
- Anorexia
- Malaise
- Nausea/vomiting
- Arthralgia
- Myalgias

———— = serious side effect ☐ = black box warning. ND = no data. NR = not recommended. s = spectrum inadequate (at site). a = activity or experience inadequate. p = tissue penetration inadequate. *based on peak serum concentration after usual adult dose. †applicable to adult uncomplicated lower UTIs (CrCl > 30 mL/min).

Rare
- Drug fever/rash
- ↑ Uric acid
- Sideroblastic anemia
- ↑ AST/ALT
- <u>Hepatotoxicity</u>

Allergic Potential: Low
Safety in Pregnancy: C

Additional Clinical Considerations:
- Avoid in patients with gout (may precipitate acute attacks).
- **TB D.O.T. dose:** 4 gm (PO) 2x/week or 3 gm (PO) 3x/week.

Cerebrospinal Fluid Penetration: 100%
Meningeal dose = usual dose.

SELECTED REFERENCE:
Website: www.pdr.net

Pyrimethamine (Daraprim)

Drug Class: Antiparasitic.
Usual Dose: 75 mg (PO) q24h (see comments).
Pharmacokinetic Parameters:
Peak serum level: 0.4 mcg/mL
Bioavailability: 90%
Excreted unchanged (urine): 25%
Serum half-life (normal/ESRD): 96/96 hrs
Plasma protein binding: 87%
Volume of distribution (V_d): 2.5 L/kg
Primary Mode of Elimination: Hepatic
Dosage Adjustments*

CrCl < 10 mL/min	Use with caution
Post–HD dose	None
Post–PD dose	25 mg (PO)

CVVH/CVVHD/CVVHDF dose	No change
Moderate hepatic insufficiency	No change
Severe hepatic insufficiency	Use with caution

Drug Interactions: Folic acid (↓ pyrimethamine effect); lorazepam (↑ risk of hepatotoxicity); sulfamethoxazole, trimethoprim, TMP–SMX (↑ risk of thrombocytopenia, anemia, leukopenia).
Adverse Effects:
Common
- Drug fever/rash

Uncommon
- Tremors
- Ataxia
- Leukopenia
- Megaloblastic anemia
- Thrombocytopenia
- Pancytopenia

Rare
- <u>Seizures</u>

Allergic Potential: Low
Safety in Pregnancy: C

Additional Clinical Considerations:
- Antacids decrease absorption.
- **Toxoplasmosis Dose:** 200 mg (PO) × 1 dose, then 50–75 mg/kg (PO) q24h (with folinic acid 20 mg PO q24h plus either sulfadiazine or clindamycin).

Cerebrospinal Fluid Penetration: 10–25%

SELECTED REFERENCE:
Website: www.pdr.net

―――― = serious side effect ☐ = black box warning. ND = no data. NR = not recommended. s = spectrum inadequate (at site). a = activity or experience inadequate. p = tissue penetration inadequate. *based on peak serum concentration after usual adult dose. †applicable to adult uncomplicated lower UTIs (CrCl > 30 mL/min).

Quinine sulfate

Drug Class: Antimalarial.
Usual Dose: 650 mg (PO) q8h (see comments).
Pharmacokinetic Parameters:
Peak serum level: 3.8 mcg/mL
Bioavailability: 80%
Excreted unchanged (urine): 5%
Serum half-life (normal/ESRD): 7/14 hrs
Plasma protein binding: 95%
Volume of distribution (V_d): 3 L/kg
Primary Mode of Elimination: Renal/Hepatic
Dosage Adjustments*

CrCl 10–50 mL/min	650 mg (PO) q12h
CrCl < 10 mL/min	650 mg (PO) q24h
Post–HD dose	None
Post–PD dose	650 mg (PO)
CVVH/CVVHD/CVVHDF dose	650 mg (PO) q24h
Mild-moderate hepatic insufficiency	No change
Severe hepatic insufficiency	325 mg (PO) q12h; use caution

Drug Interactions: Amiodarone, aluminum-based antacids (↓ quinidine absorption); astemizole, cisapride, terfenadine (↑ interacting drug levels, torsade de pointes; avoid); cimetidine, ritonavir (↑ quinidine toxicity: headache, deafness, blindness, tachycardia); cyclosporine (↓ cyclosporine levels); digoxin (↑ digoxin levels); dofetilide, flecainide (arrhythmias); mefloquine (seizures, may ↑ QT interval, torsade de pointes, cardiac arrest, ↓ mefloquine efficacy); metformin (↑ risk of lactic acidosis); pancuronium, succinylcholine, tubocurarine (neuromuscular blockade); warfarin (↑ INR).
Adverse Effects:
Common
- Cinchonism
- Lightheadedness

Uncommon
- Nausea/vomiting/diarrhea
- Drug fever/rash
- ↑ QTc
- Drug induced SLE
- Abdominal discomfort

Allergic Potential: High
Safety in Pregnancy: C

Additional Clinical Considerations:
- **PO Malaria Dose:** 650 mg (PO) q8h (plus doxycycline 100 mg PO q12h) × 3–7 days).
- **IV Malaria Dose:** quinine hydro-chloride 600 mg (IV) q8h × 3–7 days, or quinidine gluconate 10 mg/kg (IV) × 1 dose (infuse over 1–2 hours) then 0.02 mg/kg/min (IV) × 72 hours or until parasitemia < 1%.

Cerebrospinal Fluid Penetration: 2–5%

SELECTED REFERENCES:
Corpelet C, Vacher P, Coudor F, et al. Role of quinine in life-threatening Babesia divergens infection successfully treated with clindamycin. Eur J Clin Microbiol Infect Dis 24:74–75, 2005. (PMID:15616840)
Website: www.pdr.net

—— = serious side effect ☐ = black box warning. ND = no data. NR = not recommended. s = spectrum inadequate (at site). a = activity or experience inadequate. p = tissue penetration inadequate. *based on peak serum concentration after usual adult dose. †applicable to adult uncomplicated lower UTIs (CrCl > 30 mL/min).

Quinupristin/Dalfopristin (Synercid)

Drug Class: Streptogramin.
Usual Dose: 7.5 mg/kg (IV) q8h.

Moderate hepatic insufficiency	No change
Severe hepatic insufficiency	Use with caution

Spectrum Synopsis*
Hits
   Gram + : MSSA, MRSA, CoNS, VRE
   Gram – : Few GNB
   Problem pathogens:
      Listeria, Corynebacterium JK
Misses
   Gram + : VSE
   Gram – : Some GNB
   Problem pathogens:
      Nocardia, Acinetobacter,
      S. maltophilia, B. cepacia

(Full *Susceptibility Profiles* p. 208).

Resistance Potential: Low
Pharmacokinetic Parameters:
  Peak serum level: 3.2/8 mcg/mL
  Bioavailability: Not applicable
  Excreted unchanged: 20% (urine); 80%
  (feces) Serum half-life (normal/ESRD):
  [3.1/1]/[3.1/1] hrs
  Plasma protein binding: 55/15%
  Volume of distribution (V_d): 0.45/
  0.24 L/kg
Primary Mode of Elimination: Hepatic
Dosage Adjustments*

CrCl < 10 mL/min	No change
Post–HD dose	None
Post–PD dose	None
CVVH/CVVHD/ CVVHDF dose	No change

Drug Interactions: Amiodarone, amlodipine (↑ amlodipine toxicity); astemizole, cisapride (may ↑ QT interval, torsades de pointes); carbamazepine (↑ carbamazepine toxicity: ataxia, nystagmus, diplopia, headache, seizures); cyclosporine, delavirdine, indinavir, nevirapine (↑ interacting drug levels); diazepam, midazolam (↑ interacting drug effect); diltiazem, felodipine, isradipine (↑ interacting drug toxicity: dizziness, hypotension, headache, flushing); disopyramide (↑ disopyramide toxicity: arrhythmias, hypotension, syncope); docetaxel (↑ interacting drug toxicity: neutropenia, anemia, neuropathy); lidocaine (↑ lidocaine toxicity: neurotoxicity, arrhythmias, seizures); methylprednisolone (↑ methylprednisolone toxicity: myopathy, diabetes mellitus, cushing's syndrome); nicardipine, nifedipine, nimodipine (↑ interacting drug toxicity: dizziness, hypotension, flushing, headache); statins (↑ risk of rhabdomyolysis).

Adverse Effects:
Common
- Infusion site reactions
- Hyperbilirubinemia
Uncommon
- Nausea/vomiting
Rare
- <u>Myalgias</u> (severe/prolonged)
- <u>Hepatotoxicity</u>
Allergic Potential: Low
Safety in Pregnancy: B

——— = serious side effect ☐ = black box warning. ND = no data. NR = not recommended. s = spectrum inadequate (at site). a = activity or experience inadequate. p = tissue penetration inadequate. *based on peak serum concentration after usual adult dose. †applicable to adult uncomplicated lower UTIs (CrCl > 30 mL/min).

Additional Clinical Considerations:
- Requires central IV line for administration.
- *Not effective against E. faecalis (VSE).*
- *Useful for daptomycin resistant MSSA/ MRSA infections.*

Cerebrospinal Fluid Penetration: <10%

(also see *Antibiotic Pearls & Pitfalls* p. 535).

SELECTED REFERENCES:
Blondeau JM, Sanche Se. Quinupristin/dalfopristin. Expert Opin Pharmacother 3:1341–64, 2002. (PMID:12186626)
Bryson HM, Spencer CM. Quinupristin/dalfopristin. Drugs 52:406–15, 1996. (PMID:8875130)
Kim MK, Nicolau DP, Nightingale CH, et al. Quinupristin/dalfopristin: A treatment option for vancomycin-resistant enterococci. Conn Med 64:209–12, 2000. (PMID:10812767)
Website: www.pdr.net

Raltegravir (Isentress) RAL

Drug Class: HIV integrase inhibitor.
Usual Dose: 400 mg (PO) q12h.
Pharmacokinetic Parameters:
Peak serum level: 6.5 mcg/mL
Bioavailability: ~ 32% (20–43%)
Excreted unchanged: 51% (feces); 9% (urine)
Serum half-life (normal/ESRD): 9–12 hrs/ ND
Plasma protein binding: 83%
Volume of distribution (V_d): ND
Primary Mode of Elimination: Fecal/ Renal
Dosage Adjustments*

CrCl < 10 mL/min	No change
Post–HD dose	None
Post–PD dose	None
CVVH/CVVHD/ CVVHDF dose	No change
Mild/moderate hepatic insufficiency	No change
Severe hepatic insufficiency	Use with caution

Antiretroviral Dosage Adjustments

Atazanavir	No change
Atazanavir/ritonavir	No change
Efavirenz	No change
Rifampin	raltegravir 800 mg q12h
Ritonavir	No change
Tenofovir	No change
Tipranavir/ritonavir	No change

Drug Interactions: Rifampin (↓ raltegravir levels, use with caution). In-vitro, raltegravir does not inhibit CYP1A2, CYP2B6, CYP2C8, CYP2C9, CYP2C19, CYP2D6 or CYP3A and does not induce CYP3A4. In addition, raltegravir does not inhibit P-glycoprotein-mediated transport. Raltegravir is therefore not expected to affect the pharmacokinetics of drugs that are substrates of these enzymes or P-glycoprotein (e.g., protease inhibitors, NNRTIs, methadone, opioid analgesics, statins, azole antifungals, proton pump inhibitors, oral contraceptives, anti-erectile dysfunction agents).

―――― = serious side effect ☐ = black box warning. ND = no data. NR = not recommended. s = spectrum inadequate (at site). a = activity or experience inadequate. p = tissue penetration inadequate. *based on peak serum concentration after usual adult dose. †applicable to adult uncomplicated lower UTIs (CrCl > 30 mL/min).

Adverse Effects:

Common
- Nausea/vomiting/diarrhea
- Drug
- Rash

Uncommon
- Headache
- ↑ CPK
- Rhabdomyolysis

Rare
- Stevens-Johnson syndrome
- TEN

Allergic Potential: Low
Safety in Pregnancy: C

Additional Clinical Considerations:
- Use with caution in patients at increased risk for myopathy or rhabdomyolysis, e.g., statins.

Cerebrospinal Fluid Penetration: No data

SELECTED REFERENCE:
Website: www.pdr.net

Ribavirin (Rebetol, Copegus)

Drug Class: Antiviral (RSV, HCV).
Usual Dose: 600 mg (PO) q12h.
Pharmacokinetic Parameters:
Peak serum level: 0.07–0.28 mcg/mL
Bioavailability: 64%
Excreted unchanged (urine): 40%
Serum half-life (normal/ESRD): 120 hrs/ no data
Plasma protein binding: 0%
Volume of distribution (V_d): 10 L/kg

Primary Mode of Elimination: Hepatic
Dosage Adjustments*

CrCl 50–80 mL/min	No change
CrCl < 50 mL/min	Avoid
Post–HD dose	Avoid
Post–PD dose	Avoid
CVVH/CVVHD/ CVVHDF dose	Avoid
Mild-moderate hepatic insufficiency	No change
Severe hepatic insufficiency	Avoid

Drug Interactions: Ribavirin may antagonize the in vitro antiviral activity of stavudine and zidovudine against HIV. Pegylated interferon (Pegasys) in HIV patients (↓ CD_4 counts).

Adverse Effects:

Common
- Drug fever/rash
- Nausea/vomiting
- Leukopenia
- Anemia
- Hyperbilirubinemia
- ↑ Uric acid

Rare
- Hemolytic anemia may result in worsening of cardiac disease (fatal and non-fatal myocardial infarctions). Avoid if significant history of cardiac disease should not be treated with ribavirin. With interferon, adverse effects include severe depression, autoimmune/infectious disorders, pulmonary dysfunction, pancreatitis and diabetes.

Allergic Potential: Low

─── = serious side effect ☐ = black box warning. ND = no data. NR = not recommended. s = spectrum inadequate (at site). a = activity or experience inadequate. p = tissue penetration inadequate. *based on peak serum concentration after usual adult dose. †applicable to adult uncomplicated lower UTIs (CrCl > 30 mL/min).

Safety in Pregnancy: X (avoid pregnancy during therapy and for 6 months after completion of therapy in both female patients and male partners of taking ribavirin)

Additional Clinical Considerations:
- **Nebulizer dose for RSV:** 20 mg/mL aerosolized over 12 hours once daily × 3–7 days. Also as activity against Lassa fever and HPS.
- **RSV Transplant Dose:**
  Loading Dose: 30 mg/kg (IV) (not to exceed 2g), then 16 mg/kg (IV) q6h × 4 days (not to exceed 1g);
  Maintenance Dose: 8 mg/kg (IV) (not to exceed 500 mg) x 3–6 days.
- For Crimean-Congo fever give ribavirin initial **Loading Dose** 30 mg/kg (PO) × 1 then
  Maintenance Dose: 15 mg/kg (PO) q6h × 4 days, then give 7.5 mg/kg (PO) q8h × 6 days.
- If hemoglobin level falls < 10 g/dL, reduce ribavirin dose to 600 mg daily.
- If hemoglobin falls < 8.5 g/dL discontinue ribavirin

Highly active against HCV and RSV.
Some activity against, HEV, adenoviruses and arboviral hemorragic fever viruses.
No activity against EBV, CMV, HBV, HDV.

Cerebrospinal Fluid Penetration: 70%

SELECTED REFERENCE:
Website: www.pdr.net

Rifabutin (Mycobutin)

Drug Class: TB drug.
Usual Dose: 300 mg (PO) or 5 mg/kg q24h.

Pharmacokinetic Parameters:
Peak serum level: 0.38 mcg/mL
Bioavailability: 20–50%
Excreted unchanged (urine): 10%
Serum half-life (normal/ESRD): 45/45 hrs
Plasma protein binding: 85%
Volume of distribution (V_d): 9.3 L/kg
Primary Mode of Elimination: Hepatic
Dosage Adjustments*

CrCl < 30 mL/min	150 mcg (PO) q24h
CrCl < 10 mL/min	No change
Post–HD dose	None
Post–PD dose	None
CVVH/CVVHD/CVVHDF dose	None
Moderate hepatic insufficiency	No change
Severe hepatic insufficiency	No change

Drug Interactions: Atovaquone, amprenavir, indinavir, nelfinavir, ritonavir, clarithromycin, erythromycin, telithromycin, fluconazole, itraconazole, ketoconazole (↓ interactg drug levels, ↑ rifabutin levels); beta-blockers, clofibrate, cyclosporine, enalapril, oral contraceptives, quinidine, sulfonylureas, tocainide, warfarin (↓ interacting drug effect); corticosteroids (↑ corticosteroid requirement); delavirdine (↓ delavirdine levels, ↑ rifabutln levels; avoid); digoxin, phenytoin, propafenone, theophylline, zidovudine (↓ interacting drug levels); methadone (↓ methadone levels, withdrawal); mexiletine (↑ mexiletine clearance); protease inhibitors (↓ protease inhibitor levels, ↑ rifabutin levels; caution).

--- = serious side effect ⬛ = black box warning. ND = no data. NR = not recommended. s = spectrum inadequate (at site). a = activity or experience inadequate. p = tissue penetration inadequate. *based on peak serum concentration after usual adult dose. †applicable to adult uncomplicated lower UTIs (CrCl > 30 mL/min).

Adverse Effects:

Common
- Drug fever/rash
- Leukopenia
- Red/orange discoloration of body secretions

Uncommon
- Nausea/vomiting
- Abdominal pain
- Thrombocytopenia

Rare
- ↑ AST/ALT

Allergic Potential: High
Safety in Pregnancy: B

Additional Clinical Considerations:
- Avoid in leukopenic patients with WBC ≤ 1000 cells/mm³.
- Always use as part of a multi-drug regimen, never as monotherapy.
- **Rifabutin doses when co-administered with antiretrovirals:** 450 mg (PO) q24h with EFV; 150 mg (PO) q24h with AVP, IDV, NFV, FPN; 150 mg (PO) q48h with RTV/LPV combination

Cerebrospinal Fluid Penetration: 50–70%
Meningeal dose = usual dose.

SELECTED REFERENCES:

Choong K, Looke D. Cross-reaction to rifabutin after rifampicin induced flu-liked syndrome and thrombocytopenia. Scand J Infect Dis 43:238, 2011. (PIMD:20849363)

Finch CK, Chrisman CR, Baciewicz AM, et al. Rifampin and rifabutin drug Interactions: an update. Arch Intern Med 162:985–92, 2002. (PMID:11996607)

Horne DJ, Spitters C Narita M. Experience with rifabutin replacing rifampin in the treatment of tuberculosis. Int J Tuberc Lung Dis 15:1485–9, 2011. (PMID:22008761)

Website: www.pdr.net

Rifampin (Rifadin, Rimactane)

Drug Class: TB drug, antibiotic.
Usual Dose: 600 mg (PO) q24h (**TB dose**); 300 mg (PO) q12h (**Antibiotic dose**)
Resistance Potential: High (aerobic GNBs with non-TB monotherapy)
Pharmacokinetic Parameters:
  Peak serum level: 7 mcg/mL
  Bioavailability: 95%
  Excreted unchanged (urine): 15%
  Serum half-life (normal/ESRD): 3.5/11 hrs
  Plasma protein binding: 80%
  Volume of distribution (V_d): 0.93 L/kg
Primary Mode of Elimination: Hepatic
Dosage Adjustments*

CrCl < 10 mL/min	No change
Post–HD dose	None
Post–PD dose	None
CVVH/CVVHD/CVVHDF dose	No change
Moderate hepatic insufficiency	No change; use caution
Severe hepatic insufficiency	Avoid

Drug Interactions: Amprenavir, indinavir, nelfinavir (↑ rifampin levels); beta-blockers, clofibrate, cyclosporine, oral contraceptives, quinidine, sulfonylureas, tocainamide, warfarin (↓ interacting drug effect); caspofungin (↓ caspofungin levels, may ↓ caspofungin effect); clarithromycin, ketoconazole (↑ rifampin levels, ↓ interacting drug levels); corticosteroids (↑ corticosteroid requirement); delavirdine (↑ rifampin levels, ↓ delavirdine levels; avoid); disopyramide, itraconazole, phenytoin, propafenone, theophylline, methadone, nelfinavir, ritonavir, tacrolimus, drugs whose metabolism is induced by rifampin, e.g., ACE inhibitors, dapsone, diazepam, digoxin, diltiazem, doxycycline, fluconazole, fluvastatin, haloperidol, nifedipine, progestins, triazolam, tricyclics, zidovudine (↓ interacting drug levels); fluconazole, rifampin (↓ posaconazole levels) TMP–SMX (↑ rifampin levels); INH (INH converted into toxic hydrazine); mexiletine (↑ mexiletine clearance); nevirapine (↓ nevirapine levels; avoid).

Adverse Effects:

Common
- Red/orange discoloration of body secretions

Uncommon
- Dizziness
- Flu-like symptoms
- Drug fever/rash
- Thrombocytopenia
- ↑ AST/ALT

Allergic Potential: Moderate
Safety in Pregnancy: C

Additional Clinical Considerations:
- Contraindicated in HIV. For anti–TB prophylaxis/therapy. Potent CYP 3A4 inducer.
- **TB D.O.T. dose:** 10 mg/kg or 600 mg (PO) 2–3x/week.
- **Do not use as monotherapy for S. aureus.**
- **Of no proven clinical advantage when combined with another anti–MSSA/MRSA antibiotic.**
- **With another anti-staphylococcal drug dose:** 300 mg (PO) q12h.
- 300 mg (PO) q8h may be used for S. aureus PVE or Brucella SBE.
- **Nasal carriage dose:** 600 mg (PO) q5h × 72 hours.

Additional Pharmacokinetic Considerations:

Non-CSF	% of Serum Levels
Peritoneal fluid	NR(s)
Bile	100%
Synovial fluid	ND
Bone	100%
Prostate	NR(s)
CSF	
Non-inflamed meninges	1%
Inflamed meninges (ABM)	10%

Meningeal dose = usual dose (TB only)

SELECTED REFERENCES:

Czekaj J, Dinh A, Moldovan A, et al. Efficacy of a combined oral clindamycin-rifampicin regimen for therapy of staphylococcal osteoarticular infections. Scand J Infect Dis 43:962-967, 2011. (PMID:21916775)

Eisen D, Denholm JS, Recommendations for rifampicin therapy of staphylococcal infection in IDSA prosthetic joint infection guidelines are not

---

supported by available literature. Clin Infect Dis 57:159, 2013. (PMID:23537907)

Euba G, Murillo O, Fernandez-Sabe N, et al. Treatment of chronic staphylococcal osteomyelitis: intravenous or oral? how long? Antimicrob Agents Chemother 53:2672–2676, 2009. (PMID:19307356)

Gauthier TP, Rifampicin plus colistin in the era of extensively drug-resistant acinetobacter baumannii infections. Clin Infect Dis 57:359-362, 2013. (PMID:23616496)

Gomez J, Canovas E, Banos V, et al. Linezolid plus rifampin as a salvage therapy in prosthetic joint infections treated without removing the implant. Antimicrob Agents Chemother 55:4308–4310, 2011. (PMID:216900277)

Johnson JR. Rifampin and methicillin-resistant Staphylococcus aureus bone and joint infections. Clin Infect Dis 53:98–99, 2011. (PMID:21653311)

Krause PJ, Corrow CL, Bakken JS. Successful treatment of human granulocytic ehrlichiosis in children using rifampin. Pediatrics. 112:e252–3, 2003. (PMID:12949322)

Maki DG. In adults with S aureus bacteremia, adding rifampin to standard antibiotic therapy did not improve outcomes. Ann Intern Med 168:JC32, 2018. (PMID: 29554670)

Nguyen S, Pasquet A, Legout L, et al. Efficacy and tolerance of rifampin-linezolid compared with rifampin-cotrimoxazole combinations in prolonged oral therapy for bone and joint infections. Clin Microbiol Infect Dis 15:1163–1169, 2009. (PMID:19438638)

Pina JM, Clotet L, Ferrer A, et al. Cost-effectiveness of rifampin for 4 months and isoniazid for 9 months in the treatment to tuberculosis infection. Eur J Clin Microbiol Inf Dis 32:647-655, 2013. (PMID:23238684)

Velásquez GE, Brooks MB, Coit JM, et al. Efficacy and Safety of high-dose rifampin in pulmonary tuberculosis. A Randomized controlled trial. Am J Respir Crit Care Med 198:657-66, 2018. (PMID: 29954183)

Website: www.pdr.net

Rilpivirine (Edurant) RPV

Drug class: HIV NNRTI.
Usual dose: 25 mg (PO) q24h (with meal).
Pharmacokinetic Parameters:
  Peak serum level: 1 mcg/mL
  Bioavailability: ND
  Excreted unchanged: 1%
  Serum half-life (normal/ESRD): 50/50 hrs
  Plasma protein binding: 99%
  Volume of distribution (V_d): ND
Primary Mode of Elimination: Hepatic
Dosage Adjustments*

CrCl <10 mL/min	No change
Post-HD dose	None
Post-PD dose	None
CVVH/CVVHD/CVVHDF dose	No change
Mild to moderate hepatic insufficiency	No change
Severe hepatic insufficiency	Use with caution

Drug Interactions: Clarithromycin ($\downarrow$ clarithromycin levels). Any drug that induces or inhibits CYP3A may $\uparrow$/$\downarrow$ rilpivirine levels.
Contraindications: carbamazepine, oxycarbazepine, phenobarbital, phenytoin, rifabutin, rifampin, rifapentine, proton pump inhibitors, dexamethasone (except single dose), St. John's Wort.

―――― = serious side effect ☐ = black box warning. ND = no data. NR = not recommended. s = spectrum inadequate (at site). a = activity or experience inadequate. p = tissue penetration inadequate. *based on peak serum concentration after usual adult dose. †applicable to adult uncomplicated lower UTIs (CrCl > 30 mL/min).

Adverse Effects:

Common

- Headache
- Depression
- Abdominal pain

Uncommon

- Dizziness
- Insomnia
- Bad dreams
- Fatigue
- Drug fever/rash

Rare

- ↑ QTc

Allergic Potential: Low

Safety in Pregnancy: B

Additional Clinical Considerations:

- Antacid and H2 blockers should be separated.
- **Do not administer with other NNRTI's.**

SELECTED REFERENCES:

Miller CD, Crain J, Tran V, et al. Rilipivirine: A new addition to the anti-HIV-1 armamentarium. Drugs Today 47:5–15, 2011. (PMID:21373646)

Website: www.pdr.net

Rimantadine (Flumadine)

Drug Class: Antiviral (influenza A)

Usual Dose: 100 mg (PO) q12h (see comments).

Pharmacokinetic Parameters:

Peak serum level: 0.7 mcg/mL
Bioavailability: 90%
Excreted unchanged (urine): 25%

Serum half-life (normal/ESRD): 25/38 hrs
Plasma protein binding: 40%
Volume of distribution (V_d): 4.5 L/kg

Primary Mode of Elimination: Hepatic

Dosage Adjustments*

CrCl 10–50 mL/min	No change
CrCl < 10 mL/min	100 mg (PO) q24h
Post–HD dose	None
Post–PD dose	None
CVVH/CVVHD/CVVHDF dose	No change
Moderate hepatic insufficiency	No change
Severe hepatic insufficiency	100 mg (PO) q24h

Drug Interactions: Alcohol (↑ CNS effects); benztropine, trihexyphenidyl, scopolamine (↑ interacting drug effect: dry mouth, ataxia, blurred vision, slurred speech, toxic psychosis); cimetidine (↓ rimantadine clearance); CNS stimulants (additive stimulation); digoxin (↑ digoxin levels); trimethoprim (↑ rimantadine and trimethoprim levels).

Adverse Effects:

Uncommon

- Dizziness
- Headache
- Insomnia
- Anticholinergic effects: Blurry vision, dry mouth, orthostatic hypotension, urinary retention, constipation.

───── = serious side effect ☐ = black box warning. ND = no data. NR = not recommended. s = spectrum inadequate (at site). a = activity or experience inadequate. p = tissue penetration inadequate. *based on peak serum concentration after usual adult dose. †applicable to adult uncomplicated lower UTIs (CrCl > 30 mL/min).

Allergic Potential: Low
Safety in Pregnancy: C

Additional Clinical Considerations:
- Ineffective against influenza-B.
- Patients ≥ 60 years old or with a history of seizures should receive 100 mg (PO) q24h.
- **Influenza dose (prophylaxis):** 100 mg (PO) q12h for duration of exposure/outbreak.
- **Influenza dose (therapy):** 100 mg (PO) q12h × 7 days.

***Highly active** against influenza A.*
__No activity__ against other viruses.

Cerebrospinal Fluid Penetration: <10%

SELECTED REFERENCE:
Website: www.pdr.net

Ritonavir (Norvir) RTV

Drug Class: HIV protease inhibitor.
Usual Dose: 100–400 mg (PO) q12h–q24h.
Pharmacokinetic Parameters:
Peak serum level: 11 mcg/mL
Bioavailability: No data
Excreted unchanged (urine): 3.5%
Serum half-life (normal/ESRD): 4 hrs/ no data
Plasma protein binding: 99%
Volume of distribution (V_d): 0.41 L/kg
Primary Mode of Elimination: Hepatic
Dosage Adjustments*

CrCl < 10 mL/min	No change
Post–HD dose	None
Post–PD dose	None
CVVH/CVVHD/CVVHDF dose	None
Mild-moderate hepatic insufficiency	No change
Severe hepatic insufficiency	Avoid

Antiretroviral Dosage Adjustments

Atazanavir	Ritonavir 100 mg q24h + atazanavir 300 mg q24h (with food)
Delavirdine	Delavirdine: no change; ritonavir: No data
Efavirenz	Ritonavir 600 mg q12h (500 mg q12h for intolerance)
Fosamprena-vir	Fosamprenavir 1400 mg + ritonavir 200 mg q24h
Indinavir	Ritonavir 100–200 mg q12h + indinavir 800 mg q12h, or 400 mg q12h of each drug
Nelfinavir	Ritonavir 400 mg q12h + nelfinavir 500–750 mg q12h
Nevirapine	No change

——— = serious side effect ☐ = black box warning. ND = no data. NR = not recommended. s = spectrum inadequate (at site). a = activity or experience inadequate. p = tissue penetration inadequate. *based on peak serum concentration after usual adult dose. †applicable to adult uncomplicated lower UTIs (CrCl > 30 mL/min).

Saquinavir	Ritonavir 400 mg q12h + saquinavir 400 mg q12h
Ketoconazole	Caution; do not exceed ketoconazole 200 mg q24h
Rifampin	Avoid
Rifabutin	Rifabutin 150 mg q48h or 3x/week

Drug Interactions: Antiretrovirals, rifabutin, rifampin (see dose adjustment grid, above); saquinavir (↑ QTc/torsades de pointes, ↑ PR intervals) alprazolam, diazepam, estazolam, flurazepam, midazolam, triazolam, zolpidem, meperidine, propoxyphene, piroxicam, quinidine, amiodarone, encainide, flecainide, propafenone, astemizole, bepridil, bupropion, cisapride, clorazepate, clozapine, pimozide, St. John's wort, terfenadine (avoid); alfentanil, fentanyl, hydrocodone, tramadol, disopyramide, lidocaine, mexiletine, erythromycin, clarithromycin, warfarin, dronabinol, ondansetron, metoprolol, pindolol, propranolol, timolol, amlodipine, diltiazem, felodipine, isradipine, nicardipine, nifedipine, nimodipine, nisoldipine, nitrendipine, verapamil, etoposide, paclitaxel, tamoxifen, vinblastine, vincristine, loratadine, tricyclic antidepressants, paroxetine, nefazodone, sertraline, trazodone, fluoxetine, venlafaxine, fluvoxamine, cyclosporine, tacrolimus, chlorpromazine, haloperidol, perphenazine, risperidone, thioridazine, clozapine, pimozide, methamphetamine (↑ interacting drug levels); voriconazole (↓ voriconazole levels); telithromycin (↑ ritonavir levels); codeine, hydromorphone, methadone, morphine, ketoprofen, ketorolac, naproxen, diphenoxylate, oral contraceptives, theophylline (↓ interacting drug levels); carbamazepine, phenytoin, phenobarbital, clonazepam, dexamethasone, prednisone (↓ ritonavir levels, ↑ interacting drug levels; monitor anticonvulsant levels); metronidazole (disulfiram-like reaction); tenofovir, tobacco (↓ ritonavir levels); sildenafil (do not exceed 25 mg in 48 hrs); tadalafil (max. 10 mg/72 hrs); vardenafil (max. 2.5 mg/72 hrs).

Adverse Effects:
Common
- Nausea/vomiting/diarrhea
- Abdominal pain
- Circumoral/extremity parathesias
- Taste perversion
- Hyperglycemia (including worsening diabetes, new-onset diabetes, DKA)
- Hyperlipidemia
- ↑ AST/ALT
- <u>Fat redistribution</u>

Uncommon
- Anorexia
- <u>Pancreatitis</u>

────── = serious side effect ▭ = black box warning. ND = no data. NR = not recommended. s = spectrum inadequate (at site). a = activity or experience inadequate. p = tissue penetration inadequate. *based on peak serum concentration after usual adult dose. †applicable to adult uncomplicated lower UTIs (CrCl > 30 mL/min).

- Anemia
- Leukopenia
- ↑ CPK

Rare

- <u>Renal stones</u> (with ritonavir boosted atazanavir)

- Given with other ART agents. Ritonavir tablets are NOT bioequivalent to ritonavir capsules. Ritonavir capsules may experience more GI adverse effects when switching from the capsule to the tablet because of the greater maximum plasma concentration (C_{max}) with the tablet.

Allergic Potential: Low
Safety in Pregnancy: B

Additional Clinical Considerations:

- Usually used at low dose (100–400 mg/day) as pharmacokinetic "booster" of other PI's. GI intolerance decreases over time.
- Take with food if possible (serum levels increase 15%, fewer GI side effects).
- Separate dosing from ddI by 2 hours.

Cerebrospinal Fluid Penetration: <1%

SELECTED REFERENCES:

Lea AP, Faulds D. Ritonavir. Drugs 52:541–6, 1996. (PMID:8891466)

McDonald C, Uy J, Hu W, et al. Clinical significance of hyperbilirubinemia among HIV-1-infected patients treated with atazanavir/ ritonavir through 96 weeks in the CASTLE study. AIDS patient care STDS 26–259–64, 2012. (PMID:22404421)

Nishijima T, Tsukada K, Teruya K, et al. Efficacy and safety of once-daily ritonavir-based antiretroviral therapy in low-body weight treatment-naïve patients with HIV infections. AIDS 13;26:649–51 2012. (PMID:22233654)

Piliero PJ. Interaction between ritonavir and stains. Am J Med 112:510–1, 2002. (PMID:11959074)

Rockwood N, Mandalia S, Bower M, et al. Ritonavir-boosted atazanavir exposure is associated with an increased rate of renal stones compared with efavirenz, ritonavir-boosted lopinavir and ritonavir-boosted darunavir. AIDS 25:1671–3, 2011. (PMID:21716074)

Website: www.pdr.net

Spectinomycin (Spectam, Trobicin)

Drug Class: Aminocyclitol.
Usual Dose: 2 gm (IM) × 1 dose.
Pharmacokinetic Parameters:

Peak serum level: 100 mcg/mL
Bioavailability: Not applicable
Excreted unchanged (urine): 80%
Serum half-life (normal/ESRD): 1.6/16 hrs
Plasma protein binding: 20%
Volume of distribution (V_d): 0.25 L/kg

Primary Mode of Elimination: Renal
Dosage Adjustments*

CrCl < 10 mL/min	No change
Post–HD dose	None
Post–PD dose	None
CVVH/CVVHD/CVVHDF dose	None

—— = serious side effect ☐ = black box warning. ND = no data. NR = not recommended. s = spectrum inadequate (at site). a = activity or experience inadequate. p = tissue penetration inadequate. *based on peak serum concentration after usual adult dose. †applicable to adult uncomplicated lower UTIs (CrCl > 30 mL/min).

Moderate hepatic insufficiency	No change
Severe hepatic insufficiency	No change

Drug Interactions: None.
Adverse Effects:
Common
- Pain at injection site

Uncommon
- Drug fever/rash

Allergic Potential: Low
Safety in Pregnancy: B

Additional Clinical Considerations:
- **Ineffective in pharyngeal GC** (poor penetration into secretions).

Cerebrospinal Fluid Penetration: <10%

SELECTED REFERENCES:
Fiumara NJ. The treatment of gonococcal proctitis: An evaluation of 173 patients treated with 4 gm of spectinomycin. JAMA 239:735–7, 1978. (PMID:146099)
Holloway WJ. Spectinomycin. Med Clin North Am 66:169–173, 1982. (PMID:6460907)
McCormack WM, Finland M. Spectinomycin. Ann Intern Med 84:712–16, 1976. (PMID:132888)
Website: www.pdr.net

Streptomycin

Drug Class: Aminoglycoside.
Usual Dose: 1 gm (IM) q24h or 15 mg/kg (IM) q24h.
Pharmacokinetic Parameters:
Peak serum level: 25–50 mcg/mL
Bioavailability: Not applicable
Excreted unchanged (urine): 90%
Serum half-life (normal/ESRD): 2.5/100 hrs

Plasma protein binding: 35%
Volume of distribution (V_d): 0.26 L/kg
Primary Mode of Elimination: Renal
Dosage Adjustments*

CrCl 10–50 mL/min	15 mg/kg (IM) q72h or 1 gm (IM) q72h
CrCl < 10 mL/min	15 mg/kg (IM) q72h or 1 gm (IM) q96h
Post–HD dose	15 mg/kg (IM) or 1 gm (IM) 2–3 x/week
Post–PD dose	15 mg/kg (IM) or 1 gm (IM) or 20–40 mg/mL in dialysate q24h
CVVH/CVVHD/CVVHDF dose	15 mg/kg (IM) or 1 gm (IM) q96h
Mild-moderate hepatic insufficiency	No change
Severe hepatic insufficiency	No change

Drug Interactions: Amphotericin B, cephalothin, cyclosporine, enflurane, methoxyflurane, NSAIDs, polymyxin B, radiographic contrast, vancomycin (↑ nephrotoxicity); cis-platinum (↑ nephrotoxicity, ↑ ototoxicity); loop diuretics (↑ ototoxicity); neuromuscular blocking agents (↑ apnea, prolonged paralysis); non-polarizing muscle relaxants (↑ apnea).
Adverse Effects:
Common
- Drug fever/rash
- Eosinophilia

Uncommon
- Ototoxicity (cochlear and vestibular)
- Neurotoxic reactions: (Optic nerve dysfunction, peripheral neuritis,

───── = serious side effect ☐ = black box warning. ND = no data. NR = not recommended. s = spectrum inadequate (at site). a = activity or experience inadequate. p = tissue penetration inadequate. *based on peak serum concentration after usual adult dose. †applicable to adult uncomplicated lower UTIs (CrCl > 30 mL/min).

arachnoiditis, encephalopathy, respiratory paralysis secondary to neuromuscular blockage)

Allergic Potential: Low
Safety in Pregnancy: D

Additional Clinical Considerations:
- May be given IV slowly over 1 hour.
- **TB D.O.T. Dose:** 20–30 mg/kg (IM) 2–3x/week.
- **Tularemia Dose:** 1 gm (IV/IM) q12h.
- **Plague Dose:** 2 gm (IV/IM) q12h.

Cerebrospinal Fluid Penetration: 20%

SELECTED REFERENCE:
Website: www.pdr.net

Tafenoquine (Krintafel)

Drug Class: Antimalarial.
Usual Dose: 300 mg (PO) (see doses for malaria prophylaxis p. 396 and treatment p. 271).
Pharmacokinetic Parameters:
  Peak serum level: ND
  Bioavailability: ND
  Excreted unchanged: ND
  Serum half-life (normal): 15 days
  Plasma protein binding: 99.5%
  Volume of distribution (V_d): 23 L/kg
Primary Mode of Elimination: Hepatic
Dosage Adjustments*

CrCl < 50 mL/min	ND
Post-HD/Post-PD dose	ND
CVVH dose	ND
Hepatic insufficiency	ND

Drug Interactions: Dofetilide levels, metformin levels.

Adverse Effects:
Common:
- Headache
- Dizziness
- Nausea/Vomiting
- Decreased hemoglobin

Uncommon:
- Insomnia
- Hypersensitivity reactions

Rare:
- Hemolytic anemia
- Methemoglobinemia
- Photophobia
- Anxiety
- Abnormal dreams
- Somnolence

Allergic Potential: Low

Additional Clinical Considerations:
- Test for G6PD deficiency prior to starting tafenoquine
- Not indicated for monotherapy of acute malaria
- Administer with food. If vomiting occurs within 1 hour, repeat dose.
- Not indicated for children under 16 years
- Avoid during pregnancy

Cerebrospinal Fluid Penetration: No data

SELECTED REFERENCE:
Lacerda MVG, et al. Single dose tafenoquine to prevent relapse of Plasmodium vivax malaria. N Engl J Med 380:215-28, 2019. (PMID: 30550322)
Lalanos-Cuentas A, et al. Tafenoquine plus cloroquine for the treatment and relapse prevention of Plasmodium vivax malaria (DETECTIVE): a multicentre, double-blind, randomized phase 2b dose-selection study. Lancet 383:1049-58, 2014. (PMID: 24360639)
Website: www.pdr.net

——— = serious side effect ☐ = black box warning. ND = no data. NR = not recommended. s = spectrum inadequate (at site). a = activity or experience inadequate. p = tissue penetration inadequate. *based on peak serum concentration after usual adult dose. †applicable to adult uncomplicated lower UTIs (CrCl > 30 mL/min).

Tedizolid (Sivextro)

Drug Class: Oxazolidinone
Usual Dose: 200 mg (IV) q24h × 6 days; 200 mg (PO) q24h × 6 days

---

Spectrum Synopsis*
Hits
  Gram + : MSSA, MRSA, CoNS, VRE
  Gram – : None
  Problem pathogens:
    None
Misses
  Gram + : VRE
  Gram – : All aerobic GNB, B. fragilis
  Problem pathogens:
    Listeria, Nocardia,
    Acinetobacter, S. maltophilia,
    B. cepacia

Resistance Potential: Low
Pharmacokinetic Parameters:
Peak serum level: 2.2–3 mcg/mL
Bioavailability: 91%
Excreted unchanged: < 3%
Serum half-life (normal/ESRD): 11 h/11 h
Plasma protein binding: 70–90%
Volume of distribution (V_d): 1–1.14 L/kg
Primary Mode of Elimination: Hepatic
Dosage Adjustments*

CrCl < 30 mL/min	No change
Post-HD dose	No change
Post-PD dose	No change
CVVH dose	No change
Hepatic insufficiency	No change

Drug Interactions: Serotonin syndrome: fever, delerium, hypertension, tremor/clonus, hyperreflexia. Serotonergic agents, e.g., SSRIs, MAOIs, St. John's wort, ritonavir (↑ risk of serotonin syndrome).
Adverse Effects:
Uncommon
- Anemia
- Thrombocytopenia
- Pancytopenia

Allergic Potential: Low
Safety in Pregnancy: C

Additional Clinical Considerations:
- Useful for treatment of linezolid resistant staphylococci.
- ↓ incidence of thrombocytopenia compared to linezolid (2.3% vs. 4.9%).
- PO dose may be taken with or without food.
- Other anti-staphylococcal antibiotics are preferred for febrile neutropenia.

Cerebrospinal Fluid Penetration: No data

(also see ***Antibiotic Pearls & Pitfalls*** p. 535).

SELECTED REFERENCES:

Das D, Tulkens PM, Mehra P, et al. Tedizolid phosphate for the management of acute bacterial skin and skin structure infections: safety summary. Clin Infect Dis. 58;Suppl1:S51-57, 2014. (PMID:24343833)

Flanagan S, Fang E, Munoz KA, et al. Single- and multiple-dose pharmacokinetics and absolute bioavailability of tedizolid. Pharmacotherapy. 34:891-900, 2014. (PMID:24989138)

Flanagan S, Minassian SL, Morris D, et al. Pharmacokinetics of tedizolid in subjects with renal or hepatic impairment. Antimicrob Agents Chemother. 58:6471-6476, 2014. (PMID:25136024)

Kisgen JJ, Mansour H, Unger NR, et al. Tedizolid: a new oxazolidinone antimicrobial. Am J Health Syst Pharm. 71:621-633, 2014. (PMID:24688035)

—— = serious side effect ☐ = black box warning. ND = no data. NR = not recommended. s = spectrum inadequate (at site). a = activity or experience inadequate. p = tissue penetration inadequate. *based on peak serum concentration after usual adult dose. †applicable to adult uncomplicated lower UTIs (CrCl > 30 mL/min).

Moran GJ, Fang E, Corey GR, et al. Tedizolid for 6 days versus linezolid for 10 days for acute bacterial skin and skin-structure infections (ESTABLISH-2): a randomised, double-blind, phase 3, non-inferiority trial. Lancet Infect Dis. 14:696-705, 2014. (PMID:24909499)

O'Riordan W, Green S, Mehra P, et al. Tedizolid phosphate for the management of acute bacterial skin and skin structure infections: efficacy summary. Clin Infect Dis. 58;Suppl1:S43-50, 2014. (PMID:24343832)

Prokocimer P, De Anda C, Fang E, et al. Tedizolid phosphate vs linezolid for treatment of acute bacterial skin and skin structure infections: the ESTABLISH-1 randomized trial. JAMA. 309:559-569, 2013. (PMID:2340368)

Shorr AF, Lodise TP, Corey GR, et al. Analysis of the phase 3 ESTABLISH trials: Tedizolid versus linezolid in acute bacterial skin and skin structure infection. Antimicrob Agents Chemother. 59:864-871, 2015. (PMID:25421472)

Website: www.pdr.net

Telavancin (Vibativ)

Drug class: Lipoglycopeptide.
Usual dose: 10 mg/kg (IV) q24h.

Spectrum Synopsis*
Hits
  Gram + : MSSA, MRSA, CoNS, VSE
  Gram – : None
  Problem pathogens: None
Misses
  Gram + : VRE
  Gram – : All aerobic GNB, B. fragilis
  Problem pathogens:
    Listeria, Nocardia,
    Acinetobacter, S. maltophilia,
    B. cepacia

(also see **Antibiotic Pearls & Pitfalls** p. 537).

Resistance Potential: Low
Pharmacokinetic Parameters:
  Peak serum level: 93–108 mcg/mL
  Bioavailability: not applicable
  Excreted unchanged: 76%
  Serum half-life (normal/ESRD): 6–9 hrs/ no data
  Plasma protein binding: 93%
  Volume of distribution (V_d): 1.33-1.45 L/kg
Primary Mode of Elimination: Renal
Dosage Adjustments*

CrCl > 50 mL/min	No change
CrCl 30–50 mL/min	7.5 mg/kg (IV) q24h
CrCl 10–29 mL/min	10 mg/kg (IV) q48h
CrCl < 10 mL/min	Avoid
Post–HD dose	None
Post–PD dose	None
CVVH/CVVHD/ CVVHDF dose	7.5 mg/kg (IV) q24h
Mild-moderate hepatic insufficiency	No change
Severe hepatic insufficiency	Use with caution

Drug Interactions: Drugs that prolong QT_c (additive effect); PT, INR, PTT (↑ levels); other interactions unlikely because is not metabolized through CYP450 system.
Adverse Effects:
Common
• Nausea/vomiting/diarrhea

─── = serious side effect ☐ = black box warning. ND = no data. NR = not recommended. s = spectrum inadequate (at site). a = activity or experience inadequate. p = tissue penetration inadequate. *based on peak serum concentration after usual adult dose. †applicable to adult uncomplicated lower UTIs (CrCl > 30 mL/min).

- Headache
- Metallic taste

Uncommon

- Increased mortality with preexisting renal impairment (CrCl < 50 mL/min)

Rare

- C. difficile diarrhea/colitis
- Adverse developmental outcomes in pregnancy

Allergic Potential: Low
Safety in Pregnancy: C

Additional Clinical Considerations:

- Infuse over at least 60 minutes to minimize infusion-related reactions.
- Efficacy may be decreased with CrCl < 50 mL/min. Effective for MSSA/MRSA cSSSIs.

Cerebrospinal Fluid Penetration:
  Inflamed meninges: 2%
  Non-inflamed meninges: 1%

(also see *Antibiotic Pearls & Pitfalls* p. 537).

SELECTED REFERENCES:
Marcos LA, Camins BC. Successful treatment of vancomycin-intermediate Staphylococcus aureus pacemaker lead infective endocarditis with telavancin. Antimicrob Agents Chemother 54:5376–5378, 2010. (PMID:208763)
Plotkin P, Patel K, Uminski A, et al. Telavancin (Vibativ), a new option for the treatment of gram-positive infections. Pharm Ther 36:127–138, 2011. (PMID:21572764)
Saravolatz LD, Stein GE, Johnson LB. Telavancin: a novel lipoglycopeptide. Clin Infect Dis 49:1908–1914, 2009. (PMID:19911938)
Twilla JD, Gelfand MS, Cleveland KO, et al. Telvancin for the treatment of methicillin-resistant Staphylococcus aureus osteomyelitis. J Antimicrob Chemother 66:2675–2677, 2011. (PMID:21831987)
Wilson SE, O'Rierdan W, Hopkins A, et al. Telavancin versus vancomycin for the treatment of complicated skin and skin-structure infections associated with surgical procedures. Am J Surg 197:791–796, 2009. (PMID:19095213)
Website: www.pdr.net

Telithromycin (Ketek)

Drug Class: Ketolide.
Usual Dose: Acute sinusitis/AECB: 800 mg (PO) q24h × 5 days. Community-acquired pneumonia: 800 mg (PO) q24h × 7–10 days. 800 mg (PO) dose taken as two 400-mg tablets (PO).

Spectrum Synopsis*
Hits
   Gram + : Most GAS, most
      S. pneumoniae, MSSA, VSE
   Gram – : Some aerobic GNB,
      B. fragilis
   Problem pathogens:
      Bordetella, oral anaerobes
Misses
   Gram + : MRSA, VRE
   Gram – : Most aerobic GNB
   Problem pathogens:
      Listeria, Nocardia,
      Acinetobacter, S. maltophilia,
      B. cepacia

——— = serious side effect [____] = black box warning. ND = no data. NR = not recommended. s = spectrum inadequate (at site). a = activity or experience inadequate. p = tissue penetration inadequate. *based on peak serum concentration after usual adult dose. †applicable to adult uncomplicated lower UTIs (CrCl > 30 mL/min).

Resistance Potential: Low.

Pharmacokinetic Parameters:

Peak serum level: 2.27 mcg/mL

Bioavailability: 57%

Excreted unchanged (urine): 13%

Serum half-life (normal/ESRD): 9.8/11 hrs

Plasma protein binding: 65%

Volume of distribution (V_d): 2.9 L/kg

Primary Mode of Elimination: Hepatic

Dosage Adjustments*

CrCl < 30 mL/min	600 mg (PO) q24h
CrCl < 30 mL/min + hepatic impairment	400 mg (PO) q24h
Post–HD/Post–PD dose	400 mg (PO)
CVVH/CVVHD/CVVHDF dose	400 mg (PO) q24h

Drug Interactions: Digoxin (↑ inter-acting drug levels); ergot derivatives (acute ergot toxicity); itraconazole, ketoconazole (↑ telithromycin level); midazolam, triazolam (↑ interacting drug levels, sedation); oral anticoagulants (may ↑ anticoagulant effects; monitor PT/INR); simvastatin (↑ risk of rhabdo-myolysis; giving simvastatin 12h after telithromycin decreases the ↑ in simvas-tatin levels ~ 50%); theophylline (additive nausea). CYP 3A4 inhibitor/substate.

Contraindications: Cisapride and pimozie. **Patients with history of hepatitis/jaundice** (rarely fatal acute/ fulminant hepatitis or acute lever failure with pre-existing liver disease)

Adverse Effects:

Common

- Non-C. difficile diarrhea

Uncommon

- Headache
- Nausea
- Dizziness
- Syncope

Rare

- Life-threatening respiratory failure with myasthenia gravis

Allergic Potential: Low

Safety in Pregnancy: C

Additional Clinical Considerations:

- May take with or without food.

SELECTED REFERENCES:

Carbon C, Moola S, Velancsics I, et al. Telithromycin 800 mg once daily for seven to ten days is an effective and well-tolerated treatment for community-acquired pneumonia. Clin Microbiol Infect 9:691–703, 2003. (PMID:12925111)

Hagberg L, Torres A, van Rensburg D, et al. Efficacy and tolerability of once-daily telithromycin compared with high-dose amoxicillin for treatment of community-acquired pneumonia. Infection 30:378–386, 2002. (PMID:12478329)

van Rensburg D, Fogarty C, De Salvo MC, et al. Efficacy of oral telithromycin in community-acquired pneumonia caused by resistant Streptococcus pneumoniae. Journal of Infection 51:201–5, 2005. (PMID:16230211)

Website: www.pdr.net

───── = serious side effect ☐ = black box warning. ND = no data. NR = not recommended. s = spectrum inadequate (at site). a = activity or experience inadequate. p = tissue penetration inadequate. *based on peak serum concentration after usual adult dose. †applicable to adult uncomplicated lower UTIs (CrCl > 30 mL/min).

Tenofovir disoproxil fumarate (Viread) TDF

Drug Class: HIV nucleotide analogue.
Usual Dose: 300 mg (PO) q24h.
Pharmacokinetic Parameters:
  Peak serum level: 0.29 mcg/mL
  Bioavailability: 25%/39% (fasting/high fat meal)
  Excreted unchanged (urine): 32%
  Serum half-life (normal/ESRD): 17 hrs/ no data
  Plasma protein binding: 0.7–7.2%
  Volume of distribution (V_d): 1.3 L/kg
Primary Mode of Elimination: Renal
Dosage Adjustments*

CrCl 30–49 mL/min	300 mg (PO) q48h
CrCl 10–29 mL/min	300 mg (PO) 2x/week
CrCl < 10 mL/min	Avoid
Post–HD dose	300 mg q7 days
Post–PD dose	No data
CVVH/CVVHD/ CVVHDF dose	300 mg (PO) 2x/week
Moderate hepatic insufficiency	No change
Severe hepatic insufficiency	No change

Drug Interactions: Not a substrate/ inhibitor of cytochrome P-450 enzymes. Didanosine (if possible, avoid concomitant didanosine due to impaired CD_4 response and increased risk of virologic failure); valganciclovir (↑ tenofovir levels); atazanavir, lopinavir/ritonavir (↑ tenofovir levels) (↓ atazanavir levels; use atazanavir 300 mg/ritonavir 100 mg with tenofovir); telaprevir (↑ tenofovir levels).

Adverse Effects:
Common
- Nausea/vomiting/diarrhea
- Asthenia
- Headache
- Decrfeased bone density

Uncommon
- <u>Renal tubular acidosis</u>
- Fanconi-like syndrome

Rare
- <u>Immune reconstitution syndrome (IRIS)</u>

- Lactic acidosis with hepatic steatosis Lactic acidosis and severe hepatomegaly with steatosis. Severe acute exacerbations of HBV

Allergic Potential: Low
Safety in Pregnancy: B

Additional Clinical Considerations:
- Eliminated by glomerular filtration/ tubular secretion.
- May be taken with or without food.
- If possible, avoid concomitant didanosine
- ***Active against HBV***.

Cerebrospinal Fluid Penetration: No data

SELECTED REFERENCE:
Website: www.pdr.net

—— = serious side effect ☐ = black box warning. ND = no data. NR = not recommended. s = spectrum inadequate (at site). a = activity or experience inadequate. p = tissue penetration inadequate. *based on peak serum concentration after usual adult dose. †applicable to adult uncomplicated lower UTIs (CrCl > 30 mL/min).

Terbinafine (Lamisil, Daskil)

Drug Class: Antifungal.
Usual Dose: 250 mg (PO) q24h.
Pharmacokinetic Parameters:
  Peak serum level: 1 mcg/mL
  Bioavailability: 70%
  Excreted unchanged (urine): < 1%
  *Serum half-life (normal/ESRD): 24 hrs/
  no data*
  Plasma protein binding: 99%
  Volume of distribution (V_d): 13.5 L/kg
Primary Mode of Elimination: Renal/
  Hepatic
Dosage Adjustments*

CrCl ~ 50–60 mL/min	No change
CrCl < 50 mL/min	Avoid
Post–HD dose	Avoid
Post–PD dose	Avoid
CVVH/CVVHD/CVVHDF dose	Avoid
Moderate—severe hepatic insufficiency	Avoid

Drug Interactions: Cimetidine (↓ terbinafine clearance, ↑ terbinafine levels); phenobarbital, rifampin (↑ terbinafine clearance, ↓ terbinafine levels).
Adverse Effects:
Common
  • Headache
Uncommon
  • Nausea/vomiting/diarrhea
  • Abdominal pain
  • Visual disturbances
  • ↑ AST/ALT
  • Drug fever/rash
Rare
  • Leukopenia
  • Lymphopenia
Allergic Potential: Low
Safety in Pregnancy: B

Additional Clinical Considerations:
  • May cause green vision and lens/
    retina changes.
Cerebrospinal Fluid Penetration: <10%

SELECTED REFERENCES:
Abdel-Rahman SM, Nahata MC. Oral terbinafine:
  A new antifungal agent. Ann Pharmacother
  31:445–56, 1997. (PMID:9101008)
Darkes MJ, Scott LJ, Goa KL. Terbinafine: a review
  of its use in onychomycosis in adults. Am J Clin
  Dermatol 4:39–65, 2003. (PMID:12477372)
Website: www.pdr.net

Tetracycline (various)

Drug Class: Tetracycline.
Usual Dose: 500 mg (PO) q6h
(*take without food*).

Spectrum Synopsis*
Hits
  Gram + : Some S. pneumoniae
  Gram – : H. influenzae, B. fragilis
  Problem pathogens:
    Listeria, Nocardia, Bordertalla
Misses
  Gram + : GAS, GBS, MSSA, MRSA,
    VSE, VRE
  Gram – : Most GNB, Shigella

——— = serious side effect ☐ = black box warning. ND = no data. NR = not recommended. s = spectrum inadequate (at site). a = activity or experience inadequate. p = tissue penetration inadequate. *based on peak serum concentration after usual adult dose. †applicable to adult uncomplicated lower UTIs (CrCl > 30 mL/min).

Problem pathogens:
Acinetobacter, S. maltophilia,
B. cepacia

Urine Spectrum[†]

- Same as serum spectrum *plus* many GNB uropathogens including P. aeruginosa
- Optimal urinary pH = 5–6
- Urine levels = 300 mcg/mL

(Full *Susceptibility Profiles* p. 196).

Resistance Potential: High
(S. pneumoniae, MSSA)

Pharmacokinetic Parameters:
Peak serum level: 1.5 mcg/mL
Bioavailability: 60%
Excreted unchanged (urine): 60%
Serum half-life (normal/ESRD): 8/108 hrs
Plasma protein binding: 5%
Volume of distribution (V_d): 0.7 L/kg

Primary Mode of Elimination: Renal

Dosage Adjustments*

CrCl 50–80 mL/min	500 mg (PO) q12h
CrCl 10–50 mL/min	500 mg (PO) q24h
Post–HD/Post–PD dose	None
CVVH/CVVHD/ CVVHDF dose	500 mg (PO) q12h
Moderate hepatic insufficiency	No change
Severe hepatic insufficiency	≤ 1 gm (PO) q24h

Drug Interactions: Antacids, Al[++], Ca[++], Fe[++], Mg[++], Zn[++], multivitamins, sucralfate (↓ absorption of tetracycline); barbiturates, carbamazepine, phenytoin (↓ half-life of tetracycline); bicarbonate (↓ absorption and ↑ clearance of tetracycline); digoxin (↑ digoxin levels); insulin (↑ insulin effect); methoxyflurane (↑ nephrotoxicity).

Adverse Effects:

Common

- Tooth discoloration and enamel hypoplasia
- Nausea/vomiting/diarrhea

Uncommon

- Vaginal candidiasis
- Photosensitizing reactions
- Benign intracranial hypertension (pseudotumor cerebri)

Allergic Potential: Low

Safety in Pregnancy: D

Additional Clinical Considerations:

- ***Hepatotoxicity dose dependent*** (≥ 2 gm/day), especially in pregnancy/ renal failure.
- Doxycycline or minocycline preferred for all tetracycline uses.

Additional Pharmacokinetic Considerations*

Non-CSF	% of Serum Levels
Peritoneal fluid	NR(s)
Bile	1000%
Synovial fluid	NR(s)
Bone	NR(s)
Prostate	50%
CSF	
Non-inflamed meninges	5%
Inflamed meninges (ABM)	5%

——— = serious side effect ☐ = black box warning. ND = no data. NR = not recommended. s = spectrum inadequate (at site). a = activity or experience inadequate. p = tissue penetration inadequate. *based on peak serum concentration after usual adult dose. [†]applicable to adult uncomplicated lower UTIs (CrCl > 30 mL/min).

(also see **Antibiotic Pearls & Pitfalls** p. 530).

SELECTED REFERENCES:

Agwuh KN, MacGowan A. Pharmacokinetics and pharmacodynamics of the tetracyclines including glycylcyclines. J of Antimicrob Chemotherapy 58:256–265, 2006. (PMID:16816396)

Cunha BA, Comer J, Jonas M. The tetracyclines. Med Clin North Am 66:293–302, 1982. (PMID:7038336)

Smilack JD, Wilson WE, Cocerill FR 3rd. Tetracycline, chloramphenicol, erythromycin, clindamycin, and metronidazole. Mayo Clin Proc 66:1270–80, 1991. (PMID:1749296)

Website: www.pdr.net

Ticarcillin (Ticar)

Drug Class: Anti-pseudomonal penicillin.
Usual Dose: 3 gm (IV) q6h.

Spectrum Synopsis*

Hits

   Gram + : BGAS, VSE, MSSA
   Gram – : Most GNB (P. aeruginosa)
      B. fragilis
   Problem pathogens:
      None

Misses

   Gram + : MRSA, VRE
   Gram – : Some GNB
   Problem pathogens:
      Listeria, Nocardia,
      Acinetobacter, S. maltophilia,
      B. cepacia

Urine Spectrum†

• Same as serum spectrum
• Optimal urinary pH = 5–6
• Urine levels = 2500 mcg/mL

(Full **Susceptibility Profiles** p. 196).

Resistance Potential: Low

Pharmacokinetic Parameters:

   Peak serum level: 118–300 mcg/mL
   Bioavailability: Not applicable
   Excreted unchanged (urine): 95%
   Serum half-life (normal/ESRD): 1/5 hrs
   Plasma protein binding: 45%
   Volume of distribution (V_d): 0.2 L/kg

Primary Mode of Elimination: Renal

Dosage Adjustments*

CrCl 50–80 mL/min	No change
CrCl 10–50 mL/min	2 gm (IV) q8h
CrCl < 10 mL/min	2 gm (IV) q12h
Post–HD dose	2 gm (IV)
Post–PD dose	3 gm (IV)
CVVH/CVVHD/ CVVHDF dose	2 gm (IV) q8h
Moderate hepatic insufficiency	No change
Severe hepatic insufficiency	No change

Drug Interactions: Aminoglycosides (inactivation of ticarcillin in renal failure); warfarin (↑ INR); oral contraceptives (↓ oral contraceptive effect); cefoxitin (↓ ticarcillin effect).

Adverse Effects:

Common

• Drug fever/rash
• IV site thrombophlebitis

Uncommon

• Hives

Rare

• Serum sickness
• Anaphylactic reactions
• Inhibition of platelet aggregation (dose-dependent)

——— = serious side effect ⬜ = black box warning. ND = no data. NR = not recommended. s = spectrum inadequate (at site). a = activity or experience inadequate. p = tissue penetration inadequate. *based on peak serum concentration after usual adult dose. †applicable to adult uncomplicated lower UTIs (CrCl > 30 mL/min).

- Erythema multiforme/Stevens-Johnson Syndrome

Allergic Potential: High
Safety in Pregnancy: B

Additional Clinical Considerations:
- Administer 1 hour before or after aminoglycoside.

May increase LPS (endotoxin) release from GNB potentially increasing endotoxin mediated tissue damage

---

Additional Pharmacokinetic Considerations*

Non-CSF	% of Serum Levels
Peritoneal fluid	34%
Bile	20%
Synovial fluid	20%
Bone	<1%
Prostate	NR(p)
CSF	
Non-inflamed meninges	1%
Inflamed meninges (ABM)	30%

Meningeal dose = usual dose

SELECTED REFERENCE:
Website: www.pdr.net

Ticarcillin/Clavulanate (Timentin)

Drug Class: Anti-pseudomonal penicillin/β-lactamase inhibitor.
Usual Dose: 3.1 gm (IV) q6h.

Spectrum Synopsis*
Hits
  Gram + : All non-enterococcal streptococci, VSE
  Gram – : Most GNB aerobic (modest P. aeruginosa activity) B. fragilis

---

Problem pathogens:
  None
Misses
  Gram + : MRSA, VRE
  Gram – : Some GNB
  Problem pathogens:
    Acinetobacter, S. maltophilia, B. cepacia
Urine Spectrum†
- Optimal urinary pH = 5–6
- Same as serum spectrum
- Urine levels = 2500 mcg/mL

(Full **Susceptibility Profiles** p. 196).
Resistance Potential: Low
Pharmacokinetic Parameters:
Peak serum level: 330 mcg/mL
Bioavailability: Not applicable
Excreted unchanged (urine): 95/45%
Serum half-life (normal/ESRD): [1/13]/[1/2] hrs
Plasma protein binding: 45/25%
Volume of distribution (V_d): 0.2/0.3 L/kg
Primary Mode of Elimination: Renal
Dosage Adjustments*

CrCl 30–60 mL/min	3.1 gm (IV) q8h
CrCl 10–30 mL/min	3.1 gm (IV) q12h
CrCl < 10 mL/min	2 gm (IV) q12h
Post–HD dose	3.1 gm (IV)
Post–PD dose	3.1 gm (IV)
CVVH/CVVHD/CVVHDF dose	3.1 gm (IV) q8h
Moderate hepatic insufficiency	If CrCl < 10 mL/min: 2 gm (IV) q24h
Severe hepatic insufficiency	If CrCl < 10 mL/min: 2 gm (IV) q24h

---

—— = serious side effect ☐ = black box warning. ND = no data. NR = not recommended. s = spectrum inadequate (at site). a = activity or experience inadequate. p = tissue penetration inadequate. *based on peak serum concentration after usual adult dose. †applicable to adult uncomplicated lower UTIs (CrCl > 30 mL/min).

Drug Interactions: Aminoglycosides
(↓ aminoglycoside levels); methotrexate
(↑ methotrexate levels); vecuronium
(↑ vecuronium effect).
Adverse Effects:
Common
- Drug rash/fever
- IV site thrombophlebitis

Uncommon
- Eosinophilia
- ↑ AST/ALT

Rare
- <u>Serum sickness</u>
- <u>Anaphylactic reactions</u>
- <u>C. difficile diarrhea/colitis</u>
- <u>Erythema multiforme/Stevens-Johnson Syndrome</u>

Allergic Potential: High
Safety in Pregnancy: B

Additional Clinical Considerations:
- 20% of clavulanate removed by dialysis.

May increase LPS (endotoxin) release from GNB potentially increasing endotoxin mediated tissue damage

---

Additional Pharmacokinetic Considerations*

Non-CSF	% of Serum Levels
Peritoneal fluid	ND
Bile	100%
Synovial fluid	ND
Bone	ND
Prostate	NR(p)
CSF	
Non-inflamed meninges	1%
Inflamed meninges (ABM)	<10%

(also see **Antibiotic Pearls & Pitfalls** p. 530).

SELECTED REFERENCE:
Website: www.pdr.net

Tigecycline (Tygacil)

Drug Class: Glycylcycline.
Usual Dose: SDT: Loading dose: = 100
mg (IV) × 1 dose, then **Maintenance
dose:** 50 mg (IV)/q12h **HDT: Loading
dose:** = 200* – 400[†] mg (IV) × 1 dose,
then **Maintenance dose:** = 100* – 200[†]
mg (IV) q24h (see comments[†]).
SDT = standard dose tigecycline (CSSSIs,
CIAIs, CAP)
HDT = high dose tigecycline (serious systemic infectious*, MDR GNB infections[†]
including urosepsis[†])

Spectrum Synopsis*
Hits
  Gram + : All streptococci (including
PRSP, VSE, VRE), CoNS, MSSA, MRSA
  Gram – : Most GNB, B. fragilis
  Problem pathogens:
    Acinetobacter, S. maltophilia,
    B. cepacia, CRE (including
    most metallo-β-lactamases)
Misses
  Gram + : None
  Gram – : Most Proteus, P. aeruginosa
    Providencia
  Problem pathogens:
    Some MBL
Urine Spectrum[†]
- Same as serum spectrum
- Optimal urinary pH = 5–6.
- Urinary spectrum is concentration
dependent (higher than usual
systemic IV doses may be needed to
eradicate susceptible uropathogens)
- Urine levels = 10–30 mcg/mL

(Full **Susceptibility Profiles** p. 196).

——— = serious side effect ☐ = black box warning. ND = no data. NR = not recommended. s = spectrum inadequate (at site). a = activity or experience inadequate. p = tissue penetration inadequate.
*based on peak serum concentration after usual adult dose. [†]applicable to adult uncomplicated lower UTIs
(CrCl > 30 mL/min).

Resistance Potential: Low
  (Acinetobacter baumanii–dose related)

Pharmacokinetic Parameters:
  Peak serum level: 1.45 mcg/mL (100 mg
  dose); 0.87 mcg/mL (50 mg dose)
  Bioavailability: Not applicable
  Excreted unchanged (urine): 22%
  Serum half-life (normal/ESRD): 42/42 hrs
  Plasma protein binding: 89%
  Volume of distribution (V_d): 8 L/kg

Primary Mode of Elimination: Biliary

Dosage Adjustments*

CrCl < 10 mL/min	No change
Post–HD dose	None
Post–PD dose	None
CVVH/CVVHD/ CVVHDF dose	No change
Mild-moderate hepatic insufficiency	No change
Severe hepatic insufficiency (Child Pugh C)	100 mg (IV) × 1 dose, then 25 mg (IV) q12h

Drug Interactions: Warfarin
(↑ INR). Does not inhibit and is not
metabolized by CYP450.

Adverse Effects:

Common
  • Nausea/vomiting

Uncommon
  • Dizziness
  • ↑ Alkaline phosphatase
  • ↑ LDH
  • ↑ BUN
  • ↓ Fibrinogen levels
  • Thrombocytosis

Rare
  • Pancreatitis

Allergic Potential: Low

Safety in Pregnancy: D

Additional Clinical Considerations:
  • Tetracycline or doxycycline suscepti-bilities *not* predictive of tigecycline susceptibilities.
  • If any question re: tetracycline/ doxycycline susceptibility, request tigecycline susceptibilities.
  • ***Higher Loading (LD)/Maintenance Doses (MD) suggested for serious systemic infections or infections due to MDR Klebsiella pneumoniae, CRE, or MDR Acinetobacter baumanii.*§†***
  • ***Following the initial Loading Dose** (based on PK parameters) **LD, tigecycline is optimally given as a single daily (q24h) maintenance dose** (since $t_{1/2}$ = 42 hrs).*
  • ***Effective against all other GNBs, MSSA/MRSA, VSE/VRE, and B. fragilis. (misses only P. aeruginosa, most Proteus sp., and some Providencia sp.).***
  • *Tigecycline rarely causes N/V if suffi-ciently diluted and slowly infused.*
  • If N/V occurs, ↑ infusion volume and infusion time (see *p. 757*).
  • **Effective monotherapy for serious systemic infections (due to susceptible pathogens)**
  • Minimal resistance potential.
  • *Protective against C. difficile*
  • ***Effective against C. difficile diarrhea/colitis.***

—— = serious side effect ☐ = black box warning. ND = no data. NR = not recommended. s = spec-trum inadequate (at site). a = activity or experience inadequate. p = tissue penetration inadequate.
*based on peak serum concentration after usual adult dose. †applicable to adult uncomplicated lower UTIs (CrCl > 30 mL/min).

May inhibit antibiotic induced LPS (endotoxin) release from GNB potentially minimizing endotoxin mediated tissue damage.

For nausea/vomiting (↑ volume and ↑ infusion time).

Tigecycline Dose[†]	Infusion Volume	Infusion Time
100 mg	100 mL	30 min
200 mg*	250 mL	60 min
400 mg[§]	500 mL	120 min

* For systemic infections.
[§] For serious systemic infections or UTIs due to susceptible MDR GNBs.
[†] Maintence dose (MD) = half of the loading dose (LD).

Additional Pharmacokinetic Considerations*	
Non-CSF	**% of Serum Levels**
Peritoneal fluid	ND
Bile	>3000%
Synovial fluid	60%
Bone	30%
Prostate	ND
CSF	
Non-inflamed meninges	1%
Inflamed meninges (ABM)	8%

(also see **Antibiotic Pearls & Pitfalls** p. 536).

SELECTED REFERENCES:

Aldape MJ, Heeny DD, Bryant AE, et al. Tigecycline suppresses toxin A and B production and sporulation in C. difficile. J Anti Chemo 70:153–159, 2015. (PMID:25151204)

Babinchak T, Ellis-Grosse E, Dartois N, et al. The efficacy and safety of tigecycline for the treatment of complicated intra-abdominal infections: analysis of pooled clinical trial data. Clin Infect Dis 41(Suppl 5:S3):54–67, 2005. (PMID:1608007)

Baron J, Klein N, Cunha BA. Once daily high dose tigecycline is optimal: Tigecycline PK/PD Parameters Predict Clinical Effectiveness. Journal of Clinical Medicine 7: e49-56, 2018. (PMID: 29522431)

Bergallo C, Jasovich A, Teglia O, et al. Safety and efficacy of intravenous tigecycline in Treatment of community-acquired pneumonia: results from a double-blind randomized Phase 3 comparison study with levofloxacin. Diagn Microbiol Infect Dis 63:52–61, 2009. (PMID:18990531)

Betts JW, Phee LM, Woodford N, et al. Activity of colistin in combination with tigecycline or rifampicin against multidrug-resistant Stenotrophomonas maltophilia. Eur J Clin Microbiol Infect Dis 33:1565-1572, 2014. (PMID:2478100)

Bhattacharya I, Gotfried MH, Ji AJ, et al. Reassessment of tigecycline bone concentrations in volunteers undergoing elective orthopedic procedures. J Clin Pharm. 54:70-74, 2014. (PMID:24155157)

Bopp LH, Baltch AL, Ritz WJ, et al. Activities of tigecycline and comparators against Legionella pneumophila and Legionella micdadei extracellularly and in human monocytederived macrophages. Diagn Microbiol Infect Dis 69:86–93, 2011. (PMID:21146719)

Britt NS, Steed ME, Potter EM, et al. Tigecycline for the treatment of severe and severe complicated clostridium difficile infection. Inf Dis Ther, (ahead of print), 2014. (PMID:25466443)

Brust K, Evans A, Plemmons R. Favourable outcome in the treatment of carbapenem-resistant Enterobacteriaceae urinary tract infection with high-dose tigecycline. J Anti Chemo 69:2875–2876, 2014. (PMID:24879666)

Bulik CC, Wiskirchen DE, Shepard A, et al. Tissue penetration and pharmacokinetics of

──── = serious side effect ☐ = black box warning. ND = no data. NR = not recommended. s = spectrum inadequate (at site). a = activity or experience inadequate. p = tissue penetration inadequate. *based on peak serum concentration after usual adult dose. [†]applicable to adult uncomplicated lower UTIs (CrCl > 30 mL/min).

tigecycline in diabetic patients with chronic wound infections described by using in vivo microdialysis. Antimicrob Agents Chemother 54:5209–4213, 2010. (PMID:20921312)

Cheong EY, Gottlieb T. Intravenous tigecycline in the treatment of severe recurrent Clostridium difficile colitis. Med J. Aust 4:374–375, 2011. (PMID:21470094)

Conde-Estévez D, Grau S, Horcajada JP, et al. Off-label prescription of tigecycline: clinical and microbiological characteristics and outcomes. Int J Antimicrob Agents 36:471–472, 2010. (PMID:20828992)

Cunha BA, Baron J, Cunha CB. Monotherapy with High Dose Once Daily Tigecycline is Highly Effective Against Acinetobacter baumanii and other Multi-Drug Resistant (MDR) Gram-Negative Bacilli. International Journal of Antimicrobial Agents 52:199-120, 2018. (PMID:29501604)

Cunha BA, Baron J, Cunha CB. Once daily high dose tigecycline - pharmacokinetic/pharmacodynamic based dosing for optimal clinical effectiveness: dosing matters, revisited. Expert Rev Anti Infect Ther. 15:257-267, 2017. (PMID:27917692)

Cunha BA. Tigecycline dosing is critical in preventing tigecycline resistance because relative resistance is, in part, concentration dependent. Clin Microbiol Infect 21:e39–40, 2015. (PMID:25708550)

Cunha BA, McDermott B, Nausheen S. Single once daily high dose therapy of tigecycline in a urinary tract infection due to multi-drug resistant (MDR) Klebsiella pneumoniae and MDR Enterobacter agglomerans. J Chemo 19:753–754, 2008. (PMID:18230562)

Cunha BA. Once daily tigecycline therapy of multidrug-resistant and non-multidrug resistant gram-negative bacteremias. J Chemo 19:232–33, 2007. (PMID:17434836)

Cunha BA. Antimicrobial therapy of multidrug-resistant Streptococcus pneumoniae, vancomycin-resistant enterococci, and methicillin-resistant Staphlycoccus aureus. Med Clin N Am 90:1165–82, 2006. (PMID:17116442)

Curcio D. Skin and soft tissue infections due to methicillin-resistant Staphylococcus aureus:

Role of tigecycline. Clin Infect Dis 52:1468–1469, 2011. (PMID:21498390)

Dartois N, Castiang N, Gandjini H, et al. Tigecycline versus levofloxacin for the treatment of community-acquired pneumonia: European experience. J Chemother 20:28–35, 2008. (PMID:19036672)

De Pascale G, Antonelli M. Appropriate tigecycline use for extensively drug resistant infections: The standard dose may not be enough! Crit Care Med 43:e533–544, 2015. (PMID:26468725)

De Pascale G, Montini L, Pennisi M, et al. High dose tigecycline in critically ill patients with severe infections due to multidrug-resistant bacteria. Crit Care 5:18, 2014. (PMID:2487101)

Eckmann C, Heizmann W, Bodmann KF, et al. Tigcycline in the treatment of patients with necrotizing skin and soft tissue infections due to multiresistant bacteria. Surg Infect 16:618–625, 2015. (PMID:26115414)

Falagas ME, Vardakas KZ, Tsiveriotis KP, et al. Effectiveness and safety of high-dose tigecycline containing regimens for the treatment of severe bacterial infections. Int J Anti Agents 44:1–7, 2014. (PMID:24602499)

Fraise AP. Tigecycline: The answer to beta-lactam and fluoroquinolone resistance? Journal of Infection 53:293–300, 2006. (PMID:16876253)

Geerlings SE, van Donselaar-van der Pant KA, Keur I. Successful treatment with tigecycline of two patients with complicated urinary tract infections caused by extended-spectrum betalactamase-producing Escherichia coli. J Antimicrob Chemother 65:2048–2049, 2010. (PMID:20554566)

Kuo SC, Wang FD, Fung CP, et al. Clinical experience with tigecycline as treatment for serious infections in elderly and critically ill patients. J Microbiol Immunol Infect 44:45–51, 2011. (PMID:21531352)

Larson KC, Belliveau PP, Spooner LM. Tigecycline for the treatment of severe Clostridium difficile infection. Ann Pharm 45:1005–1010, 2011. (PMID:21730279)

Lauf L, Ozsvar Z, Mitha I, et al. Phase 3 study comparing tigecycline and ertapenem in patients with diabetic foot injections with and without osteomyelitis. Diag Microbiol Infect Dis. 78:469-480, 2014. (PMID:24439136)

——— = serious side effect ☐ = black box warning. ND = no data. NR = not recommended. s = spectrum inadequate (at site). a = activity or experience inadequate. p = tissue penetration inadequate. *based on peak serum concentration after usual adult dose. †applicable to adult uncomplicated lower UTIs (CrCl > 30 mL/min).

Marchaim D, Pogue JM, Tzuman O, et al. Major variation in MICs of tigecycline in gram-negative bacilli as a function of testing method. J Clin Microbiol. 52:1617–1621, 2014. (PMID:24599978)

McKeage K, Keating GM. Tigecycline: in community-acquired pneumonia. Drugs 68:2633–2644, 2008. (PMID:19093704)

Meagher AK, Ambrose PG, Grasela TH, et al. The pharmacokinetic and pharmacodynamic profile of tigecycline. Clin Infect Dis 41(Suppl 5):S333–40, 2005. (PMID:16080071)

Metan G, Alp E, Yildiz O, et al. Clinical experience with tigecycline in the treatment of carbapenem-resistant Acinetobacter infections. J Chemother 22:110–114, 2010. (PMID:20435570)

Nilsson LE, Frimodt-Moller N, Vaara M, et al. Comparative activity of tigecycline and tetracycline on Gram-negative and Gram-positive bacteria revealed by a multicentre study in four North European countries. Scand J Infect Dis 43:707–713, 2011. (PMID:21619494)

Nix DE, Matthias KR. Should tigecycline be considered for urinary tract infections? A pharmacokinetic re-evaluation. J Antimicrob Chemother 65:1311–1312, 2010. (PMID:20378673)

Noviello S, Ianniello F, Leone S, et al. In vitro activity of tigecycline: MICs, MBCs, time-kill curves and post-antibiotic effect. J Chemotherapy 20:577–580, 2008. (PMID:19028619)

Pai M. Serum and urine pharmacokinetics of tigecycline in obese class III and normal weight adults. J Antimicrob Chemo. 69:190-199, 2014. (PMID:23883872)

Pallotto C, Fiorio M, D'Avolio A, et al. Cerebrospinal fluid penetration of tigecycline. Scand J Infect Dis. 46:69-72, 2014. (PMID:24131423)

Pankey GA. Tigecycline. J Antimicrob Chemother 53:470–80, 2005. (PMID:16040625)

Polidori M, Nuccorini A, Tascini C, et al. Vancomycin-resistant Enterococcus faecium (VRE) bacteremia in infective endocarditis successfully treated with combination daptomycin and tigecycline. J Chemother 23:240–241, 2011. (PMID:21803704)

Qvist N, Warren B, Leister-Tebbe H, et al. Efficacy of tigecycline versus ceftriaxone plus metronidazole for the treatment of complicated intra-abdominal infections: results from a randomized, controlled trail. Surg Infect 13:102–3, 2012. (PMID:22439781)

Raad I, Hanna H, Jiang Y, et al. Comparative activities of daptomycin, linezolid, and tigecycline against catheter-related methicillin-resistant Staphylococcus bacteremic isolates embedded in biofilm. Antimicrob Agents Chemother 51:1656–1660, 2007. (PMID:17353249)

Rodvold K, Gotfried M, Cwik M, et al. Serum, tissue and body fluid concentrations of tigecycline after a single 10 mg dose. J of Anti Chemo 58:1221-1229, 2006. (PMID: 17012300)

Routsi C, Kokkoris S, Douka E, et al. High-dose tigecycline associated alterations in coagulation parameters in critically ill patients with severe infections. International Journal of Antimicroial Agents 45:84-85, 2015. (PMID:25241261)

Schwab KS, Hahn-Ast C, Heinz WJ, et al. Tigecycline in febrile neutropenic patients with haematological malignancies: a retrospective case documentation in four university hospitals. Infection 42:97-104, 2014. (PMID:23979853)

Stein GE, Craig WA. Tigecycline: A Critical Analysis. Clin Infect Dis 43:518–24, 2006. (PMID:16838243)

Swoboda S, Ober M, Hainer C, et al. Tigecycline for the treatment of patients with severe sepsis or septic shock: a drug use evaluation in a surgical intensive care unit. J Antimicrob Chemother 61:729–733, 2008. (PMID:18222953)

Valve K, Vaalasti A, Anttila VJ, et al. Disseminated Legionella pneumophila infection in an immunocompromised patient treated with tigecycline. Scand J Infect Dis 42:152–155, 2010. (PMID:19916901)

Xie J, Wang T, Sun J, et al. Optimal tigecycline dosage regimen is urgently needed: results from a pharmacokinetic/pharmacodynamic analysis of tigecycline by Monte Carlo simulation. Int J Infect Dis. 18:62-67, 2014. (PMID:24246741)

Zhang Q, Zhou S, Zhou J. Tigecycline treatment causes a decrease in fibrinogen levels.

Anti Agents Chemo 59:1650–1655, 2015. (PMID:25547356)
Zinner SH. Overview of antibiotic use and resistance: setting the stage for tigecycline. Clin Infect Dis 41(Suppl 5):S289–92, 2005. (PMID:16080067)
Website: www.pdr.net

Tobramycin (Nebcin)

Drug Class: Aminoglycoside.
Usual Dose: 240 mg or 5 mg/kg (IV) q24h (preferred over q8h dosing)

Spectrum Synopsis*
Hits
  Gram + : MSSA
  Gram – : Most GNB (most P. aeruginosa)
  Problem pathogens: Some Acinetobacter
Misses
  Gram + : MRSA, VSE, VRE
  Gram – : Many P. aeruginosa, B. fragilis
  Problem pathogens: S. maltophilia, B. cepacia, most Acinetobacter
Urine Spectrum†
  • Same as serum spectrum
  • Optimal urinary pH = 6–7

(Full *Susceptibility Profiles* p. 208).

Resistance Potential: High (P. aeruginosa, aerobic GNBs)
Pharmacokinetic Parameters:
*Peak serum levels: 4–8 mcg/mL (q8h dosing);
16–24 mcg/mL (q24h dosing)
Bioavailability: Not applicable
Excreted unchanged (urine): 95%
Serum half-life (normal/ESRD): 2.5/56 hrs
Plasma protein binding: 10%*

Volume of distribution (V_d): 0.24 L/kg
Primary Mode of Elimination: Renal
Dosage Adjustments*

CrCl 50–80 mL/min	120 mg (IV) q24h or 2.5 mg/kg (IV) q24h
CrCl 10–50 mL/min	120 mg (IV) q48h or 2.5 mg/kg (IV) q48h
CrCl < 10 mL/min	60 mg (IV) q48h or 1.25 mg/kg (IV) q48h
Post–HD dose	80 mg (IV) or 1 mg/kg (IV)
Post–HFHD dose	120 mg (IV) or 2.5 mg/kg (IV)
Post–PD dose	40 mg (IV) or 0.5 mg/kg (IV) or 2–4 mg/L in dialysate q24h
CVVH/CVVHD/CVVHDF dose	120 mg (IV) q48h or 2.5 mg/kg (IV)
Mild-moderate hepatic insufficiency	No change
Severe hepatic insufficiency	No change

Drug Interactions: Amphotericin B, cyclosporine, enflurane, methoxyflurane, NSAIDs, polymyxin B, radiographic contrast, vancomycin (↑ nephrotoxicity); cis-platinum (↑ nephrotoxicity, ↑ ototoxicity); loop diuretics (↑ ototoxicity); neuromuscular blocking agents (↑ apnea, prolonged paralysis); non-polarizing muscle relaxants (↑ apnea).

——— = serious side effect ▭ = black box warning. ND = no data. NR = not recommended. s = spectrum inadequate (at site). a = activity or experience inadequate. p = tissue penetration inadequate. *based on peak serum concentration after usual adult dose. †applicable to adult uncomplicated lower UTIs (CrCl > 30 mL/min).

Adverse Effects:
Uncommon

- Ototoxicity associated with prolonged/extremely high peak serum levels (usually irreversible), Cochlear toxicity (1/3 of ototoxicity) manifests as decreased high frequency hearing, but deafness is unusual.
  Vestibular toxicity (2/3 of ototoxicity) develops before ototoxicity (typically manifests as tinnitus).
- Neuromuscular blockade with rapid infusion/ansorption
- Nephrotoxicity only with prolonged/ extremely high serum trough levels
- Reversible non-oliguric renal failure (ATN)

Allergic Potential: Low
Safety in Pregnancy: D

Additional Clinical Considerations:

- **Single daily dosing greatly reduces nephrotoxic/ototoxic potential.**
- IV infusion should be given slowly over 1 hour. May be given IM.
- *Avoid intraperitoneal infusion due to risk of neuromuscular blockade.*
- *Avoid intratracheal/aerosolized intrapulmonary instillation, which predisposes to antibiotic resistance.*
- V_d increases with edema/ascites, trauma, burns, cystic fibrosis; may require ↑ dose. V_d decreases with dehydration, obesity; may require ↓ dose.
- **Renal cast counts are the best indicator of aminoglycoside nephrotoxicity, not serum creatinines.**
- Dialysis removes ~ 1/3 of tobramycin from serum.
- **Tobramycin Nebulizer Dose:** 300 mg via nebulizer q12h *(not recommended due to ↑ risk of resistance).*
- **CAPD dose:** 2–4 mg/L in dialysate (IP) with each exchange.
- **Therapeutic Serum Concentrations** (for therapeutic efficacy, *not toxicity*):
  Peak levels (q24h/q8h dosing) = 16–24/8–10 mcg/ mL
  Trough levels (q24h/q8h dosing) = 0/1–2 mcg/mL
- **Synergy Dose:** 120 mg (IV) q24h or 2.5 mg/kg (IV) q24h
- **Intrathecal (IT) dose:** 5 mg (IT) q24h (always give with septimic IV therapy)

May inhibit antibiotic induced LPS (endotoxin) release from GNB potentially minimizing endotoxin mediated tissue damage.

Additional Pharmacokinetic Considerations*

Non-CSF	% of Serum Levels
Peritoneal fluid	40%
Bile	20%
Synovial fluid	NR(a)
Bone	ND
Prostate	NR(p)
Urine†	>500%
CSF	
Non-inflamed meninges	<1%
Inflamed meninges (ABM)	20%

Meningeal dose:
  Intrathecal dose: 5 mg (IT) q24h
  (always give with systemic IV therapy)

――― = serious side effect ☐ = black box warning. ND = no data. NR = not recommended. s = spectrum inadequate (at site). a = activity or experience inadequate. p = tissue penetration inadequate. *based on peak serum concentration after usual adult dose. †applicable to adult uncomplicated lower UTIs (CrCl > 30 mL/min).

(also see **Antibiotic Pearls & Pitfalls** p. 531).

SELECTED REFERENCES:

Buijk SE Mouton JW, Gyssens IC, et al. Experience with a once-daily dosing program of aminoglycosides in critically ill patients. Intensive Care Med 28:936–42, 2002. (PMID:12122533)

Cheer SM, Waugh J, Noble S. Inhaled tobramycin (TOBI): a review of its use in the management of Pseudomonas aeruginosa infections in patients with cystic fibrosis. Drugs 63:2501–20, 2003. (PMID:14609360)

Cunha BA. Aminoglycosides: Current role in antimicrobial therapy. Pharmacotherapy 8:334–50, 1988. (PMID:3146747)

Edson RS, Terrel CL. The aminoglycosides. Mayo Clin Proc 74:519–28, 1999. (PMID:10319086)

Geller DE, Pistlick WH, Nardella PA, et al. Pharmacokinetics and bioavailability of aerosolized tobramycin in cystic fibrosis. Chest 122:219–26, 2002. (PMID:12114362)

Gilbert DN. Once-daily aminoglycoside therapy. Antimicrob Agents Chemother 35:399–405, 1991. (PMID:2039189)

Kahler DA, Schowengerdt KO, Fricker FJ, et al. Toxic serum trough concentrations after administration of nebulized tobramycin. Pharmacotherapy 23:543–5, 2003. (PMID:12680485)

Lortholary O, Tod M, Cohen Y, et al. Aminoglycosides. Med Clin North Am 79:761–87, 1995. (PMID:7791422)

Whitehead A, Conway SP, Etherington C, et al. Once-daily tobramycin in the treatment of adult patients with cystic fibrosis. Eur Respir J 19:303–9, 2002. (PMID:11866010)

Wood GC, Chapman JL, Boucher BA, et al. Tobramycin bladder irrigation for treating a urinary tract infection in a critically ill patient. Ann Pharmacother 38:1318–9, 2004. (PMID:15173558)

Website: www.pdr.net

Trimethoprim (Proloprim, Trimpex) TMP

Drug Class: Folate antagonist.
Usual Dose: 100 mg (PO) q12h (see comments).

Spectrum Synopsis*
Hits
  Gram + : GAS, GBS, MSSA, some CA-MRSA
  Gram – : Most GNB
  Problem pathogens: Listeria, Nocardia, PCP, Toxoplasma
Misses
  Gram + : HA-MRSA, VSE, VRE
  Gram – : P. aeruginosa, B. fragilis
  Problem pathogens: Acinetobacter, S. maltophilia, B. cepacia
Urine Spectrum†
- Same as serum spectrum
- Optimal urinary pH = 6–7
- Urine level = 100 mcg/mL

(see **Susceptibility Profiles** p. 196).
Resistance Potential: High
  (S. pneumoniae, E. coli)
Pharmacokinetic Parameters:
Peak serum level: 2–8 mcg/mL
Bioavailability: 98%
Excreted unchanged (urine): 67%
Serum half-life (normal/ESRD): 8/24 hrs
Plasma protein binding: 44%
Volume of distribution (V_d): 1.8 L/kg
Primary Mode of Elimination: Renal
Dosage Adjustments*

———— = serious side effect ☐ = black box warning. ND = no data. NR = not recommended. s = spectrum inadequate (at site). a = activity or experience inadequate. p = tissue penetration inadequate. *based on peak serum concentration after usual adult dose. †applicable to adult uncomplicated lower UTIs (CrCl > 30 mL/min).

CrCl 10–30 mL/min	50 mg (PO) q12h
CrCl < 10 mL/min	Avoid (except for PCP, see TMP–SMX)
Post–HD dose	Avoid (except for PCP, see TMP–SMX)
Post–PD dose	100 mg (PO)
CVVH/CVVHD/ CVVHDF dose	50 mg (PO) q12h
Moderate— severe hepatic insufficiency	No change

Drug Interactions: Azathioprine (leukopenia); amantadine, dapsone, digoxin, methotrexate, phenytoin, rifampin, zidovudine ($\uparrow$ interacting drug levels, nystagmus with phenytoin); diuretics ($\uparrow$ serum K^+ with K^+-sparing diuretics, $\downarrow$ serum Na^+ with thiazide diuretics); warfarin ($\uparrow$ INR, bleeding).
Adverse Effects:
Uncommon
- Nausea/vomiting
- Leukopenia
- Thrombocytopenia
- Hyperkalemia
- Hyponatremia
- Folate deficiency

Allergic Potential: Low
Safety in Pregnancy: C

Additional Clinical Considerations:
- **Useful in sulfa-allergic patients unable to take TMP–SMX.**
- **PCP dose:** 5 mg/kg (PO) q8h plus dapsone 100 mg (PO) q24h.
- TMP is lipid soluble and penetrates most tissues well.

Additional Pharmacokinetic Considerations*

Non-CSF	% of Serum Levels
Peritoneal fluid	NR(s)
Bile	100%
Synovial fluid	NR(p)
Bone	30%
Prostate	300%
CSF	
Non-inflamed meninges	10%
Inflamed meninges (ABM)	40%

Meningeal dose = 300 mg or 5 mg/kg (PO) q6h.

(also see **Antibiotic Pearls & Pitfalls** p. 533).

SELECTED REFERENCES:
Brogden RN, Carmine AA, Heel RC, et al. Trimethoprim: A review of its antibacterial activity, pharmacokinetics and therapeutic use in urinary tract infections. Drugs 23:405–30, 1982. (PMID:7049657)

Friesen WT, Hekster YA, Vree TB. Trimethoprim: clinical use and pharmacokinetics. Drug Intelligence & Clinical Pharmacy 15:325–30, 1981. (PMID:7023899)

Neu HC. Trimethoprim alone for treatment of urinary tract infection. Rev Infect Dis 4:366–71, 1982. (PMID:7051236)

Website: www.pdr.net

Trimethoprim– Sulfamethoxazole (Bactrim, Septra) TMP–SMX

Drug Class: Folate antagonist/ sulfonamide.
Usual Dose: 2.5–5 mg/kg (IV/PO) q6h.

―――― = serious side effect ☐ = black box warning. ND = no data. NR = not recommended. s = spectrum inadequate (at site). a = activity or experience inadequate. p = tissue penetration inadequate. *based on peak serum concentration after usual adult dose. †applicable to adult uncomplicated lower UTIs (CrCl > 30 mL/min).

Spectrum Synopsis*

Hits

Gram + : MSSA, some CA-MRSA

Gram – : Most aerobic GNB

Problem pathogens:
Listeria, Nocardia, PCP,
Toxoplasma

Misses

Gram + : HA-MRSA, GAS, GBS, VSE,
VRE

Gram – : P. aeruginosa, B. fragilis

Problem pathogens:
Acinetobacter, S. maltophilia,
B. cepacia

Urine Spectrum†

- Same as serum spectrum
- Optimal urinary pH = 6–7

(Full *Susceptibility Profiles* p. 196).

Resistance Potential: High
(S. pneumoniae, E. coli)

Pharmacokinetic Parameters:
Peak serum level: 2–8/40–80 mcg/mL
Bioavailability: 98%
Excreted unchanged (urine): 67/85%
*Serum half-life (normal/ESRD): (10/8)/
40–80 hrs*
Plasma protein binding: 44–70%
Volume of distribution (V_d): 1.8/0.3 L/kg

Primary Mode of Elimination: Renal

Dosage Adjustments*

CrCl 15–30 mL/min	1.25 2.5 mg/kg (IV/PO) q6h
CrCl < 15 mL/min	Avoid (except for PCP use 1.25–2.5 mg/kg [IV/PO] q8h)
Post–HD dose	2.5 mg/kg (IV/PO)
Post–PD dose	0.16 mg/kg (IV/PO)
CVVH/CVVHD/CVVHDF dose	2.5 mg/kg (IV/PO) q6h
Moderate—severe hepatic insufficiency	No change

Drug Interactions: *TMP component:*
Azathioprine (leukopenia); amantadine,
dapsone, digoxin, methotrexate,
phenytoin, rifampin, zidovudine
(↑ interacting drug levels, nystagmus
with phenytoin); diuretics (↑ serum K^+
with K^+-sparing diuretics, ↓ serum Na^+
with thiazide diuretics); warfarin (↑ INR,
bleeding). *SMX component:* Cyclosporine
(↓ cyclosporine levels); phenytoin
(↑ phenytoin levels, nystagmus, ataxia);
methotrexate (↑ antifolate activity);
sulfonylureas, thiopental (↑ interacting
drug effect); warfarin (↑ INR, bleeding).

Adverse Effects:

Common

- Nausea/vomiting/diarrhea

Uncommon

- Leukopenia
- Hemolytic anemia ± G6PD deficiency
- Thrombocytopenia
- Hyperkalemia
- Hyponatremia
- Folate deficiency
- ↑ AST/ALT
- Drug fever/rash
- Phototoxic skin emptions
- <u>Drug induced aseptic meningitis</u>

———— = serious side effect ☐ = black box warning. ND = no data. NR = not recommended. s = spectrum inadequate (at site). a = activity or experience inadequate. p = tissue penetration inadequate.
*based on peak serum concentration after usual adult dose. †applicable to adult uncomplicated lower UTIs (CrCl > 30 mL/min).

Rare
- Hypoglycemia
- Aplastic anemia
- Stevens-Johnson Syndrome
- TEN
- C. difficile diarrhea/colitis

Allergic Potential: Very high (SMX); none (TMP)

Safety in Pregnancy: C

Additional Clinical Considerations:
- Drug fever/rash (SMX only)
- TMP-SMX falsely ↑ serum creatinine (does not ↓ renal function)
- Excellent bioavailability (IV = PO).

TMP–SMX IV and PO Equivalence:

- **TMP-SMX** (TMP component) **10 mg/kg (IV) q24h** (70 kg patient)

  = 2 SS† tablets (PO) q6h

  or

  = 1 DS†† tablet (PO) q6h

- **TMP-SMX** (TMP component) 20 mg/kg (IV) q24h (70 kg patient)

  = 4 SS tablets (PO) q6h

  or

  = 2 DS tablets (PO) q6h

† 1 SS tablet = TMP 80 mg + SMX 400 mg.
†† 1 DS tablet = TMP 160 mg + SMX 800 mg.

In sulfa allergic patients, use TMP (SMX is the allergic component) which is equally effective as TMP–SMX.

Additional Pharmacokinetic Considerations*

Non-CSF	% of Serum Levels
Peritoneal fluid	NR(s)
Bile	NR(p/s)
	1000%
Synovial fluid	NR(p)
Bone	30%
Prostate	300/0
	(TMP/SMX)

CSF

Non-inflamed meninges	10%
Inflamed meninges (ABM)	40%

Urine spectrum
- Urinary spectrum same as serum spectrum
- Optimal urinary pH:
  Urine acidification: ↑ TMP urine/no effect on SMX excretion
  Urine alkalization: ↓ TMP/↑ SMX excretion
- Urinary levels = 60 (TMP)/150 (SMX) mcg/mL

Meningeal dose = 5 mg/kg (IV/PO) q6h.

(also see ***Antibiotic Pearls & Pitfalls*** p. 533).

SELECTED REFERENCES:
Chetchotisakd P, Chierakul W, et al. Trimethoprim-sulfamethoxazole versus trimethoprim-sulfamethoxazole plus doxycycline as oral eradicative treatment for melioidosis: a multicentre, double-blind, non-inferiority, randomized controlled trial. Lancet. 1:807-814, 2014. (PMID:24284287)
Cockerill FR, Edson RS. Trimethoprim-sulfamethoxazole. Mayo Clin Proc 66:1260–9, 1991. (PMID:1749295)
Cunha BA. Minocycline often forgotten but preferred to trimethoprim-sulfamethoxazole (TMP-SMX) or doxycycline for the treatment of community associated methicillin-resistant S. aureus skin & soft tissue infections. Int

—— = serious side effect ☐ = black box warning. ND = no data. NR = not recommended. s = spectrum inadequate (at site). a = activity or experience inadequate. p = tissue penetration inadequate. *based on peak serum concentration after usual adult dose. †applicable to adult uncomplicated lower UTIs (CrCl > 30 mL/min).

Antimicrob Agents. 42:497-799, 2013. (PMID:24126085)

Cunha BA. Prophylaxis for recurrent urinary tract infections: nitrofurantoin, not trimethoprim-sulfamethoxazole or cranberry juice. Arch Intern Med 172:82–3, 2012. (PMID:22232158)

Gelfand MS, Cleveland KO, Ketterer DC. Susceptibility of Streptococcus pyogenes to trimethoprim-sulfamethoxazole. J Clin Micro 51:1350-1351, 2013. (PMID:23509241)

Masters PA, O'Bryan TA, Zurlo JM, et al. Trimethoprim-sulfamethoxazole revisited. Arch Intern Med 163:402–10, 2003. (PMID:13588198)

Muhammed SA, Rolain JM, Le Poullain MN. Orally administered trimethoprim-sulfamethoxazole for deep staphylococcal infections. J Antimicrob Chemother. 69:757-760, 2014. (PMID:24123429)

Nayak SU, Simon GL, Myocarditis after trimethoprim-sulfamethoxazole treatment for ehrlichiosis. Emerg Inf Dis 19:1975-1977, 2013. 24274783)

Pallin DJ, Binder WD, Allen MB, et al. Clinical trial: Comparative effectiveness of cephalexin plus trimethoprom-sulfamethaxazole versus cephalexin: treatment of uncomplicated celiulitis: randomized controlled trial. Clin Infect Dis 56:1754-1762, 2013. (PMID:23457080)

Sanchez GV, Master RN, Bordon J. Trimethoprim-sulfamethoxazole may no longer be acceptable for the treatment of acute uncomplicated cystitis in the United States. Clin Infect Dis 53:316–7, 2011. (PMID:21765092)

Website: www.pdr.net

Valacyclovir (Valtrex)

Drug Class: Antiviral (HSV, VZV).
Usual Dose:
HSV-1/2: Herpes labialis: *Initial therapy:* 2 gm (PO) q12h × 1 day. *Recurrent/intermittent therapy:* 1 gm (PO) q12h × 3 days.
Genital herpes: *Initial therapy:* 1 gm (PO) q12h × 3 days. *Recurrent/intermittent therapy (< 6 episodes/year):* normal host: 500 mg (PO) q24h × 5 days; HIV-positive: 1 gm (PO) q12h × 7–10 days. *Chronic suppressive therapy (> 6 episodes/year):* normal host: 1 gm (PO) q24h × 1 year; HIV-positive: 500 mg (PO) q12h × 1 year.
HSV-1 late onset VAP: 1 gm (PO) q8h × 10 days.
Meningitis/encephalitis:
1 gm (PO) q8h × 10 days.*
VZV: Chickenpox: 1 gm (PO) q8h × 5 days.
VZV pneumonia: 1–2 gm (PO) q8h × 10 days.
Herpes zoster (shingles) (dermatomal/disseminated): 1 gm (PO) q8h × 7–10 days.
VZV meningitis/encephalitis:
2 gm (PO) q6h × 10 days.*
Pharmacokinetic Parameters:
Peak serum level: 3.7–5 mcg/mL
Bioavailability: 55%
Excreted unchanged (urine): 1%
Serum half-life (normal/ESRD): 3/14 hrs
Plasma protein binding: 15%
Volume of distribution (V_d): 0.7 L/kg
Primary Mode of Elimination: Renal
Dosage Adjustments* (based on 1 gm q8h)

CrCl 30–50 mL/min	1 gm (PO) q12h
CrCl 10–30 mL/min	1 gm (PO) q24h
CrCl < 10 mL/min	500 mg (PO) q24h

Post–HD dose	1 gm (PO)
Post–PD dose	500 mg
CVVH/CVVHD/ CVVHDF dose	500 mg (PO) q24h
Moderate hepatic insufficiency	No change
Severe hepatic insufficiency	No change

Drug Interactions: Cimetidine, probenecid ($\uparrow$ acyclovir levels).
Adverse Effects:
Common
- Headache
- Nausea/vomiting/diarrhea

Uncommon
- $\uparrow$ AST/ALT

Rare
- Drug fever/rash
- HUS/TTP (HIV only)
- Encephalopathy (without dose $\downarrow$ in ARF/CRF)

Allergic Potential: Low
Safety in Pregnancy: B

Additional Clinical Considerations:
- Converted to acyclovir in liver.
- VZV IC_{90} ~ 2 × HSV.

Highly active against HSV > VZV.
Some activity against CMV.
No activity against EBV, RSV or
adenoviruses.

Additional Pharmacoknetic considerations:
Meningitis/Encephalitis dose =
　HSV: 1 gm (PO) q8h

VZV: 2 gm (PO) q6h

Cerebrospinal Fluid Penetration: 54%

SELECTED REFERENCES:
Acosta EP, Fletcher CV. Valacyclovir. Ann Pharmacotherapy 31:185–91, 1997. (PMID:9034421)
Cunha BA, Baron J. Oral valacyclovir treatment of herpes simplex virus (HSV) or varicella zoster virus (VZV) meningitis, Meningoencephalitis or encephalitis: A Pharmacokinetic Perspective. Journal of Chemotherapy 29:122-125, 2017. (PMID: 29522431)
Kotton CN, Kumar D, Caliendo AM, et al. International consensus guidelines on the management of cytomegalovirus in solid organ transplantation. Transplantation 89:779–795, 2010. (PMID:20224515)
Pouplin T, Pouplin JN, Van Toi P, et al. valacyclovir for Herpes simplex encephalitis. Antimicrob Agents Chemother 55:3624–3626, 2011. (PMID:21576427)
Vigil KJ, ChemalyRF. Valacyclovir: approved and off-label uses for the treatment of herpes virus infections in immunocompetent and immunocompromised adults. Expert Opin Pharmacother 11:1901–1913, 2010. (PMID:20536295)
Website: www.pdr.net

Valganciclovir (Valcyte)

Drug Class: Antiviral (CMV, HSV, HHV-6)
Usual Dose: *Induction dose:* 900 mg (PO) q12h × 21 days, then ***Maintanance dose:*** 900 mg (PO) q24h (*Normal hosts*: until cured. *Compromised hosts*: chronic suppressive therapy). 900 mg dose taken as two 450 mg tablets once daily.

―――― = serious side effect ☐ = black box warning. ND = no data. NR = not recommended. s = spectrum inadequate (at site). a = activity or experience inadequate. p = tissue penetration inadequate. *based on peak serum concentration after usual adult dose. †applicable to adult uncomplicated lower UTIs (CrCl > 30 mL/min).

Pharmacokinetic Parameters:
Peak serum level: 5.6 mcg/mL
Bioavailability: 59.4%
Excreted unchanged (urine): 90%
Serum half-life (normal/ESRD): 4.1/ 67.5 hrs
Plasma protein binding: 1%
Volume of distribution (V_d): 15.3 L/kg
Primary Mode of Elimination: Renal
Dosage Adjustments*

CrCl 40–60 mL/min	450 mg (PO) q12h (induction), then 450 mg (PO) q24h (maintenance)
CrCl 25–40 mL/min	450 mg (PO) q24h (induction), then 450 mg (PO) q48h (maintenance)
CrCl 10–25 mL/min	450 mg (PO) q48h (induction), then 450 mg (PO) 2x/week (maintenance)
CrCl < 10 mL/min	Avoid
Post–HD dose	Avoid
Post–PD dose	Use same dose as CrCl 25–40 mL/min
CVVH/CVVHD/ CVVHDF dose	Use same dose as CrCl 25–50 mL/min
Mild-moderate hepatic insufficiency	No change
Severe hepatic insufficiency	Use with caution

Drug Interactions: Cytotoxic drugs (may produce additive toxicity: stomatitis, bone marrow depression, alopecia); imipenem (↑ risk of seizures); probenecid (↑ valganciclovir levels); zidovudine (↓ valganciclovir levels, ↑ zidovudine levels, possible neutropenia); didanosine (↑ didanosine); cyclosporine amphotericin, (↑ nephrotoxicity); mycophenolate mofetil (↑ mycophenolate mofetil and gangcyclovir levels in renal insufficiency); tenofovir (↑ tenofovir, gangcyclovir levels).

Adverse Effects:
Common
- Nausea/vomiting/diarrhea
- Drug fever/rash
- Graft rejection
- Retinal detachment
- ↑ Creatinine
- Hypertension
- Severe leukopenia, anemia, thrombo-cytopenia, pancytopenia
- Bone marrow aplasia and aplastic anemia

Uncommon
- Paresthesias
- Peripheral neuropathy

Rare
- Inhibition of spermatogenesis
- Birth defects
- Malignancies

Allergic Potential: Low
Safety in Pregnancy: C

= serious side effect ☐ = black box warning. ND = no data. NR = not recommended. s = spectrum inadequate (at site). a = activity or experience inadequate. p = tissue penetration inadequate. *based on peak serum concentration after usual adult dose. †applicable to adult uncomplicated lower UTIs (CrCl > 30 mL/min).

Additional Clinical Considerations:
- Tablets should be taken with food.
- Valganciclovir is rapidly hydrolyzed to ganciclovir.
- Not interchangeable on a tablet-to-tablet basis with oral ganciclovir.
- Serum concentration equivalent to IV ganciclovir.
- Indicated for induction/maintenance therapy of CMV infection.

Highly active against CMV, HHV-6, and HSV.

Some activity against VZV, EBV and adenoviruses.

No activity against RSV.

Cerebrospinal Fluid Penetration: 70%
Meningeal dose = usual dose.

SELECTED REFERENCES:

Avery RK. Low-dose valganciclovir for cytomegalovirus phylaxis in organ transplantation: is less really more? Clin Infect Dis 52:322–324, 2011. (PMID:21190935)

Asberg A, Rollag H, Hartmann A. Valganciclovir for the prevention and treatment of CMV in solid organ transplant recipients. Expert Opin Pharmacother 11:1159–1166, 2010. (PMID:20367273)

Czock D, Scholle C, Rasche FM, et al. Pharmacokinetics of valganciclovir and ganciclovir in renal impairment. Clin Pharmacol Ther 72:142–50, 2002. (PMID:12189361)

Humar A, Limaye AP, Blumberg EA, et al. Extended valganciclovir prophylaxis in D+/R- kidney transplant recipients is associated with long-term reduction in cytomegalovirus disease: two-year results of the IMPACT study. Transplantation 90:1427–1431, 2010. (PMID:21197713)

Kalil AC, Midru C, Florescu DF. Effectiveness of valganciclovir 900 mg versus 450 mg for cytomegalovirus prophylaxis in transplantation: direct and indirect treatment comparison

meta-analysis. Clin Infect Dis 52:313–321, 2011. (PMID:21189424)

Kotton CN, Kumar D, Caliendo AM, et al. International consensus guidelines on the management of cytomegalovirus in solid organ transplantation. Transplantation 89:779–795, 2010. (PMID:20224515)

Lopau K, Greser A, Wanner C. Efficacy and safety of preemptive anti-CMV therapy with valganciclovir after kidney transplantation. Clin Transplant 21:80–85, 2007. (PMID:17302595)

Luan, FL, Kommareddi M, Ojo AO. Impact of cytomegalovirus disease in D+/R- kidney transplant patients receiving 6 months low-dose valganciclovir prophylaxis. Am J Transplant 11:1936–1942, 2011. (PMID:21827608)

Razonable RR, Paya CV. Valganciclovir for the prevention and treatment of cytomegalovirus disease in immunocompromised hosts. Expert Rev Anti Infect Ther 2:27–41, 2004. (PMID:15482169)

Website: www.pdr.net

Vancomycin (Vancocin)

Drug Class: Glycopeptide.
Usual Dose: 1 gm (IV) q12h (see comments).

Spectrum Synopsis*
Hits
  Gram + : MSSA, MRSA, VISA, CoNS, VSE (with gentamicin)
  Gram – : None
  Problem pathogens:
    C. difficile (PO only)
Misses
  Gram + : VRSA, VRE
  Gram – : All GNB, B. fragilis
  Problem pathogens:
    Listeria, Nocardia, Acinetobacter, S. maltophilia, B. cepacia

(Full **Susceptibility Profiles** p. 208).

———— = serious side effect ⬜ = black box warning. ND = no data. NR = not recommended. s = spectrum inadequate (at site). a = activity or experience inadequate. p = tissue penetration inadequate. *based on peak serum concentration after usual adult dose. †applicable to adult uncomplicated lower UTIs (CrCl > 30 mL/min).

Resistance Potential: Low
(MSSA, MRSA, VSE; ↑ prevalence of VRE)
Pharmacokinetic Parameters:
Peak serum level: 63 mcg/mL
Bioavailability: IV (not applicable)/PO
(0%)
Excreted unchanged (urine): 90%
Serum half-life (normal/ESRD): 6/180 hrs
Plasma protein binding: 55%
Volume of distribution (V_d): 0.7 L/kg
Primary Mode of Elimination: Renal
Dosage Adjustments*

CrCl 50–80 mL/min	1 gm (IV) q12h
CrCl 10–50 mL/min	1 gm (IV) q24h
CrCl < 10 mL/min	1 gm (IV) q week
Post–HD dose	None
Post–HFHD dose	500 mg (IV)
Post–PD dose	None
CVVH/CVVHD/ CVVHDF dose	1 gm (IV) q24h
Moderate hepatic insufficiency	No change
Severe hepatic insufficiency	No change

Drug Interactions: Aminoglycosides,
amphotericin B, polymyxin B
(↑ nephrotoxicity).
Adverse Effects:
Common
- Hypotension
- Red Man/red neck syndrome
- Nausea/vomiting/diarrhea (oral formulation)
- Hypokalemia (oral formulation)

Uncommon
- Leukopenia
- Thrombocytopenia
Rare
- Cardiac arrest
Allergic Potential: Low
Safety in Pregnancy: C

Addition Clinical Considerations:
- Not nephrotoxic.
- "Red man/neck syndrome" can be prevented/minimized by infusing IV vancomycin slowly over 1–2 hours.
- Intraperitoneal absorption = 40%.
- **IV vancomycin increases VRE prevalence.**
- **C. difficile diarrhea dose:** oral vancomycin 250 mg (PO) q6h. *If no response in 72 hours ↑ dose to 500 mg (PO) q6h to complete therapy.*
- **C. difficile diarrhea relapse dose:** 500 mg (PO) q6h × 1 month and reevaluate.
- **Do *not* taper dose.** Should C. difficile recur, treat × 2 or 3 months with 500 mg (PO) q6h.
- **C. difficile colitis:** *Oral vancomycin ineffective for C. difficile colitis.*
- **Therapeutic Serum Concentrations** (for therapeutic efficacy only, *not toxicity*):
  Peak level = 25–40 mcg/mL
  Trough level = 5–12 mcg/mL
- There are **no convincing data that vancomycin is ototoxic or nephrotoxic. CrCl, not serum**

—— = serious side effect ☐ = black box warning. ND = no data. NR = not recommended. s = spectrum inadequate (at site). a = activity or experience inadequate. p = tissue penetration inadequate. *based on peak serum concentration after usual adult dose. †applicable to adult uncomplicated lower UTIs (CrCl > 30 mL/min).

levels, should be used to adjust vancomycin dosing.

- **Prolonged/high dose vancomycin (60 mg/kg/day or 2 gm [IV] q12h) has been useful without toxicity.** In treating S. aureus osteomyelitis, S. aureus infections with high MICs (VISA), and infections in difficult-to-penetrate tissues.

- In bone, vancomycin tissue concentrations are ~ 25% of serum levels.

- **With S. aureus, vancomycin (IV) use predisposes to permeability mediated resistance (due to cell wall thickening** recognized as ↑ MICs, i.e., "MIC creep" for vancomycin and other anti-S. aureus antibiotics.

Additional Pharmacokinetic Considerations:

Non-CSF	% of Serum Levels
Peritoneal fluid§	15%
Bile	NR(p) <10%
Synovial fluid	NR(p) 15%
Bone	25%
Prostate	NR(s,p)
CSF	
Non-inflamed meninges	<1%
Inflamed meninges (ABM)	15%

Intrathecal (IT) dose = 20 mg (IT) q24h (always give with systemic IV therapy: 1g (IV) q12h)

Meningeal dose = 2 gm (IV) q12h

(also see **Antibiotic Pearls & Pitfalls** p. 534).

SELECTED REFERENCES:

Ajao AO, Harris AD, Roghmann MC, et al. Systematic review of measurement and adjustment for colonization pressure in studies of methicillin-resistant Staphylococcus aureus, vancomycin-resistant enterococci, and clostridium difficile acquisition. Infect Control Hosp Epidemiol 32:481–489, 2011. (PMID:21515979)

Black E, Lau TT, Ensom MH. Vancomycin-induced neutropenia: is it dose- or duration-related? Ann Pharmacother 45:629–638, 2011. (PMID:21521866)

Cantu TG, Yamanaka-Yuen NA, Lietman PS. Serum vancomycin concentrations: Reappraisal of their clinical value. Clin Infect Dis 18:533–43, 1994. (PMID:8038306)

Cruciani M, Gatti G, Lazzarini L, et al. Penetration of vancomycin into human lung tissue. Journal of Antimicrobial Chemotherapy 38:865–69, 1996. (PMID:8961057)

Cunha BA, Cunha CB. Vancomycin ineffective in eliminating MRSA colonization of respiratory secretions in ventilated ICU Patients: A clinical and pharmacokinetic perspective. Clinical infectious disease 66:981-982, 2018. (PMID: 29088403)

Cunha BA, Jaber N, Blum S. Antibiotic stewardship implications of empiric vancomycin or linezolid for ventilator associated pneumonia: MRSA coverage has no effect on outcomes. International Journal of Antimicrobial Agents 13:27-28, 2018. (PMID: 29909171)

Cunha BA, Sessa J, Blum S. Enhanced efficacy of high dose oral vancomycin therapy: Shortened duration of clostridium difficile diarrhea in hospitalized adults not responding to conventional oral vancomycin therapy. Journal of Clinical Medicine 7:e75-81, 2018. (PMID: 29642570)

Cunha BA. Vancomycin revisited: a reappraisal of clinical use. Critical Care Clinics of North America 24:394–420, 2008. (PMID:18361953)

Cunha BA, Mohan SS, Hamid N, McDermott GP, Daniels P. Cost ineffectiveness of serum vancomycin levels. Eur J Clin Microbiol Infect Dis 13:509–511, 2007. (PMID:17534676)

Cunha BA. Vancomycin. Med Clin North Am 79:817–31, 1995. (PMID:7791425)

Deresinski S. Vancomycin: does it still have a role as an antistaphylococcal agent? Expert Rev Anti Infect Ther 5:393–401, 2007. (PMID:17547504)

El Amari EB, Vuagnat A, Stern R, et al. High versus standard dose vancomycin for osteomyelitis. Scand J Infect Dis 36:712–7, 2004. (PMID:15513395)

Hidayat LK, Hsu DI, Quist R, et al. High-dose vancomycin therapy for methicillin-resistant Staphylococcus aureus infections. Arch Inter Med 166:2138–44, 2006. (PMID:17060546)

Huttner A, Harbarth S: Guidelines for vancomycin use. Clin Infect Dis 50:616, 2010. (PMID:20095831)

Moellering RC Jr. Monitoring serum vancomycin levels: climbing the mountain because it is there? Clin Infect Dis 18:544–6, 1994. (PMID:8038307)

Okamoto H. Vancomycin-induced immune thrombocytopenia. N Engl J Med 356:2537–2538, 2007. (PMID:17575587)

Ricard JD, Wolff M, Lacerade JC, et al. Levels of vancomycin in cerebrospinal fluid of adult patients receiving adjunctive corticosteroids to treat pneumococcal meningitis: a prospective multicenter observational study. Clin Infect Dis 44:250–255, 2007. (PMID:17173226)

Rybak MJ. The pharmacokinetic and pharmacodynamic properties of vancomycin. Clin Infect Dis 42:S35–9, 2006. (PMID:16323118)

Saribas S, Bagdatli Y. Vancomycin tolerance in enterococci. Chemotherapy 50:250–4, 2004. (PMID:15528891)

Stevens DL. The role of vancomycin in the treatment paradigm. Clin Infect Dis 42:S51–7, 2006. (PMID:16323121)

Vandecasteele SJ, De Vriese AS. Vancomycin dosing in patients on intermittent hemodialysis. Semin Dial 24:50–55, 2011. (PMID:21338394)

Wang G, Hindler JF, Ward KW, et al. Increased vancomycin MICs for Staphylococcus aureus clinical isolates from a university hospital during a 5-year period. Journal of Clinical Microbiology 44:3883–86, 2006. (PMID:16957043)

Website: www.pdr.net

Voriconazole (Vfend)

Drug Class: Triazole antifungal.
Usual Dose: <u>IV dosing</u>: **Loading dose:** 6 mg/kg (IV) q12h × 1 day, then **Maintenance dose:** 4 mg/kg (IV) q12h. *Can switch to weight-based PO maintenance dosing anytime while on maintenance IV dose* (see comments). <u>PO dosing</u>: *Weight ≥ 40 kg*: Loading dose of 400 mg (PO) q12h × 1 day, then maintenance dose of 200 mg (PO) q12h. *If response is inadequate, the dose may be increased to 300 mg (PO) q12h. Weight < 40 kg:* Loading dose of 200 mg (PO) × 1 day, then maintenance dose of 100 mg (PO) q12h. If response is inadequate, the dose may be increased to 150 mg (PO) q12h. (*Take without food*).
<u>For chronic/non-life-threatening infections</u>: PO loading dose may be given (see comments).

Pharmacokinetic Parameters:
  Peak serum level: 2.3–4.7 mcg/mL
  Bioavailability: 96%
  Excreted unchanged (urine): 2%
  Serum half-life (normal/ESRD): 6/6 hrs
  Plasma protein binding: 58%
  Volume of distribution (V$_d$): 4.6 L/kg

Primary Mode of Elimination: Hepatic

Dosage Adjustments*

CrCl 50–80 mL/min	No change
CrCl 10–50 mL/min	No change PO; avoid IV
CrCl < 10 mL/min	No change PO; avoid IV
Post–HD dose	Usual dose PO; avoid IV
Post–PD dose	No data
CVVH/CVVHD/ CVVHDF dose	4 mg/kg (PO) q12h; avoid (IV)
Moderate hepatic insufficiency	6 mg/kg (IV) q12h × 1 day or 200 mg (PO) q12h × 1 day, then 2 mg/kg (IV) q12h or 100 mg (PO) q12h (> 40 kg)
Severe hepatic insufficiency	Use with caution

Drug Interactions: Benzodiazepines, vinca alkaloids (↑ interacting drug levels); carbamazepine, ergot alkaloids, rifampin, rifabutin, sirolimus, long-acting barbiturates (contraindicated with voriconazole); cyclosporine, ↓ (cyclosporine by 1/2 and monitor); efavirenz (↑ maintence dose of voriconazole to 400 mg (PO) q12h and

decrease efavirenz dose to 300 mg (PO) q12h while on voriconazole); omeprazole (↑ interacting drug levels, ↓ interacting drug dose by 50%); tacrolimus (↑ tacrolimus levels, ↓ tacrolimus dose by 66%); phenytoin (↓ voriconazole levels); ↑ voriconazole dose from 4 mg/kg [IV] to 5 mg/kg [IV] and from 200 mg [PO] to 400 mg [PO]; warfarin (↑ INR); statins (↑ risk of rhabdomyolysis); dihydro-pyridine calcium channel blockers (hypotension); tacrolimus (reduce tacrolimus dose by 1/3 and monitor while on voriconazole); sulfonylureas (hypoglycemia). Voriconazole has not been studied with protease inhibitors or NNRTIs, but ↑ voriconazole levels are predicted (↑ hepatotoxicity/adverse effects); ↑ voriconazole levels with meningeal meropenem (↓ voriconazole).

Adverse Effects:
Common
• Visual disturbances:.blurry blue colored brightness
• Hallucinations
• ↑ Creatinine
Uncommon
• Nausea/vomiting
• Headache
• Photophobia
• Drug fever/rash
• Hypokalemia
• ↑ AST/ALT
Rare
• Hypoglycemia
• Squamous cell carcinomas (with chronic therapy)
• Melanoma (with chronic therapy)
• ↑ QTc
• Stevens-Johnson syndrome

------- = serious side effect [   ] = black box warning. ND = no data. NR = not recommended. s = spectrum inadequate (at site). a = activity or experience inadequate. p = tissue penetration inadequate. *based on peak serum concentration after usual adult dose. †applicable to adult uncomplicated lower UTIs (CrCl > 30 mL/min).

Allergic Potential: High
Safety in Pregnancy: D

Additional Clinical Considerations:

- If intolerance to therapy develops, the IV maintenance dose may be reduced to 3 mg/kg and the PO maintenance dose may be reduced in steps of 50 mg/d to a minimum of 200 mg/d q12h (weight ≥ 40 kg) or 100 mg q12h (weight < 40 kg).
- Non-linear kinetics (doubling of oral dose = 2.8-fold increase in serum levels).
- 10–15% of patients have serum levels >6 mcg/mL.
- Food decreases bioavailability; take 1 hour before or after meals.
- Do not use IV voriconazole if CrCl < 50 mL/min to prevent accumulation of voriconazole IV vehicle, sulphobutyl ether cyclodextrin (SBECD); instead use oral formulation, which has no SBECD.
- Loading dose may be given PO for chronic/non-life-threatening infections.
- Because of visual effects, do not drive or operate machinery.
- Monitor LFTs before and during therapy.
- Suspension contains sucrose.

Highly active against C. albicans, non-albicans Candida, Aspergillus, Cryptococcus, Hansenula and Pseudallescheria/Scedosporium.

Some activity against Fusaria, Fluconazole/Itraconazole resistant C. albicans, Coccidiomycosis, and Penicillium marneffei.

No activity against Rhizopus or Mucor.

Cerebrospinal Fluid Penetration: 90%
Meningeal dose = usual dose.

SELECTED REFERENCES:

Aypar E, Kendirli T, Tutar E, et al. Voriconazole-induced QT interval prolongation and torsades de pointes. Pediatr Int 53: 761–763, 2011. (PMID:21955009)

Camuset J, Nunes H, Dombret MC, et al. Treatment of chronic pulmonary aspergillosis by voriconazole in nonimmunocompromised patients. Chest 131:1435–1441, 2007. (PMID:17400661)

Capitano B, Potoski BA, Husain S, et al. Intrapulmonary penetration of voriconazole in patients receiving an oral prophylactic regimen. Antimicrob Agents Chemother 50:1878–80, 2006. (PMID:16641467)

Cowen EW, Nguyen JC, Miller DD, et al. Chronic phototoxicity and aggressive squamous cell carcinoma of the skin in children and adults during treatment with voriconazole. J Am Acad Dermatol 62:31–37, 2010. (PMID:19896749)

den Hollander JG, van Arkel C, Rijnders BJ, et al. Incidence of voriconazole hepatotoxicity during intravenous and oral treatment for invasive fungal infections. J Antimicrob Chemother 57:1248–50, 2006. (PMID:16556632)

Denes E, Boumediene A, Durox H, et al. Voriconazole concentrations in synovial fluid and bone tissues. J Antimicrob Chemother 59:818–819, 2007. (PMID:17329266)

Denning DW, Ribaud P, Milpied N, et al. Efficacy and safety of voriconazole in the treatment of acute invasive aspergillosis. Clin Infect Dis 34:563–71, 2002. (PMID:11807679)

Elter T, Sieniawski M, Gossmann A, et al. Voriconazole brain tissue levels in rhinocerebral aspergillosis in a successfully treated young woman. Int J Antimicrob Agents 28:262–5, 2006. (PMID:16908120)

Hicheri Y, Cook G, Cordonnier C. Antifungal prophylaxis in haematology patients: the role voriconazole. Clin Microbiol Infect 18:1–15, 2012. (PMID:22409648)

Hoffman HL, Rathbun RC. Review of the safety and efficacy of voriconazole. Expert Opin Investig Drugs 11:409–29, 2002. (PMID:11866669)

Kim MM, Vikram HR, Kusne S, et al. Treatment of refractory coccidioidomycosis with voriconazole or posaconazole. Clin Infect Dis, 53:1060–6, 2011. (PMID:22045955)

——— = serious side effect ⬜ = black box warning. ND = no data. NR = not recommended. s = spectrum inadequate (at site). a = activity or experience inadequate. p = tissue penetration inadequate. *based on peak serum concentration after usual adult dose. †applicable to adult uncomplicated lower UTIs (CrCl > 30 mL/min).

Leveque D, Nivoix Y, Jehl F, Herbrecht R. Clinical pharmacokinetics of voriconazole. Int J Antimicrob Agents 27:274–84, 2006. (PMID:16563707)

Miller DD, Cown EW, Ngugen JC, et al. Melanoma associated with long-term voriconazole therapy: a new manifestation of chronic photosensitivity. Arch Dermatol 146:300–304, 2010. (PMID:20083676)

Poza G, Montoya J, Redondo C, et al. Meningitis caused by Pseudallescheria boydii treated with voriconazole. Clin Infect Dis 30:981–2, 2000. (PMID:10880322)

Radaj J, Krouzecky A, Stehlik P, et al. Pharmacokinetic evaluation of voriconazole treatment in critically ill patients undergoing continuous venovenous hemofiltration. Ther Drug Monit 33:393–397, 2011. (PMID:21654349)

Rondeau S, Couderu L, Dominique S, et al. High Frequency of voriconazole-related phototoxicity in cystic fibrosis patients. Eur Respir J 39:782–4, 2012. (PMID:22379155)

Solis-Munoz P, Lopex JC, Bernal W, et al. Voriconazole hepatotoxicity in severe liver dysfunction. J of Inf 66:80-86, 2013. (PMID:23041040)

Tan K, Brayshaw N, Tomaszewski K, et al. Investigation of the potential relationships between plasma voriconazole-concentrations and visual adverse events or liver function test abnormalities. J Clin Pharmacol 46:235–43, 2006. (PMID:16432276)

Walsh TJ, Anaissie EJ, Denning DW, et al. Treatment of Aspergillosis. Clin Infect Dis 46:327–360, 2008. (PMID:18177225)

Website: www.pdr.net

Zidovudine (Retrovir) ZDV Azidothymidine AZT

Drug Class: HIV NRTI (nucleoside reverse transcriptase inhibitor).
Usual Dose: 300 mg (PO) q12h or 200 mg (PO) q8h (see comments). IV solution 10 mg/mL (dose 1 mg/kg 5–6 x/day).

Pharmacokinetic Parameters:
Peak serum level: 1.2 mcg/mL
Bioavailability: 64%
Excreted unchanged (urine): 16%
Serum half-life (normal/ESRD): 1.1/ 1.4 hrs
Plasma protein binding: < 38%
Volume of distribution (V_d): 1.6 L/kg
Primary Mode of Elimination: Hepatic
Dosage Adjustments*

CrCl < 15 mL/min	100 mg (PO) q8h or 300 mg (PO) q24h
Post–HD/PD dose	100 mg or 300 mg
CVVH/CVVHD/ CVVHDF dose	300 mg (PO) q24h
Moderate—severe hepatic insufficiency	Use with caution

Drug Interactions: Acetaminophen, atovaquone, fluconazole, methadone, probenecid, valproic acid (↑ zidovudine levels); clarithromycin, nelfinavir, rifampin, rifabutin (↓ zidovudine levels); dapsone, flucytosine, ganciclovir, interferon alpha, bone marrow suppressive/ cytotoxic agents (↑ risk of hematologic toxicity); indomethacin (↑ levels of zidovudine toxic metabolite); phenytoin (↑ zidovudine levels, ↑ or ↓ phenytoin levels); ribavirin (↓ zidovudine effect; avoid).
Adverse Effects:
Common
- Headache
- Nausea/vomiting/diarrhea
- Anorexia
- Malaise
- Macrocytosis

―――― = serious side effect ☐ = black box warning. ND = no data. NR = not recommended. s = spectrum inadequate (at site). a = activity or experience inadequate. p = tissue penetration inadequate. *based on peak serum concentration after usual adult dose. †applicable to adult uncomplicated lower UTIs (CrCl > 30 mL/min).

Uncommon
- Insomnia
- Myalgias
- Leukopenia
- <u>Anemia</u>
- Thrombocytopenia
- Asthenia
- Blue/black nail discoloration
- ↑ AST/ALT

Rare
- Myositis/myopathy
- Lactic acidosis with hepatic steatosis
- Zidovudine has been associatged with hematologic toxicity including

neutropenia and severe anemia. Prolonged used of zidovudine has been associated with symptomatic myopathy as well as lactic acidosis and severe hepatomegaly with steatosis, including fatal cases.

Allergic Potential: Low
Safety in Pregnancy: C

Additional Clinical Considerations:
- Antagonized by ganciclovir or ribavirin.

Cerebrospinal Fluid Penetration: 60%

SELECTED REFERENCE:
Website: www.pdr.net

REFERENCES

Ambrose P, Nightingale AT (eds). Principles of Pharmacodynamics. Marcel Dekker, Inc., New York, 2001.

Arikan S Rex JH (eds). Antifungal Drugs in Manual of Clinical Microbiology (8th Ed), 2003.

Baddour L, Gorbach SL (eds). Therapy of Infectious Diseases. Saunders, Philadelphia, 2003.

Bennet JE, Dolin R, Blaser MJ (eds). Mandell, Douglas, and Bennett's Principles and Practice of Infectious Diseases (9th Ed). Philadelphia Elsevier Churchill Livingstone, 2019.

Bennet WM, Aronoff GR, Golper TA, Morrison G, Brater DC, Singer I (eds). Drug Prescribing in Renal Failure (2nd Ed), American College of Physicians, Philadelphia, 2000.

Bodey GP, Feinstein V (eds). Candidiasis. New York, Raven Press, 1985.

Bope ET, Kellerman RD (eds). Conn's Current Therapy, Elsevier, Philadelphia, PA, 2019.

Bowden RA, Ljungman P, Snydman DR (eds). Transplant Infections (3rd Ed), Lippincott Williams & Wilkins, Philadelphia, PA, 2010.

Brandstetter R, Cunha BA, Karetsky M (eds). The Pneumonias. Mosby, Philadelphia, 1999.

Brook I (ed). Sinusitis. Taylor & Francis Group, New York, New York, 2006.

Brusch JL Endocarditis Essentials. Jones & Bartlett, Sudbury, MA, 2010.

Brusch, JL. Infective Endocarditis: Management in the Era of Intravascular Devices. Informa Healthcare, New York 2007.

Bryskier A (ed). Antimicrobial Agents. ASM Press, Washington, D.C., 2005.

Calderone RA (ed). Candida and Candidiasis. ASM Press, Washington DC, 2002.

Cimolai N (ed). Laboratory Diagnosis of Bacterial Infections. New York, Marcel Dekker, 2001.

Cohen J, Powderly WG, Opal S (Eds). Infectious Diseases (4th Ed). Elsevier, Philadelphia 2016.

Cunha BA (ed). Infectious Disease in the Elderly. John Wright & Co., London, 1988.

Cunha BA (ed). Tick-Borne Infectious Diseases. Marcel Dekker, New York, 2005.

Cunha CB, Cunha BA (eds). Infectious Disease in Critical Care Medicine (4th Ed), CRC Press, Boca Raton, 2020.

Cunha CB, Schlossberg D (eds). Clinical Infectious Disease (3rd Ed), Cambridge University Press, Cambridge, 2020.

Despommier DD, Gwadz RW Hotez PJ, Knirsh CA (eds). Parasitic Diseases (5th Ed), Apple Tree Productions, LLC, New York, New York, 2005.

Faro S, Soper DE (eds). Infectious Diseases in Women. WB Saunders Company, Philadelphia, 2001.

Farrar J (ed). Manson's Tropical Diseases (23rd Ed). Elsevier Saunders, London, 2014.

Finch RG, Greenwood D, Norrby SR, Whitley RJ (eds). Antibiotic and Chemotherapy. Churchill Livingstone, United Kingdom, 2003.

Glauser MP, Pizzo PA (eds). Management of Infection in Immunocompromised Patients. W.B. Saunders, London, 2000.

Gorbach SL, Bartlett JG, Blacklow NR (eds). Infectious Diseases (3rd Ed), Philadelphia, Lippincott, Williams & Wilkins, 2004.

Grayson ML (ed). Kucers' The Use of Antibiotics (6th Ed), ASM Press, Washington, DC, 2010.

Guerrant RL, Walker DH, Weller PF (eds). Tropical Infectious Disease: Principles, Pathogens & Practice (3rd Ed), Elsevier, Philadelphia, 2011.

Halperin JJ. Encephalitis: Diagnosis and Treatment. Informa Healthcare, New York, 2008.

Hauser AR, Rello J (eds). Severe Infections Caused by Pseudomonas Aeruginosa. Kluwer Academic Publishers, Boston, Massachusetts, 2003.

Koff RS Hepatitis Essentials, Jones & Bartlett, Sudbury, MA, 2011.

Madkour MM (ed). Tuberculosis. Springer-Verlag, Berlin Germany, 2004.

Maertens JA, Marr KA. Diagnosis of Fungal Infections. Informa Healthcare, New York, 2007.

McMillan A, Young H, Ogilvie MM, Scott GR (eds). Clinical practice in Sexually Transmissible Infections, Saunders, London, England, 2002.

O'Grady F, Lambert HP, Finch RG, Greenwood D (eds). Antibiotic and chemotherapy (2nd Ed). Churchill Livingston, New York, 1997.

Pai MP, Momary KM, Rodvold KA. Antibiotic Drug Interactions. Med Clin N Am 90:1223–55, 2006.

Pilch RF, Ziliinskas RA (eds). Encyclopedia of Bioterrorism Defense. Wiley-Liss, Hoboken, New Jersey, 2005.

Piscitelli SC, Rodvold KE (eds). Drug Interactions in Infectious Diseases. Humana Press, Totowa, 2001.

Raoult D, Parola P. Rickettsial Diseases. Informa Healthcare, New York, 2007.

Ristuccia AM, Cunha BA (eds). Antimicrobial Therapy. Raven Press, New York, 1984.

Rom WN, Garay SM (eds). Tuberculosis. Lippincott Williams & Wilkins, Philadelphia, Pennsylvania, 2004.

Sax PE, Cohen CJ. HIV Essentials (7th Ed), Jones & Bartlett, Sudbury, MA, 2017.

Scheld W, Whitley R, Marra C (eds). Infections of the Central Nervous System (3rd Ed), Lippincott Williams & Wilkins, Philadelphia, 2005.

Schlossberg D (ed). Tuberculosis & Nontuberculous Mycobacterial Infections (7th Ed), ASM Press, New York, 2017.

Schlossberg D (ed). Current Therapy of Infectious Disease (3rd Ed), Mosby-Yearbook, St. Louis, 2008.

Scholar EM, Pratt WB (eds). The Antimicrobial Drugs (2nd Ed), Oxford University Press, New York, 2000.

Wormser GP (ed). AIDS (4th Ed), Elsevier, Philadelphia, 2004.

Yoshikawa TT, Rajagopalan S (eds). Antibiotic Therapy for Geriatric Patients. Taylor & Francis, New York, 2006.

Yu VL, Merigan, Jr. TC, Barrier SL (eds). Antimicrobial Therapy and Vaccines (2nd Ed), Williams & Wilkins, Baltimore, 2005.

Zinner SH, Young LS, Acar JF, Ortiz-Neu C (eds). New Considerations for Macrolides, Azalides, Streptogramins, and Ketolides. Marcel Dekker, New York, 2000.

APPENDIX

PK/PD Clinical Considerations

Debra Willner, PharmD
Samad Tirmizi, PharmD
Cheston B. Cunha, MD
Burke A. Cunha, MD

Appendix-1

PK/PD: Clinical Correlations

Clinically relevant antibiotic penetration.
- Antibiotics must bind to bacteria's target site
  - Must penetrate the outer membrane of the organism (penetration resistance) eg vancomycin induces cell wall thickening resulting in ↑ MICs to vancomycin as well as other antibiotics
  - Must avoid being pumped out of the organism (efflux resistance) eg quinolones, tetracyclines
  - Antibiotic must remain intact to be effective (resistance hydrolysis by β-lactamases) eg cephalosphorins.
- Effective Antibiotic Concentrations
  - After absorption into serum, antibiotics are reversibly bound to serum albumin.
  - After albumin sites are saturated, the excess/free antibiotic increases in the serum
  - Along a concentration gradient, the free (unbound) antibiotic penetrates into the interstitial space and into tissue.
  - The free (unbound) antibiotic penetrates into the interstitial space and into tissue.
  - The free (unbound) drug after entering tissues becomes reversibly bound to tissue proteins.
  - Only the remaining (unbound) is available to radicate bacteria at the site of infection
  - Important to get steady state rapidly in ill patients.

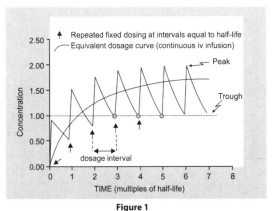

Figure 1
Adapted from: http://slideplayer.com/slide/9262832/27/images/22/steady+state+level

Appendix-1: *(cont'd)*

PK/PD: Clinical Correlations

In figure, the straight line represents a medication administered as a continuous infusion, while the triangular lines represent repeated fixed doses. Dosing intervals for antibiotics reflect the half-life of the medication—the time it takes for 50% of the drug to be eliminated from the body. When the concentration of the antibiotic stabilizes, steady state is achieved, and the concentration of drug remains constant in the body. *Steady state concentration is achieved after 3-5 half-lives.* This correlates with the doses in which the infusion curve reaches a plateau. When monitoring drug levels, in order to obtain a true steady state trough concentration, blood samples should be taken 30 minutes prior to the 4th dose.

Appendix-2: Concentration vs. Time Dependent Kinetics

Concentration Dependent Kinetics (Aminoglucosides)	Time Dependent Kinetics (β-lactams)
• Killing increases ~ to peak concentration (up to 10x MIC optimal, if no toxicity) • No further killing with higher doses	• Killing constant with concentration 2–4x MIC above the MIC • Higher levels do not result in enhanced killing • With β-lactams, levels should be above the MIC for ≥ 50% of the dosing interval.

Time, Concentration and AUC/MIC-Dependent Antibiotic Pharmacodynamics

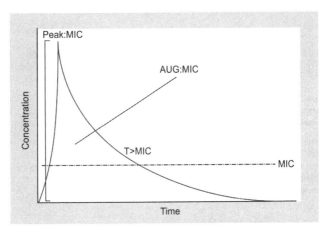

Figure 2
Adapted from: Bolus J. Prolonged-Infusion Dosing of Beta-Lactam Antibiotics. US Pharmacist
https://www.uspharmacist.com/article/prolongedinfusion-dosing-of-betalactam-antibiotics.

With regard to pharmacodynamics, antibiotics display their effect through various relationships with the drug's minimum inhibitory concentration (MIC). Concentration-dependent antibiotics, such as aminoglycosides, display maximal antimicrobial effects the when the concentrations are at their highest concentration above the MIC peak. Time-dependent antibiotics, such as beta-lactams, display antimicrobial effect if their concentrations are above the MIC, regardless of the concentration. Antibiotics which display properties of both concentration and time-dependent antibiotics, such as vancomycin, have their antimicrobial effects measured through 24-hour AUC:MIC ratios.

Intermittent versus Once Daily Dosing of Aminoglycosides

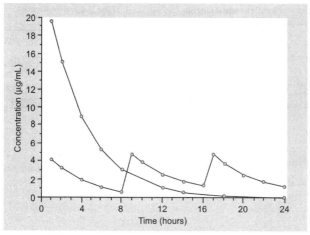

Figure 3

Adapted from: Nicolau DP, Freeman CD, Belliveau PP, Nightingale CH, Ross JW, Quintillant R. Experience with a once-daily aminoglycoside program administered to 2,184 adult patients. Antimicrobial Agents and Chemotherapy. 39:650-655, 1995. doi:10.1128/aac.39.3.650.

Since aminoglycosides demonstrate concentration-dependent killing by maximizing at their peak concentration, they are optimally administered as a once-daily dosing, vs. their traditional interval dosing-every 8 or 12 hours. Once daily dosing has virtually eliminated nephrotoxicity and ototoxicity, this graph depicts the concentration of gentamicin when administered once daily versus every 8 hours. (P. aeruginosa MIC = 4 mcg/mL)

Appendix-3

PAE Post-antibiotic Effect (The Eagle Effect)

- Continued suppression of bacterial growth after antibiotic exposure with levels falling below the organism's MIC is called the PAE.
- Differs from the initial suppression with sub-inhibitory antibiotic concentrations
- PAEs are related to the antibiotic's mechanism of action eg protein synthesis, cell wall synthesis
- PAEs may effect Gram + or – organisms.
- PAEs explain efficacy of intermittent dosing with antibiotics with short half lives (t½).

Appendix 4: Post-Antibiotic Effects (PAEs) for Selected Antibiotics

Mechanism of Action	Antimicrobial Agent	Gram Positive Organisms				
		MSSA	MRSA	S. pneumoniae	Enterococcus sp.	GAS
Cell wall agents	Penicillins	2–3h	–	3h	–	4h
	Cephalosporins	–	–	3–5h	–	–
	Carbapenems	3h	–	–	1–2h	–
	Monobactams (Aztreonam)	–	–	–	–	–
	Vancomycin	2–3h	2h	–	2h	–
	Telavancin	4–5h	4–5h	–	–	–
	Daptomycin	1–6h	1–6h	1–2h	–	–
Protein synthesis	Aminoglycosides	–	–	–	–	–
	Macrolides	4h	–	3–4h	–	3–4h
	Tetracyclines	1–2h	–	3h	–	3h
	Tigecycline	3–5h	3–5h	2–5h	3–6h	–
	Linezolid	2–3h	2–3h	3h	2–3h	–
	Quinipristin/ Dalfopristin	1–3h	1–3h	2–3h	2–7h	–
DNA alteration	Fluoroquinolones	1–2h	1h	–	–	–
Anti-folate	TMP–SMX	–	–	–	–	–
		E.coli	Klebsiella sp.	Proteus sp.	Enterobacter sp.	Pseudomonas sp.
Cell wall agents	Penicillins	0–1h	0–1h	0–1h	–	–
	Cephalosporins	0–1h	0–1h	0–1h	–	–
	Carbapenems	2–4h	2–4h	2–3h	2–3h	3–5h
	Monobactams (Aztreonam)	–	–	–	–	–
	Vancomycin	–	–	–	–	–

(h) = hours
(–) = no data/no activity

Appendix 4: Post-Antibiotic Effects (PAEs) for Selected Antibiotics *(cont'd)*

Mechanism of Action	Antimicrobial Agent	Gram Positive Organisms				
		E. coli	*Kleb-siella sp.*	*Proteus sp.*	*Entero-bacter sp.*	*Pseudo-monas sp.*
	Telavancin	–	–	–	–	–
	Daptomycin	–	–	–	–	–
Protein synthesis	Aminoglycosides	3–5h	3h	–	3–5h	3–5h
	Macrolides	–	–	–	–	–
	Tetracyclines	3–5h	–	–	–	–
	Tigecycline	2h	1–2h	–	1h	–
	Linezolid	–	–	–	–	–
	Quinipristin/ Dalfopristin	–	–	–	–	–
DNA alteration	Fluoroquinolones	2–4h	–	–	–	2–4h
Anti-folate	TMP–SMX	0–1h	1–2h	1–2h	–	–

• PAEs with Protein Synthesis/DNA Inhibitors.

Antibiotic Examples	Gram + Organisms	Gram – Organisms
Aminoglycosides, macrolides Tetracyclines Chloramphenicol Quinolones	Long PAEs : 1–5 hrs	Short PAEs: 1 h

• PAE with Cell Wall Synthesis Inhibitors.

β-lactams Glycopeptides Carbapenems	No PAEs	No PAEs 1–5 hrs*

• PAE explain efficacy of intermittent dosing with antibiotics with short half lives (t½_.

* P. aeruginosa

Malaria in Adults (United States)

Clinical Diagnosis/ Plasmodium species	Region Acquired	Recommended Adult Drug Doses
Severe malaria[1,2,3,4]	**All regions**	**Quinidine gluconate**[2] *plus* **either: Doxycycline or Clindamycin** **Quinidine gluconate:** 6.25 mg base/ kg (=10 mg salt/kg) (IV over 1–2 hrs) then 0.0125 mg base/kg/min (=0.02 mg salt/kg/min) continuous infusion for at least 24 hours. An alternative regimen is 15 mg base/kg (=24 mg salt/kg) loading dose IV infused over 4 hours, followed by 7.5 mg base/kg (=12 mg salt/kg) infused over 4 hours q8h, starting 8 hours after the loading dose. Once parasite density <1% and patient can take oral medication, complete treatment with oral quinine, dose as above. Quinidine/quinine course = 7 days in Southeast Asia; = 3 days in Africa or South America. **Doxycycline:** Treatment as above, give 100 mg (IV/PO) q12h × 7 days. **Clindamycin:** Treatment as above. If patient not able to take oral medication, give 10 mg base/kg (IV) then 5 mg base/kg (IV/PO) q8h × 7 days.
Uncomplicated malaria/ ***P. falciparum*** or Species not identified (If "species not identified" is subsequently diagnosed as *P. vivax* or *P. ovale:* see *P. vivax* and *P. ovale* treat with primaquine)	**Chloroquine resistant or unknown resistance**[5] (All malarious regions except those specified as chloroquine-resistant listed in box below)	**A. Atovaquone-proguanil (Malarone)**[6] *Adult tab = 250 mg atovaquone/ 100 mg proguanil* 4 adult tabs (PO) q24h × 3 days **or**

Malaria in Adults (United States) *(cont'd)*

Clinical Diagnosis/ *Plasmodium* species	Region Acquired	Recommended Adult Drug Doses
Uncomplicated malaria/ *P. falciparum* (cont'd)	**Chloroquine resistant or unknown resistance** (cont'd)	**B. Artemether/lumefantrine (Coartem)[6]** *1 tablet = 20 mg artemether/120 mg lumefantrine* A 3-day treatment schedule with a total of 6 oral doses is recommended based on weight. The patient should receive the initial dose, followed by the second dose 8 hours later, then 1 dose (PO) q12h × 2 days. ≥ 35 kg: 4 tablets per dose **or** **C. Quinine sulfate *plus* either: Doxycycline[9] or Clindamycin** **Quinine sulfate[8]:** 542 mg base (=650 mg salt)[7] (PO) q8h × 3 or 7 days **Doxycycline:** 100 mg (PO) q12h × 7 days **Clindamycin:** 20 mg base/kg/day (PO) divided q8h × 7 days **or** **D. Mefloquine (Lariam)[10]** 684 mg base (=750 mg salt) (PO) as initial dose, followed by 456 mg base (=500 mg salt) (PO) given 6–12 hours after initial dose Total dose = 1,250 mg salt
Uncomplicated malaria/ *P. falciparum* or *Species not identified*	**Chloroquine sensitive** (Central America west of Panama Canal; Haiti; the Dominican Republic; and most of the Middle East)	**Chloroquine phosphate (Aralen)** 600 mg base (=1,000 mg salt) (PO) immediately, followed by 300 mg base (=500 mg salt) (PO) at 6, 24, and 48 hours Total dose: 1,500 mg base (=2,500 mg salt) **or** **Hydroxychloroquine (Plaquenil)** 620 mg base (=800 mg salt) (PO) immediately, followed by 310 mg base (=400 mg salt) (PO) at 6, 24, and 48 hours Total dose: 1,550 mg base (=2,000 mg salt)

Malaria in Adults (United States) *(cont'd)*

Clinical Diagnosis/ *Plasmodium* species	Region Acquired	Recommended Adult Drug Doses
Uncomplicated malaria/ *P. malariae* or *P. knowlesi*	**All regions**	**Chloroquine phosphate:** Treatment as above **or** **Hydroxychloroquine:** Treatment as above
Uncomplicated malaria/ *P. vivax* or *P. ovale*	**All regions** (for suspected chloroquine-resistant *P. vivax*, see below)	**Chloroquine phosphate** *plus* **Primaquine phosphate**[11] **Chloroquine phosphate:** Treatment as above **Primaquine phosphate:** 30 mg base (PO) q24h × 14 days **or** **Hydroxychloroquine** *plus* **Primaquine phosphate**[11] **Hydroxychloroquine:** Treatment as above **Primaquine phosphate:** 30 mg base (PO) q24h × 14 days
Uncomplicated malaria/ *P. vivax*	**Chloroquine resistant**[12] (Papua New Guinea and Indonesia)	**A. Quinine sulfate** *plus* **either: Doxycycline** *plus* **Primaquine phosphate**[11] **Quinine sulfate:** Treatment as above **Doxycycline:** Treatment as above **Primaquine phosphate:** Treatment as above **or** **B. Atovaquone/proguanil** *plus* **Primaquine phosphate** **Atovaquone/proguanil:** Treatment as above **Primaquine phosphate:** Treatment as above **or** **C. Mefloquine**[10] *plus* **Primaquine phosphate**[11] **Mefloquine:** Treatment as above **Primaquine phosphate:** Treatment as above

Malaria in Adults (United States) *(cont'd)*

Clinical Diagnosis/ Plasmodium species	Region Acquired	Recommended Adult Drug Doses
Uncomplicated malaria: alternatives for pregnant women[13,14,15,16]	**Chloroquine sensitive** (see uncomplicated malaria sections above for chloroquine-sensitive species by region)	**Chloroquine phosphate:** Treatment as above **or** **Hydroxychloroquine:** Treatment as above
Uncomplicated malaria: alternatives for pregnant women *(cont'd)*	**Chloroquine resistant** *P. falciparum*[1] (see sections above for regions with chloroquine resistant *P. falciparum*)	**Quinine sulfate** *plus* **Clindamycin** **Quinine sulfate:** Treatment as above **Clindamycin:** Treatment as above
	Chloroquine resistant *P. vivax* (see uncomplicated malaria sections above for regions with chloroquine-resistant *P. vivax*)	**Quinine sulfate** **Quinine sulfate**[7]: 650 mg salt (PO) q8h × 7 days

1. Persons with a positive blood smear or history of recent possible exposure and no other recognized pathology who have one or more of the following clinical criteria (impaired consciousness/coma, severe normocytic anemia, renal failure, pulmonary edema, acute respiratory distress syndrome, circulatory shock, disseminated intravascular coagulation, spontaneous bleeding, acidosis, hemoglobinuria, jaundice, repeated generalized convulsions, and/or parasitemia of >5%) are considered to have manifestations of more severe disease. Severe malaria is most often caused by *P. falciparum*.

2. Patients diagnosed with severe malaria should be treated aggressively with parenteral antimalarial therapy. Treatment with IV quinidine should be initiated as soon as possible after the diagnosis has been made. Patients with severe malaria should be given an intravenous loading dose of quinidine unless they have received more than 40 mg/kg of quinine in the preceding 48 hours or if they have received mefloquine within the preceding 12 hours. Consultation with a cardiologist and a physician with experience treating malaria is advised when treating malaria patients with quinidine. During administration of quinidine, blood pressure monitoring (for hypotension) and cardiac monitoring (for widening of the QRS complex and/or lengthening of the QTc interval) should be monitored continuously and blood glucose (for hypoglycemia) should be monitored periodically. Cardiac complications, if severe, may warrant temporary discontinuation of the drug or slowing of the intravenous infusion.

3. Consider exchange transfusion if the parasite density (i.e. parasitemia) is >10% OR if the patient has altered mental status, non-volume overload pulmonary edema, or renal complications. The parasite density can be estimated by examining a monolayer of red blood cells (RBCs) on the thin smear under oil immersion magnification. The slide should be examined where the RBCs are more or less touching (approximately 400 RBCs per field). The parasite density can then be

estimated from the percentage of infected RBCs and should be monitored every 12 hours. Exchange transfusion should be continued until the parasite density is <1% (usually requires 8–10 units). IV quinidine administration should not be delayed for an exchange transfusion and can be given concurrently throughout the exchange transfusion.

4. Pregnant women diagnosed with severe malaria should be treated aggressively with parenteral antimalarial therapy.

5. There are 4 options (A, B, C, or D) available for treatment of uncomplicated malaria caused by chloroquine-resistant *P. falciparum*. Options A, B, and C are equally recommended. Because of a higher rate of severe neuropsychiatric reactions seen at treatment doses, option D (mefloquine) not recommend unless the other options cannot be used. For option C, because there is more data on the efficacy of quinine in combination with doxycycline, these treatment combinations preferred to quinine with clindamycin.

6. Take with with food or whole milk. If patient vomits within 30 minutes of taking a dose, then they should repeat the dose.

7. US manufactured quinine sulfate capsule is in a 324 mg dosage; therefore 2 capsules should be sufficient for adult dosing. Pediatric dosing may be difficult due to unavailability of non-capsule forms of quinine.

8. For infections acquired in Southeast Asia, quinine treatment should continue for 7 days. For infections acquired elsewhere, quinine treatment should continue for 3 days.

9. Doxycycline are not indicated for use in children less than 8 years old. For children less than 8 years old with chloroquine-resistant *P. falciparum*, atovaquone-proguanil and artemether-lumefantrine are recommended treatment options; mefloquine can be considered if no other options are available. For children less than 8 years old with chloroquine-resistant *P. vivax*, mefloquine is the recommended treatment. If it is not available or is not being tolerated and if the treatment benefits outweigh the risks, atovaquone-proguanil or artemether-lumefantrine should be used instead.

10. Treatment with mefloquine is not recommended in persons who have acquired infections from Southeast Asia due to drug resistance.

11. Primaquine is used to eradicate any hypnozoites in the liver, to prevent relapses, in *P. vivax* and *P. ovale* infections. Because primaquine can cause hemolytic anemia in G6PD-deficient persons, G6PD screening must occur prior to starting treatment with primaquine. For persons with borderline G6PD deficiency or as an alternate to the above regimen, primaquine may be given 45 mg orally one time per week for 8 weeks; consultation with an expert in infectious disease and/or tropical medicine is advised if this alternative regimen is considered in G6PD-deficient persons. Primaquine must not be used during pregnancy.

12. There are three options (A, B, or C) available for treatment of uncomplicated malaria caused by chloroquine-resistant *P. vivax*. High treatment failure rates due to chloroquine-resistant *P. vivax* have been well documented in Papua New Guinea and Indonesia. Rare case reports of chloroquine-resistant *P. vivax* have also been documented in Burma (Myanmar), India, and Central and South America. Persons acquiring *P. vivax* infections outside of Papua New Guinea or Indonesia should be started on chloroquine. If the patient does not respond, the treatment should be changed to a chloroquine-resistant P. vivax regimen and CDC should be notified (Malaria Hotline number listed below). For treatment of chloroquine-resistant *P. vivax* infections, options A, B, and C are equally recommended.

13. For pregnant women diagnosed with uncomplicated malaria caused by chloroquine-resistant *P. falciparum* or chloroquine-resistant *P. vivax* infection, treatment with doxycycline is generally not indicated. However, doxycycline may be used in combination with quinine (as recommended for non-pregnant adults) if other treatment options are not available or are not being tolerated, and the benefit is judged to outweigh the risks.

14. Atovaquone-proguanil and artemether-lumefantrine are generally not recommended for use in pregnant women, particularly in the first trimester due to lack of sufficient safety data. For pregnant women diagnosed with uncomplicated malaria caused by chloroquine-resistant *P. falciparum* infection, atovaquone-proguanil or artemether/lumefantrine may be used if other treatment options are not available or are not being tolerated, and if the potential benefit is judged to outweigh the potential risks.

15. Because of a possible association with mefloquine treatment during pregnancy and an increase in stillbirths, mefloquine is generally not recommended for treatment in pregnant women. However, mefloquine may be used if it is the only treatment option available and if the potential benefit is judged to outweigh the potential risks.

16. For *P. vivax* and *P. ovale* infections, primaquine phosphate for radical treatment of hypnozoites should not be given during pregnancy. Pregnant patients with *P. vivax* and *P. ovale* infections should be maintained on chloroquine prophylaxis for the duration of their pregnancy. The chemoprophylactic dose of chloroquine phosphate is 300 mg base (=500 mg salt) orally once per week. After delivery, pregnant patients who do not have G6PD deficiency should be treated with primaquine.

Based on CDC Recommendations for Malaria in the US
CDC Malaria Hotline: weekdays 9 am – 5 pm EST: (770) 488-7788 or (855) 856–4713
after hours, weekends and holidays: (770) 488-7100

Malaria in Children (United States)

Clinical Diagnosis/ *Plasmodium* species	Region Acquired	Recommended Drugs and Pediatric Dose (*pediatric dose should not exceed adult dose*)
Severe malaria[1,2,3]	**All regions**	**Quinidine gluconate**[2] ***plus* either: Doxycycline**[8] **or Clindamycin** **Quinidine gluconate:** Same mg/kg dosing and recommendations as for adults. **Doxycycline:** Treatment as above. For children <45 kg, give 2.2 mg/kg (IV) q12h and then switch to (PO) doxycycline (dose as above) as soon as patient can take oral medication. For children >45 kg, use same dosing as for adults. Treatment × 7 days. **Clindamycin:** Treatment as above. 10 mg base/kg loading dose (IV) followed by 5 mg base/kg (IV/PO) q8h. Treatment × 7 days.
Uncomplicated malaria/ ***P. falciparum*** or Species not identified[4]	**Chloroquine resistant or unknown resistance**[11] (All Malarious regions except those specified as chloroquine-resistant listed in box below)	**A. Atovaquone proguanil (Malarone)**[5] *Adult tab = 250 mg atovaquone/ 100 mg proguanil* *Peds tab = 62.5 mg atovaquone/ 25 mg proguanil* 5–8 kg: 2 peds tabs (PO) q24h × 3d 9–10 kg: 3 peds tabs (PO) q24h × 3d 11–20 kg: 1 adult tab (PO) q24h × 3d 21–30 kg: 2 adult tabs (PO) q24h × 3d 31–40 kg: 3 adult tabs (PO) q24h × 3d > 40 kg: 4 adult tabs (PO) q24h × 3d **or**

Malaria in Children (United States) *(cont'd)*

Clinical Diagnosis/ *Plasmodium* species	Region Acquired	Recommended Drugs and Pediatric Dose *(pediatric dose should not exceed adult dose)*
If "species not identified" is subsequently diagnosed as *P. vivax* or *P. ovale*: see *P. vivax* and *P. ovale* (below) re. treatment with primaquine		**B. Artemether-lumefantrine (Coartem)[5]** *1 tablet = 20 mg artemether/120 mg lumefantrine* A 3-day treatment schedule with a total of 6 oral doses is recommended for both adult and pediatric patients based on weight. The patient should receive the initial dose, followed by the second dose 8 hours later, then 1 dose (PO) q12h × 2 days. 5–15 kg: 1 tablet per dose 15–25 kg: 2 tablets per dose 25–35 kg: 3 tablets per dose ≥ 35 kg: 4 tablets per dose **or** **C. Quinine sulfate[3] *plus* either: Doxycycline[8] or Clindamycin** **Quinine sulfate[6,7]:** 8.3 mg base/kg (=10 mg salt/kg) (PO) tid × 3 or 7 days **Doxycycline:** 2.2 mg/kg (PO) q12h × 7 days **Clindamycin:** 20 mg base/kg/day (PO) divided q8h × 7 days **or** **D. Mefloquine (Lariam)[9]** 13.7 mg base/kg (=15 mg salt/kg) (PO) as initial dose, followed by 9.1 mg base/kg (=10 mg salt/kg) (PO) given 6–12 hours after initial dose. Total dose = 25 mg salt/kg

Malaria in Children (United States) *(cont'd)*

Clinical Diagnosis/ *Plasmodium* species	Region Acquired	Recommended Drugs and Pediatric Dose (*pediatric dose should not exceed adult dose*)
Uncomplicated malaria **P. falciparum** or *Species not identified*	**Chloroquine sensitive** (Central America west of Panama Canal; Haiti; the Dominican Republic; and most of the Middle East)	**Chloroquine phosphate (Aralen)** 10 mg base/kg (PO) immediately, followed by 5 mg base/kg (PO) at 6, 24, and 48 hours Total dose: 25 mg base/kg **or** **Hydroxychloroquine (Plaquenil and generics)** 10 mg base/kg (PO) immediately, followed by 5 mg base/kg (PO) at 6, 24, and 48 hours Total dose: 25 mg base/kg
Uncomplicated malaria/ **P. malariae** or **P. knowlesi**	**All regions**	**Chloroquine phosphate:** Treatment as above **or** **Hydroxychloroquine:** Treatment as above
Uncomplicated malaria/ **P. vivax** or **P. ovale**	**All regions** For suspected chloroquine-resistant *P. vivax*, see below	**Chloroquine phosphate *plus* Primaquine phosphate**[10] **Chloroquine phosphate:** Treatment as above **Primaquine:** 0.5 mg base/kg (PO) qd × 14 days **or** **Hydroxychloroquine *plus* Primaquine phosphate**[10] **Hydroxychloroquine:** Treatment as above **Primaquine phosphate:** 0.5 mg base/kg (PO) qd × 14 days

Malaria in Children (United States) *(cont'd)*

Clinical Diagnosis/ Plasmodium species	Region Acquired	Recommended Drugs and Pediatric Dose (*pediatric dose should not exceed adult dose*)
Uncomplicated malaria/ P. vivax	**Chloroquine resistant[11]** (Papua New Guinea and Indonesia)	**A. Quinine sulfate** *plus* **either Doxycycline[8]** *plus* **Primaquine phosphate[10]** **Quinine sulfate:** Treatment as above **Doxycycline** Treatment as above **Primaquine phosphate:** Treatment as above
		or
		B. Atovaquone proguanil *plus* **Primaquine phosphate** **Atovaquone proguanil:** Treatment as above **Primaquine phosphate:** Treatment as above
		or
		C. Mefloquine *plus* **Primaquine phosphate[10]** **Mefloquine:** Treatment as above **Primaquine phosphate:** Treatment as above

1. Persons with a positive blood smear or history of recent possible exposure and no other recognized pathology who have one or more of the following clinical criteria (impaired consciousness/ coma, severe normocytic anemia, renal failure, pulmonary edema, acute respiratory distress syndrome, circulatory shock, disseminated intravascular coagulation, spontaneous bleeding, acidosis, hemoglobinuria, jaundice, repeated generalized convulsions, and/or parasitemia of >5%) are considered to have manifestations of more severe disease. Severe malaria is most often caused by P. falciparum.

2. Patients diagnosed with severe malaria should be treated aggressively with parenteral antimalarial therapy. Treatment with IV quinidine should be initiated as soon as possible after the diagnosis has been made. Patients with severe malaria should be given an intravenous loading dose of quinidine unless they have received more than 40 mg/kg of quinine in the preceding 48 hours or if they have received mefloquine within the preceding 12 hours. Consultation with a cardiologist and a physician with experience treating malaria is advised when treating malaria patients with quinidine. During administration of quinidine, blood pressure monitoring (for hypotension) and cardiac monitoring (for widening of the QRS complex and/ or lengthening of the QTc interval) should be monitored continuously and blood glucose (for hypoglycemia) should be monitored periodically. Cardiac complications, if severe, may warrant temporary discontinuation of the drug or slowing of the intravenous infusion.

3. Consider exchange transfusion if the parasite density (i.e. parasitemia) is >10% OR if the patient has altered mental status, non-volume overload pulmonary edema, or renal complications. The parasite density can be estimated by examining a monolayer of red blood cells (RBCs) on the thin smear under oil immersion magnification. The slide should be examined where the RBCs are more or less touching (approximately 400 RBCs per field). The parasite density can then be estimated from the percentage of infected RBCs and should be monitored every 12 hours. Exchange transfusion should be continued until the parasite density is <1% (usually requires 8–10 units). IV quinidine administration should not be delayed for an exchange transfusion and can be given concurrently throughout the exchange transfusion.

4. There are 4 options (A, B, C, or D) available for treatment of uncomplicated malaria caused by chloroquine-resistant *P. falciparum*. Options A, B, and C are equally recommended. Because of a higher rate of severe neuropsychiatric reactions seen at treatment doses, we do not recommend option D (mefloquine) unless the other options cannot be used. For option C, because there is more data on the efficacy of quinine in combination with doxycycline or tetracycline, these treatment combinations are generally preferred to quinine in combination with clindamycin.

5. Take with with food or whole milk. If patient vomits within 30 minutes of taking a dose, then they should repeat the dose.

6. US manufactured quinine sulfate capsule is in a 324 mg dosage; therefore 2 capsules should be sufficient for adult dosing. Pediatric dosing may be difficult due to unavailability of non-capsule forms of quinine.

7. For infections acquired in Southeast Asia, quinine treatment should continue for 7 days. For infections acquired elsewhere, quinine treatment should continue for 3 days.

8. Doxycycline is not indicated for use in children less than 8 years old. For children less than 8 years old with chloroquine-resistant *P. falciparum*, atovaquone-proguanil and artemether-lumefantrine are recommended treatment options; mefloquine can be considered if no other options are available. For children less than 8 years old with chloroquine-resistant *P. vivax*, mefloquine is the recommended treatment. If it is not available or is not being tolerated and if the treatment benefits outweigh the risks, atovaquone-proguanil or artemether-lumefantrine should be used instead.

9. Treatment with mefloquine is not recommended in persons who have acquired infections from Southeast Asia due to drug resistance.

10. Primaquine is used to eradicate any hypnozoites that may remain dormant in the liver, and thus prevent relapses, in *P. vivax* and *P. ovale* infections. Because primaquine can cause hemolytic anemia in G6PD-deficient persons, G6PD screening must occur prior to starting treatment with primaquine. For persons with borderline G6PD deficiency or as an alternate to the above regimen, primaquine may be given 45 mg orally one time per week for 8 weeks; consultation with an expert in infectious disease and/or tropical medicine is advised if this alternative regimen is considered in G6PD-deficient persons. Primaquine must not be used during pregnancy.

11. There are three options (A, B, or C) available for treatment of uncomplicated malaria caused by chloroquine-resistant *P. vivax*. High treatment failure rares due to chloroquine-resistant *P. vivax* have been well documented in Papua New Guinea and Indonesia. Rare case reports of chloroquine-resistant *P. vivax* have also been documented in Burma (Myanmar), India, and Central and South America. Persons acquiring *P. vivax* infections outside of Papua New Guinea or Indonesia should be started on chloroquine. If the patient does not respond, the treatment should be changed to a chloroquine-resistant *P. vivax* regimen and CDC should be notified (Malaria Hotline number listed above). For treatment of chloroquine-resistant *P. vivax* infections, options A, B, and C are equally recommended.

Based on CDC Recommendations for Malaria in the US
CDC Malaria Hotline: weekdays 8 am – 4:30 pm EST: (770) 488-7788 or (855) 856-4713
after hours, weekends and holidays: (770) 488-7100

INDEX